Melanoma Antigens and Antibodies

Melanoma Antigens and Antibodies

Edited by

Ralph A. Reisfeld

Scripps Clinic and Research Foundation
La Jolla, California

and

Soldano Ferrone

Columbia University
New York, New York

PLENUM PRESS • NEW YORK AND LONDON

Library of Congress Cataloging in Publication Data

Main entry under title:

Melanoma antigens and antibodies

Includes bibliographical references and index.
1. Melanoma—Immunological aspects. 2. Tumor antigens. 3. Immunoglobulins.
I. Reisfeld, Ralph A. II. Ferrone, Soldano, 1940—   . [DNLM: 1. Melanoma—
Immunology. QZ 200 M517]

RC280.S5M38	616.99′4	82-5288
ISBN-13: 978-1-4684-4081-2 e-ISBN-13: 978-1-4684-4079-9		AACR2
DOI: 10.1007/978-1-4684-4079-9		

© 1982 Plenum Press, New York
Softcover reprint of the hardcover 1st edition 1982

A Division of Plenum Publishing Corporation
233 Spring Street, New York, N.Y. 10013

Contributors

ROBERTO S. ACCOLLA, Unit of Human Cancer Immunology, Lausanne Branch, Ludwig Institute for Cancer Research, 1066 Epalinges, Switzerland

RONALD T. ACTON, Departments of Microbiology and Epidemiology, University of Alabama in Birmingham, Birmingham, Alabama 35294

CHARLES M. BALCH, Departments of Microbiology and Surgery; Cellular Immunobiology Unit, Comprehensive Cancer Center; Veterans Hospital, University of Alabama in Birmingham, Birmingham, Alabama 35294

BRUCE O. BARGER, Department of Microbiology and Epidemiology, University of Alabama in Birmingham, Birmingham, Alabama 35294

JOSEF BRÜGGEN, Department of Experimental Dermatology, Universitäts-Hautklinik, 4400 Münster, West Germany

BRUCE BUDOWLE, Department of Microbiology, University of Alabama in Birmingham, Birmingham, Alabama 35294

JEAN-CLAUDE BYSTRYN, Department of Dermatology, New York University School of Medicine, New York, New York 10016

STEFAN CARREL, Unit of Human Cancer Immunology, Lausanne Branch, Ludwig Institute for Cancer Research, 1066 Epalinges, Switzerland

RENATO CAVALIERE, Istituto Regina Elena, 00161 Rome, Italy

ALISTAIR J. COCHRAN, Division of Surgical Oncology and Departments of Surgery and Pathology, UCLA School of Medicine, University of California, Los Angeles, California 90024

PETER B. DENT, Departments of Pediatrics and Pathology, McMaster University; The Ontario Cancer Treatment & Research Foundation (Hamilton Clinic), Hamilton, Ontario, L8N 3Z5 Canada

SOLDANO FERRONE, Department of Pathology, College of Physicians and Surgeons, Columbia University, New York, New York 10032

D. R. GALLOWAY, Department of Molecular Immunology, Scripps Clinic and Research Foundation, La Jolla, California 92037

DOUGLAS M. GERSTEN, Department of Pathology and National Biomedical Research Foundation, Georgetown University, Washington, D.C. 20007

RODNEY C. P. GO, Department of Epidemiology, University of Alabama in Birmingham, Birmingham, Alabama 35294

NICOLE GROSS, Unit of Human Cancer Immunology, Lausanne Branch, Ludwig Institute for Cancer Research, 1066 Epalinges, Switzerland

RISHAB K. GUPTA, Division of Oncology, Department of Surgery, UCLA School of Medicine, University of California, Los Angeles, California 90024; and Surgical Service, V.A. Medical Center, Sepulveda, California 91343

W. J. HALLIDAY, Department of Microbiology, University of Queensland, Brisbane, Australia 4067

INGEGERD HELLSTRÖM, Division of Tumor Immunology, Fred Hutchinson Cancer Research Center, Seattle, Washington 98104; Departments of Microbiology/Immunology and Pathology, University of Washington, Seattle, Washington 98195

KARL ERIK HELLSTRÖM, Division of Tumor Immunology, Fred Hutchinson Cancer Research Center, Seattle, Washington 98104; Departments of Microbiology/Immunology and Pathology, University of Washington, Seattle, Washington 98195

PETER HERSEY, Medical Research Department, Kanematsu Memorial Institute, Sydney Hospital, Sydney, N.S.W. 2000, Australia

ARIEL HOLLINSHEAD, Division of Hematology and Oncology, Department of Medicine, The George Washington University Medical Center, Washington, D.C. 20037

KOHZOH IMAI, Department of Molecular Immunology, Scripps Clinic and Research Foundation, La Jolla, California 92037

YOSHIFUMI ISHII, Department of Developmental Therapeutics, M.D. Anderson Hospital and Tumor Institute, Houston, Texas 77030

NEIL E. KAY, Department of Pathology, College of Physicians and Surgeons, Columbia University, New York, New York, 10032

PETER J. KELLEHER, Department of Medicine, National Jewish Hospital and Research Center, Denver, Colorado 80206

HILARY KOPROWSKI, The Wistar Institute of Anatomy and Biology, Philadelphia, Pennsylvania 19104

W. DANIEL KUNDIN, Division of Hematology and Oncology, Department of Medicine, The George Washington University Medical Center, Washington, D.C. 20037

M. G. LEWIS, Department of Pathology, Stritch School of Medicine, Loyola University, Maywood, Chicago, Illinois 60153

SHUEN-KUEI LIAO, Departments of Pediatrics and Pathology, McMaster University; The Ontario Cancer Treatment & Research Foundation (Hamilton Clinic), Hamilton, Ontario, L8N 3Z5 Canada

JEAN-PIERRE MACH, Unit of Human Cancer Immunology, Lausanne Branch, Ludwig Institute for Cancer Research, 1066 Epalinges, Switzerland

Egon Macher, Department of Experimental Dermatology, Universitäts-Hautklinik, 4400 Münster, West Germany

John J. Marchalonis, Department of Biochemistry, Medical University of South Carolina, Charleston, South Carolina 29403

Giora M. Mavligit, Department of Developmental Therapeutics, M. D. Anderson Hospital and Tumor Institute, Houston, Texas 77030

R. P. McCabe, Department of Molecular Immunology, Scripps Clinic and Research Foundation, La Jolla, California 92037

William H. McCarthy, Melanoma Unit, Department of Surgery, University of Sydney, Sydney Hospital, Sydney, N.S.W. 2000, Australia

Percy Minden, Department of Medicine, National Jewish Hospital and Research Center, Denver, Colorado 80206

Kenneth F. Mitchell, The Wistar Institute of Anatomy and Biology, Philadelphia, Pennsylvania 19104

Alton C. Morgan, jr., Department of Molecular Immunology, Scripps Clinic and Research Foundation, La Jolla, California 92037

Donald L. Morton, V. A. Medical Center, Sepulveda, California 91343; and Division of Oncology, Department of Surgery, UCLA School of Medicine, University of California, Los Angeles, California 90024

Pier-Giorgio Natali, Istituto Regina Elena, 00161 Rome, Italy

Michele A. Pellegrino, Department of Pathology, College of Physicians and Surgeons, Columbia University, New York, New York, 10032

T. M. Phillips, Department of Medicine, George Washington Medical Center, Washington, D.C. 20037

W. D. Queen, Department of Medicine, George Washington Medical Center, Washington, D.C. 20037

R. A. Reisfeld, Department of Molecular Immunology, Scripps Clinic and Research Foundation, La Jolla, California 92037

Jeffrey M. Roseman, Department of Epidemiology, University of Alabama in Birmingham, Birmingham, Alabama 35294

Charles Scott, Paul M. Aggeler Memorial Laboratory, Department of Medicine, Children's Hospital, University of California Medical Center, San Francisco, California 94122

Seng-Jaw Soong, Department of Biostatistics, University of Alabama in Birmingham, Birmingham, Alabama 35294

Clemens Sorg, Department of Experimental Dermatology, Universitäts-Hautklinik, 4400 Münster, West Germany

Lynn E. Spitler, Paul M. Aggeler Memorial Laboratory, Department of Medicine, Children's Hospital, University of California Medical Center, San Francisco, California 94122

Zenon Steplewski, The Wistar Institute of Anatomy and Biology, Philadelphia, Pennsylvania 19104

LUDWIG SUTER, Department of Experimental Dermatology, Universitäts-Hautklinik, 4400 Münster, West Germany

KEITH TANNER, Division of Hematology and Oncology, Department of Medicine, The George Washington University Medical Center, Washington, D.C. 20037

DOROTHEA TERBRACK, Department of Experimental Dermatology, Universitäts-Hautklinik, 4400 Münster, West Germany

D. M. P. THOMSON, The Montreal General Hospital Research Institute, The Montreal General Hospital, Quebec, Canada H3G 1A4

ARABELLA B. TILDEN, Departments of Microbiology and Surgery; Cellular Immunobiology Unit, Comprehensive Cancer Center; Veterans Hospital, University of Alabama in Birmingham, Birmingham, Alabama 35294

FEREYDOUN VAKILZADEH, Department of Experimental Dermatology, Universitäts-Hautklinik, 4400 Münster, West Germany

BARRY S. WILSON, Department of Pathology, University of Michigan Medical School, Ann Arbor, Michigan 48109

LINDA K. WOODS, Surgical Oncology Laboratory, Denver General Hospital, Denver, Colorado 80204

Preface

The ever-expanding research on human cancer has resulted in numerous technical and conceptual advances during the last few years. Serological, structural, and biological characterization of human melanoma constitutes one area of research that has received considerable attention from researchers and clinicians and has generated new and exciting information. In this volume, we have attempted to assemble work on topics that produced some of the most recent advances. We asked each author to describe and interpret his most current research and, whenever possible, to compare and contrast it with work of other investigators in the field. We have been careful not to impose our viewpoints except in contributions from our own laboratories, since we want to provide the reader with as many divergent and sometimes opposing viewpoints as feasible. Therefore, we have not been overly concerned with overlaps in some individual topics. We hope that this volume will provide the reader with a well-balanced overview of current problems and ideas in a particular area of cancer research.

We wish to express our thanks to all contributors for their timely and very interesting manuscripts, and we sincerely hope that the reader will enjoy this volume and benefit as much from it as we did.

R. A. Reisfeld
S. Ferrone

La Jolla

PREFACE

Contents

CHAPTER 7

Protein Antigens of Mouse Melanomas

DOUGLAS M. GERSTEN AND JOHN J. MARCHALONIS

CHAPTER 8

Clinical Significance of Tumor-Associated Antigens and Antitumor Antibodies
in Human Malignant Melanoma

RISHAB K. GUPTA AND DONALD L. MORTON

CHAPTER 9

Specificity of Cell-Mediated Immunoreactivity in Melanoma and Comments on
the Nature of Serum Blocking Factors

W. J. HALLIDAY

CHAPTER 10

Antigens in Human Melanomas Detected by Using Monoclonal Antibodies as Probes

KARL ERIK HELLSTRÖM AND INGEGERD HELLSTRÖM

CHAPTER 11

The Nature and Significance of Melanoma Antigens Recognized by Human Subjects

PETER HERSEY AND WILLIAM H. MCCARTHY

CHAPTER 12

Cellular and Humoral Studies of Malignant Melanoma

ARIEL HOLLINSHEAD, KEITH TANNER, AND W. DANIEL KUNDIN

CHAPTER 13

Immunodiagnosis of Human Melanoma: Detection of Circulating Melanoma-Associated Antigens by Radioimmunoassay

YOSHIFUMI ISHII AND GIORA M. MAVLIGIT

CHAPTER 14

The Association between Antigens of Human Malignant-Melanoma Cells and
Mycobacterium bovis (BCG)

PERCY MINDEN, PETER J. KELLEHER, AND LINDA K. WOODS

CHAPTER 15

Monoclonal Antibodies to Human Melanoma-Associated Antigens: Elicitation
and Evaluation with Immunochemically Defined Antigen Preparations

ALTON C. MORGAN, JR.

CHAPTER 16

The Significance of Circulating Immune Complexes in Patients with Malignant
Melanoma

T. M. PHILLIPS, W. D. QUEEN, AND M. G. LEWIS

1

Immunogenetics of Melanoma

RONALD T. ACTON, CHARLES M. BALCH, BRUCE BUDOWLE,
RODNEY C. P. GO, JEFFREY M. ROSEMAN, SENG-JAW SOONG,
AND BRUCE O. BARGER

1. Introduction

Human melanoma of the skin is a disease that has received a great deal of attention from basic scientists and clinicians over the last several years. One reason for this increased interest is that the incidence of the disease is rapidly increasing in the United States as well as in other countries (Crombie, 1979; Cutler and Young, 1975; Elwood and Lee, 1974; Magnus, 1977; Ohsumi and Seiji, 1977). In attempting to understand the etiology of melanoma, one must consider two major factors: the genetic makeup of the host and environmental insults (Clark *et al.*, 1977; Klepp and Magnus, 1979; McGovern, 1977). Ultimately, one would like to be able to identify highly susceptible individuals in the population early in life and provide measures to minimize or prevent insult by environmental agents. With this in mind, we will attempt to review the current state of knowledge with regard to the immunogenetics of melanoma in order to establish whether this goal is in sight. The authors have taken the liberty of selecting data by others that illustrate the current level of understanding in this area rather than attempting an all-encompassing review. Since the highest melanoma mortality rate in the United States is found in Alabama (Mason and McKay, 1974), we will review the immunogenetic data collected from patients mainly residing in the state of Alabama treated at the Melanoma Clinic of the University of Alabama in Birmingham. The clinical and pathological characteristics of this patient group have previously been published (Balch *et al.*, 1978, 1979a,b, 1980, 1981; Balch, 1980).

RONALD T. ACTON • Departments of Microbiology and Epidemiology   CHARLES M. BALCH • Departments of Microbiology and Surgery   BRUCE BUDOWLE • Department of Microbiology   BRUCE O. BARGER • Department of Microbiology and Epidemiology   RODNEY C. P. GO AND JEFFREY M. ROSEMAN • Department of Epidemiology • SENG-JAW SOONG   Department of Biostatistics, University of Alabama in Birmingham, Birmingham, Alabama 35294.

1

2. Genetic Factors

The role of genetic factors in the onset of melanoma has to be evaluated by reference to data from four areas. First, there are animal models that have been used to identify the role of specific genes in the onset of the disease. Second, the data on families in which more than one member is affected with the disease have been interpreted to suggest different possible modes of inheritance of the susceptibility gene(s). Whether the gene(s) responsible for the disease in multiply affected families account(s) for a significant proportion of the overall population incidence will also be discussed. Third, the genetically determined variables associated with the disease in various racial and ethnic groups will be reviewed. Of particular interest are the genetic-marker results, which are relatively limited, but because they point to the possibility of identifying individuals in the population at higher risk for the disease will receive broader coverage. Fourth, the evidence that progression of the tumor may be influenced by the host's immune response, which is known to be under genetic control (Benacerraf and Germain, 1978; Clark et al., 1977; Ferrone and Pellegrino, 1978; Gutterman et al., 1975; Lewis et al., 1979) will be reviewed.

2.1. Animal Models

Several investigators reported concurrently that a fraction of the F_1 hybrids generated by crossing the platyfish (Platypoecilus maculatus) and the swordtail (Xiphophorus helleri) developed spontaneous melanoma (Gordon, 1927; Häussler, 1972; Kosswig, 1927). As hypothesized by Anders et al. (1979), the development of melanomas in these hybrids is due to the interaction of a Mendelian inherited tumor gene, which can bring about transformation of melanophore precursor cells to a malignant state, and other epistatic genes. The expression of the tumor gene is therefore controlled by other genes that repress the neoplastic transformation event or those that regulate the growth of the transformed cell. This model illustrates how the presence or absence of a certain combination of genes can bring about neoplastic transformation in the apparent absence of a known inducer.

Strafuss et al. (1968) were the first to observe melanoma in a breed of Sinclair miniature swine. They estimated the lifetime incidence of cutaneous melanomas in this breed to be 21%. Further studies by Millikan et al. (1974) revealed that the melanocytic tumors develop spontaneously and that the incidence in newborn offspring of two affected parents was 62%. A more recent study by Hook et al. (1979) demonstrated an incidence of 54% in newborn progeny of two affected parents and an incidence of 85% by 1 year of age. The incidence of melanoma in progeny from matings where only the male was affected was 22%, and 21% where only the female was affected, suggesting no sex linkage. The incidence was only 2% when both parents were normal. Since the swine were all kept in the same facility and fed the same diet, these data suggest that the development of melanoma in these animals is largely influenced by genetic mechanisms. The specific gene or genes involved with predisposing an animal to this disease are not known. Since the tumor is often found in newborns, it is not likely that immune-response (Ir) genes are involved in this form.

2.2. Familial Melanoma

It has been some 30 years since Cawley (1952) and Greifelt (1952) reported on the familial occurrence of malignant melanoma. Subquently, there have been several reports documenting the occurrence of familial melanoma (Anderson *et al.*, 1967; Anderson, 1971; Kopf *et al.*, 1976; Lynch and Krush, 1968; Lynch *et al.*, 1975, 1977, 1978; Schoch, 1963; Turkington, 1965; Wallace *et al.*, 1971, 1973). The frequency of familial melanoma reported from these studies is 1–6% of all cases. The clinical characteristics of 106 probands from multiply affected families and 2128 probands from simplex families were compared by Anderson (1971). The patients from familial cases were found to have a younger age distribution, an earlier average age at first diagnosis, a higher frequency of multiple primary melanomas, and a higher survival rate than nonfamilial patients. Several possible modes of inheritance have been suggested from familial data. The observation that the frequency of melanoma is higher among children whose mothers were affected (17%) compared to the frequency in children whose fathers were affected (9%) led Anderson (1971) to suggest that the inheritance involved a maternal cytoplasmic component in addition to the inheritance of certain genes. Several investigations have suggested that the data best fit an autosomal dominant mode of inheritance with incomplete penetrance (Anderson *et al.*, 1967; Lynch and Krush, 1968; Lynch *et al.*, 1975; Reimer *et al.*, 1978; Sutherland *et al.*, 1975). However, Wallace *et al.* (1971, 1973) felt that the data from 113 familial cases of melanoma in Queensland, Australia, which has the highest incidence in the world, fit a polygenic mode of inheritance. Clark *et al.* (1978), Greene *et al.*, (1978), and Reimer *et al.* (1978) have described various heritable precursor lesions in seven cases of familial melanoma. Clark *et al.* (1978) observed in six of these melanoma families that 15 of 17 patients with melanoma and 22 of 41 of their relatives without melanoma had unique moles. According to the investigators, these moles histologically reveal "typical melanocytic hyperplasia, lymphocytic infiltration, delicate fibroplasia and new blood vessels that occur within a compound nevus or *de novo*." Two of these moles were shown to develop into malignant melanoma through photographs taken over a period of time. These moles were designated the "B-K mole syndrome." This group of investigators subsequently observed in seven melanoma-prone families that 18 of 20 melanoma patients and 24 of 43 first-degree relatives had the B-K mole syndrome (Reimer *et al.*, 1978). The moles were shown to progress to melanoma in 6 family members. Therefore, these investigators suggest that this syndrome could be used to identify individuals at high risk for developing melanoma. The heritable nature of this syndrome appeared to represent an autosomal dominant trait.

Lynch and co-workers (Lynch and Krush, 1968; Lynch *et al.*, 1975, 1977) have observed in five melanoma families an excess of other histological varieties of cancer. The types of tumors found in association with melanoma were carcinoma of the breast, gastrointestinal tract, lymphoreticular system, and sarcoma. Lokich (1975), during a 12-year period when 107 cases of melanoma and 261 cases of breast cancer were seen, observed 5 patients with both these malignant diseases. It may be that there are regulatory gene defects that permit the development of multiple tumor types. Such a defect might lead to inadequate immune surveillance for malignant cells or an inappropriate type of immune response to such cells.

As can be seen from these reports, the familial incidence of melanoma is well documented, but proof that most of these familial cases have a genetic etiology has not been formally demonstrated. It should now be possible to conduct a formal segregation analysis, taking into account physiological, immunological, and genetic heterogeneity, in order to determine the mode(s) of inheritance for this disease. Perhaps the reported association of various genetic polymorphisms with melanoma that will be discussed in the next section will point the way for more formal analyses, such as linkage analysis.

2.3. Genetic Polymorphisms

There have been several reports wherein the population association of various genetic polymorphisms with melanoma were investigated. The increased frequency of blood group O has been reported in numerous population samples of melanoma patients. Jörgensen (1967) observed a higher frequency of blood group O in melanoma patients from Göttingen, Germany, compared with controls. Walter *et al.* (1979) examined the frequency of ABO, MNSs, Rh, P, Kell, Duffy, Kidd, Hp, Gc, Gm, Inv, ACP, PGM, EsD, and 6-PGD in 191 malignant melanoma patients and controls from the Rhineland–Palatinate area of Germany. An increased frequency of blood group O was found in patients with melanoma compared to controls. Moreover, when the German data on the OA ratio were combined with those of Ikonopisov and Tsanov (1974) from Bulgaria, the O group was found to be statistically ($p < 0.001$) increased in the melanoma population. There was also an increase in the incidence of O in patients relative to controls when comparing the OB ratio. However, this increase in blood group O was significant only for the Bulgarian data. Not all studies have reported the association with blood group O. Lamm *et al.* (1974b), in an investigation of 212 patients from Aarhus, Denmark, with melanoma, did not find any difference in ABO phenotype frequencies when compared with 562 healthy controls. Studies by Jörgensen and Lal (1972) sought an association between blood groups ABO and Rh, serum groups Gm^1, Gm^2, Inv_1, Hp, and Gc, and melanoma in 164 patients from around Göttingen, Germany. Although there were slight increases in melanoma patients compared to controls for all the markers investigated, only Gm^2 was significantly increased. Gm^2 was found in 55.49% of the patients with melanoma compared with 21.85% of normal controls ($\chi^2 = 67.8113$, $p < 0.001$). Walter *et al.* (1979) also found a higher frequency of $Gm(-1)$ in the German melanoma-patient population, although it was not statistically significant. In another study, Schultheis *et al.* (1975) evaluated the association of Gm allotypes in 71 patients with melanoma from Hanover, Germany. These investigators found no significant difference between the frequency of Gm allotypes in patients and that in controls.

The data dealing with the association of genes at the major histocompatibility complex (MHC) and melanoma are of such importance for future studies that some pertinent features of this genetic system will be discussed in some detail. The term MHC refers to a region on the short arm of chromosome 6, as diagrammatically shown in Fig. 1. Within the MHC are the loci that code for the human leukocyte antigen (*HLA*) system, which have been designated in order from the centromeric end outward *D/DR, B, C,* and *A*. These highly polymorphic genes code for cell-surface glycoproteins that can be detected by two methods. The genes at the *A, B, C,* and *DR* loci code for serologically defined cell-surface antigens that can be detected using the original microcytotoxicity technique (Terasaki and

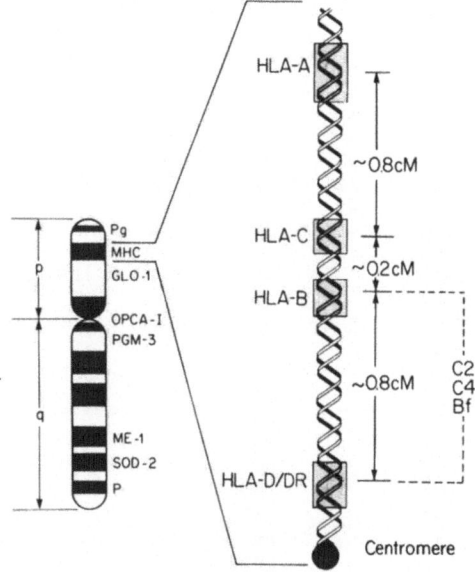

FIGURE 1. Diagrammatic representation of the gene map of chromosome 6 with an expanded view of the major histocompatibility complex (MHC) located on the short arm (p) between the genes for pepsinogen (Pg) and glyoxalase-1 (GLO-1) (Bakker *et al.*, 1979; Lamm *et al.*, 1974a). The relative distances between the four loci, i.e., *D/DR, B, C,* and *A,* are defined by a unit termed the centimorgan (cM), which represents a crossover value of 1%. The genes that code for complement components C2 and C4 are also found within this region, but their exact order or location has not been determined (Rittner and Mauff, 1978). Properdin factor B (Bf) has been reported to be situated somewhere in the region between *HLA-B* and *D/DR* (Schreuder *et al.*, 1980).

McCelland, 1964) or modifications thereof (Amos *et al.*, 1970; Mittal, 1978; Terasaki *et al.*, 1978). The *HLA-A-, -B-,* and *-C*-locus antigens are found on the cells of most tissues, while *-DR* (*D*-related) antigens are detected on B lymphocytes and macrophages using special serological methods (Terasaki *et al.*, 1978). The *HLA-D* gene products are termed lymphocyte-defined antigens (LD antigens) and are detected using cellular typing methods such as mixed-lymphocyte culture (MLC) or a refinement of this method that utilizes homozygous typing cells (HTC) (Leeuwen *et al.*, 1973; Bach and Hirschhorn, 1964). The genes that code for D antigens are closely associated with those that code for DR. There is evidence to suggest that they may be two independent but tightly linked loci (Balner, 1979). The D/DR antigens are felt to correspond to immune-region-associated antigens described in mice. Also within the MHC region are loci that code for the polymorphic variants of certain complement components, C2 and C4, and properdin factor B (Bf) (Rittner, 1976; Rittner and Mauff, 1978; Schreuder *et al.*, 1980). In addition to the aforementioned genes, the genes that control immune responsiveness, immune surveillance, susceptibility to disease, and possibly morphogenesis either have been mapped at the MHC or their location at this region has been inferred from studies in mice (Bach and van Rood, 1976; Bodmer and Bodmer, 1978; McDevitt and Bodmer, 1974). Thus, on the basis of these data, one can hypothesize how genes within the MHC might also be involved in susceptibility or resistance to melanoma.

As shown in Fig. 2, there are at present 20 *A*-locus, 40 *B*-locus, 8 *C*-locus, 10 *DR*-locus, and 12 *D*-locus specificities approved by the HLA nomenclature committee that met under the auspices of the World Health Organization (WHO) and the International Union of Immunology Societies after the Eighth International Histocompatibility Testing Workshop (Albert *et al.*, 1980). The frequencies of the genes that code for HLA specificities vary for different racial and ethnic groups, which is an important consideration in disease-asso-

HLA-A	HLA-C	HLA-B	HLA-D	HLA-DR
A1	Cw1	B5	Dw1	DR1
A2	Cw2	B7	Dw2	DR2
A3	Cw3	B8	Dw3	DR3
A9	Cw4	B12	Dw4	DR4
A10	Cw5	B13	Dw5	DR5
A11	Cw6	B14	Dw6	DRw6
Aw19	Cw7	B15	Dw7	DR7
Aw 23(9)	Cw8	Bw16	Dw8	DRw8
A24(9)		B17	Dw9	DRw9
A25(10)		B18	Dw10	DRw10
A26(10)		Bw21	Dw11	
A28		Bw22	Dw12	
A29		B27		
Aw30		Bw35		
Aw31		B37		
Aw32		Bw38(w16)		
Aw33		Bw39(w16)		
Aw34		Bw40		
Aw36		Bw41		
Aw43		Bw42		
		Bw44(12)		
		Bw45(12		
		Bw46		
		Bw47		
		Bw48		
		Bw49(w21)		
		Bw50(w21)		
		Bw51(5)		
		Bw52(5)		
		Bw53		
		Bw54(w22)		
		Bw55(w22)		
		Bw56(w22)		
		Bw57(17)		
		Bw58(17)		
		Bw59		
		Bw60(40)		
		Bw61(40)		
		Bw62(15)		
		Bw63(15)		

FIGURE 2. Nomenclature for the HLA specificities recognized by the 1980 HLA nomenclature committee. Each antigen is identified by a letter for the locus that controls it followed by a number defining the particular specificity, i.e., A1. Some of the antigens also bear a "w" designation (e.g., Aw19), which is a provisional designation identifying antigens that are not fully accepted specificities and must be subjected to further analysis before being accepted. When a specificity is followed by a number in parentheses, e.g., A24(9), this indicates that the specificity A24 was split from the specificity originally defined as A9. The A24 is a narrow specificity that, due to the discovery of more specific antisera, was split from the broad specificity A9.

ciation studies. As judged from population genetic studies, most of the alleles for A and B specificities in the Caucasian population have been accounted for. This is not the case for the *C* and *D/DR* genes, wherein there still remains a large frequency of "blanks." Blanks are the absence of a detectable specificity on the cells of a given individual by the currently available antisera due presumably to an undetected or unidentified allelic product. Thus, it is important that studies to determine the association of HLA specificities with a given disease utilize a control group of the same racial and ethnic background as the diseased group and ideally from the same geographic area.

The malignant diseases were one of the first to be investigated for associations with *HLA*. Therefore, there is a substantial amount of literature on this subject (reviewed by Acton and Barger, 1980; Murphy *et al.*, 1977). For the purpose of this review, we will limit ourselves to a discussion of those studies wherein an association of *HLA* with malignant melanoma in Caucasians has been investigated. Table I is a compilation of ten such studies from around the world. As noted in the table, we calculated the χ^2, p value, and relative risk for some of the data if exact values were not given in the original reports. As was seen in Fig. 2, there are 78 HLA-A, -B, -C, and -DR specificities that can be assessed in association studies, thus leading to the possibility that some of these will deviate significantly at the 0.05 probability level by chance alone. A common way of correcting for this possibility is to multiply the p value by the number of HLA specificities that were analyzed in the study. Svejgaard et al. (1974) have noted that this is a conservative approach and tends to obviate false associations that might appear. Cole (1979) has presented sound arguments as to the fallacy of the reputed need to correct the first study. Even if necessary, this conservative correction could be required only in the first study showing an association, since in subsequent studies the hypothesis would be that the previously reported deviation of a specific antigen was replicable, and not as with the first study that any HLA antigen frequency deviates from control. We have chosen to present uncorrected as well as corrected p values.

As can be seen in Table I, only a couple of investigators have reported the same antigen to be deviated in melanoma patients compared with healthy controls. Bergholtz et al. (1977) and Singal et al. (1974) both reported an increase in B27 in their malignant-melanoma patient population as compared to healthy controls. Lamm et al. (1974b) and Tarpley et al. (1975) both reported a decrease of B7 in their patient population. These were the only instances in which investigators from different geographic areas of the world found the same HLA antigen deviations in their patient populations. The most statistically significant finding was that of Pelligris et al. (1980), who observed a significant increase in B40 and a decrease in Bw35 in their malignant-melanoma patient population. This deviation remained when the patient population was broken down into those with and without present clinical evidence of melanoma. Although the increase of B40 and decrease of Bw35 was essentially the same in these two groups, an excess of HLA blanks was observed at both A and B loci in the group with clinical evidence of malignant melanoma. However, because Clark et al. (1973, 1974) reported the masking of B5 in individuals with metastatic melanoma, the increase in HLA blanks by the Italian group needs further confirmation. The largest patient population to be investigated has come from Terasaki's group in California (Nathanson et al., 1980; Terasaki et al., 1977). These investigators originally looked at the frequencies of 25 HLA-A, -B, and -C antigens in 226 melanoma patients compared with 575 healthy controls. The expression of these antigens in the patient population was essentially the same as in healthy controls. The frequencies of these antigens were also analyzed in the patient population when stratified for sex and stage of disease. Again, there were no significant differences observed. These latter two investigators made one point that is important to remember when evaluating the data summarized in Table I, i.e., the difficulty of demonstrating an HLA association with melanoma in patient populations with various European ancestral origins. The fact that several of the aforementioned investigators were studying heterogeneous populations might have been a factor in their not finding a significant difference in expression of HLA antigens in the melanoma-patient population as compared to healthy controls. Likewise, those investigators who have demonstrated an increase or decrease in HLA specificities in the patient population may have been fortunate to have been looking at a relatively homongeneous subracial group of Caucasians. This is an important aspect of such studies to bear in mind, since epidemiological data suggest that

TABLE I

Summary of Studies on the Association of HLA with Melanoma in Caucasians

Geographic area	HLA antigens studied (number)	HLA type ↑ Inc.	HLA type ↓ Dec.	Antigen frequency — Patients Total	Patients % Pos.	Controls Total	Controls % Pos.	Significance[a] χ^2	p	p^c	RR[b]	Reference
Oslo, Norway	32	B27	—	54	24	215	11	5.39	2.0×10^{-2}	6.4×10^{-1}	2.5	
	8	LD108	—	43	21	209	9	4.82	2.8×10^{-2}	2.2×10^{-1}	2.8	Bergholtz *et al.* (1977)
Ontario, Canada	23	B27	—	33	24	200	9	5.08	1.5×10^{-2}	3.5×10^{-1}	3.5	Singal *et al.* (1974)
Aarhus, Denmark	25	—	B7	212	26	562	35	4.80	2.1×10^{-1}	5.3	0.7	Lamm *et al.* (1974b)
Maryland, U.S.	21	B8	—	87	31	389	17	8.18	4.2×10^{-3}	8.8×10^{-2}	2.2	
	21	—	B7	87	18	389	30	6.31	1.2×10^{-2}	2.5×10^{-1}	0.5	Tarpley *et al.* (1975)
London, England	23	Bw18	—	54	15	107	3	7.60	5.8×10^{-3}	1.3×10^{-1}	6.0	Cordon (1973)
Liege, Belgium	18	A9	—	33	36	830	21	3.67	4.3×10^{-2}	7.7×10^{-1}	2.2	Van Wijck and Bouillenne (1973)
Milan, Italy	37	B40	—	140	15	904	4	23.61	5.6×10^{-7}	2.0×10^{-5}	4.1	
Montreal Canada	37	—	Bw35	140	13	853	28	13.69	1.6×10^{-6}	5.9×10^{-3}	0.4	Pelligris *et al.* (1980)
	32	0	0	31	—	160	—	—	—	—	—	Espinoza *et al.* (1979)
California, U.S.	8	0	0	236	—	575	—	—	—	—	—	Nathanson *et al.* (1980)
	25	0	0	226	—	3896	—	—	—	—	—	Terasaki *et al.* (1977)

[a] χ^2 and p values when underlined were calculated by the authors and were not taken from the references cited. All corrected p values (p^c) were calculated by the authors.

[b] (RR) Relative risk, calculated by the authors using the cross-products or incidence-ratio formula of Woolf (1955); $RR = (a \times d)/(c \times b)$ where a is the number of patients possessing the particular HLA antigen, b is the number of patients lacking the particular HLA antigen, c is the number of controls possessing the particular HLA antigen, and d is the number of controls lacking the particular HLA antigen. The relative risk of developing melanoma for a person possessing B27 living in Norway would be: $(13 \times 191)/(24 \times 41) = 2.52$.

only certain subgroups of Caucasoids are at an increased risk for developing malignant melanoma (Lane Brown and Melia, 1973; McGovern, 1977; Segi, 1963).

In a recent report, Hersey et al. (1979b) made mention of unpublished data where the frequencies of HLA antigens were analyzed in familial-melanoma patients. They reported a higher frequency of A2 in the patient population compared to normal controls. Moreover, the family segregation of HLA in 13 families did not reveal linkage of the sus-ceptibility gene(s) for melanoma to the MHC. Since this was an unpublished observation, no evidence for a formal linkage analysis was given. To our knowledge, this is the only study of HLA in familial melanoma and the only attempt to demonstrate linkage of one or more melanoma-susceptibility genes with genes at the MHC.

2.4. The Immune Response

Studies mainly in mice and guinea pigs have demonstrated that genes at the MHC are involved in control of several immune functions (Benacerraf and Germain, 1978). There is also considerable evidence for the existence of MHC *Ir* genes in man (C. E. Buckley et al., 1973; Spencer et al., 1976; Cunningham-Rundles et al., 1978; Haverkorn et al., 1975; G. E. Buckley III and Roseman, 1976). Numerous reports in this volume as well as other sources document an immune response to transformed melanocytes (Ferrone and Pellegrino, 1978; Gutterman et al., 1975; Spitler, 1976). It is suspected that the appearance or spontaneous regression of melanoma may in fact be due to, respectively, a deficient or adequate host immune response to the transformed melanocyte (Lewis, 1972; Lewis et al., 1979; Nathanson, 1976).

Evidence that the host's immune response to melanoma is under genetic control can be sought in studies of immune reactivity in familial-melanoma patients and their relatives. Dean et al. (1979) investigated 60 members of four families prone to melanoma and observed a diminished response to pooled alloantigens by one-way MLC. Not only the melanoma patients but also patients with precursor nevi, unaffected blood relatives, and spouses demonstrated a diminished response. The fact that unrelated family members (spouses) had a diminished response led these authors to suggest that environmental factors such as viruses, rather than specific genes, may be involved. This interpretation of the data is consistent with the reports of Roy et al. (1976) and Spitler et al. (1977), who reported that tumor-specific immune reactivity is due to contact with melanoma patients. Vanden-bark et al. (1979) have measured the immune reactivity to melanoma extracts by the leu-kocyte-adherence inhibition test in 40 members of three melanoma-prone families and also found that the responses were not genetically determined but correlated to length of expo-sure to melanoma patients. Thus, these reports do not offer evidence for the segregation of immune-response capability in melanoma-prone families.

There is one preliminary report that suggests that a specific expression of the immune response is associated with the occurrence of melanoma and that the depression is under genetic control. Hersey et al. (1979b) found an association between natural-killer (NK) cell activity and melanoma in 13 families with 18 melanoma patients and 53 relatives. There was low NK activity in a high proportion of melanoma patients and their families. This was not associated with a general depression of the immune response. Although a formal analysis was not conducted, these investigators suggested that NK activity was inherited in an autosomal dominant mode. An association of HLA antigens or ABO blood group with melanoma and NK activity was not observed. Preliminary observations also did not reveal in these families the segregation of HLA haplotypes with the disease or NK activity. A low incidence of the Rh-negative phenotype was observed in the patients. This observation was not significant, but was of interest in view of the previous finding by Hersey *et al.* (1979a) that Rh-negative subjects have higher NK activity than Rh-positive subjects. In summary, although there is a paucity of evidence to suggest that *Ir* genes contribute to the susceptibility to melanoma, only a few family studies have been reported, and these investigators have evaluated only a few measures of immune responsiveness.

3. An Immunogenetic Analysis of Melanoma Patients in Alabama

We will now draw attention to the immunogenetic data that have been collected on the Caucasian patients treated at the Melanoma Clinic at the University of Alabama in Birmingham (UAB). As previously pointed out, Alabama has the highest melanoma mortality rate of any state in the United States (Mason and McKay, 1974). We therefore began a study in 1978 to evaluate genetic and epidemiological factors in this patient population. This study was enhanced by the UAB Melanoma Registry, which is an ongoing retrospective–prospective analysis of all patients with melanoma treated at the UAB. Since initiation of the study, the data collected on 105 patients have been evaluated. There were 40 male and 65 female patients, as can be seen in Table II, which also summarizes the place of birth of these patients and continuity of domicile in Alabama. We found that 71.4% of all the patients were born in Alabama, 13.3% in a surrounding state, and only 15.3% from outside the southern United States. Moreover, 70.5% of the patients had lived all their lives in Alabama.

TABLE II

Place of Birth and Continuity of Domicile of Melanoma Patients Treated at the UAB Melanoma Clinic

Variable	Total		Male		Female	
	Number	%	Number	%	Number	%
Birthplace						
Alabama	75	71.4	29	72.5	46	70.8
Surrounding states	14	13.3	5	12.5	9	13.9
Other	16	15.3	6	15.0	10	15.3
TOTALS:	105	100	40	100	65	100
Continuity of domicile in Alabama						
Uninterrupted	74	70.5	29	72.5	45	69.2
Interrupted	31	29.5	11	27.5	20	30.8

TABLE III

Familial Characteristics of Melanoma Patients Treated at the UAB Melanoma Clinic

Familial occurrence	Patients (96)		Male (41)		Female (55)	
	Number	%	Number	%	Number	%
Cancer						
First-degree relatives only	31	32.3	11	26.8	20	36.4
First- and second-degree relatives	21	21.9	8	19.5	13	23.6
First- and/or second-degree relatives	75	78.1	29	70.7	46	83.6
Skin cancer or melanoma or both						
First-degree relatives only	15	15.6	7	17.1	8	14.5
First- and/or second-degree relatives	23	24.0	9	22.0	4	25.5
Melanoma only						
First-degree relatives only	4	4.2	3	7.3	1	1.8
First- and/or second-degree relatives	8	8.4	4	9.8	4	7.3

Table III summarizes the familial variables for our patient population. Perhaps the most striking finding is the high frequency of all types of cancer reported in the relatives of our probands. The probands reported that 32.3% of their first-degree relatives, 21.9% of their first- and second-degree relatives, and 78.1% of their first- and/or second-degree relatives had cancer. Lynch *et al.* (1977, 1978) have observed a similar incidence of cancer in the relatives of probands reporting with melanoma. Further, in our patient population, almost 16% of first-degree relatives of probands and 24% of their first- and/or second-degree relatives had skin cancer or melanoma or both. When this was broken down for melanoma only, the probands reported that 4% of their first-degree relatives and 8% of their first- and/or second-degree relatives were affected. This incidence is in agreement with the 1–6% familial cases of all cases of melanoma estimated by other investigators. Anderson (1971) has observed up to 44% familial occurrence of those with several primary melanomas. Reimer *et al.* (1978) have found what they term precursor lesions in 56% of first-degree relatives.

A sample of the patients presenting to the UAB Melanoma Clinic during 1978–1981 have been evaluated for the frequencies of HLA antigens and Bf phenotype. A full report of these investigations has been submitted for publication, and only the key findings will be presented here (Acton *et al.*, 1980; Barger *et al.*, 1982; Budowle *et al.*, 1982). The frequencies of the aforementioned polymorphisms in the melanoma-patient population were compared with those in controls randomly selected from the local Caucasian population. Only those controls who did not report a family or personal history of cancer or an HLA-associated disease and were at least third-generation Americans were chosen.

For a comparison of HLA-A, -B, and -C antigens, 217 controls and 98 melanoma patients were typed. We observed an increase of B27 and a decrease of B7 and Bw35 in our patient population compared to normal controls. These deviations in antigen frequencies were not statistically significant. However, as shown in Table I, other investigators have noted deviation of these same antigens. Table IV summarizes those HLA antigens and Bf phenotypes that were found to deviate significantly between melanoma patients and controls. No significant deviations were observed between controls and patients for the *A-*

TABLE IV

Frequencies (%) of HLA Antigens and Properdin Factor B Found to Deviate Significantly between Melanoma Patients and Controls[a]

	Phenotype frequencies				
Polymorphism	Controls	Patients	p	p^c	RR
Bw42	0.0	4.1	0.002	0.091	—
DR4	16.0	37.8	0.001	0.021	2.8
Bf-F	52.0	32.3	0.025	0.100	0.4
Bf-S	83.3	98.4	0.005	0.020	12.2

[a]Symbols: (p) Level of statistical significance; (p^c) corrected p value; (RR) relative risk computed by the odds-ratio method of Woolf (1955).

and *C-* locus antigens. However, as can be seen in Table IV, Bw42 was significantly increased in the patient population (p = 0.002). Since this *B*-locus antigen has not been previously reported associated with melanoma, we applied the Bonferroni inequality by multiplying the p values by the number of antigens (45) tested. The resultant p value is no longer significant (p = 0.091). When the frequency of DR antigens in 69 melanoma patients was compared with that in 106 controls, DR4 was found to be significantly increased even after the p value was corrected (p = 0.021). Individuals who possess DR4 have a 2.8-fold greater risk of developing melanoma than those who do not possess this antigen. This is the first report demonstrating a significant increase in the frequency of DR4 in melanoma patients compared to healthy controls. Bergholtz *et al.* (1977) observed an increased frequency of the *D*-locus antigen LD108 in their patient population that was not statistically significant after the p value was corrected for the number of antigens tested (Table I). The only other study in which *DR*-locus antigens have been investigated in melanoma patients is that by Nathanson *et al.* (1980), who did not find significant deviations in the patient population. However, these investigators stressed that their Los Angeles patient population was heterogeneous. Alabama has a relatively nonmigratory population with very few people leaving the state. Moreover, there is a preponderance of individuals with a Celtic background (Scotch-Irish) as determined by surnames and declaration of ancestral origin. The melanoma-patient population studied in Alabama is most likely a relatively homogeneous group. Further investigations must be conducted to assure that the association is truly disease-related and not secondary to ethnic differences between cases and controls.

To date, the frequencies of the Bf alleles have been determined for 102 healthy controls and 62 melanoma patients. The Bf-F allele was carried by 32.3% of our melanoma patients compared to 52% of healthy controls (p < 0.05, uncorrected only). Individuals carrying this allele would appear to have a relative risk of less than 1.0 for developing melanoma. There is a significant increase of individuals carrying the Bf-S allele among melanoma patients (97.4%) compared to healthy controls (83.3%) (p < 0.05, corrected). Those individuals possessing this gene have a 12.2-fold greater risk for melanoma. This is the first report we are aware of demonstrating an association of Bf with melanoma. However, these data have to be viewed with caution for the moment. The fact that 83.3% of the normal population is Bf-S-positive makes this marker of limited use to predict who is at risk. Moreover, the fact that there was only one Bf-FF individual in the sample of melanoma patients assessed—the other patients typed being either SS, FS, SS, or F1S—accounts in part for the high relative risk (12.2) for those who are phenotypically Bf-S. Individuals who are Bf-F homozygous are at low risk for melanoma, which could be of some use as a marker, particularly among melanoma-prone families. The typing of additional patients and controls would permit more stable estimates of the Bf-FF frequencies. The difficulty in interpreting the present data is due to the low frequency of the Bf-F1 and Bf-S1 alleles in our population, which makes the Bf system essentially a two-allele system. Therefore, where one component is overrepresented in a sample, the other one will be underrepresented. This is indeed the case in our sample of the melanoma population. The Bf-F allele is present in low frequency in the patient population, while the Bf-S is increased. One way to separate these effects is to compare haplotype frequencies using other MHC markers. This can be done only by assessing family members.

In view of the association of DR4 with melanoma in our patient population, it is not surprising that there is also a deviation in the frequency of the Bf alleles, since the loci for DR and Bf have been reported in linkage disequilibrium (Baur and Danilovs, 1980). We therefore sought to analyze which of the DR and Bf polymorphisms reported to be in linkage disequilibrium were most strongly associated with melanoma. Table V is a compilation of four 2 × 2 contingency tables evaluating the association of DR4 vs. Bf-S with melanoma. When the presence or absence of either Bf-S or DR4 is held constant and the presence or absence of the other allele in the melanoma population is compared vs. the healthy controls, both polymorphisms appear associated with the disease. For some of the cells analyzed, the numbers are small, and the proportions of those with and without the allele were not statistically significantly different. However, there is an increased relative risk for both DR4 and Bf-S when analyzed alone in the patient population in the absence of the other. Table VI is a similar analysis for DR3 and Bf-F. As can be seen, the decrease of DR3 in the patient population seems to occur only in the presence of Bf-F. Again, more patients and controls need to be typed to confirm these preliminary observations.

TABLE V
Stratified Association of HLA-DR4 and Bf-S with Melanoma

Polymorphism	Bf-S$^+$				Bf-S$^-$			
	Melanoma	Controls	RR	p	Melanoma	Controls	RR	p
DR4$^+$	21	14			1	3		
			2.6	<0.01			5.0	NS[a]
DR4$^-$	40	70			1	15		
	DR4$^+$				DR4$^-$			
Bf-S$^+$	21	14			40	70		
			4.5	NS			8.6	<0.025
Bf-S$^-$	1	3			1	15		

[a](NS) Not significant.

Table VI
Stratified Association of HLA-DR3 and Bf-F with Melanoma

Polymorphism	Bf-F⁺				Bf-F⁻			
	Melanoma	Controls	RR	p	Melanoma	Controls	RR	p
DR3+	3	21			13	11		
			0.3	NS[a]			1.6	NS[a]
DR3⁻	17	32			29	38		

	DR3⁺				DR3⁻			
Bf-F⁺	3	21			17	32		
			0.1	<0.005			0.5	NS
Bf-F⁻	13	11			29	38		

[a](NS) Not significant.

One particularly interesting observation made on our patient population was the association of DR antigens with state of disease. A significant association ($p = 0.0025$) of DR4 with Stage I melanoma was found when compared to controls for a relative risk of 3.4. The numbers of Stage II and III patients were too small to compare each group separately with the control group. When these two stages were pooled into a single group, there were sufficient numbers for analysis. When the Stage II–III group was compared to controls, a significant decrease ($p = 0.0132$) in DR3 was observed. When this group was compared to Stage I patients, a significant decrease ($p = 0.0205$) of DR3 was also observed. When the p values were corrected for the number of antigens tested, the difference in DR3 frequency was no longer significant. It could well be that the death rate is increased among DR3 Stage I patients and that they would therefore be less likely to appear in the Stage II–III group in a cross-sectional study. Alternatively, DR3 could be a marker predicting a more favorable prognosis in that Stage I patients with this HLA antigen may be less likely to progress to Stage II or Stage III. A longitudinal study needs to be conducted wherein patients are typed on initial presentation with disease and their cases followed. We are currently involved in such a study. These observations on our melanoma population are consistent with a large body of data that suggest that HLA antigens can indeed be used to predict survival and outcome of therapy for individuals affected with various types of malignancies (Acton et al., 1980).

4. Implications and Future Direction

In this review, we have examined the evidence for an immunogenetic role in the occurrence or natural history of melanoma. The animal results provide evidence that genetic mechanisms are indeed involved in the etiology of melanoma. In addition, none of the genes that have been identified appear to be involved in immune responsiveness. On the surface, it would appear that the best case for immunogenetic involvement in humans comes from the familial-melanoma data. However, unequivocal documentation that genetic mechanisms are involved in the etiology of familial melanoma is lacking. There is great need for a formal segregation analysis, taking into account apparent heterogeneity, to be conducted on these families as a means of establishing the mode(s) of inheritance. The possibility of using certain clinical syndromes such as the B-K mole syndrome to identify family members at risk for developing melanoma (Clark et al., 1978; Reimer et al., 1978) is exciting. However, the usefulness of this syndrome as a high-risk marker needs to be more fully established by other investigators in a larger number of families. Moreover, these families should be evaluated with regard to the inheritance of the various genetic polymorphisms shown to be associated with melanoma in population studies. This would allow one to determine whether the melanoma-susceptibility gene or genes are linked to the genes that code for these polymorphisms, assuming these population associations are caused by linkage disequilibrium. The HLA antigens would be key in an evaluation of this kind due to the documented use of this polymorphic system in other disease studies of multiply affected families (Dausset and Svejgaard, 1977; Terasaki, 1980) and to the known linkage between the histocompatibility genes and Ir genes from animal studies and the suggested linkage in man. The association of HLA antigens with melanoma could be explained by their being in linkage disequilibrium with these Ir genes. It is therefore very likely that multiple genes are involved in protecting or predisposing an individual to melanoma. The Italian (Pellegris et al., 1980) as well as the Alabama study demonstrated a significant increase in certain HLA specificities in the respective melanoma samples compared with controls. One could speculate that this was due to the ethnic homogeneity of the respective samples of patients. Additional studies are needed using both familial and nonfamilial cases before the full potential of this and other polymorphic markers can be realized. Using genetic markers to predict outcome after onset of melanoma is another potentially important area that needs further study. There are several reports indicating that HLA will be useful in this regard for a number of malignant diseases (Acton and Barger, 1980). For example, those individuals presenting with acute lymphocytic leukemia who are A2 have a greater likelihood of survival than those lacking this HLA specificity (Harris et al., 1978).

More information relative to the immune competence of melanoma-prone families is needed. If these family studies revealed an association between HLA haplotypes, for example, and measures of immune competence, one could then examine their cosegregation in families to discern whether the immune capability is linked to the MHC or melanoma susceptibility or both. At the moment, the preliminary studies along this line reported by Hersey et al. (1979b) are not encouraging, but the amount of data is so limited that more detailed analyses on a large number of families are warranted. Ideally, a longitudinal study in high-risk families could answer some of these questions.

There are several reports that subracial groups of Caucasians such as those who are of Celtic or Scandinavian heritage are more at risk for melanoma particularly after migration to areas of higher UV intensity (Lane Brown et al., 1971; Magnus, 1977; Segi, 1963). To identify those at high risk, we need to determine the relative risk of melanoma of different subracial groups at different UV intensities. In the past, such a study would have had to depend on the vagueness of family trees to assess the contribution of a particular ethnic heritage. It is now possible if enough alleles in an individual are identified to assess the degree of genetic difference with respect to possible parental populations within certain confidence limits. This would confer on such studies a degree of validity not previously possible.

It would be particularly important to consider the epidemiology of the disease to fully understand the involvement of genes in the etiology. For example, there is a need to examine the genetic–environmental interaction in order to understand the role of UV light as an inducer of melanoma. As previously alluded to, the epidemiology data reveal that Caucasians are more at risk for melanoma than blacks, with identifiable subgroups of Caucasians at greater risk. Melanoma patients have lighter skin and eyes, do not tolerate the sun as well, do not tan easily, and due to dress, work, or recreational habits or latitude of domicile, may have been exposed to the sun for longer duration or greater intensities than normal controls (Clark *et al.*, 1977; Kleep and Magnus, 1979; McGovern, 1977). As one can readily appreciate, the problem is not easy, for it requires determining the level at which genetic mechanisms are involved to render an individual susceptible to an environmental insult. The data presented herein suggest that susceptibility differs in racial and ethnic groups—being most pronounced in individuals and families with certain phenotypic characteristics—could be explained by one or more sets of genes related to melanocyte development, replication, differentiation, growth, metabolism, or regulation. Given that melanoma patients can respond to their tumors, one has to speculate that there are genes that control or modulate this latter immune response. Depending on the alleles inherited, one could be highly susceptible or resistant to melanoma. Since the frequencies of specific alleles differ among the many racial and ethnic groups, one would expect to see different genetic associations in melanoma patients from various parts of the world (Baur and Danilovs, 1980. Familial melanoma may be explained by the fact that certain matings result in the presence of multiple-susceptibility genes governing, for example, melanin production and immune-response capability.

One way to test the validity of these speculations and help define the etiology of melanoma is to conduct large-scale case–control studies wherein multiple variables including the following are assessed: racial and ethnic heritage; phenotypic characteristics (e.g., hair, eye, skin color, sensitivity to the sun, ability to tan, family history of disease); genotypic characteristics (e.g., HLA, Bf, ABO, Rh, Gm^1, Gm^2); dress, work, and recreational habits; place(s) and duration of domicile prior to presenting with melanoma. Obviously, detailed assessment of the immune-response capabilities (particularly to melanoma-tumor antigens) of the subjects and family members should be a part of the protocol. For comparison, these variables should also be evaluated in a large healthy control sample from a well-defined population. It is important to recall that the odds ratio, which can be calculated from a case–control study in a relatively rare disease like melanoma, is a good estimate of the relative risk, which can be measured directly only in a prospective study. Persons with different clinical and pathological forms of melanoma should probably be analyzed separately.

If designed and conducted properly, this type of study would allow one the opportunity to analyze together all the many known variables that may influence onset of the disease or survival, or both. From such a study, one could estimate the relative contribution of each of the factors to the occurrence of melanoma. Additionally, such a study would yield the capability of predicting with a high degree of sensitivity and specificity those individuals at risk in the population for malignant melanoma. This would allow preventive and early-detection measures to be effected that should counter the increase of this disease in our society.

ACKNOWLEDGMENTS. The authors would like to express appreciation to Dr. John R. Durant for his support and encouragement as well as to Mss. Sandra Boyd and Mary Estock for secretarial assistance. The authors' research cited herein was supported in part by PHS Grant Nos. CA 15338, CA 09128, CA 18609, CA 27197, and CA 13148 awarded by the National Cancer Institue, DHHS.

References

Acton, R. T., and Barger, B. O., 1980 The potential use of HLA to predict risk of malignant diseases and outcome of therapy, in: *Pediatric Oncology* (G. B. Humphrey, L. P. Dehner, and G. B. Grindey, eds.), pp. 47–77, Martin Nijhoff, The Hague.

Acton, R. T., Barger, B. O., Murphy, C. C., Roseman, J. M., Ingalls, A. L., and Balch, C. M., 1980, Apparent association of HLA antigens with melanoma; *Proc. Am. Assoc. Cancer Res. 21:49.*

Albert, E., Amos, D. B., Bodmer W. F., Ceppellini, R., Dausset, J., Kissmeyer-Nielsen, F. Mayr, W., Payne, R., van Rood, J. J., Terasaki, P. I., and Walford, R. L., 1980, Nomenclature for factors of the HLA system 1980; *Tissue Antigens* 16:113.

Amos, D. B., Bashir, H., Boyle, W., MacQueen, M., and Tijlikainen, F., 1970, A simple microcytotoxicity test; *Transplantation* 7:220.

Anders, F., Diehl, H., Schwab, M., and Anders, A., 1979, Contributions to an understanding of the cellular origin of melanoma in the Gordon–Kosswig Xiphorine fish tumor system, *Pigm. Cell* 4:142.

Anderson, D. E., 1971, Clinical characteristics of the genetic variety of cutaneous melanoma in man; *Cancer* 21:721.

Anderson, D. E., Smith, L., and McBride, C. M., 1967, Hereditary aspects of malignant melanoma, *J. Am. Med. Assoc.* 200:741.

Bach, F. H., and Hirschhorn, K., 1964, Lymphocyte interaction: A potential histocompatibility test *in vitro,* *Science* 143:813.

Bach, F. H., and van Rood, J. J., 1976, The major histocompatibility complex—genetics and biology, *N. Engl. J. Med.* 295:806, 872, 927.

Bakker, E., Pearson, P. L., Khan, P. M., Schreuder, G. M., and Madau, K., 1979, Orientation of major histocompatibility (MHC) genes relative to the centromere of human chromosome 6, *Clin. Genet.* 15:198.

Balch, C. M., 1980, Surgical management of regional lymph nodes in cutaneous melanoma, *J. Am. Acad. Dermatol.* 3:511.

Balch, C. M., Murad, T. M., Soong, S., Ingalls, A. L., Halpern, N. B., and Maddox, W. A., 1978, A multifactoral analysis of melanoma. I. Prognostic histopathological features comparing Clark's and Breslow's staging methods, *Ann. Surg.* 188:732.

Balch, C. M., Murad, T., Soong, S., Ingalls, A. L., Richards, P. C., and Maddox, W. A., 1979a, Tumor thickness as a guide to surgical management of clinical Stage I melanoma patients, *Cancer* 43:883.

Balch, C. M., Soong, S., Murad, T., Ingalls, A. L., and Maddox, W. A., 1979b, A multifactorial analysis of melanoma. II. Prognostic factors of clinical Stage I disease, *Surgery* 86:343.

Balch, C. M., Wilkerson, J. A., Murad, T. J., Soong, S. J., Ingalls, A. L., and Maddox, W. A., 1980, The prognostic significance of ulceration of cutaneous melanoma, *Cancer* 45:3012.

Balch, C. M., Soong, S. J., Murad, T. M., Ingalls, A. L., and Maddox, W. A., 1981, A multifactorial analysis of melanoma. III. Prognostic factors in melanoma patients with lymph node metastases (Stage II), *Ann. Surg.* 193:377.

Balner, H., 1979, Are D and DR antigens identical? A review of available data for man and the rhesus monkey, *Transplant. Proc.* 11:657.

Barger, B. O., Acton, R. T., Soong, S. J., Roseman, J. M., and Balch, C. M., 1982, Increase of HLA-DR4 in melamona patients from Alabama, *Cancer Res.* (in press).

Baur, M. P., and Danilovs, J. A., 1980, Reference tables of two and three locus haplotype frequencies for HLA-A, B, C, DR, Bf and GLO, in: *Histocompatibility Testing 1980* (P. I. Terasaki, ed.), pp. 994–1210, UCLA Tissue Typing Laboratory, Los Angeles.

Benacerraf, B., and Germain, R. N., 1978, The immune response genes of the major histocompatibility complex, *Transplant. Rev.* **38**:70.

Bergholtz, B., Brennhovd, I., Klepp, O., Kaakinen, A., and Thorsby, E., 1977, HLA antigens in malignant melanoma, in: *HLA and Malignancy* (G. P. Murphy, E. Cohen, J. E. Fitzpatrick, and D. Pressman, eds.), pp. 175–180, Alan R. Liss, New York.

Bodmer, W. F., and Bodmer, J. G., 1978, Evolution and function of the HLA system, *Br. Med. Bull* **34**:309.

Buckley, C. E., Dorsey, F. C., Corley, R. B., Ralph, W. B., Woodburh, M. A., and Amos, D. B., 1973, HLA linked human immune response genes, *Proc. Natl. Acad. Sci. U.S.A.* **70**:2157.

Buckley, G. E., III, and Roseman, J. M., 1976, Immunity and survival, *J. Am. Geratr. Soc.* 24:241.

Budowle, B., Barger, B., Balch, C. M., Go, R. C. P., Roseman, J. M., and Acton, R. T., 1982, Associations of properdin factor B with melanoma, *Cancer Genetics and Cytogenetics* (in press).

Cawley, E. P., 1952, Genetic aspects of malignant melanoma, *Arch. Dermatol.* **65**:440.

Clark, D. A., Necheles, T., Nathanson, L., and Silverman, E., 1973, Apparent HLA-A5 deficiency in malignant melanoma, *Transplantation* **15**:326.

Clark, D. A., Necheles, T. F., Nathanson, L., Whitten, D., Silverman, E., and Flavers, A., 1974, Apparent HLA-A5 deficiency in human malignant melanoma. II. HL-A5 masking activity in sera of patients with progressing disease. *Isr. J. Med. Sci.* 10:836.

Clark, W. H., Jr., Mastrangelo, M. J., Ainsworth, A. M., Berd, D., Bellet, R. E., and Bernardino, E. A., 1977, Current concepts of the biology of human cutaneous malignant melanoma, *Adv. Cancer Res.* **24**:267.

Clark, W. H., Reimer, R. R., Greene, M., Ainsworth, A. M., and Mastrangelo, M. J., 1978, Origin of familial malignant melanomas from heritable melanocytic lesions: The B-K syndrome, *Arch. Dermatol.* **114**:732.

Cole, P., 1979, The evolving case control study, *J. Chron. Dis.* **32**:15.

Codron, A. L., 1973, HL-A and malignant melanoma, *Lancet* 1:938.

Crombie, I. K., 1979, Racial differences in melanoma incidence with latitude in North American and Europe, *Br. J. Cancer* **40**:774.

Cunningham-Rundles, S., Cunningham-Rundles, C., Pollack, M. S., Good, R. A., and Dupont, B., 1978, Response to wheat antigen in *in vitro* lymphocyte transformation among HLA-B8 positive normal donors, *Transplant. Proc.* 10:4.

Cutler, S. J., and Young, J. L., Jr., 1975, Third National Cancer Survey: Incidence Data, National Cancer Institute Monograph 41, DHEW Publication No. (NIH) 75-487.

Dausset, J., and Svejgaard, A. (eds), 1977, *HLA and Disease*, Munksgaard, Copenhagen.

Dean J. H., Greene, M. H., Reimer, R. R., LeSane,R. V., McKeen, E. A., Mulvihill, J. J., Blattner, W. A., Herberman, R. B., and Fraumeni, J. F., Jr., 1979, Immunologic abnormalities in melanoma-prone families, *J. Natl. Cancer Inst.* **63**:1139.

Elwood, J. M., and Lee, J. A. H., 1974, Trends in mortality from primary tumours of the skin in Canada, *Can. Med. Assoc. J.* **110**:913.

Espinoza, L. R., Dorval, G., and Osterland, C. K., 1979, Levamisole-induced adverse reactions and histocompatibility testing in malignant melanoma, *Tissue Antigens* 13:236.

Ferrone, S., and Pellegrino, M. A., 1978, Antigens and antibodies in malignant melanoma, in: *The Handbook of Cancer Immunology*, Vol. 6 (H. Waters, ed.), pp. 291–327, Garland STPM Press, New York.

Gordon, M., 1972, The genetics of viviparous top-minnow *Platypoecilus*: The inheritance of two kinds of melanophores, *Genetics* **12**:253.

Greene, M. H., Reimer, R. R., Clark, W. H., Jr. and Mastrangelo, M. J., 1978, Precursor lesions in familial melanoma, *Semin. Oncol.* **5**:85.

Greifelt, A., 1952, Malignes Melanom: Beziehungen zu Schwangerschaft, Pubertät, Kindheit: Familiäre maligne Melanome, *Arztliche Wochenschr.* 7:676.

Gutterman, J. V., Mavbigit, G., Reed, R., Richman, S., McBride, C. E., and Hersh, E. M., 1975, Immunology and immunotherapy of human-malignant melanoma: Historic review and perspectives for the future, *Semin. Oncol.* **2**:155.

Harris, R., Lawler, S. D., and Oliver, R. T. D., 1978, The HLA system in acute leukaemia and Hodgkin's disease, *Br. Med. Bull.* **34**:301.

Häussler, G., 1927, Über Melanombildung bei Bastarden von *Xiphophorus helleri* and *Ptalypoecilus maculatus var rubra, Klin. Wochenschr.* 7:1561.

Haverkorn, M. T., Hofman, B., Masurel, N., and Van Rood, J. J., 1975, HLA linked genetic control of immune response in man, *Transplant. Rev.* 22:120.

Hersey, P., Edwards, A., Trilivas, C., Shaw, H., and Melton, G. W., 1979a, Relationship of natural killer-cell activity to rhesus antigens in man, *Br. J. Cancer* 39:234.

Hersey, P., Edwards, A., Honeyman, M., and McCarthy, W. H., 1979b, Low natural-killer-cell activity in familial melanoma patients and their relatives, *Br. J. Cancer* 40:113.

Hook, R. R., Jr., Auttman, M. D., Adelstein, E. H., Oxenhandler, R. W., Millikan, L. E., and Middleton, C. C., 1979, Influence of selective breeding on the incidence of melanoma in Sinclair miniature swine, *Int. J. Cancer* 24:668.

Ikonopisov, R. L., and Tsanov, T. I., 1974, Blood groups in patients with malignant melanoma of the skin, *Tumori* 60:361.

Jörgensen, G., 1967, The ABO blood group-polymorphism in the multifactorial genetic system, *Humangenetik* 3:264.

Jörgensen, G., and Lal, V. B., 1972, Serogenetic investigations on malignant melanomas with reference to the incidence of ABO system, Rh system, Gm, INV, Hp and Gc systems, *Humangenetik* 15:227.

Klepp, O., and Magnus, K., 1979, Some environmental and bodily characteristics of melanoma patients: A case-control study, *Int. J. Cancer* 23:482.

Kopf, A. W., Mintzis, M., Grier, R. N., Silvers, D. N., and Bart, R. S., 1976, Familial malignant melanoma, *Curtis* 17:873.

Kosswig, C., 1927, Über Bastarde der Teleostier *Platypoecilus* and *Xiphophorus, Z. Indukt. Abstamm.-Vererbungsl.* 44:253.

Lamm, L. U., Friedrich, U., Petersen, G. B. Jørgensen, J., Nielsen, J., Therkelsen, A. J., and Kissmeyer-Nielsen, F., 1974a, Assignment of the major histocompatibility complex to chromosome No. 6 in a family with a pericentric inversion, *Hum. Hered.* 24:273.

Lamm, L. U., Kissmeyer-Nielsen, F., Kjerbye, K. E., Mogensen, B., and Petersen, N. C., 1974b, HL-A and ABO antigens in malignant melanoma: A study of 212 cases, *Cancer* 33:1458.

Lane Brown, M. M., and Melia, D. F., 1973, Celticity and cutaneous malignant melanoma in Massachusetts, in: *Pigment Cell: Mechanisms in Pigmentation* (V. J. McGovern and P. Russell, eds.), pp. 229–235, S. Karger, Basel

Lane Brown, M. M., Sharpe, C. A. B., Macmillan, D. S., and McGovern, V. J., 1971, Genetic predisposition to melanoma and other skin cancer in Australians, *Med. J. Aust.* 1:852.

Leeuwen, A. V., Schruit, H. R. E., and Rood, J. J. V., 1973, Typing for MLC (LD). II. The selection of non-stimulator cells by the MLC inhibition tests using SD identical stimulator cells (MISTS) and fluorescent antibody studies, *Transplant. Proc.* 5:1539.

Lewis, M. G., 1972, Immunology of human malignant melanoma, *Ser. Haematol.* 5:44.

Lewis, M. G., Phillips, T. M., Noble, P. B., and Hartmann, D. P., 1979, Immune derangement in patients with malignant melanoma, *J. Cut. Pathol.* 6:201.

Lokich, J. J., 1975, Malignant melanoma and carcinoma of the breast, *J. Surg. Oncol.* 7:199.

Lynch, H. T., and Krush, A. J., 1968, Heredity and malignant melanoma: Implications for early cancer detection, *Can. Med. Assn. J.* 99:17.

Lynch, H. T., Frichot, B. C., Lynch, P., Lynch, J., and Guirgis, H. A., 1975, Family studies of malignant melanoma and associated cancer, *Surg. Gynecol. Obstet.* 141:517.

Lynch, H. T., Guirgis, H. A., Lynch, P. M., Lynch, J. F., and Harris, R. E., 1977, Familial cancer syndromes: A survey, *Cancer* 39:1867.

Lynch, H. T., Organ, C. H., Jr., Harris, R. E., Guirgis, H. A., Lynch, P. M., and Lynch, J. F., 1978, Familial cancer: Implications for surgical management of high-risk patients, *Surgery* 83:104.

Magnus, K., 1977, Incidence of malignant melanoma of the skin in the five Nordic countries: Significance of solar radiation, *Int. J. Cancer* 20:477.

Mason, T. J., and McKay, F. W., 1974, U.S. cancer mortality by county: 1950–1969, DHEW Publication No. (NIH) 74–615.

McDevitt, H. O., and Bodmer, W. F., 1974, HL-A, immune response genes and disease, *Lancet* 1:1269.

McGovern, V. J., 1977, Epidemiological aspects of melanoma: A review, *Pathology* 9:233.

Millikan, L. E., Boylon, J. L., Hook, R. R., Jr., and Manning, P. J., 1974, Melanoma in Sinclair swine: A new animal model, *J. Invest. Dermatol.* **62**:20.

Mittal, K. K., 1978, Standardization of the HLA typing method and reagents, *Vox Sang.* **34**:58.

Murphy, G. P., Cohen, E., Fitzpatrick, J. E., and Pressman, D. (eds), 1977, *HLA and Malignancy, Progress in Clinical and Biological Research,* Vol. 16, Alan R. Liss, New York.

Nathanson, L., 1976, Spontaneous regression of malignant melanoma: A review of the literature on incidence, clinical features and possible mechanisms, *Natl. Cancer Inst. Monogr.* **44**:67.

Nathanson, S. D., Park, M. S., Drew, S. I., Morton, D. L., and Terasaki, P. I., 1980, First and second B-lymphocyte antigen expression in malignant melanoma, *Transplant. Proc.* **12**:118.

Ohsumi, T., and Seiji, M., 1977, Statistical study on malignant melanoma in Japan (1970–1976), *Tohoku J. Exp. Med.* **121**:355.

Pellegris, G., Illeni, M. T., Vaglini, M., Rovini, D., Cascinelli, N., and Masserini, C., 1980, HLA antigens in malignant melanoma patients, *Tumori* **66**:51.

Reimer, R. R., Clark, W. H., Jr., Greene, M. H., Ainsworth, A. M., and Fraumeni, J. F., 1978, Precursor lesions in familial melanoma: A new genetic preneoplastic syndrome, *J. Am. Med. Assoc.* **239**:744.

Rittner, C., 1976, Genetic loci of components of the classical and alternate pathway of complement activation: A new dimension of the immunogenetic linkage group (HLA) on chromosome 6 in man, *Hum. Genet.* **35**:1.

Rittner, C., and Mauff, G., 1978, MHC-associated complement genes in man and animals, *Behring Inst. Mitt.* **62**:100.

Roy, C., Lewis, M. G., Capek, A., Shibata, H., and Jerry, L. M., 1976, Lymphocytotoxicity against melanoma cells from individuals with varying exposure to melanoma tissue, *Proc. Am. Assoc. Cancer Res.* **17**:153.

Schoch, E. P., 1963, Familial malignant melanoma: A pedigree and cytogenetic study, *Arch. Dermatol.* **88**:445.

Schreuder, I., Meo, T., Termijtelen, A., and Meera Khan, P., 1980, The Bf locus is between HLA-B and D/DR, in: *Histocompatibility Testing 1980* (P. I. Terasaki, ed.), pp. 931–932, UCLA Tissue Typing Laboratory, Los Angeles.

Schultheis, W., Peter, H. H., and Deicher, H., 1975, Gm(1) and Gm(2) immunoglobulin allotypes in patients with malignant melanoma, *Humangenetik* **28**:177.

Segi, M., 1963, World incidence and distribution of skin cancer, *Natl. Cancer Inst. Monogr.,* No. 16, p. 245.

Singal, D. P., Bent, P. B., McCulloch, P. B., Blajchman, M. H., and MacLaren, R. G. C., 1974, HL-A antigens in malignant melanoma, *Transplantation* **18**:186.

Spencer, M. J., Cherry, J. D., and Terasaki, P. I., 1976, HLA antigens and antibody response after influenza A vaccine, *N. Engl. J. Med.* **294**:13.

Spitler, L. E., 1976, Malignant melanoma, *J. Invest. Dermatol.* **67**:435.

Spitler, L. E., Littovy, R. N., and Sagebiel, R. W., 1977, Cellular immunity in patients with malignant melanoma and their household contacts, *Cancer Immunol. Immunother.* **2**:69.

Strafuss, A. C., Dommert, A. R., Tumbleson, M. E., and Middleton, C. C., 1968, Cutaneous melanoma in miniature swine, *Lab. Anim. Care* **18**:165.

Sutherland, E. M., Kloepper, H. W., Mansell, P. W. A., and Krementz, E. T., 1975, Familial melanoma, *Pigment Cell* **2**:421.

Svejgaard, A., Jersild, C., Nielsen, L., Stuab, Nielsen L., Bodmer, W. F., 1974, HL-A antigens and disease: Statistical and genetical considerations, *Tissue Antigens* **4**:95.

Tarpley, J. L., Chretien, P. B., Rogentine, N., Jr., Twomey, P. L., and Dellon, A. L., 1975, Histocompatibility antigens and solid malignant neoplasms, *Arch. Surg.* **110**:269.

Terasaki, P. I., and McCelland, J. D., 1964, Microdroplet assay of human serum cytotoxins, *Nature (London)* **204**:998.

Terasaki, P. I., Perdue, S. T., and Mickey, M. R., 1977, HLA frequencies in cancer: A second study, in: *Genetics of Human Cancer* (J. J. Mulvilhill, R. W. Miller, and J. F. Fraumoni, Jr., eds.), pp. 321–328, Raven Press, New York.

Terasaki, P. I., Bernoco, D., Park, M. S., Ozturk, G., and Iwaki, Y., 1978, Microdroplet testing for HLA-A, -B, -C and -D antigens: The Philip Levine Award Lecture, *Am. J. Clin. Histopathol.* **69**:103.

Terasaki, P. I. (ed.), 1980, *Histocompatibility Testing 1980,* UCLA Tissue Typing Laboratory, Los Angeles.

Turkington, R. W., 1965, Familial factors in malignant melanoma, *J. Am. Med. Assoc.* **192**:85.

Vandenbark, A. A., Greene, M. H., Burger, P. R., Vetto, R. M., and Reimer, R. R., 1979, Immune response to melanoma extracts in three melanoma-prone families, *J. Natl. Cancer Inst.* **63**:1147.

Van Wijck, R., and Bouillenne, C., 1973, HL-A antigen and susceptibility to malignant melanoma, *Transplantation* **16**:371.

Wallace, D. C., Exton, L. A., and McLeod, G. R. C., 1971, Genetic factors in malignant melanoma, *Cancer* **27**:1262.

Wallace, D. C., Beardmore, G. L., and Exton, L. A., 1973, Familial malignant melanoma, *Ann. Surg.* **177**:15.

Walter, H., Brachtel, R., and Hilling, M., 1979, On the incidence of blood group O and Gm(-1) phenotypes in patients with malignant melanoma, *Hum. Genet.* **49**:71.

Woolf, B., 1955, On estimating the relationship between blood group and disease, *Ann. Hum. Genet.* **19**:251.

2

Indomethacin, Prostaglandin, and Immune Regulation in Melanoma

CHARLES M. BALCH AND ARABELLA B. TILDEN

1. Introduction

Melanoma patients exhibit decreased immunocompetence as measured by a variety of *in vitro* and *in vivo* immunological responses (Golub *et al.*, 1974; Eilber *et al.*, 1975; Zembala *et al.*, 1977). It has been assumed that this decreased immunocompetence is due to a deficiency of effector-cell function (e.g., antibody-forming B lymphocytes, cytotoxic T lymphocytes). Such a concept led to a strategy of immunotherapy manipulations with the goal of *stimulating* the immune system to correct the deficit. However, information obtained in recent years has demonstrated that the tempo, intensity, and even the choice of effector cells may be regulated in part by suppressor cells and by helper cells (also called amplifying cells, accessory cells, or inducer cells). Thus, the observation that melanoma patients exhibit decreased immunocompetence should be examined in the context of helper and suppressor lymphocytes or macrophages or both, for the immunosuppressed state in some patients might be due to too little "help" or too much suppression. Furthermore, this concept may partially explain the failure of immunotherapy to improve survival rates, since there is some experimental evidence that immunotherapy agents may have a dual effect by stimulating both effector cells and suppressor cells with the result that there is no *net* change in immune balance.

Immune regulation can take place by cell–cell contact between regulatory cells and effector cells as well as by release of soluble mediators. This chapter will focus on one important group of mediators: prostaglandin (PG) and other metabolic products of arachidonic acid that can regulate certain cellular immune responses. Such immunopharmacol-

CHARLES M. BALCH AND ARABELLA B. TILDEN • Departments of Surgery and Microbiology; Cellular Immunobiology Unit, Comprehensive Cancer Center; Veterans Hospital, University of Alabama in Birmingham, Birmingham, Alabama 35294

23

ogy assays involving the PG system often utilize indomethacin because it can inhibit PG synthesis. It should be emphasized, however, that indomethacin has other effects on cellular function independent of PG production.

2. Prostaglandin and Indomethacin

PGs are important regulatory hormones that influence cellular immune functions in their microenvironment rather than via a systemic effect. They have been proposed as intercellular soluble mediators, since they have been demonstrated to both stimulate and inhibit lymphoid cells and their immune functions, depending on the response being tested (Goodwin and Webb, 1980; Stenson and Parker, 1980). PG metabolism may represent an important pathogenetic mechanism in tumor immunology, since this hormone can suppress a number of cellular immune responses. PGs have been demonstrated to inhibit T-lymphocyte proliferative response to mitogens and alloantigens (Goodwin et al., 1977a; Darrow and Tomar, 1980), lymphokine production (Gordon et al., 1976; Koopman et al., 1973), natural and antibody-dependent cellular cytotoxicity (Droller et al., 1978b; Brunda et al., 1980), cell-mediated cytolysis (Henney et al., 1972; Schultz et al., 1978), and antibody production (Braun and Ishizuka, 1971; Webb and Osheroff, 1975; Plescia et al., 1975; Fulton and Levy, 1980). Macrophages and monocytes are the primary lymphoid-cell types that synthesize PGs (Goodwin et al., 1977a; Kurland and Bockman, 1978). Numerous stimuli have been used to stimulate PG production by macrophages, including immune complexes and immune stimulants such as bacillus Calmette Guérin (BCG) and Corynebacterium parvum. PG may therefore contribute to certain aspects of the decreased immunocompetence in cancer patients.

Stenson and Parker (1980) and other investigators have emphasized certain pitfalls and limitations associated with PG-related experiments. They have pointed out, for example, that contaminating cells such as granulocytes and platelets also contain PGs and may therefore influence results of macrophage assays. Moreover, even purified macrophage populations are heterogeneous, with different subpopulations discernible by physical properties that vary considerably in their ability to synthesize PGs (Picker et al., 1980). Dose–response relationships are also important, since PG may have varying effects at different concentrations. Another problem in interpreting PG data is the diversity of arachidonic acid metabolites produced by macrophages that may have different effects on cellular metabolism. Finally, there are several shortcomings of in vitro immune studies involving PG as models for in vivo events, especially since PGs are metabolized rapidly and excreted.

Indomethacin is a commonly used antiinflammatory drug the primary effect of which is to block the synthesis of arachidonic acid into PGs by inhibiting PG synthetase (also termed cyclooxygenase). Here again, the doses of indomethacin used may influence metabolic pathways of arachidonic acid. At higher doses, some of its selective effects for cyclooxygenase products are diminished and other systems are influenced. For example, it is known that indomethacin has direct effects on cellular function such as: (1) uncoupling of oxidative phosphorylation, (2) stabilization of lysosomes, (3) membrane stabilization, and (4) inhibition of a number of enzymes (Shen and Winter, 1977). One of its important effects in terms of a cellular proliferation is the perturbation of cyclic AMP (cAMP) levels through inhibition of phosphodiesterase (Weiss and Hart, 1977) and the inhibition of AMP-dependent protein kinases (Kantor and Hampton, 1978). Although it is generally assumed that indomethacin effects are the result of PG synthetase inhibition, it is important to distinguish this effect from the non-PG-related effects of indomethacin.

3. Helper- and Suppressor-Cell Function in Tumor-Bearing Mice

PG-mediated immune suppression has been found to influence several parameters of immune function in animals bearing both viral and chemically induced tumors. For example, PG has been shown in tumor-bearing mice to inhibit natural killer (NK) activity (Droller *et al.*, 1978b; Brunda *et al.*, 1980) and to suppress the plaque-forming cell responses (Fulton and Levy, 1980). The administration of indomethacin *in vitro* and *in vivo* enhances both mitogen responses and NK activity in mice bearing either fibrosarcoma, mammary adenocarcinoma, or Cloudman melanoma (Pelus and Strausser, 1976; Droller *et al.*, 1978a; Brunda *et al.*, 1980). Pelus and Bockman (1979) found that splenic macrophages from animals bearing methylcholanthrene (MCA)-induced fibrosarcomas or Maloney-sarcoma-virus-induced tumors produced significantly more PG than macrophages from normal non-tumor-bearing littermates.

Some animal tumors have been shown to elaborate high levels of PG relative to normal tissues (Plescia *et al.*, 1975; Karim, 1976; Trevisani *et al.*, 1980). Grinwich and Plescia (1977) reported that PG produced by mouse fibrosarcoma cells suppressed antibody production *in vitro* and that indomethacin blocked this immunosuppression. They and others have also made the important observation that *in vivo* administration of indomethacin retarded growth of the chemically induced fibrosarcoma tumors (Plescia *et al.*, 1975; Grinwich and Plescia, 1977; Lynch and Salomon, 1979) and hepatoma tumors (Trevasani *et al.*, 1980).

PG may also have an important influence on the therapeutic effectiveness of immunotherapy in these animal tumor models. It has been assumed that immunotherapy acts by exerting a positive effect on lymphocyte and macrophage function. However, there is increasing evidence that biological response modifiers, such as *C. parvum* and BCG, may have a dual effect by enhancing the activity of both effector cells and suppressor cells (Kirchner *et al.*, 1975; Scott, 1972). Immunotherapy might therefore cause offsetting increases in both positive and negative regulatory functions so that there is no net change in immune balance. In fact, there is experimental evidence that PG-mediated and other forms of suppression are actually enhanced by BCG and *C. parvum* immunotherapy (Humes *et al.*, 1977; Grimm *et al.*, 1978; Savary and Lotzova, 1978; Ojo *et al.*, 1978; Murahata and Zighelboim, 1979; Tracey and Adkinson, 1980) and that the oral administration of indomethacin increases the therapeutic effectiveness of these immune stimulants in sarcoma-bearing mice (Grimm *et al.*, 1978; Lynch and Salomon, 1979). It is therefore possible that the combination of indomethacin and immunotherapy might have a more positive therapeutic benefit.

An opposite relationship of PG and indomethacin has been demonstrated in the mouse B16 melanoma mode. Both PGD_2 and PGE_2 decrease the growth rate of metastatic B16 melanoma *in vivo,* while indomethacin actually enhances B16 tumor growth (Santoro *et al.,* 1976; Stringfellow and Fitzpatrick, 1979; Favalli *et al.,* 1980). Furthermore, the combination of chemotherapy plus PGE_2 had a synergistic antitumor effect (Hofer *et al.,* 1980). These diametric results from experiments in the MCA-induced-sarcoma mice may represent different biological features of the tumor itself, the immune response to it, and/or the differences in doses of PG used by different investigators.

4. Helper- and Suppressor-Cell Function in Cancer Patients

Depressed immune responses in patients with cancer and other diseases may be related to abnormalities of immune regulation with imbalances of suppressor- and helper-cell function. A relative excess of suppressor-cell activity has been demonstrated in patients with head and neck carcinomas (Balch *et al.,* 1981a), lung carcinoma (Jerrells *et al.,* 1978; Han and Takita, 1980), osteogenic sarcoma (Yu *et al.,* 1977), bladder-cell carcinoma (Bean *et al.,* 1977), Hodgkin's lymphoma (Goodwin *et al.,* 1977b; Engleman *et al.,* 1978), acute leukemia (Broder *et al.,* 1978), and multiple myeloma (Broder *et al.,* 1975). Furthermore, there is some indirect evidence that immunotherapy in cancer patients might activate suppressor-cell function. Such an event would explain the transient decrease in mitogen response and other parameters of immune function observed in cancer patients for 1–7 days after receiving immunotherapy injections (Thatcher *et al.,* 1979; Gill *et al.,* 1980).

A number of suppressor-cell systems have been identified in man. These include suppressor lymphocytes and suppressor monocytes. Monocytes have been shown to suppress lymphocyte responses by several mechanisms including the elaboration of PGE_2 (Goodwin *et al.,* 1977a; Kurland and Bockman, 1978; Metzger *et al.,* 1980). The mitogen response to phytohemagglutimin (PHA) and concanavalin A (Con A) is an excellent *in vitro* model to analyze in this context, since accessory or helper monocytes are an absolute requirement for T-lymphocyte proliferation and the rate of proliferation can be decreased by suppressor monocytes. Furthermore, this particular *in vitro* assay coordinates well with *in vivo* measures of immunocompetence in melanoma patients (Golub *et al.,* 1974).

Goodwin *et al.* (1977a) first showed that PGE_2 inhibited T-cell mitogenesis in normal humans and further that the addition of PG synthetase inhibitors to PHA cultures would result in increased [³H]thymidine incorporation. An increased PHA and Con A mitogen response with indomethacin has been demonstrated in patients with Hodgkin's lymphoma (Goodwin *et al.,* 1977b), head and neck epidermoid carcinomas (Balch *et al.,* 1981a), and lung carcinomas (Han and Takita, 1980). Han and Takita (1980) observed a greater enhancement of lymphocyte response by indomethacin in weak responders as compared to strong responders in 26 lung-cancer patients and 17 healthy controls. A greater enhancement was also noted in lung-cancer patients with active disease as compared to those in clinical remission. Balch *et al.* (1981a) have found that both indomethacin and the experimental drug R0-205720 (the only known effect of which is to inhibit PG synthesis) enhanced the PHA and Con A responses of 23 head and neck carcinoma patients to a greater degree than the responses of 19 normal subjects. They also demonstrated excessive PGE_2 production by blood mononuclear cells from the head and neck cancer patients compared to the normal controls (11.7 $\pm$ 1.3 vs. 4.2 $\pm$ 0.9 ng/ml; $p < 0.001$). Goodwin *et al.* (1977b) found that the depressed mitogen response in Hodgkin's-disease patients could be corrected by inhibiting PGE synthesis with either indomethacin or R0-205720 and that the hyporesponsiveness to mitogens was due to a measured increase in the production of PGE_2.

In light of this information, we performed a series of experiments on 33 melanoma patients and 29 normal subjects to determine whether their mitogen response to PHA and Con A was decreased to any significant degree and whether this immune suppression was related to the PG system.

5. Mitogen Response in Melanoma Patients and Normal Subjects

The lymphocyte responses to Con A and PHA were used as a measure of immunocompetence in 33 melanoma patients compared to that of 29 normal individuals. Of the melanoma patients, 21 had localized melanoma (Stage I) and 8 had regional node metastases (Stage II), while 4 had distant metastases (Stage III). Eight patients were receiving nonspecific immunotherapy (BCG or *C. parvum*) at the time of this study. None was receiving chemotherapy.

Total monuclear cells were separated from heparinized blood by Ficoll-Hypaque density centrifugation as previously described (Balch *et al.*, 1977). The peripheral-blood mononuclear cells (PBMC) were washed and suspended in tissue-culture medium with 20% fetal calf serum (FCS) and gentamycin. By Wright stain analysis, the average number of monocytes was the same for both normal subjects (24 $\pm$ 12%) and melanoma patients (24 $\pm$ 11%). PBMC, 1 $\times$ 10^5, were suspended in 20% FCS plus gentamycin and cultured in microtiter plates with different doses of PHA or Con A. The cells were incubated at 37°C in 5% CO_2 for a total of 96 hr. Cultures were pulsed with [^{14}C]thymidine (0.0125 μCi/well) 16 hr before being harvested. The net counts per minute of triplicate cultures were calculated as counts per minute of cells with mitogen minus counts per minute of cells without mitogen.

The results demonstrated that the mitogen response from the melanoma patients was significantly depressed compared to normal control values for all three concentrations of Con A and PHA (Table I). Thus, in 32 of the 33 melanoma patients, the responses to one

TABLE I

Mitogen Responses to Concanavalin A and Phytohemagglutinin Comparing Melanoma Patients and Normal Controls

Mitogen	Dose (μg/ml)	Melanoma patients[a]	Normal controls[a]	p Value
Con A	1	1433 $\pm$ 193	2,545 $\pm$ 351	0.03
	5	4525 $\pm$ 546	7,010 $\pm$ 492	< 0.0001
	10	4949 $\pm$ 438	8,558 $\pm$ 549	< 0.0001
PHA	20	6227 $\pm$ 438	10,961 $\pm$ 725	< 0.0001
	100	6804 $\pm$ 491	10,276 $\pm$ 606	< 0.0001
	200	6370 $\pm$ 559	8,798 $\pm$ 511	0.007

[a]Mean counts per minute [^{14}C]thymidine $\pm$ S.E.

or both of the two mitogens was below the normal range. These results confirmed numerous observations that lymphocytes from cancer patients have decreased mitogen responses (Hersh and Oppenheim, 1965; Golub *et al.*, 1974; Wanebo *et al.*, 1975; Zembala *et al.*, *1977). There were no significant differences in the 8 patients who were receiving immunotherapy compared to those who were not.*

6. Effects of Indomethacin on Mitogen Response

Aliquots of PBMC from the same subjects were also tested in parallel with indomethacin to determine whether this drug might enhance the mitogen response observed in melanoma patients, either by inhibiting PGE_2-mediated suppression or by other actions on the lymphoid cells. Dose–response curves of indomethacin demonstrated that a 1 $\mu g/ml$ dose (approximately 10^{-6} M) was the most appropriate dose, while lower concentrations (down to 10^{-8} M) had gradually diminishing effects. The concentration of 1 $\mu g/ml$ dose was therefore used throughout these experiments.

Indomethacin caused a significant increase in the proliferative responses to PBMC from melanoma patients at all doses of PHA and Con A, whereas it caused a much lower change in the response of PBMC from normal subjects (Table II). The percentage increase in mitogen response with indomethacin was more pronounced at lower doses, and the differences were statistically significant. At a 1 $\mu g/ml$ dose of Con A, the mean response of melanoma patients increased from 56 to 81% of normal response, while at the lowest PHA dose used (20 $\mu g/ml$), the mitogen response increased from 57 to 77% of normal when the PBMC were incubated with indomethacin. Goodwin *et al.* (1978) had previously shown that PGE_2 inhibition of lymphocyte proliferation is higher with submitogenic doses of lectins and, conversely, that the indomethacin effect is usually greater at lower mitogen doses. Differences were also detectable at the highest doses used, but they were not statistically significant due to sample variability (Table II).

TABLE II

Percentage Enhancement of Mitogen Response When Blood Mononuclear Cells Were Incubated with Indomethacin

Mitogen[a]	Dose ($\mu g/ml$)	Melanoma patients[b]	Normal controls[b]	p Value
Con A	1	86 ± 17	17 ± 9	0.0001
	5	46 ± 10	16 ± 6	0.012
	10	47 ± 16	21 ± 5	0.130
PHA	20	50 ± 11	11 ± 5	0.0017
	100	41 ± 11	8 ± 5	0.0089
	200	33 ± 12	10 ± 5	0.088

[a] Plus indomethacin (1 $\mu g/ml$) in all cultures.
[b] Mean percentage increase ± S.E.

TABLE III
TABLE III
Indomethacin Enhancement in Melanoma Patients Comparing Their Stage of Disease

Mitogen[a]	Dose (μg/ml)	Localized melanoma (Stage I)[b]	Metastatic melanoma (Stages II and III)[b]
Con A	1	81 ± 23 (18)	95 ± 24 (11)
	5	38 ± 14 (18)	58 ± 13 (11)
	10	34 ± 11 (21)	69 ± 40 (11)
PHA	20	38 ± 12 (19)	69 ± 22 (12)
	100	38 ± 11 (21)	46 ± 22 (12)
	200	25 ± 9 (21)	47 ± 29 (12)

[a]Plus indomethacin (1 μg/ml) in all cultures.
[b]Mean percentage increase ± S.E. Number of patients tested in parentheses.

7. Correlation with Clinical Status of Melanoma Patients

The prognostic factors that influence survival rates include: the stage of disease, the tumor thickness, the patient's age and sex, and tumor location (Balch *et al.*, 1978, 1979a,b, 1981b). It is important in this type of immunological study to correlate the observed results with clinical characteristics of the melanoma patients to ensure that the immunological effect was not a secondary one.

The melanoma-patient data were subdivided by stage of disease to determine how the indomethacin effect might be related to the extent of tumor dissemination. At all doses of Con A and PHA, the level of [14C]thymidine incorporation was lower for patients with regional and distant metastatic disease (Stages II and III) than for those with localized disease (Stage I). Furthermore, the increase in mitogen response in the presence of indomethacin was greater in patients with metastatic disease than in those with localized disease (Table III). These differences, however, were not statistically significant.

Age of the individual was also examined as a separate variable, since it is known that older patients have a lower survival rate and thicker tumors (Balch *et al.*, 1979b) and since it has been shown by Goodwin and Messner (1979) that PGE_2-mediated suppression increases as a function of age. Although there was a tendency for the indomethacin effect to increase with age in both the control and patient groups, the magnitude of increase within each age group was significantly greater for the melanoma patients (data not shown).

8. Indomethacin Effects on Purified Lymphocytes and Monocytes

It is known that both accessory monocytes and suppressor monocytes modulate the degree of lymphocyte-proliferation response to PHA and Con A. Moreover, the monocyte has shown to be the major PG-producing cell in normal human PBMC (Goodwin *et al.*, 1977a; Kurland and Bockman, 1978; Picker *et al.*, 1980). To confirm this observation in melanoma patients, we isolated erythrocyte-rosette-positive (ER^+) T lymphocytes to determine whether the indomethacin effect would be abrogated when monocytes were depleted. Aliquots (1 ml) of Ficoll-Hypaque-purified PBMC [at 1×10^7/ml in Roswell Park Memorial Institute (RPMI) 1640 medium with 10% FCS] were mixed with 1 ml 5% sheep red blood cells (SRBC) treated with 2-aminoethylisothiouronium bromide (Pellegrino *et al.*, 1975; Balch *et al.*, 1977). The ER^+ T lymphocytes were isolated by a double-rosetting technique, and SRBC were removed by treatment with ammonium chloride lysing buffers. More than 98% of the purified lymphocytes formed E rosettes.

In a sample of eight melanoma patients and four normal controls, the mitogen response for blood mononuclear cells (both lymphocytes and monocytes) was enhanced by indomethacin for the melanoma patients, but not for the normal subjects. In contrast, when the monocytes were depleted, the purified T lymphocytes (ER^+) exhibited no differences in their PHA responses for the melanoma patients compared to normal controls (Table IV). Thus, the *in vitro* defect in immune competence for these melanoma patients was related to an abnormality in regulatory monocyte function. There are at least two explanations for this observed defect. First, the melanoma patients might have an abnormality in PG-mediated suppression that was blocked by indomethacin. Alternatively, they might have a defect in monocyte helper activity or suppressor activity that was directly influenced by indomethacin and was independent of PG metabolism. Experiments were next performed to examine these two possibilities.

9. Are the Indomethacin Effects Related to Prostaglandin?

Three experiments were performed to determine whether the indomethacin effect was due to inhibition of PGE_2-mediated suppression by monocytes. We expected that the indomethacin effect would be due to inhibition of PGE_2 production by suppressor monocytes, since Goodwin *et al.* (1977b) had clearly demonstrated this mechanism of action for the depressed mitogen responses observed in patients with Hodgkin's lymphoma and we had observed this abnormality in patients with head and neck carcinomas (Balch *et al.*, 1981a).

First, PGE_2 production by monocytes from melanoma patients was directly measured and compared to that obtained for normal subjects. Supernatants from PBMC cultures

TABLE IV

Phytohemagglutinin Response of Monocyte-Depleted Er^+ T Lymphocytes Incubated with and without Indomethacin

Patients[a]	Without indomethacin[b]	With indomethacin[b]
Normal (4)	5128 ± 910	5019 ± 714
Melanoma (8)	5140 ± 764	5593 ± 966

[a]Number of patients studied in parentheses.
[b]Mean counts per minute [^{14}C]thymidine ± S.E.

TABLE V

T-Lymphocyte Suppression of Mitogen Response by Exogenous PGE_2

PGE$_2$ dose (moles)	Con A (1 μg/ml)[a]		PHA (20 μg/ml)[a]	
	Melanoma patients	Normal controls	Melanoma patients	Normal controls
3×10^{-9}	19 ± 7	26 ± 5	11 ± 6	18 ± 4
3×10^{-8}	30 ± 5	46 ± 3	42 ± 6	43 ± 5
3×10^{-7}	52 ± 4	57 ± 2	57 ± 5	60 ± 4
3×10^{-6}	59 ± 4	65 ± 3	65 ± 5	65 ± 4

[a] Percentage inhibition of the mitogen response ± S.E.

were tested in a competitive-inhibition radioimmunoassay to quantitate PGE_2 production (Jaffe *et al.*, 1973). In a group of 12 melanoma patients and 11 normal controls, the amount of PGE_2 produced by cultured PBMC was the same for patients and controls (3.92 ± 0.69 vs. 3.22 ± 0.46 ng/ml).

Second, the suppressive effects of exogenous PGE_2 were compared using PBMC from patients and from normal controls. In these experiments, we examined the magnitude of PHA and Con A response in the presence of various doses of PGE_2 to determine whether lymphocyte function in melanoma patients might be more easily suppressed by equivalent PGE_2 doses. Aliquots of PBMC were first preincubated with indomethacin at doses known to block endogenous production of PG and then stimulated with mitogens in the presence of PGE_2 at different doses. The results showed that PGE_2 dose–response curves for PBMC from melanoma patients did not differ significantly from that obtained for normal controls (Table V).

Finally, another drug (R0-205720, Roche) was used to determine whether it could mimic the effects observed for indomethacin, since the only known action of R0-205720 is to inhibit PG synthetase. The results showed that R0-205720 did not increase the mitogen response of PBMC from six melanoma patients. Thus, the PHA response for the melanoma patients was increased by 61% with indomethacin, but only 11% with R0-205720. The Con A response increased by 64% with indomethacin, while it actually decreased by 12% with R0-205720. Appropriate controls with the alcohol diluent alone showed no significant effect on these results.

These three experiments thus indicated that the indomethacin enhancement of mitogen response in melanoma patients was clearly not related to PGE_2 production.

10. Summary

These experiments were designed to test a hypothesis that abnormalities in immune regulation exist in melanoma patients. Monocyte regulation of T-lymphocyte responses to the mitogens PHA and Con A were chosen as *in vitro* models of immune competence. A significantly depressed response to one or both of these mitogens was observed in 32 of 33 melanoma patients compared to that of 29 normal individuals. This abnormality could be partially corrected by incubating the PBMC with the drug indomethacin. The indomethacin enhancement of the mitogen responses was not related to the melanoma patients' age, stage of disease, or treatment. Its primary effect appeared to be related to an abnormal monocyte function, since monocyte depletion of blood lymphoid cells eliminated the differences in the mitogen response for melanoma patients compared to normal controls. Furthermore, there was no longer any enhancement of T-lymphocyte proliferation after indomethacin treatment.

Our initial interpretation of these data was that indomethacin was blocking PGE_2-mediated suppression by monocytes. However, the indomethacin effect was not related to PGE_2 by three criteria: (1) PGE_2 production by monocytes was not increased in melanoma patients compared to controls; (2) the magnitude of lymphocyte suppression with equivalent doses of exogenous PGE_2 was the same for melanoma patients as compared to normal controls; and (3) another drug (R0-205720) the only known effect of which is to inhibit PG synthetase did not increase the mitogen response in melanoma patients. These findings illustrate the pitfalls in overinterpreting experimental results using indomethacin.

Since indomethacin has multiple pharmacological effects, it is important to directly prove whether any drug-related effects are due to PG production or some other mechanism. Alternative hypotheses now being tested include the following: (1) indomethacin may be blocking the activity of suppressor monocytes by some mechanism other than PGE_2 production or (2) indomethacin may be enhancing the activity of helper (accessory)-monocyte populations. Identifying these cellular participants and their interactions with greater precision in the future may provide challenging and exciting prospects about immunological regulation that in turn may lead to more effective treatment approaches involving the immunological subsystem.

Note Added in Proof We have since performed further experiments on the effect of indomethacin on isolated ER^+ T lymphocytes and adherent cells (AC). Purified ER^+ T lymphocytes were pretreated with indomethacin ($1\mu g/ml$) for four hours and washed extensively. The indomethacin-treated ER^+ cells and AC were recombined in a 10:1 ratio and assayed for Con A response. The AC were added back to the ER^+ T cells to determine whether indomethacin might have a direct effect on T lymphocytes in the presence of optimal accessory cell numbers. Pretreatment of the T lymphocytes with indomethacin was sufficient to enhance the proliferative response of the reconstituted cells. There was no enhancement when adherent monocytes were pre-incubated with indomethacin. Thus, indomethacin may have a direct effect on T lymphocytes when these cells are provided with adequate accessory cell function. (A. B. Tilden and C. M. Balch, 1982, Immune modulatory effects of indomethacin in melanoma patients is not related to prostaglandin-mediated suppression (submitted for publication).

References

Balch, C. M., Dougherty, P. A., Dagg, M. K., Diethelm, A. G., and Lawton, A. R., 1977, Detection of human T cells using anti-monkey thymocyte antisera, *Clin. Immunol. Immunopathol.* **8**:448.

Balch, C. M., Murad, T. M., Soong, S., Ingalls, A. L., Halpern, N. B., and Maddox, W. A., 1978, A multifactorial analysis of melanoma. I. Prognostic histopathological features comparing Clark's and Breslow's staging methods, *Ann. Surg.* **188**:732.

Balch, C. M., Murad, T. M., Soong, S. J., Ingalls, A. L., Richards, P. C., and Maddox, W. A., 1979a, Tumor thickness as a guide to surgical management of clinical stage I melanoma patients, *Cancer* **43**:883.

Balch, C. M., Soong, S. J., Murad, T. M., Ingalls, A. L., and Maddox, W. A., 1979b, A multifactorial analysis of melanoma. II. Prognostic factors in patients with State I (localized) melanoma, *Surgery* **86**:343.

Balch, C. M., Dougherty, P. A., and Tilden, A. B., 1981a, Excessive prostaglandin E_2 production by suppressor cells in head and neck cancer patients, Proceedings ASCO/AACR (in press).

Balch, C. M., Soong, S. J., Murad, T. M., Ingalls, A. L., and Maddox, W. A., 1979b, A multifactorial analysis of melanoma. II. Prognostic factors in patients with Stage I (localized) melanoma, *Surgery* **86**:343.

Balch, C. M., Dougherty, P. A., and Tilden, A. B., 1981a, Excessive prostaglandin E_2 production by suppressor cells in head and neck cancer patients, Proceedings ASCO/AACR **23**:310.

cell activity in man, *J. Exp. Med.* **146**:1455.

Braun, W., and Ishizuka, M., 1971, Antibody formation: Reduced responses after administration of excessive amounts of nonspecific stimulators, *Proc. Natl. Acad. Sci. U.S.A.* **68**:114.

Broder, S., Humphrey, R., Durm, M., Blackman, M., Meade, B., Goldman, C., Strober, W., and Waldmann, T., 1975, Impaired synthesis of polyclonal (non-paraprotein) immunoglobulins by circulating lymphocytes from patients with multiple myeloma—role of suppressor cells, *N. Engl. J. Med.* **293**:887.

Broder, S., Poplack, D., Whang-Peng, J., Durm, M., Goldman, C., Muul, L. and Waldmann, T. A., 1978, Characterization of a suppressor-cell leukemia: Evidence for the requirement of an interaction of two T cells in the development of human suppressor–effector cells, *N. Engl. J. Med.* **298**:66.

Brunda, M. J., Herberman, R. B., and Holden, H. T., 1980, Inhibition of murine natural killer cell activity by prostaglandins, *J. Immunol.* **124**:2682.

Darrow, T. L., and Tomar, R. H., 1980, Prostaglandin-mediated regulation of the mixed lymphocyte culture and generation of cytotoxic cells, *Cell. Immunol.* **56**:172.

Droller, M. J., Perlmann, P., and Schneider, M. U., 1978a, Enhancement of natural and antibody-dependent lymphocyte cytotoxicity by drugs which inhibit prostaglandin production by tumor target cells, *Cell. Immunol.* **39**:154.

Droller, M. J., Schneider, M. U., and Perlmann, P., 1978b, A possible role of prostaglandins in the inhibition of natural and antibody-dependent cell-mediated cytotoxicity against tumor cells, *Cell. Immunol.* **39**:165.

Eilber, F. R., Nizze, J. A., and Morton, D. L., 1975, Sequential evaluation of general immune competence in cancer patients: Correlation with clinical course, *Cancer* **35**:660.

Engleman, E. G., Hoppe, R., and Kaplan, H., 1978, Suppressor cells of the mixed lymphocyte reaction in healthy subjects and patients with Hodgkin's disease and sarcoidosis, *Clin. Res.* **26**:513.

Favalli, C., Garaci, E., Etheredge, E., Santoro, M. G., and Jaffe, B. M., 1980, Influence of PGE on the immune response in melanoma-bearing mice, *J. Immunol.* **125**:897.

Fulton, A. M., and Levy, J. G., 1980, The possible role of prostaglandins in mediating immune suppression by nonspecific T suppressor cells, *Cell. Immunol.* **52**:29.

Gill, P. G., Waller, C. A., MacLennan, I. C. M., and Morris, P. J., 1980, Effect of intravenous *Corynebacterium parvum* on peripheral-blood effector cells of cancer patients, *Br. J. Cancer* **41**:782.

Golub, S. H., O'Connell, T. X., and Morton, D. L., 1974, Correlation of *in vivo* and *in vitro* assays of immunocompetence in cancer patients, *Cancer Res.* **34**:1833.

Goodwin, J. S., and Messner, R. P., 1979, Sensitivity of lymphocytes to prostaglandin E_2 increases in subjects over age 70, *J. Clin. Invest.* **64**:434.

Goodwin, J. S., and Webb, D. R., 1980, Regulation of the immune response by prostaglandins, *Clin. Immunol. Immunopathol.* **15**:106.

Goodwin, J. S., Bankhurst, A. D., and Messner, R. P., 1977a, Suppression of human T-cell mitogenesis by prostaglandin, *J. Exp. Med.* **146**:1719.

Goodwin, J. S., Messner, R. P., Bankhurst, A. D., Peake, G. T., Saiki, J. H., and Williams, R. C., Jr., 1977b, Prostaglandin-producing suppressor cells in Hodgkin's disease, *N. Engl. J. Med.* **297**:963.

Goodwin, J. S., Messner, R. P., and Peake, G. T., 1978, Prostaglandin suppression of mitogen-stimulated lymphocytes: *In vitro* changes with mitogen dose and preincubation, *J. Clin. Invest.* **62**:753.

Gordon, D., Bray, M., and Morley, J., 1976, Control of lymphokine secretion by prostaglandins, *Nature (London)* **262**:401.

Grimm, W., Seitz, M., Kirchner, H., and Gemsa, D., 1978, Prostaglandin synthesis in spleen cell cultures of mice injected with *Corynebacterium parvum*, *Cell. Immunol.* **40**:419.

Grinwich, K. D., and Plescia, O. J., 1977, Tumor-mediated immunosuppression: Prevention by inhibitors of prostaglandin synthesis, *Prostaglandins* **14**:1175.

Han, T., and Takita, H., 1980, Indomethacin-mediated enhancement of lymphocyte response to mitogens in healthy subjects and lung cancer patients, *Cancer* **46**:2416.

Henney, C. S., Bourne, H.R., and Lichtenstein, L. M., 1972, The role of cyclic 3',5' adenosine monophosphate in the specific cytolytic activity of lymphocytes, *J. Immunol.* **108**:1526.

Hersh, E. M., and Oppenheim, J. J., 1965, Impaired *in vitro* lymphocyte transformation in Hodgkin's disease, *N. Engl. J. Med.* **273**:1006.

Hofer, D., Dubitsky, A., and Jaffe, B., 1980, Prostaglandin potentiation of the effect of chemotherapy on B-16 melanoma, *Surg. Forum* **31**:417.

Humes, J. L., Bonney, R. J., Pelus, L. M., Dahlgren, M. E., Sadowski, F. A., Kuehl, F. A., Jr., and Davies, P., 1977, Macrophages synthesize and release prostaglandins in response to inflammatory stimuli, *Nature (London)* **269**:149.

Jaffe, B. M., Behrman, H. R., and Parker, C. W., 1973, Radioimmunoassay measurement of prostaglandin E, A, and F in human plasma, *J. Clin. Invest.* **52**:398.

Jerrells, T. R., Dean, J. H. Richardson, G. L., McCoy, J. L., and Herberman,R. B., 1978, Role of suppressor cells in depression of *in vitro* lymphoproliferative responses of lung and breast cancer patients, *J. Natl. Cancer Inst.* **61**:1001.

Kantor, H. S., and Hampton, M., 1978, Indomethacin in submicromolar concentrations inhibit cyclic AMP-dependent protein kinase, *Nature (London)* **276**:841.

Karim, S. M. M., 1976, Prostaglandins and tumors, *Adv. Prostaglandin Res.* **2**:303.

Kirchner, H., Glaser, M., and Herberman, R. B., 1975, Suppression of cell-mediated tumor immunity by *Corynebacterium parvum*, *Nature (London)* **257**:396.

Koopman, W. J., Gillis, M. H., and David J. R., 1973, Prevention of MIF activity by agents known to increase cellular cyclic AMP, *J. Immunol.* **110**:1609.

Kurland, J. L., and Bockman, R., 1978, Prostaglandin E production by human monocytes and mouse macrophages, *J. Exp. Med.* **147**:95.

Lynch, N. R., and Salomon, S. C., 1979, Tumor growth inhibition and potentiation of immunotherapy by indomethacin in mice, *J. Natl. Cancer Inst.* **69**:97.

Metzger, Z., Hoffeld, J. R., and Oppenheim, J. J., 1980, Macrophage mediated suppression. I. Evidence for participation of both hydrogen peroxide and prostaglandins in suppression of murine lymphocyte proliferation, *J. Immunol.* **124**:983.

Murahata, R. I., and Zighelboim, J., 1979, Inhibition of cell-mediated cytotoxicity to tumor alloantigens by systemic administration of *Corynebacterium parvum*, *Cancer Immunol. Immunother.* **6**:101.

Ojo, E., Haller, O., Kimura, A., and Wigzell, H., 1978, An analysis of conditions allowing *Corynebacterium parvum* to cause either augmentation or inhibition of natural killer cell activity against tumor cells in mice, *Int. J. Cancer* **21**:444.

Pellegrino, M. A., Ferrone, S., Dierich, M. P., and Reisfeld, R. A., 1975, Enhancement of sheep red blood cell human lymphocyte rosette formation by the sulfhydryl compound 2-amino ethylisothiouronium bromide, *Clin. Immunol. Immunopathol.* **3**:324.

Pelus, L., and Bockman, R., 1979, Increased prostaglandin synthesis by macrophages from tumor-bearing mice. *J. Immunol.* **123**:2118.

Pelus, L. M., and Strausser, H. R., 1976, Indomethacin enhancement of spleen-cell responsiveness to mitogen stimulation in tumorous mice, *Int. J. Cancer* **18**:653.

Picker, L. J., Raff, H. V., Goldyne, M. E., and Stobo, J. D., 1980, Metabolic heterogeneity among human monocytes and its modulation by PGE_2, *J. Immunol.* **124**:2557.

Plescia, O. J., Smith, A. H., and Grinwich, K., 1975, Subversion of immune system by tumor cells and role of prostaglandins, *Proc. Natl. Acad. Sci. U.S.A.* **72**:1848.

Santoro, M. G., Philpott, G. W., and Jaffe, B. M., 1976, Inhibition of tumor growth *in vitro* by prostaglandin E_2, *Nature (London)* **263**:777.

Savary, C. A., and Lotzova, E., 1978, Suppression of natural killer cell cytotoxicity by splenocytes from *Corynebacterium parvum*-injected, bone marrow-tolerant, and infant mice, *J. Immunol.* **120**:239.

Schultz, R. M., Pavlidis, N. A., Stylos, W. A., and Chirigos, M. A., 1978, Regulation of macrophage tumoricidal function: A role for prostaglandins of the E series, *Science* **202**:320.

Scott, M. T., 1972, Biological effects of the adjuvant *Corynebacterium parvum*. I. Inhibition of PHA, mixed lymphocyte and GVH reactivity, *Cell. Immunol.* **5**:459.

Shen, T. -Y., and Winter, C. A., 1977, Chemical and biological studies on indomethacin, sulindac and their analogs, *Adv. Drug Res.* **12**:89.

Stenson, W. F., and Parker, C. W., 1980, Prostaglandins, macrophages, and immunity, *J. Immunol.* **125**:1.

Stringfellow, D., and Fitzpatrick, F., 1979, Prostaglandin D_2 controls pulmonary metastasis of malignant melanoma cells, *Nature (London)* **282**:76.

Thatcher, N., Swindell, R., and Crowther, D., 1979, Effect of *Corynebacterium parvum* and BCG therapy on immune parameters in patients with disseminated melanoma: A sequential study over 28 days. II. Changes in non-specific (NK, K and T cell) lymphocytoxicity and delayed hypersensitivity skin reactions, *Clin. Immunol.* **35**:171.

Tracey, D. E., and Adkinson, N. F., Jr., 1980, Prostaglandin synthesis inhibitors potentiate the BCG-induced augmentation of natural killer cell activity, *J. Immunol.* **125**:136.

Trevisani, A., Ferretti, E., Capuzzo, A., and Tomasi, V., 1980, Elevated levels of prostaglandin E_2 in Yoshida hepatoma and the inhibition of tumour growth by non-steroidal anti-inflammatory drugs. *Br. J. Cancer* **41**:341.

Wanebo, H. J., Jun, M. Y., Strong. E. W., and Oettgen, H., 1975, T-cell deficiency in patients with squamous cell cancer of the head and neck, *Am. J. Surg.* **130**:445.

Webb, D. R., and Osheroff, P. L., 1975, Antigen stimulation of prostaglandin synthesis and control of immune responses, *Proc. Natl. Acad. Sci. U.S.A.* **73**:1300.

Weiss, B., and Hait, W. N., 1977, Selective cyclic nucleotide phosphodisterase inhibitors as potential therapeutic agents, *Annu. Rev. Pharmacol. Toxicol.* **17**:441.

Yu, A., Watts, H., Jaffe, N., and Parkman, R., 1977, Concomitant presence of tumor-specific cytotoxic and inhibitor lymphocytes in patients with osteogenic sarcoma, *N. Engl. J. Med.* **297**:121.

Zembala, M., Mytar, B., Popiela, T., and Asherson, G. L., 1977, Depressed *in vitro* peripheral blood lymphocyte response to mitogens in cancer patients: The role of suppressor cells, *Int. J. Cancer* **19**:605.

3

Shedding and Degradation of Cell-Surface Macromolecules and Melanoma-Associated Antigens by Human Melanoma

JEAN-CLAUDE BYSTRYN

1. Introduction

Tumor antigens, particularly those expressed on the surface of cells, are believed to have a critical though complex effect on tumor growth. They may stimulate immune responses and thus increase resistance to cancer. Conversely, alone or in complex with antibodies, they may interfere with humoral and cellular immune destruction of malignant cells and thus may enhance tumor growth. Since these effects can be mediated by soluble tumor antigens, the factors that influence their accumulation in body fluids may have an important impact on tumor growth.

For this reason, we have conducted a number of studies, using malignant melanoma as a model, that have elucidated some of the factors that influence tissue levels of soluble tumor antigens. As described subsequently, at least two factors appear to be of importance. The first, and most important, is the ability of tumor cells to rapidly release tumor antigens. The second is the susceptibility of these antigens to degradation.

JEAN-CLAUDE BYSTRYN • Department of Dermatology, New York University School of Medicine, New York, New York 10016.

2. Release of Tumor Antigens

2.1. Antigen Release by Tumor Cells

Soluble tumor antigens have been found in various body fluids of tumor-bearing animals and man (Thomson *et al.,* 1973; Baldwin *et al.,* 1973; Currie and Basham, 1972) and in the media of cells in tissue culture (Currie and Basham, 1972). In melanoma, tumor antigens have been found in the fluid of cystic tumors (Jehn *et al.,* 1970), in the urine of patients with this cancer (Carrel and Theilkaes 1973), in the kidneys of mice with B16 melanoma (Poskitt *et al.,* 1974), and in the media of murine (Bystryn *et al.,* 1974a) and human melanoma cells in culture (Bystryn, 1977; Grimm *et al.,* 1976; Gupta *et al.,* 1979; Stuhlmiller and Seigler, 1977; Leong *et al.,* 1978; McCabe *et al.,* 1978).

Two mechanisms can account for the presence of soluble antigens in body fluids. One is autolysis and release from dying cells; the other is release from viable cells. The evidence to date indicates that tumor antigens, as well as unrelated macromolecules, are rapidly released by viable tumor cells. The rate of release is such as to suggest that this process accounts for the bulk of soluble antigens found in patients with malignancies.

2.2. Release of Tumor-Associated Antigens by Murine Melanoma Cells

Release of tumor antigens by viable tumor cells was first demonstrated in B16 melanoma, a murine model of human melanoma (Bystryn *et al.,* 1974c). Macromolecules and antigens associated with this cancer were radiolabeled by incubating replicate plates of cells in culture with [^{3}H]leucine. After 72 hr, the cells were thoroughly washed and incubated in fresh media. At intervals thereafter, media and cells were collected from individual plates and the cells lysed in the nonionic detergent Nonidet P-40 (NP-40). Newly synthesized macromolecules in media and lysates were quantitated from the radioactivity precipitated by trichloroacetic acid and melanoma-associated antigens (MAAs) by a sensitive and quantitative double-antibody antigen-binding assay (Bystryn *et al.,* 1974a, b). It was found that approximately 44% of newly synthesized MAAs and 36% of unrelated macromolecules were released in 48 hr (Bystryn, 1976). Release of MAAs did not result solely from cell death, since it was much greater than that of ^{51}Cr-labeled cytoplasmic molecules and cell viability was over 98% at the beginning and end of all experiments.

MAAs released by melanoma cells were biologically active. This was evidenced by their ability to induce specific melanoma antibodies in syngeneic mice and to increase their resistance to otherwise lethal doses of B16 melanoma (Bystryn, 1978). Thus, 50% of a group of 91 mice immunized to MAAs partially purified from material released into media (Bystryn *et al.,* 1974a) survived over 6 weeks, whereas there were no survivors in a group of 114 mice immunized in a similar fashion to purified antigens prepared from the media of syngeneic fibroblasts. The immunity was specific, since the growth of an unrelated syngeneic tumor (BW 10232 mammary adenocarcinoma) was similar in mice immunized to MAAs or control antigens.

These findings indicate that biologically active tumor antigens and other macromolecules can be released by viable tumor cells.

2.3. Release of Cell-Surface Macromolecules and Antigens by Human Melanoma Cells

To determine whether the same phenomenon occurred in man, we have studied the release of tumor antigens and unrelated macromolecules by human melanoma (Bystryn, 1977). We have been particularly interested in the release of cell-surface antigens, since these are more likely to be biologically relevant.

Cell-surface macromolecules, including MAAs, on human melanoma cells in culture were radioiodinated by the lactoperoxidase technique. Extensive control studies confirmed that this procedure labeled only macromolecules present on the surface of the cells (Bystryn and Smalley, 1977). MAAs were quantitated by a sensitive double-antibody antigen-binding assay (Bystryn, 1977). They accounted for approximately 4–8% of the radioactivity associated with cell-surface macromolecules. Release of radioiodinated macromolecules and MAAs was studied as described above for murine melanoma cells.

Cell-surface molecules and MAAs were readily released by melanoma cells and could be detected in media within 5 min. In four experiments, on the average, 42% of MAAs and 60% of iodinated macromolecules were released in 3 hr (Fig. 1). Release was not solely the result of cell death, since cell viability was over 98% before and at the end of the experiments. Furthermore, only 1.2% of [^{3}H]leucine-labeled and 18% of ^{51}Cr-labeled cytoplasmic macromolecules were released in the same time in parallel experiments. Nor was release an artifact of the radioiodination procedure, since the amount of protein (measured by the Lowry method) released per 10^6 radioiodinated cells into fetal calf serum (FCS)-free medium in 3 hr (14.6 μg) did not differ significantly from that released by untreated cells (15.5 μg) or by cells that had been mock-iodinated by substituting sodium iodide for ^{125}I (11.7 μg) or exposed to ^{125}I (14.3 μg).

While it is known that FCS protein can adhere to melanoma cells and be subsequently released (Irie *et al.*, 1974), extensive control experiments have shown that radioiodinated FCS proteins account for only a small fraction (9–14%) of the radioactivity associated with surface macromolecules shed by these cells. Several other investigators have recently also shown that melanoma cells can release tumor-associated antigens, though the proportion released and the rate at which release occurred were not determined (Grimm *et al.*, 1976; Gupta *et al.*, 1979; Leong *et al.*, 1978; Stuhlmiller and Seigler, 1977; McCabe *et al.*, 1978).

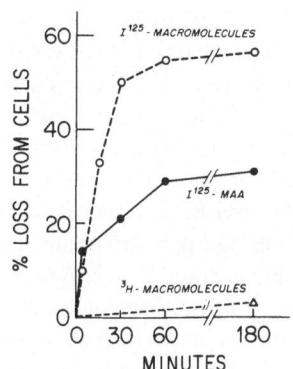

FIGURE 1. Release of radioiodinated cell-surface macromolecules and MAAs, and of [^{3}H]leucine-labeled cytoplasmic macromolecules, by viable human melanoma cells in tissue culture.

These experiments indicate that viable human melanoma cells can rapidly release cell-surface MAAs as well as unrelated macromolecules. The half-life of the process is such as to suggest that a single cell may release the equivalent of several times the amount of MAAs expressed on its surface in a single day. The rapidity of release suggests that it, rather than cell death, accounts for the bulk of soluble tumor antigens in patients with malignancies.

2.4. Release of Surface Macromolecules by Normal Cells

To determine whether the rapid release of surface macromolecules by melanoma was a phenomenon associated with malignant transformation, it was compared to the release of surface macromolecules by normal human cells.

In experiments similar to those described above, replicate confluent monolayers of normal human allogeneic fibroblasts for keratinocytes were radioiodinated, washed, and incubated in fresh media. All experiments were done on duplicate plates. In several separate experiments, it was found that the average proportion of labeled surface macromolecules released by fibroblasts (42.2 $\pm$ 11.1% S.D.) or keratinocytes (56.0 $\pm$ 10.0% S.D.) in 3 hr did not differ significantly from that released by melanoma cells (60.0 $\pm$ 9.9% S.D.) in the same time. In additional experiments, the rate of release of radioiodinated surface macromolecules by confluent monolayers of murine B16 melanoma cells (36% in 3 hr) was less than that by normal syngeneic fibroblasts (56% in 3 hr) (Bystryn et al., 1981).

These results indicate that a large proportion of externally disposed surface macromolecules is rapidly released by both malignant and normal cells and that the rate of release is similar in both instances. Thus, this process is not an expression of malignant transformation, but rather is one of the major pathways for the turnover of cell-membrane components on normal and tumor cells.

2.5. Character of Released Melanoma-Associated Antigens

A number of MAAs released into culture medium have been partially purified. In our own studies, we found that one MAA was initially released as a high-molecular-weight product that on Sephacryl S-200 chromatography (Fig. 2) ran close to the exclusion volume of the column and thus had a molecular weight of over 160,000 (Bystryn and Smalley, 1977). On further purification, the apparent molecular weight of the MAA decreased. This was probably due to MAA being released, as described subsequently, in association with fragments of the plasma membrane or as aggregates that dissociate during subsequent purification steps. Thus, following sequential chromatography on DEAE–Sephadex, phenyl sepharose, concanavalin A, and Sephadex G-150, the molecular weight of the MAA decreased to approximately 120,000 (Smalley and Bystryn, 1978). The MAA accounted for over 85% of the radioactivity associated with macromolecules in the antigen active fraction. On polyacrylamide gel electrophoresis, only a single labeled protein was present in this fraction. The MAA was a glycoprotein and appeared to be a periphereal rather than a structural component of the cell membrane, since it could be dissociated from cells by high-ionic-strength solutions and was soluble in aqueous buffers.

More recently, several other MAAs that are released by melanoma cells have been

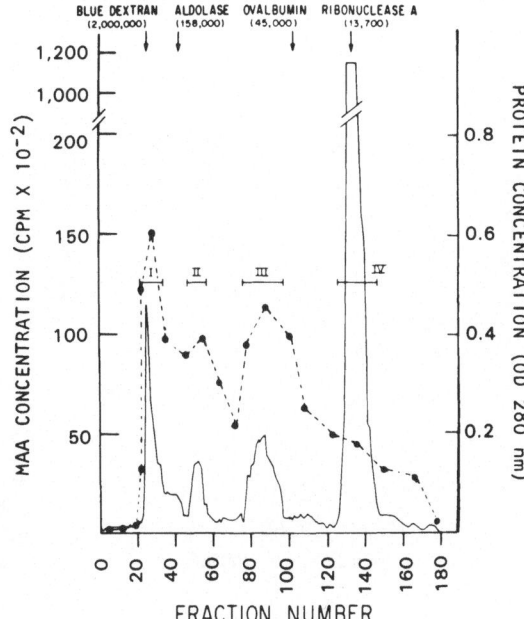

FIGURE 2. Sephacryl S-200 elution profile of radioiodinated human melanoma cell-surface macromolecules shed into culture media (___). MAA is present only in fraction 1. (. . . . . .) Elution profile of proteins measured by optical density.

partially characterized. Gupta *et al.* (1979) found two distinct antigens in spent medium of melanoma cells. One, called oncofetal antigen (OFA), was a fetal antigen also expressed on fetal brain cells and other human cancers. The other was a tumor antigen distinct from HLA and OFA. Leong *et al.* (1978) detected in media an MAA the molecular weight of which on Sephadex G-200 chromatography was in the region of 80,000–150,000. Most recently, Reisfeld *et al.* (1980) have identified two distinct antigens shed by melanoma cells. Both were glycoproteins. MPG-1 had a molecular weight of approximately 240,000 and appeared to be unique for melanoma, whereas MPG-2 had a molecular weight of 94,000 and was also expressed on fetal cells and on unrelated cancers.

2.6. Selectivity of Release

Release of cell-surface MAAs and other macromolecules appears to be selective. This is suggested by the rate of release of MAAs, which is slower than that of other macromolecules. Furthermore, by Sephadex G-200 analysis of radiolabeled macromolecules on cells and in media, relatively more low-molecular-weight macromolecules are released into media (46% of total radiolabeled macromolecules have molecular weights below 50,000) than are present on cells (22% of total). Last, polyacrylamide gel electrophoresis of labeled material on melanoma cells and released into media clearly shows that a number of macromolecules that are expressed on the surface of these cells are not released (Fig. 3). Selective release of different classes of surface macromolecules probably explains the differences in turnover rate of melanoma membrane macromolecules when alternate methods of labeling these are used. Thus, Rahman *et al.* (1977) found that the turnover rate of membrane

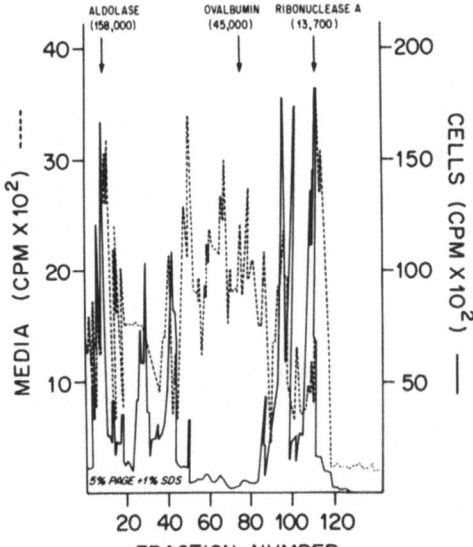

FIGURE 3. Profile of labeled macromolecules present on the surface of radioiodinated human melanoma cells (. . . . . . .) and shed (——) into culture medium in 3 hr. Analyzed by electrophoresis on 1% sodium dodecyl sulfate–5% polyacrylamide gels.

macromolecules metabolically labeled with [³H]glucosamine was much slower than those observed in our experiment, with 50% of the labeled material requiring 96 hr for release. Cell-surface macromolecules on other cells are also released selectively. Murine thymocytes release Thy-1 but not H-2 alloantigens (Vitetta *et al.*, 1974), and human lymphoid cells release β_2-microglobulins but not HLA antigens (Cresswell *et al.*, 1974).

2.7. Factors That Influence Release

To understand the mechanisms involved in the release of cell-surface components, the effect of various pharmacological agents, temperature, and cell replication on this process was studied.

The rate of release was slightly decreased at 4°C. Release was not affected by a variety of pharmacological agents that inhibit metabolic activity (iodoacetamide, antimycin A, dinitrophenol, puromycin, cycloheximide), proteolytic activity (soybean trypsin inhibitors, phenylmethylsulfonylfluoride, animocaproic acid), or cell-surface activity (sodium azide, cytochalasin B, colchicine). These findings suggest that release is independent of protein synthesis, does not require energy, is not due to degradation of surface proteins by proteolytic enzymes in FCS or released by the melanoma cells, and does not require cap formation, endocytosis, or other surface-membrane phenomena mediated by microfilaments or microtubules.

Release was influenced by the rate of cell growth. MAA release was considerably faster during the stationary phase of growth (average 40.2% released in 3 hr in four experiments) than during logarithmic growth (23.5% released in 3 hr). The converse was true for unrelated surface macromolecules, the release of which was faster during logarithmic than during stationary growth (51.5 vs. 31.7% released in 3 hr). The expression of MAAs on melanoma cell surfaces, in terms of the percentage of total acid-precipitable radioactivity associated with MAAs, was also greater during stationary than during logarithmic growth. As a result of these influences, the concentration of MAAs in culture media was from 2 to 3 times greater in confluent than in logarithmic growing cells. These findings suggest that both the expression and the release of MAAs are influenced by the rate of cell growth and thus may be cell-cycle-related phenomena. The same is true for cytoplasmic MAAs of murine B16 melanoma (Bystryn, 1976).

2.8. Mechanisms of Release

The observations discussed above and the experiments summarized below suggest that MAAs are shed in association with fragments of the plasma membrane rather than released by other mechanisms that can be envisioned, such as secretion, degradation by proteolytic enzymes outside the cells, or endocytosis followed by degradation in lysosomes and regurgitation outside the cells of the degraded material. The last three possibilities are unlikely, since release does not require energy (necessary for secretion) nor is affected by inhibitors of proteases or endocytosis. On the other hand, MAAs do appear to be released in aggregates or in association with fragments of the plasma membrane. Treatment of material released by melanoma cells with NP-40, a nonionic detergent that dissociates cell membranes, caused a loss of over 40% in the radioactivity associated with MAAs. This loss was not due to an effect of the detergent on the assay, since NP-40 did not change the amount of an unrelated antigen bound in a similar assay. Rather, it suggests that NP-40 dissociated from MAAs nonantigenic labeled membrane material adhering to them. This was confirmed by the finding that ultracentrifugation of media decreased by 57% the amount of radioactivity associated with MAAs, indicating that a large proportion of these antigens were sedimented and consequently released as large fragments or aggregates. Ultracentrifugation of NP-40-treated material caused no further reduction in radioactivity associated with MAAs, indicating that NP-40 could break up these fragments.

Recently, Morgan et al. (1980) have reported that release of some MAAs is suppressed by inhibitors of glycosylation, i.e., tunicamycin, 2-D-deoxyglucose, and glucosamine. The expression of one of these antigens on the surface of melanoma cells was unaltered by treatment with tunicamycin. These observations suggest that the carbohydrate moieties of the antigens may be required for shedding but not for expression on the cell surface.

2.9. Biological Implications

It has been proposed that antigen release is a characteristic feature of malignant cells (Alexander, 1974) and that there is a relationship between the lability of cell-surface components as a whole and the ability of tumor cells to metastasize (Currie and Alexander, 1974; Davey et al., 1976; Kim et al., 1975). However, the results of our studies indicate that surface macromolecules on melanoma cells are on the average no more labile than those on a variety of normal cells and that tumor antigens specifically are released more slowly than unrelated macromolecules. Thus, rapid release of surface material appears to be one of the normal pathways of turnover of membrane components, and no gross abnor-malities in this process accompany malignant transformation.

Rapid release of cell-surface antigens has a number of implications. By influencing the amount of antigen available to stimulate the immune system, the rate of release may influence the development of immunity or tolerance to tumor antigens. As examples, the continuous release of large amounts of soluble tumor antigens by malignant cells could lead to immune tolerance or to the "blocking" of tumor-specific antibodies or immune cells and thus enhance tumor growth. Since normal cells also rapidly release normal antigens expressed on their surface, the same mechanisms could play a role in tolerance to self antigens. Furthermore, rapid antigen shedding may also interfere with effective attachment of immune cells or antibodies or both to tumor cells and consequently after their resistance to immune destruction. Consequently, agents that influence antigen release by tumor cells may be therapeutically useful. Antigen release may also interfere with *in vitro* assays of tumor immunity. The prolonged incubation periods required for many assays may permit shed antigens to combine with and thus mask the presence of specific antibodies or immune cells. Since the amount of antigen released may be incluenced by the rate of cell growth, this phenomenon may account for the cyclical fluctuations in results of assays of tumor immunity that have been reported (Carey *et al.,* 1976). Last, the rapid release of antigens by tumor cells indicates that culture media can serve as a ready source of soluble antigens for biochemical or immunotherapeutic studies.

3. Degradation of Shed Tumor Antigens

It is obvious that the ultimate amount of tumor antigen that accumulates in body fluids will depend not only on the rate of their release but also on that of their degradation or clearance or both from extracellular fluids. From the observations that we have made to date, it appears that the most important of these two processes is release, which occurs more rapidly than degradation. However, MAAs can be degraded by a variety of normal human cells as well as by the melanoma cells themselves, so that this process will also have an impact on antigen accumulation in body fluids.

3.1. Degradation of Membrane Macromolecules on Melanoma Cells

As described earlier, a major pathway for the turnover of macromolecules on the sur-face of human melanoma cells is their release to the outside of the cells. Very little of the external membrane macromolecules that are radioiodinated is lost to degradation while still associated with cells. Of the labeled material that is lost by cells in 3 hr, 80% can be recovered as soluble macromolecules in media. For this reason, we have been interested in the fate of membrane material following its release from cells.

The methods we have used to study the susceptibility to degradation of shed membrane macromolecules and MAAs has been to collect soluble labeled material released by radio-iodinated cells into media in 3 hr. The labeled material was then incubated with unlabeled cells and the amount of radioactivity remaining associated with macromolecules or MAAs in the media determined at intervals thereafter. We have found that soluble surface material

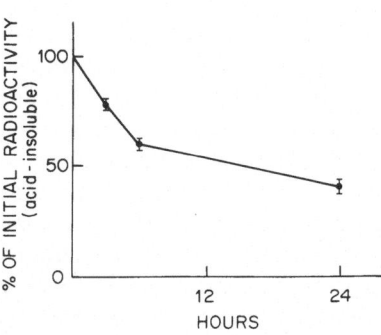

FIGURE 4. Degradation of surface macromolecules shed by human melanoma cells. Labeled surface macromolecules released by radioiodinated melanoma cells were collected and incubated with unlabeled cells. Aliquots of medium were collected following various intervals of incubation at 37°C, and the amount of labeled acid-insoluble macromolecules remaining was determined. Each point represents the average of three experiments ± S.D.

released by melanoma cells can be degraded by a variety of cells, including the melanoma cells themselves (Bystryn *et al.*, 1978; Boctor and Bystryn, 1980). The results of several experiments are illustrated in Fig. 4. There was a steady decline in acid-insoluble radioactivity with time when labeled macromolecules released by melanoma cells were reincubated with these cells, so that after 24 hrs approximately 60% had been lost. Approximately 5–10% of the loss was due to adhesion of macromolecules to cells or to the plastic surface of the culture dishes. The remainder of the loss was due to degradation of material to acid-soluble fragments. The actual amount of material degraded was probably greater than that, since some macromolecules were only partially degraded and remained as large fragments that were still acid-insoluble. The rate at which melanoma cells degrade material that they released is significantly slower than that of release, since it takes approximately 24 hr for cells to degrade half the material that they release in 3 hr. However, soluble melanoma surface macromolecules can be degraded much more quickly by other types of cells (Boctor and Bystryn, 1980). As can be seen in Table I, normal human fibroblasts and macrophages degraded this material approximately 2–3 times more rapidly than did melanoma cells.

As illustrated in Fig. 4, the rate at which shed melanoma macromolecules were degraded was biphasic, suggesting that different macromolecules are degraded at different rates. This was confirmed by several additional experiments. In the first, approximately 26% of acid-insoluble radioactivity was lost in the 3-hr period immediately following the

TABLE I

Degradation of Cell-Surface Macromolecules and Melanoma-Associated Antigens Shed by Human Melanoma Cells

| Degrading cells | Expt. No. | Degradation (%)[a] | | p[b] |
		Macromolecules	MAAs	
Fibroblasts	5	17.6 ± 3.0	51.0 ± 15.5	0.025
Macrophages	4	8.1 ± 2.2	19.5 ± 4.8	0.025
Lymphocytes	1	1.9	2.5	
Colon cancer	1	1.7	3.8	
Melanoma	4	3.4 ± 0.6	1.2 ± 0.5	0.01

[a]Per 10^6 cells/24 hr ± S.E.   [b]By Student's T test.

addition of shed labeled macromolecules to unlabeled cells, whereas 24 hr later on 4–5% of the acid-insoluble radioactivity still present was lost in 3 hr of incubation. In a second set of experiments, labeled medium was successively transferred from one confluent plate of melanoma cells to another for consecutive 6-hr incubations. The decrease in acid-insoluble radioactivity during the first 6-hr incubation was over twice as great as that during the second incubation, even though both plates had a similar number of cells. Last, the possibility that spontaneous autocatabolism of molecules already partially degraded by cells was responsible for the slow terminal phase of degradation was excluded by the following experiment: Labeled medium was incubated with melanoma cells for 6 hr, collected, and aliquots subsequently reincubated at 37°C with or without cells. Of the labeled macromolecules, 45% were degraded during the initial 6-hr incubation with cells. An additional 10% was degraded when reincubated for 18 hr with cells, whereas no further degradation occurred when reincubated in the absence of cells for a similar period of time.

3.2. Degradation of Shed Melanoma-Associated Antigens

Surface MAAs are also degraded following release, though the rate of this process is complex and depends on both the nature of the MAAs and the cells involved. Several important observations can be deduced from the studies summarized in Table I.

MAAs, at least the one we have studied, can be degraded by a wide variety of allogeneic cells including normal macrophages and lymphocytes prepared by Ficoll-Hypaque separation of fresh whole blood, cultured fibroblasts and color carcinoma cells, and the melanoma cells themselves. However, the rate of this process varied widely. MAAs were degraded most readily by fibroblasts and most poorly by melanoma. There was a 40-fold difference in degradation between these two types of cells. This was not simply a result of the poor catabolic activity of melanoma cells. Though the catabolic activity of these cells was low, as measured by their ability to degrade surface macromolecules unrelated to MAAs, it was still greater than that of lymphocytes and colon carcinoma cells, which both degraded MAAs more rapidly.

MAAs are particularly susceptible to degradation. MAAs were degraded by a variety of cells 2–3 times more rapidly than were unrelated surface macromolecules shed concurrently by melanoma cells.

Last, melanoma cells appear to have a selective defect in their ability to degrade MAAs. Though MAAs were more easily degraded by a variety of cells than were unrelated surface macromolecules shed by melanoma, the melanoma cells themselves degraded the unrelated macromolecules more rapidly than the MAAs. This was not because melanoma cells had difficulty handling "foreign" surface material, since they degraded surface material released by allogeneic fibroblasts as rapidly as their own.

While the causes for these phenomena have not been elucidated, they may have an important impact on tumor growth, which is discussed subsequently.

3.3. Selectivity of Degradation

The biphasic degradation of membrane macromolecules, and the differences in degradation between MAAs and unrelated membrane macromolecules, suggest that different

TABLE II
Selectivity of Degradation

Labeled Proteins	Concentration (μg/ml)[a]	Degradation at 24 hr (%)[b]
Albumin, bovine[c]	5.0	1.08
IgG, human[c]	2.5	0
IgM, human[c]	5.0	0.45
Released by autochthonous melanoma		
Cytoplasmic macromolecules[d]	—	1.6
Surface macromolecules[e]	15.0	42.06

[a]The indicated concentrations of labeled proteins were added with 5 ml FCS-free growth medium to confluent monolayers of melanoma cells and incubated at 37°C.
[b]Average of 2–4 experiments. Each experiment was performed in duplicate.
[c]Labeled with ^{125}I by the chloramine T technique.
[d]Metabolically labeled with [^{3}H]leucine.
[e]Labeled with ^{125}I by the lactoperoxidase technique.

types of macromolecules are degraded at different rates. To further study this question, the ability of melanoma cells to degrade a variety of labeled macromolecules was studied. As shown in Table II, melanoma cells degraded their shed surface macromolecules much more rapidly than [^{3}H]leucine-labeled macromolecules (which are predominantly of cytoplasmic origin) that they had released. Surface macromolecules were also degraded much more rapidly than soluble extracellular proteins such as human immunoglobulin G (IgG) and IgM or bovine serum albumin. In subsequent experiments, surface macromolecules released by allogeneic fibroblasts were degraded by melanoma cells at the same rate as their own surface material, and the converse was also true, indicating that the susceptibility of surface material to degradation is not related to malignant transformation.

These observations indicate that though membrane macromolecules are degraded at different rates, as a class they appear to be particularly susceptible to degradation. Why this is so has not been elucidated. One possibility is that soluble macromolecules can selectively adhere to the membrane of intact cells, leading to enhanced uptake and degradation inside lysosomes in a process similar to that described for the catabolism of lipoproteins by fibroblasts (Basu *et al.*, 1977). Alternatively, selective degradation could be mediated by enzymes that preferentially act on cell-surface macromolecules or to an increased susceptibility of such macromolecules to proteolytic or glycolytic action.

3.4. Mechanisms of Degradation

Degradation requires the presence of cells. As can be seen in Fig. 5, there was little or no degradation when labeled macromolecules released into FCS-free medium were incubated alone or with 10% FCS at 37°C, indicating that degradation was not an artifact due to dissociation of the label from macromolecules or due to proteases in the serum. Nor was there significant degradation when shed labeled macromolecules were incubated with spent media collected from unlabeled cells, indicating that even though melanoma cells are

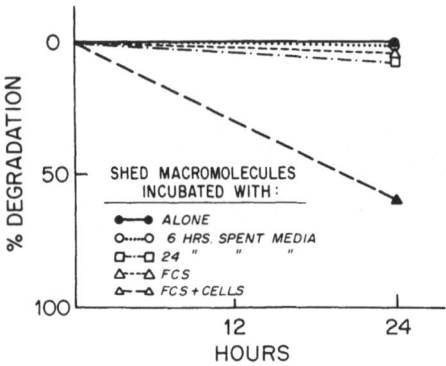

FIGURE 5. Cellular requirement for degradation. Labeled surface macromolecules shed by radioiodinated melanoma cells into FCS-free medium were collected and incubated at 37°C: (1) alone, (2) in a final concentration of 10% FCS, (3) with an equal volume of spent complete culture medium collected from melanoma cells after 6 to 24 hr incubation, and (4) with confluent monolayers of unlabeled melanoma cells. The amount of acid-insoluble macromolecules present in the samples was determined at 0 time and 24 hr later. Each point represents the average value of 2–4 experiments.

known to release proteases (Rifkin *et al.,* 1974), these enzymes were not involved in degradation.

Degradation was, at least in part, an active process requiring cell-surface and metabolic activity. It was partially inhibited by cytochalasin B at a concentration (10 μg/ml) that interferes with microfilament function and pinocytosis (Wessels *et al.,* 1971) and by iodoacetamide (10^{-4} M) or a combination of 2-deoxyglucose (18 mg/ml) and dinitrophenyl (10^{-4} M), which inhibit energy production and macromolecule metabolism. Degradation was almost completely suppressed at 4°C, a temperature that depresses metabolic activity and inhibits all endocytic activity (Silverstein *et al.,* 1977). Colchicine at a concentration (10^{-5} M) that interferes with microtubular function (Allison and Davies, 1974) had no effect on degradation, indicating that these structures were not involved in the process. Degradation was associated with uptake of shed material back into the cells, though there is as yet no direct evidence that there is a causal relation between the two processes. When unlabeled melanoma cells were incubated with labeled surface material shed by radioiodinated melanoma cells, it was found that the amount of labeled macromolecules associated with cells gradually increased with time, so that after 24 hrs approximately 7% of the macromolecules were cell-associated. Approximately two thirds of them could be removed from the cells by trypsin treatment, indicating that these molecules were absorbed to the cell's surface. The remainder of the acid-insoluble radioactivity, approximately 3% of that initially present in the medium, was resistant to trypsin treatment and presumably represents labeled macromolecules taken up by the cells.

These observations suggest that one of the mechanisms of degradation may be similar to that by which most exogenous proteins are degraded by cells, namely, endocytosis followed by degradation in lysosomes (Basu *et al.,* 1977; Carpenter and Cohen, 1976; Ehrenreich and Cohn, 1967; Gregoriadis, 1975). The ability of melanoma cells to take up surface macromolecules that they release supports this possibility. The relatively small amount of labeled macromolecules present inside the cells at any given time suggests that if degradation does occur intracellularly, it takes place rapidly once the material is taken up. Other mechanisms that may be involved in degradation but about which no information is available include cell-surface proteases that may be present on normal (Kenny *et al.,* 1976; Lavie *et al.,* 1978) and malignant cells (Quigley, 1976) including melanoma (Hatcher *et al.,* 1976) and active proteases formed as a result of interactions between FCS and cells as occur when serum plasminogen is activated to plasmin by cell-surface plasminogen activator (Christman *et al.,* 1975; Rifkin *et al.,* 1974).

3.5. Biological Implications

The autocatabolism of surface macromolecules including tumor antigens following their release from cells has a number of implications for our understanding of the normal turnover of cell membranes and tumor immunology.

The ability of cells to degrade their own surface macromolecules after they have been released outside the cells adds another pathway to the several that have been suggested to account for the turnover of surface macromolecules. Beside shedding of external material to the outside of the cells, these include proteolysis of molecules still attached to the cell membrane (Schimke, 1975), dissociation from the membrane and reentry into the cytoplasm of the cell (Schimke, 1975), and ingestion of membrane macromolecules forming the wall of endocytic vacuoles during pinocytosis followed by their digestion within lysosomes (Hubbard and Cohn, 1975; Schimke, 1975). These processes are not mutually exclusive and may indeed be occurring simultaneously. The relative contribution of these processes to the total turnover of surface macromolecules is not known. However, shedding appears to be the major pathway for the turnover of those macromolecules that can be radioiodinated and that consequently are the most external on the cell membrane. This is evidenced by the fact that approximately 80% of the radioiodinated material that is lost from melanoma cells in 3 hr can be recovered as macromolecules in media. The ability of cells to autocatabolize material that they released accounts for the degradation of even a small fraction of the material released by cells *in vitro.* However, since macromolecules are degraded at different rates, it may account for a significant proportion of the more rapidly degraded species. Furthermore, *in vivo,* the three-dimensional stacking of cells may impose restrictions on the diffusion of released molecules that might favor their degradation locally at the site of release.

The implications of these findings for tumor immunology are complex. It is evident that the amount of soluble tumor antigen that accumulates in body fluids will depend on the balance between the rate of their release and that of their degradation. Distal to tumors, the rapid degradation of MAAs by normal cells should result in faster clearance from body fluids. The rapid clearance of this potential blocking factor should have a favorable impact on host immune defenses. However, this effect will be minimized by its occurrence away from tumors. At the tumor site itself, the poor catabolic activity of the predominant cells, i.e., melanoma cells, and the selective defect in their ability to degrade MAAs, should result in local accumulation of MAAs around tumors. This should favor blocking of, and escape from, host immune defenses.

4. Conclusion

Viable human melanoma cells rapidly release cell-surface antigens and unrelated macromolecules. The rate of release is similar to that of surface macromolecules on normal cells, indicating that this process is not related to malignant transformation, but is rather one of the major pathways for the normal turnover of membrane material. The process is influenced by the rate of cell growth. MAAs released by murine tumors are biologically active. The release of MAAs by viable melanoma cells is so rapid as to suggest that this phenomenon, rather than cell death, is the major cause of the presence of soluble tumor antigens in tumor-bearing animals and man.

Soluble MAAs and unrelated surface macromolecules can be degraded by melanoma and normal human cells following their release. MAAs are in general more easily degraded than unrelated surface macromolecules released by melanoma cells. However, melanoma cells appear to have a selective defect in their ability to degrade MAAs.

Thus, the ultimate amount of tumor antigen that accumulates in body fluids will depend on the balance between the rate of their release and that of their degradation. The rapid release of MAAs, and their poor degradation locally by melanoma cells, suggest that there may be a selective accumulation of these antigens immediately around tumors, an event that favors tumor escape from host immune defenses.

ACKNOWLEDGMENT. The author's research cited herein was supported in part by USPHS Research Grant No. 13844-08.

References

Alexander, P., 1974, Escape from immune destruction by the host through shedding of surface antigens: Is this a characteristic shared by malignant and embryonic cells? *Cancer Res.* **34**:2077.

Allison, A. C., and Davies, P., 1974, Mechanisms of encodytosis and exocytosis, *Symp. Soc. Exp. Biol.* **28**:419.

Baldwin, R. W., Bowen, J. G., and Price, M. R., 1973, Detection of circulating hepatoma D23 antigen and immune complexes in tumor bearer serum, *Br. J. Cancer* **28**:16.

Basu, S. K., Anderson, R. G., Goldstein, J. L., and Brown, J. S., 1977, Metabolism of cationized lipoproteins by human fibroblasts, *J. Cell Biol.* **74**:119.

Boctor, A. M., and Bystryn, J.-C., 1980, Degradation of cell-surface melanoma associated antigens shed by human melanoma cells, *Proc. Am. Assoc. Cancer Res.* **21**:250.

Bystryn, J.-C., 1976, Release of tumor-associated antigens by murine melanoma cells, *J. Immunol.* **116**:1302.

Bystryn, J.-C., 1977, Release of cell-surface tumor-associated antigens by viable melanoma cells from humans, *J. Natl. Cancer Inst.* **59**:325.

Bystryn, J.-C., 1978, Antibody response and tumor growth in syngeneic mice immunized to partially purified B16 melanoma-associated antigens, *J. Immunol.* **120**:96.

Bystryn, J.-C., and Smalley, J. R., 1977, Identification and solubilization of iodinated cell surface human melanoma-associated antigens, *Int. J. Cancer* **20**:165.

Bystryn, J.-C., and Smalley, J. R., 1978, Purification of a cell-surface human melanoma associated antigen, *Clin. Res.* **26**:432A.

Bystryn, J.-C., Schenkein, I., Baur, S., and Uhr, J. W., 1974a, Partial isolation and characterization of antigen(s) associated with murine melanoma, *J. Natl. Cancer Inst.* **52**:1263.

Bystryn, J.-C., Schenkein, I., and Uhr, J. W., 1974b, Double-antibody radioimmunoassay for B16 melanoma antibodies, *J. Natl. Cancer Inst.* **52**:911.

Bystryn, J.-C. Bart, R. S., Livingston, P., and Kopf, A. W., 1974c, Growth and immunogenicity of B16 murine melanoma, *J. Invest. Dermatol.* **63**:369.

Bystryn, J.-C., Smalley, J. R., and Pearlstein, J., 1978, Degradation of shed cell-surface macromolecules and melanoma associated antigens (MAA) by human melanoma cells, *Proc. Am. Assoc. Cancer Res.* **19**:128.

Bystryn, J.-C., Tedholm, C. A., and Heaney-Kieras, J., 1981, Release of surface macromolecules by human melanoma and normal cells, *Cancer Res.* **41**:910.

Carey, T. E. Takahashi, T., Resnick, L. A., Oettgen, H. F., and Old, L. J., 1976, Cell surface antigens of human malignant melanoma: Mixed hemadsorption assays for humor immunity to cultured autologous melanoma cells, *Proc. Natl. Acad Sci. U.S.A.* **73**:3278.

Carpenter, G., and Cohen, S., 1976, ^{125}T-labelled human epidermal growth factor: Binding, internalization and degradation in human fibroblasts, *J. Cell Biol.* **71**:159.

Carrel, S. and Theilkaes, L., 1973, Evidence of a tumor-associated antigen in human malignant melanoma, *Nature London* **242**:609.

Christman, J. K., Acs, G., Silagi, S., and Silverstein, S. C., 1975, Plasminogen activator: Biochemical characterization and correlation with tumorigenicity, in: *Proteases and Biological Control* (E. Reich, D. B. Rifkin, and E. Shaw, eds.), pp. 827–839, Cold Spring Harbor Laboratory, Cold Spring Harbor, New York.

Cresswell, P., Springer, T., Strominger, J. L., Turner, M. J., Grey, H. M., and Kubo, R. T., 1974, Immunological identity of the small subunit of HL-A antigens and B2-microglobulin and its turnover on the cell membrane, *Proc. Natl Acad Sci. U.S.A.* **71**:2123.

Currie, G. A., and Alexander, P., 1974, Spontaneous shedding of TSTA by viable sarcoma cells: Its possible role in facilitating metastatic spread, *Br. J. Cancer* **29**:72.

Currie, G. A., and Basham, C., 1972, Serum-mediated inhibition of immunological reactions of the patient to his own tumor: A possible role for circulating antigen, *Br. J. Cancer* **26**:427.

Davey, G. C., Currie, G. A., and Alexander, P., 1976, Spontaneous shedding and antibody induced modulation of histocompatibility antigens on murine lymphomata: Correlation with metastatic capacity, *Br. J. Cancer* **33**:9.

Ehrenreich, B. A., and Cohn, Z. A., 1967, The uptake and digestion of iodinated human serum albumin by macrophages *in vitro, J. Exp. Med.* **126**:941.

Gregoriadis, G., 1975, The catabolism of glycoproteins, in: *Lysosomes in Biology and Pathology,* Vol. 4 (J. T. Dingle and R. T. Dean, eds.), pp. 265–294, North-Holland, Amsterdam.

Grimm, E. A., Silver, H. K. B., Roth, J. A., Chee, D. O., Gupta, R. K., and Morton, D. L., 1976, Detection of tumor-associated antigen in human melanoma cell line supernatants, *Int. J. Cancer* **17**:559.

Gupta, R. K., Irie, R. F., Chee, D. O., Kern, D. H., and Morton, D. L., 1979, Demonstration of two distinct antigens in spent tissue culture medium of human malignant melanoma cells, *J. Natl. Cancer Inst.* **16**:347.

Hatcher, V., Werthein, M. S., Rhee, C. Y., Tsien, G., and Burk, P. G., 1976, Relationship between cell surface protease activity and doubling time in various normal and transformed cells, *Biochim. Biophys. Acta* **451**:499.

Hubbard, A. L., and Cohn, Z. A., 1975, Externally disposed plasma membrane proteins. II. Metabolic fate of iodinated polypeptides of mouse L cells, *J. Cell Biol.* **64**:461.

Irie, R. F., Irie, K. L., and Morton, D. L., 1974, Characteristics of heterologous membrane antigen on cultured human cells, *J. Natl. Cancer Inst.* **53**:1545.

Jehn, U. W., Nathanson, L., Schwartz, R. S., and Skinner, M., 1970, *In vitro* lymphocyte stimulation by a soluble antigen from malignant melanoma, *N. Engl. J. Med.* **283**:329.

Kenny, J., Booth, A. G., George, S. G., Ingram, J., Kershaw, D., and Wood, E. J., 1976, Dipeptidyl peptidase. IV. A kidney brush border serine peptidase, *Biochem. J.* **157**:169.

Kim, U., Baumer, A., Carruthers, C., and Bielat, K., 1975, Immunological escape mechanism in spontaneously metastasizing mammary tumors, *Proc. Natl. Acad. Sci. U.S.A.* **72**:1012.

Lavie, G., Zucker-Franklin D., and Franklin E., 1978, Degradation of serum amyloid A protein by surface-associated enzymes of human blood monocytes, *J. Exp. Med.* **148**:1020.

Leong, S. P. L., Cooperband, S. R., Sutherland, C. M., Krementz, E. T., and Deckers, P. J., 1978, Detection of human melanoma antigens in cell-free supernatants, *J. Surg. Res.* **24**:245.

McCabe, R. P., Ferrone, S., Pellegrino, M. A., Kern, D. H., Holmes, E. C., and Reisfeld, R. A., 1978, Purification and immunologic evaluation of human melanoma-associated antigens, *J. Natl. Cancer Inst.* **60**:773.

Morgan, A. C., Galloway, D. M., Imai, K., Ferrone, S., and Reisfeld, R. A., 1980, The effect of inhibitors of glycosylation on the shedding and cell surface expression of human melanoma-associated antigens, *Fed. Proc. Fed. Am. Soc. Exp. Biol.* **39**:351.

Poskitt, P. K. F., Poskitt, T. R., and Wallace, H. J., 1974, Renal deposition of soluble immune complexes in mice bearing B16 melanoma: Characterization of complexes and relationship to tumor progresses, *J. Exp. Med.* **140**:410.

Quigley, J. P., 1976, Association of protease (plasminogen activator) with a specific membrane fraction isolated from transformed cells, *J. Cell Biol.* **71**:472.

Rahman, A. F. R., Liao, S. K., and Dent, P., 1977, Characterization of human malignant melanoma cell lines. VII. Glycoprotein synthesis and shedding as revealed by [³H]glucosamine labelling, *In Vitro* **13**:580.

Reisfeld, R. A., Galloway, D., Imai, K., Ferrone, S., and Morgan, A. C., 1980, Molecular profile of human melanoma associated antigens, *Fed. Am. Soc. Exp. Biol.* **39**:351.

Rifkin, D. B., Loeb, J. N., Moore, G., and Reich, E., 1974, Properties of plasminogen activators formed by neoplastic human cell cultures, *J. Exp. Med.* **139**:1317.

Schimke, R. T., 1975, Turnover of membrane proteins in animal cells, in: *Methods in Membrane Biology,* Vol. 3 (E. D. Korn, ed.), pp. 201–236, Plenum Press, New York.

Silverstein, S. C., Steinman, R. M., and Cohn, Z. A., 1977, Endocytosis, *Annu. Rev. Biochem.* **46**:669.

Smalley, J. R., and Bystryn, J.-C., 1978, Purification of a cell-surface glycoprotein from human melanoma, *Fed. Proc.* **37**:1595.

Stuhlmiller, G. M., and Seigler, H. F., 1977, Enzymatic susceptibility and spontaneous release of human melanoma tumor-associated antigens, *J. Natl. Cancer Inst.* **58**:215.

Thomson, D. M. P., Sellens, V., Eccles, S., and Alexander, P., 1973, Radioimmunoassay of tumour-specific transplantation antigen of a chemically induced rat sarcoma: Circulating soluble tumour antigen in tumour bearers, *Br. J. Cancer* **28**:377.

Vitetta, E. S., Uhr, J. W., and Boyse, E. A., 1974, Metabolism of H-2 and Thy-1 alloantigens in murine thynocytes, *Eur. J. Immunol.* **4**:276.

Wessels, N. K., Spooner, B. S., Ash, J. F., Bradley, M. D., Luduena, M. A., Taylor, E. L., Wrenn, J. T., and Yamada, K. M., 1971, Microfilaments in cellular and developmental processes: Contractile microfilament machinery of many types is reversibly inhibited by cytochalasin B, *Science* **171**:135.

4

Monoclonal Antibodies as a Tool to Detect Melanoma-Associated Antigens

STEFAN CARREL, ROBERTO S. ACCOLLA, JEAN-PIERRE MACH, AND NICOLE GROSS

1. Introduction

The existence of common serologically defined tumor-associated antigen(s) on human melanoma cells has been suggested by several studies in which human allogeneic or autologous sera have been used (Gupta and Morton, 1975; Lewis *et al.*, 1979; Carey *et al.*, 1976; Liao *et al.*, 1978; Shiku *et al.*, 1976, 1977; Cornain *et al.*, 1975; Ferrone and Pellegrino, 1977; Hersey *et al.*, 1976; Morton *et al.*, 1968; Muna *et al.*, 1969). In addition, immunization of rabbits, guinea pigs, and monkeys with human melanoma cells has led to the production of several xenoantisera that after absorption reacted preferentially with melanoma cells from primary or long-term cultures (Bystryn, 1977; Carrel *et al.*, 1980a; Fritze *et al.*, 1976; Liao *et al.*, 1979; McCabe *et al.*, 1978; Metzgar *et al.*, 1973; Sorg *et al.*, 1978; Stuhlmiller and Seigler, 1975; Viza and Phillips, 1975). The major drawback of such antisera is, however, the overwhelming number of contaminating antibodies that have to be removed by extensive absorption before any tumor specificity can be demonstrated.

The method of Köhler and Milstein (1975) allowing the production of monoclonal antibodies against single antigenic determinants represents a great improvement for the selection of antibodies reacting with tumor-associated antigens. Recently, several investigators have produced monoclonal antibodies against various human tumor antigens and markers, including neuroblastoma (Kennett and Gilbert, 1979), colon carcinoma (Herlyn *et al.*, 1979), melanoma (Koprowski *et al.*, 1978; Steplewski *et al.*, 1979; Yeh *et al.*, 1979; Woodbury *et al.*, 1980; Carrel *et al.*, 1980b,c), glioblastoma (Schnegg *et al.*, 1981), and carcinoembryonic antigen (CEA) (Accolla *et al.*, 1980).

STEFAN CARREL, ROBERTO S. ACCOLLA, JEAN-PIERRE MACH, AND NICOLE GROSS • Unit of Human Cancer Immunology, Lausanne Branch, Ludwig Institute for Cancer Research, 1066 Epalinges, Switzerland.

Koprowski et al. (1978) reported on the production of several hybrids secreting antibodies binding to melanoma cells. The antigens recognized by these antibodies appeared to be expressed only on some melanomas tested. Yeh et al. (1979) described three monoclonal antibodies that seemed to be more or less restricted to an autologous melanoma antigen. Woodbury et al. (1980) reported on a hybridoma product that bound to the majority of the melanomas tested and also to some other tumor cells, but not to normal fibroblasts or to B cells. Recently (Carrel et al., 1980b), we analyzed the specificity of three monoclonal antibodies that appeared to have a restricted reactivity toward melanoma cells.

In this chapter, we will summarize the characteristics of nine monoclonal antibodies secreted by hybrids obtained from five fusions between two distinct mouse myeloma cell lines, P3-NS1/1Ag4 (Köhler et al., 1976) and P3 × 63/Ag8 (Köhler and Milstein, 1975), and spleen cells from mice immunized with membrane-enriched fractions from two melanoma cell lines, Me43 and IGR-3. It will be shown that these antibodies have a reactivity preferential toward melanoma cells as assessed by an indirect antibody-binding radioimmunoassay (RIA) (Klinman, 1972; Williams, 1977). Our results further indicate that these antibodies recognize different antigenic determinants expressed on melanomas; however, some of them cross-react with structures present on glioblastomas. The last finding is of interest, since Schnegg et al. (1981) have produced a series of hybrids secreting antibodies against glioblastoma cells, one of which displays a unique cross-reactivity for melanoma cells. By comparing the reactivity spectrum of these cross-reacting antibodies for the panel of tumor cell lines tested, it will appear that they react with distinct antigenic determinants located on different molecules.

2. Materials and Methods

2.1. Cell Lines

All human cells used in this study were grown in Roswell Park Memorial Institute (RPMI) 1640 medium supplemented with 10% fetal calf serum (FCS). The principal characteristics of the two melanoma cell lines used for immunization, Me43 and IGR-3, are summarized in Tables I and II. The BALB/c myeloma cell lines used for fusion, P3-NSl/l Ag 4 and P3 × 63/Ag 8, were both maintained in RPMI 1640 medium containing 10% horse serum. These two cell lines are resistant to 8-azaguanine (20 µg/ml) and do not

TABLE I

Characteristics of the Me43 Cell Line

Line:	Established 1976 in our laboratory.	
Origin:	Nodular melanoma from a 52-year-old Caucasian male (primary tumor).	
Cells:	Grow as a monolayer in 10% FCS.	
	Melanin granules:	Present
	Fibronectin [large external transformation-sensitive (LETS) protein]:	Positive
	Tumorigenicity in nude mice:	Yes
	Immune-associated (Ia) antigen(s):	Absent

Table II

Characteristics of the IGR-3 Cell Line

Line:	Established 1973 (Aubert *et al.*, 1976).	
Origin:	Primary nodular-type melanoma from a 60-year-old Caucasian male	
Cells:	Grow as a monolayer in 10% FCS.	
	Melanin granules:	Present
	Fibronectin (LETS) proteins:	Positive
	Tumorigenicity in nude mice:	Yes
	Ia antigen(s):	Present (DR 1, 7)

grow in hypoxanthine–aminopterin–thymidine (HAT) selective medium (Cowan *et al.*, 1974; Köhler and Milstein, 1975).

2.2. Preparation of Crude Membrane Fractions

Membrane fractions from the two melanoma cell lines, Me43 and IGR-3, were prepared by nitrogen cavitation (Schmidt-Ulrich *et al.*, 1974). Briefly, washed cells at a minimal concentration of 5×10^7 cells/ml in 0.075 M KCl, 0.065 M NaCl, 0.25 mM $MgCl_2$, and 0.01 mM HEPES (pH 7.4) were exposed to 10 atm N_2 for 20 min at 4°C while stirring gently. After return to normal atmospheric pressure, the disrupted cells were collected and centrifuged at 4000 g for 15 min and finally at 20,000 g for 30 min. The pellet obtained after the 20,000 g spin was used to immunize the recipient animals. The protein concentration in this fraction was determined by the microbiuret method.

2.3. Immunization

BALB/C mice 3–4 months old were immunized intraperitoneally by two injections of membrane-enriched fractions from the melanoma cell line Me43 or IGR-3 (0.1 mg membrane protein in 0.2 ml 0.9% NaCl solution) in complete Freund's adjuvant. After 20 days, the mice were boosted intravenously with the same amount of membrane proteins in 0.9% NaCl. Three days later, the mice were killed and their spleen cells used for fusion.

2.4. Cell Fusion

Cell fusion was performed by incubating 10^7 mouse myeloma cells (P3-NSI/lAg4 or P3 $\times$ 63/Ag8) with 10^8 mouse spleen cells in 0.3 ml 40% polyethylene glycol (PEG) (molecular weight 1000) for 3 min at 37°C (Pontecorvo, 1975). The cells were centrifuged for 5 min at 200g; then 5 ml serum-free RPMI 1640 medium was added dropwise to dilute the PEG. After fusion, the cells were washed and resuspended in 100 ml HAT medium and distributed in four 96-well plates of 0.6-cm diameter (for a schematic representation of the fusion protocol, see Fig. 1).

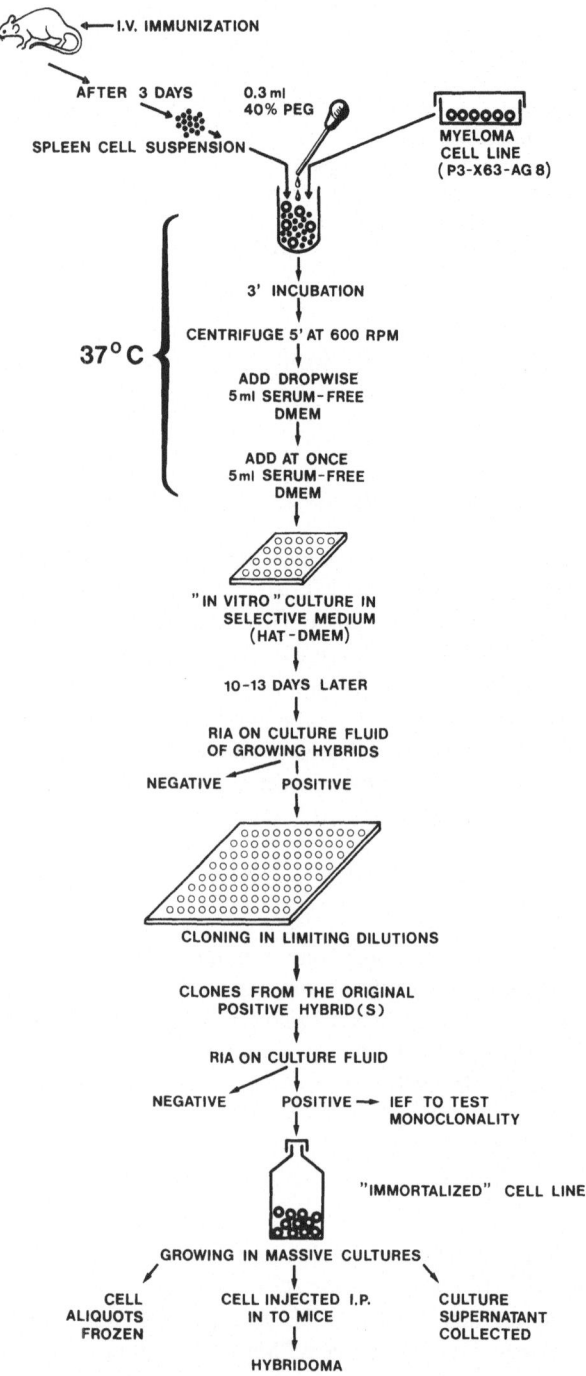

FIGURE 1. Schematic representation of the fusion protocol used for the production of monoclonal antimelanoma antibodies. (DMEM) Dulbecco's Modified Eagle's Medium; (IEF) isoelectric focusing.

TABLE III
Antibody-Detection Radioimmunoassay

Number of target cells per well[a] (U-type)	First incubation		Supernatant (μl)	Second incubation		Counts per minute per test[b] ($\times 10^{-6}$)	Background counts[c] (%)
	Time (min)	Temp (°C)		Time (min)	Temp (°C)		
5×10^5	120	20	100	60	20	0.1	2–3
25×10^4	60	4	100	60	4	0.1	1–3
5×10^4	90	4	100	90	4	0.1	1–2

[a]Cells were brought into suspension by the use of trypsin–EDTA.
[b]Second antibody ^{125}I-labeled IgG rabbit anti-mouse F(ab')$_2$.
[c]Counts detected by using, as control, P3 × 63/Ag8 culture supernatant.

2.5. Antibody-Detection Radioimmunoassay

Culture fluids of growing hybrids were tested for the presence of specific antibodies by an antibody-binding RIA essentially as described by Williams (1977). Briefly, 5×10^4 target cells, in 100 μl medium, were incubated for 90 min at 4°C with 100 μl culture fluid from the different hybrids in U-bottomed microtest plates. The plates were centrifuged at 100 g for 3 min, and the supernatants were removed. After four washings with 100 μl medium, 100 μl ^{125}I-labeled purified rabbit anti-mouse F(ab')$_2$ (10 ng protein corresponding to about 100,000 cpm) was added and incubated for 90 min at 4°C. The cells were then washed three times with medium and transferred to tubes for gamma counting. The positive hybrids detected by this method were then cloned by a limiting dilution system (Accolla *et al.*, 1980) in a 96-well plate, and a representative clone of each specificity was chosen for further studies. In some experiments, the number of target cells as well as the incubation time were different from the standard conditions (see Table III) described here.

2.6. ^{51}Cr Labeling of Target Cells

Target cells were labeled with ^{51}Cr by a modification of the method of Brunner *et al.* (1968). Target cells were adjusted to 5×10^6/ml in Tris–phosphate buffered saline containing 5% FCS. To 0.2 ml of the cell suspension (10^6 cells), 100 μCi/μg ^{51}Cr in 100 μl was added. After incubation for 30 min at 37°C with occasional shaking, the labeled target cells were washed three times with 5 ml medium plus 5% FCS.

2.7. Cytotoxicity Assay

Complement-dependent cytotoxicity (CDC) was measured by the ^{51}Cr-release assay as described previously (Carrel *et al.*, 1977). Briefly, 10^4 labeled target cells in 25-μl volumes were distributed into plastic tubes and incubated with 25 µl culture fluid or ascitic fluid (1 : 1000 dilution) for 30 min at 37°C before 50 µl fresh rabbit serum was added as a source of complement. The tubes were then incubated for 3 hr at 37°C. Cold medium was then added to stop the reaction, the tubes were centrifuged, and the radioactivity in the supernatant was counted. Specific lysis was determined as follows:

$$\text{Specific lysis } (\%) = \frac{TR - SR}{MR - SR} \times 100$$

where TR (test release) represents the radioactivity released by target cells incubated with hybridoma product and complement, SR (spontaneous release) represents the radioactivity released by target cells incubated with complement alone, and MR (maximum release) is the total amount of radioactivity released by incubation of target cells with 1 ml distilled water.

2.8. Quantitative Absorption Tests

Suspensions containing different numbers of cells ($2.5–40 \times 10^5/100$ µl) were added to equal volumes of culture fluid or ascites and incubated for 1 hr at room temperature. Cells were centrifuged and the remaining binding activity of the culture fluid or ascites tested in a radioactive binding assay as described above.

2.9. Reciprocal Binding-Inhibition Tests

Antibodies from the various clones were internally labeled by the addition of 10 µCi [³H]leucine to cultures of 10^6 hybrid cells in 1 ml leucine-free medium. After 24 hr of incubation at 37°C, culture fluids were harvested and 25 µl of each ³H-labeled antibody was incubated for 2 hr with 5×10^5 melanoma cells. The cells were centrifuged and counted in a β-liquid scintillation counter. For competition analysis, 25 µl unlabeled antibodies of the various hybridoma was allowed to react for 10 min with the target cells before the addition of 25 µl ³H-labeled antibodies from each hybrid. After 3 hr, the cells were washed and counted.

2.10. Isotype Assay

The immunologobulin (Ig) class of the positive hybrid culture fluids was determined as follows: 4×10^5 cells were incubated with culture fluid in U plates (Falcon). After centrifugation and washing, goat antisera specific for either mouse IgM, IgG$_1$, IgG$_2$, or IgA (Meloy, Springfield, Virginia) were added. After washing, ^{125}I-labeled rabbit anti-goat IgG was added. All incubation steps, lasting 2 hr each, were done at 4°C.

3. Results

3.1. Screening for Antibody-Secreting Hybrids

From five fusions between spleen cells from mice immunized with melanoma membranes and mouse myeloma cells, we obtained a total of 193 growing hybrids. In an initial screening, 55 of them were found to produce antibodies binding to one of the immunizing cell lines as determined by RIA (Table IV).

From the first fusion, we obtained a total of 26 growing hybrids, 7 of which were producing antibodies directed against the immunizing melanoma cells, Me43. As a first screening for specificity, culture fluid from these 7 hybrids was tested against two nonmelanoma cell lines, a myeloid line, K562 (Lozzio and Lozzio, 1975), and an endometrial carcinoma line, END-1 (Carrel et al., 1979). Of 7 hybrid products, 4 reacted with either one of the two control cell lines. The reactivity of the 3 hybrids secreting antibodies that did not react with these two control cell lines was then further analyzed.

From the second fusion, we obtained 8 growing hybrids, none of which secreted antibodies binding to the immunizing cell line IGR-3. From the third fusion, 14 growing hybrids were obtained, and 4 of them produced antibodies binding to the immunizing cells Me43. Of these 4 antibodies, 2 bound to the control nonmelanoma cells K562 and were discarded. The reactivity of the remaining clones was then further analyzed. The fourth fusion resulted in 87 growing hybrids with 39 secreting antibodies that bound to the immunizing cells IGR-3. After a first screening for specificity, it was found that 36 hybrid products bound to either one of the control cell lines tested and were therefore discarded. The 3 remaining clones were chosen for further specificity analysis. From the fifth fusion, we obtained a total of 58 growing hybrids, 5 of which were secreting antibodies that bound to the immunizing cells Me43. After the first screening against K562 cells, 4 of them were discarded and the specificity of the remaining hybridoma product further investigated.

TABLE IV

Somatic-Cell Hybrids Producing Monoclonal Antibodies Against Melanoma

Fusion code	Immunizing antigen[a]	Myeloma strain used	Number of growing hybrids	Number of positive hybrids for the immunizing cells	Number of hybrids with restricted reactivity for melanoma
Me I	Me43	P3-NSl/Ag4	26	7	3
Me II	Me43	P3-NSl/Ag4	8	0	—
Me III	IGR-3	P3 × 63/Ag8	14	4	2
Me IV	IGR-3	P3 × 63/Ag8	87	39	3
Me V	Me43	P3 × 63/Ag8	58	5	1
	TOTALS (five fusions):		193	55	9

[a]Mice immunized with membrane-enriched fractions.

The 9 positive hybrids selected from these five fusions, after this preliminary screening, were then cloned by limiting dilution and a representative clone for each hybrid chosen for further specificity analysis.

3.2. Specificity Analysis

The 3 selected positive clonal products from that first fusion were designated as Mel-5, Mel-7 and Mel-14. Table V summarizes the binding results obtained with these reagents on 18 different melanoma cell lines. The results are expressed as a binding ratio (BR) that represents the total number of cell-bound counts using as control culture fluid of the mouse myeloma P3 $\times$ 63/Ag8 producing an IgG_1 (κ) immunoglobulin of unknown specificity. The background counts varied for each cell line tested, ranging between 59 and 158 cpm. The results obtained with 27 nonmelanoma tumor cell lines—including 5 colon carcinomas, 4 breast carcinomas, 3 cervical carcinomas, 13 glioblastomas, 2 neuroblastomas, and 12 T- and B-cell lines as well as normal skin fibroblasts, normal spermatozoa,

TABLE V

Binding of Hybridoma Antimelanoma Antibodies to Melanoma Cell Lines

Melanoma cell lines	BR of hybridoma product[a]			Background[b] (cpm)
	Mel-5	Mel-7	Mel-14	
Me43	22	7	23	110
Me47	6	1	7	59
Me33	6	1	8	138
MP-6	13	2	12	158
Mel-57[c]	9	4	11	85
Mel-67	8	2	9	75
IGR-3[c]	20	2	23	88
Mel-2AM[c]	10	3	15	79
A-375	3	1	4	78
Mel-2AP	5	1	6	143
SK-ME1-1	6	3	8	65
SK-Mel-25	6	4	5	76
MP-8	4	1	4	85
Mel-Ei-78	25	2	24	105
Me85	5	1	4	90
Me8[c]	10	2	13	110
Me25-1	1	1	3	74
Daudel[c]	8	5	12	113

[a]Total number of cell-bound counts divided by the number of cell-bound counts using P3$\times$63/Ag8 culture fluid.
[b]Background counts bound by P3$\times$63/Ag8 culture fluid.
[c]Cell line expressing HLA-D-related (HLA-DR) antigens.

TABLE VI

Binding of Hybridoma Antimelanoma Antibodies to Various Nonmelanoma Cells

Antibody secreted by clone	Human cell lines[a]								
	Colon carcinoma	Breast carcinoma	Cervical carcinoma	Glioblas-tomas	Neuro-blastomas	B and T cells	Normal skin fibroblasts[b]	Normal sperma-tozoa[c]	Normal PBL
Me1-5	0/5	0/4	0/3	4/13	0/2	0/12	0/3	0/7	0/5
Me1-7	0/5	0/4	0/3	0/13	0/2	0/12	0/3	0/7	0/5
Me1-14	0/5	0/4	0/3	5/13	0/2	0/12	0/3	0/7	0/5

[a]Number of cell lines positive/total number of cell lines tested.
[b]Short-term cultures.
[c]Frozen samples.

seen that Me1-5 antibodies gave a BR of 3 or more on all 18 melanoma cell lines tested except for Me25-1 (Table V). The highest BR was obtained for the three melanoma lines Me43, IGR-3, and Me1-Ei-78, with values ranging from 20 to 25. Among the 27 non-melanoma lines tested (see Table VI), Me1-5 hybridoma product reacted with only 4 of 13 glioblastoma cell lines. No reactivity was observed for the 12 lymphoid cell lines or for normal skin fibroblasts, normal spermatozoa, or normal PBL. Antibodies secreted by clone Me1-7 showed a restricted specificity for a limited number of melanoma cell lines with a BR ranging from 3 to 7 for 6 melanoma lines (Table V). No binding was observed with all control cell lines tested. Hybridoma product from clone Me1-14 gave a BR ranging from 3 to 24 with all the 18 melanoma cell lines tested (Table V), with no significant binding for the 27 nonmelanoma tumor lines tested, except for 5 of 13 glioblastomas (Table VI).

Cells from the three hybridomas Me1-5, Me1-7, and Me1-14 were injected intraperitoneally (4×10^7 cells per mouse) into pristane-primed BALB/c mice, where they grew as an ascites tumor. The ascites fluid was collected 2 weeks after tumor inoculation. It contained antibody that gave a significant binding to melanoma cells, up to a dilution of 1:10,000 in the binding assay. The titration curves obtained with serial dilutions of these ascites fluids for binding to IGR-3 melanoma cells as targets are shown in Fig. 2. BR values greater than 20 were obtained for each hybridoma product at a 1:1000 dilution. No binding was seen when the same ascites fluids were tested against nonmelanoma control cell lines.

The two selected clones from the third fusion were designated as Me3-TB7 and Me3-NE4. Table VII summarizes the binding results obtained with these reagents on 6 different melanoma cell lines. It can be seen that Me3-TB7 antibodies bound to 6 of 6 melanoma lines tested, with BR values ranging from 7 to 22. Antibodies from clone Me3-NE4 bound to 4 of 6 melanoma lines, with BR values ranging from 16 to 39. The results obtained with these two hybridoma products on 13 nonmelanoma control cell lines are summarized in Table VIII. As can be seen, Me3-TB7 antibodies bound to none of the control cell lines tested, while Me3-NE4 antibodies bound to 5 of 13 lines tested, with BR values ranging from 12 to 26. Interestingly, Me3-NE4 antibodies bound only to cell lines expressing

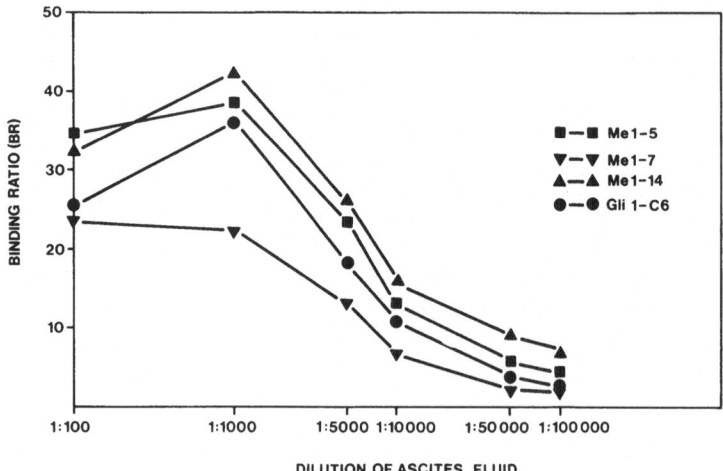

FIGURE 2. Binding assay of monoclonal antimelanoma antibodies to IGR-3 melanoma target cells. Ascites fluid of the different hybridomas was serially diluted with RPMI 1640 medium containing 10% FCS. Results are expressed as binding ratio (BR). The test was done with 50,000 target cells (see Table III). Monoclonal antimelanoma: Me1-5, Me1-7, Me1-14; monoclonal antiglioblastoma: Gli1-C6.

HLA-DR antigens, suggesting that they are directed against this particular antigen. Immunoprecipitation analysis performed with ^{125}I-labeled membrane proteins solubilized from the B-cell line Raji and run on sodium dodecyl sulfate–polyacrylamide gel electrophoresis revealed by autoradiography the presence of the two typical precipitation bands for the Ia molecule at molecular weights of 28,000 and 33,000.

From the fourth fusion, the 3 selected clones were designated as Me4-H3, Me4-F8, and Me4-H4. Table VII summarizes the binding results obtained with these reagents on 6 different melanoma lines. All 3 hybridoma products reacted with 6 of 6 melanoma lines,

TABLE VII
Binding of Hybridoma Antimelanoma Antibodies to Melanoma Cell Lines

Melanoma cell lines	Hybridoma product[a]						
	Me3-TB7	Me3-NE4	Me4-H3	Me4-F8	Me4-H4	Me5-D5	Gli1-C6[b]
IGR-3[c]	16	39	5	9	4	5	17
Me43	22	1	4	11	12	9	21
Me1-57[c]	13	26	4	12	5	3	29
Me1-2AM[c]	18	16	5	10	8	4	20
Me1-67	7	2	6	7	14	8	15
Daudel[c]	21	27	5	6	4	6	16

[a]Values are expressed as BR = total number of cell-bound counts divided by the number of cell-bound counts using P3 × 63/Ag8 culture fluid.
[b]Monoclonal antiglioblastoma antibody.   [c]Cell line expressing HLA-DR antigens.

TABLE VIII

Binding of Hybridoma Antimelanoma Antibodies to Various Nonmelanoma Cells

Target cell lines[b]	Hybridoma product[a]						
	Me3-TB7	Me4-NE4	Me4-H3	Me4-F8	Me4-H4	Me5-D5	Gli1-C6[c]
END-1	1	18	1	1	2	1	2
HT-29	1	1	1	2	1	2	1
CO-115	2	3	1	2	1	2	2
Me-180	1	1	2	1	2	1	1
IMR-32	2	1	1	2	1	1	5
LN-135	1	12	1	2	1	2	1
G-18	2	2	2	1	2	1	11
LN-215	1	1	1	2	1	2	5
K562	1	1	1	1	1	1	1
6410	1	23	1	2	2	1	2
8402	1	1	1	1	2	2	1
Raji	2	26	2	2	2	1	1
LIK	1	18	1	1	1	1	2

[a] Results are expressed in BR = total number of cell-bound counts divided by the number of cell-bound counts using P3 × 63/Ag8 culture fluid.
[b] Endometrial carcinoma (END-1); colon carcinoma (HT-29, CO-115); cervical carcinoma (Me-180); neuroblastoma (IMR-32); glioblastoma (LN-135, G-18, LN-215); myeloid line (K562); B-cell lines (6410, Raji, LIK); T-cell line (8402).
[c] Monoclonal antiglioblastoma antibody.

with BR values ranging from 4 to 6 for Me4-H3 antibodies, from 6 to 12 for Me4-F8, and from 4 to 14 for Me4-H4 antibodies. None of these hybridoma products bound to either one of the 13 control cell lines tested (see Table VIII). The selected clone from the fifth fusion was designated Me5-D5. Antibodies from this clone bound to 6 of 6 melanoma lines tested (see Table VII), with BR values ranging from 3 to 9. No reactivity for the 13 control cell lines tested was observed (see Table VIII).

3.3. Complement-Dependent Cytotoxicity of Hybridoma Products

The reactivity of the 9 selected hybridoma products was tested by CDC on ^{51}Cr-labeled target cells using ascites fluid of each clone at a 1:1000 dilution in the presence of rabbit complement. The results obtained are summarized in Table IX. None of the 3 clones selected from the first fusion secreted cytolytic antibodies, while antibodies from the 2 clones of the third fusion were able to lyse labeled target cells. The results are expressed as percentage of specific lysis of the ^{51}Cr-labeled cells. As shown in Table IX, a significant lysis was observed with Me3-TB7 antibodies for 5 of 6 melanoma cell lines tested, the percentage of lysed cells varying from 21 to 51%. No significant lysis was obtained for the 4 control cell lines tested. Antibodies from clone Me3-NE4, shown to be directed against HLA-DR antigens, were cytolytic for all cell lines expressing DR antigens. Up to 65% specific lysis was obtained for melanoma cells IGR-3 and 74% lysis for the B-cell line Raji. A similar

TABLE IX
Cytotoxic Activity of Monoclonal Antimelanoma Antibodies

Cell line used as target[b]	Hybridoma product[a]										
	Me1-5	Me1-7	Me1-14	Me3-TB7	Me3-NE4	Me4-H3	Me4-F8	Me4-H4	Me5-D5	Gli1-C6[c]	D1-12[d]
IGR-3[e]	0	0	0	46	65	0	41	0	0	0	78
Me-43	0	0	0	34	0	0	28	0	0	0	0
Me1-57[e]	0	0	0	21	38	0	27	0	0	0	31
Daudel[e]	0	0	0	0	19	0	0	0	0	0	28
Me1-67	0	0	0	44	0	0	35	0	0	0	0
Me1-2AM[e]	0	0	0	51	39	25	43	21	0	0	35
IMR-32	0	0	0	0	0	0	0	0	0	0	0
CO-115	0	0	0	0	0	0	0	0	0	0	0
END-1[e]	0	0	0	0	81	0	0	0	0	0	93
Raji[e]	0	0	0	0	74	0	0	0	0	0	78

[a]Values are expressed as percentage of specific lysis of ^{51}Cr labeled-target cells.
[b]Melanomas (IGR-3, Me-43, Me1-57, Daudel, Me1-67, Me1-2AM); neuroblastoma (IMR-32); colon carcinoma (CO-115); endometrial carcinoma (END-1); B-cell line (Raji).
[c]Monoclonal antiglioblastoma.   [d]Monoclonal anti-DR.   [e]Cell line expressing HLA-DR.

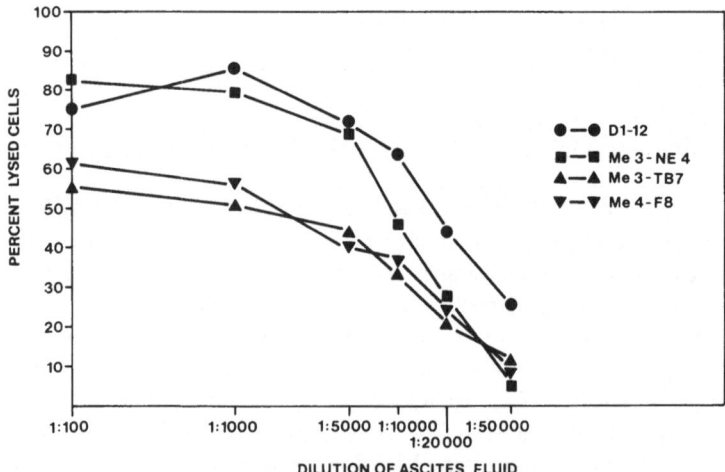

FIGURE 3. Cytotoxic activity of monoclonal antimelanoma antibodies against ^{51}Cr-labeled IGR-3 target cells. Ascites fluid of the different hybridomas was serially diluted with RPMI 1640 medium containing 10% FCS. Results are given as percentage specific lysis (see Section 2.7 for the method of calculation).

percentage of lysed cells was obtained with another monoclonal anti-DR antibody, D1-12 (Carrel *et al.*, 1981). Among the three selected hybridoma products from the fourth fusion, Me4-F8 was cytolytic for 5 of 6 melanoma lines tested, the percentage of lysed cells varying from 27 to 43%. None of the control cell lines was significantly lysed. Surprisingly, antibodies from clones Me4-H3 and Me4-H4 were cytolytic only for melanoma cells from line Me1-2AM. The hybridoma product from the fifth fusion was noncytolytic. Representative titration curves of the cytolytic antibodies are shown in Fig. 3. More than 50% of IGR-3 cells were lysed at a 1:1000 dilution for all ascites fluids tested, and even at 1:20,000 a significant percentage of lysed cells was still obtained.

3.4. Quantitative Absorption Experiments

The specificity of the three hybridoma products Me1-5, Me1-14, and Me3-TB7 for melanoma cells was further demonstrated by quantitative absorption experiments. Increasing numbers of cells from three melanoma lines (Me1-67, Me1-57, IGR-3) and from two control tumor lines (CO-115, END-1) were added to 200 μl culture fluid from hybrids Me1-5 (at 1:5 dilution), Me1-14, and Me3-TB7 (at 1:10 dilution). The remaining binding activity to IGR-3 melanoma cells in the supernatant was then tested in the binding assay (RIA). Figure 4A shows that cells from the three melanoma lines Me1-67, Me1-57, and IGR-3 absorbed the binding of Me1-5 antibodies, while as many as 16×10^6 colon-carcinoma cells (CO-115) or endometrial-carcinoma cells (END-1) gave no significant inhibition. Similarly, Fig. 4B shows that between 10 and 20×10^5 cells from the three melanoma lines were sufficient to absorb out 50% of the reactivity of Me1-14, while 16×10^6 colon-carcinoma cells (CO-115) or endometrial-carcinoma cells (END-1) gave no significant reduction of binding. Figure 4C shows that as for Me1-5 and Me1-14, only melanoma cells were able to inhibit the binding of Me3-TB7 antibodies. No inhibition was observed with the two control cell lines used.

3.5. Reciprocal Binding-Inhibition Experiments

To determine whether the three monoclonal antibodies Me1-5, Me1-14, and Me3-TB7 were directed against identical or different antigenic determinants, we performed a series of binding inhibition experiments. In these experiments, [^{3}H]leucine-labeled antibodies from the three clones were tested for their binding capacity to IGR-3 melanoma cells in the presence of an excess of unlabeled antibodies from the same or different clones. As shown in Fig. 5a, the binding of labeled Me1-5 antibodies was inhibited by unlabeled antibodies from the same clone, but not by Me1-14 or Me3-TB7 antibodies. As a control, unlabeled Me3-NE4 antibodies (anti-HLA-DR), even when used as 20-times-concentrated culture fluid, were ineffective in inhibiting the binding of labeled Me1-5. Figure 5b shows the converse experiment, where the binding of labeled Me1-14 antibodies was inhibited only by unlabeled Me1-14 and not by Me1-5 or Me3-TB7 antibodies. Figure 5c shows that the binding of labeled Me3-TB7 antibodies was inhibited only by unlabeled Me-TB7. These results clearly indicate that the antibodies from these three clones, Me1-5, Me1-14, and Me3-TB7, react with different antigenic determinants present on the same melanoma cells.

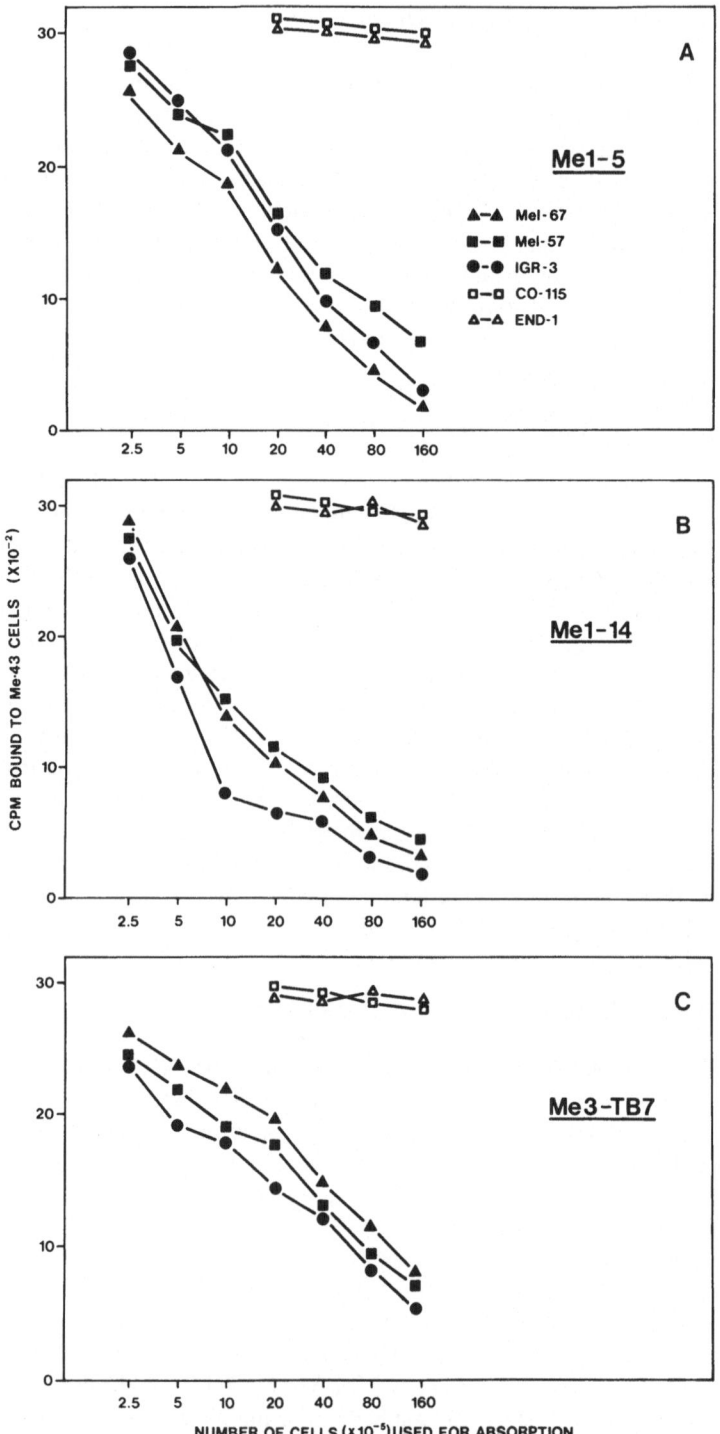

FIGURE 4. Quantitative absorption of monoclonal antimelanoma hybridoma products: (A) Me1-5; (B) Me1-14; (C) Me3-TB7. Binding assay using Me43 melanoma cells as targets. Each point represents counts per minute bound by the various culture fluids after absorption of 50 μl with the number of cells indicated. Melanoma cells: Me1-67, Me1-57, IGR-3; colon carcinoma: CO-115; endometrial carcinoma: END-1.

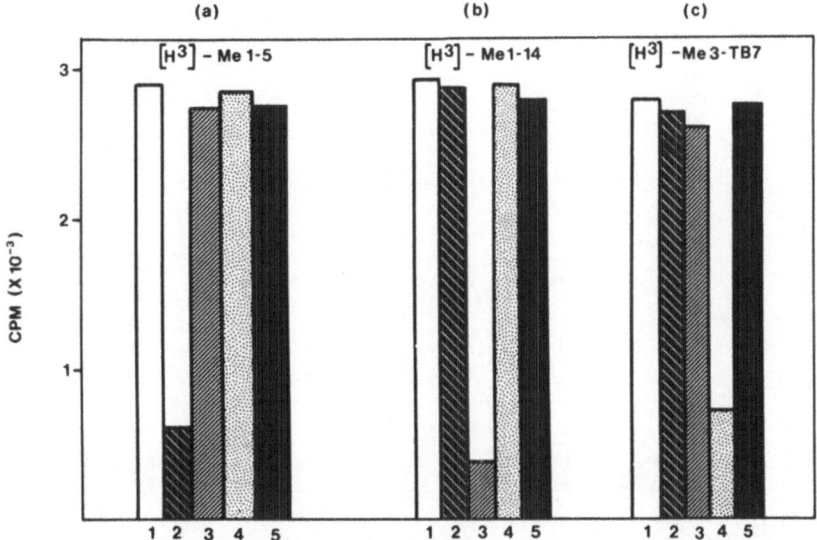

FIGURE 5. Competition of binding to IGR-3 melanoma cells among Me1-5, Me1-14, and Me3-TB7 antibodies. Antibodies from these three clones were internally labeled with [H³]leucine. Labeled Me1-5 (a), Me1-14 (b), and Me3-TB7 (c): without unlabeled culture fluid (1); after addition of unlabeled Me1-5 (2); after addition of unlabeled Me1-14 (3); after addition of unlabeled Me3-TB7 (4); after addition of unlabeled Me3-NE4 (5).

3.6. Isotype Assay

The results obtained from the isotype analysis of the antibodies produced by the five clones selected from the first and the third fusion are shown in Fig. 6. The two cytolytic clones Me3-TB7 and Me3-NE4 secrete antibodies of the IgG_2 subclass, whereas the three noncytolytic clones secrete IgG_1 (Me1-5), IgM (Me1-7), and IgG_2 (Me1-14) antibodies. Even though Me1-7 and Me1-14 seem to belong to a complement-binding class of immunoglobulins, they were not lytic for melanoma cells, even when used at very high concentrations.

3.7. Binding Assay to Fibronectin

The melanoma cells, Me-43 and IGR-3, used for immunization were shown to produce large amounts of fibronectin (LETS protein). It was important to determine whether one of the monoclonal antibodies was directed against this protein. This was carried out using a solid-phase RIA as described by Zardi et al. (1980). Unlabeled fibronectin (0.01 mg/well) was adsorbed to the wells of a polyvinyl plate. Culture fluid was then incubated for 2 hr, before ^{125}I-labeled rabbit antimouse antibodies were added. As shown in Fig. 7, none of the four hybridoma products (Me1-5, Me1-7, Me1-14, and Me3-TB7) or of two other monoclonal antibodies, anti-CEA and antiglioblastoma, bound to fibronectin. As positive control, a monoclonal antifibronectin antibody was used (Zardi et al., 1980).

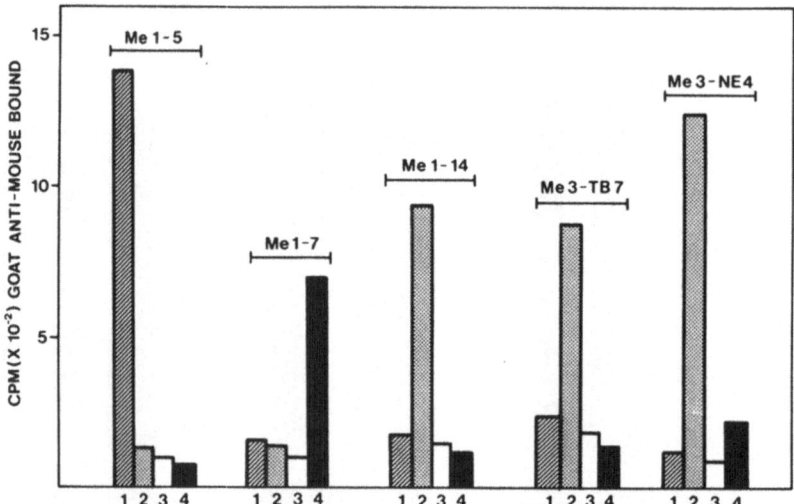

FIGURE 6. Determination of immunoglobulin class of hybridoma antibodies. Culture fluid from hybridomas Me1-5, Me1-7, Me1-14, Me3-TB7, and Me3-NE4 was tested on IGR-3 melanoma target cells. Goat antisera specific for mouse IgG_1 (1), IgG_2 (2), IgA_4 (3), or IgM (4) (100 μl diluted 1 : 5000) were used in the second incubation. The results are expressed as ^{125}I-labeled rabbit antibodies against goat IgG (100 μl containing 5 ng of antibodies representing 25,000 cpm) bound.

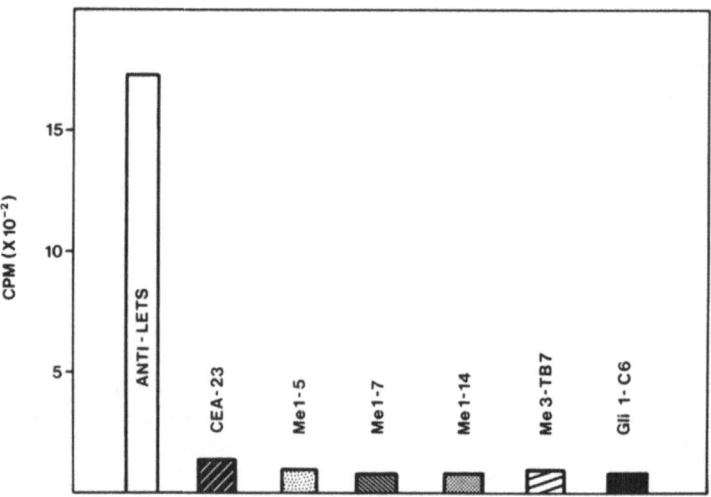

FIGURE 7. Solid-phase RIA for fibronectin. Unlabeled fibronectin (0.01 mg/well) was adsorbed to wells of a polyvinyl plate. Culture fluid was then incubated for 2 hr before ^{125}I-labeled rabbit antimouse antibodies were added. As positive control, monoclonal antifibronectin (LETS protein) was used (Zardi *et al.*, 1980). Binding of monoclonal anti-CEA (Accolla *et al.*, 1980) was taken as background. Monoclonal antimelanomas: Me1-5, Me1-7, Me1-14, Me3-TB7; monoclonal antiglioblastoma: Gli1-C6.

3.8. Reactivity of Monoclonal Antimelanoma Antibodies for Glioblastoma

During the specificity analysis of the three hybridoma products selected from the first fusion, it was observed that two of them cross-reacted with several glioblastoma cell lines. A similar cross-reactivity was also observed with one clone of the third fusion, Me3-TB7. As shown in Table X, antibodies from this clone were found to bind 5 of 13 glioglastoma lines tested. The reactivity spectrum of the three monoclonal antimelanoma antibodies, Me1-5, Me1-14, and Me3-TB7, further confirmed that these antibodies are not directed against the same antigenic determinants because they share binding capacity for only two glioblastoma lines (LN-121 and LN-229), whereas the other three glioblastoma lines, LN-181, 251-MG, and 181-SF, are bound only by Me3-TB7, Me1-14, and Me1-5, respectively. The reactivity spectrum of the monoclonal antiglioblastoma antibody, Gli1-C6, cross-reacting with melanomas, suggests that the antigenic determinant recognized by this antibody is different from those detected by the cross-reacting antimelanoma antibodies. In fact, Gli1-C6 bound 7 of 13 gliomas, particularly 118-MG cells, which were not recognized by the antimelanoma antibodies. Table X also shows that antibodies from clone Me3-NE4, as expected, bound only to HLA-DR-expressing glioma cell lines.

4. Discussion

From a total of five fusions between spleen cells from mice immunized with crude membrane fractions of two different melanoma cell lines, Me43 and IGR-3, and cells from

TABLE X

Binding of Hybridoma Antimelanoma Antibodies to Glioma Cell Lines

Glioma cell line used as target	Hybridoma product[a]					
	Me1-5	Me1-7	Me1-14	Me3-TB7	Me3-NE4	Gli1-C6[b]
LN-181	1	1	1	7	1	11
118-MG	2	2	2	1	2	12
251-MG	2	2	5	2	1	2
LN-71	1	1	2	6	2	9
LN-121[c]	4	1	6	5	15	2
LN-135[c]	2	2	9	2	7	1
LN-18	9	1	13	1	1	11
563-MG	2	2	2	2	2	2
LN-235	2	1	2	1	2	2
LN-94	2	2	2	2	2	5
MG-1073	2	1	2	6	2	3
LN-229[c]	11	1	33	5	18	5
181-SF	7	2	2	1	2	1

[a] Results are expressed as BR = total number of cell-bound counts divided by the number of cell-bound counts using P3 × 63/Ag8 culture fluid.
[b] Monoclonal antiglioblastoma antibody. [c] Cell line expressing HLA-DR antigens.

the two mouse myeloma lines P3-NSl/Ag4 and P3 × 63/Ag8, we obtained a total of 55 hybrids secreting antibodies that bound to either one of the immunizing cell lines: 12 coming from two fusions with spleen cells of mice immunized with Me43 cells and 43 from three fusions with spleen cells from mice immunized with IGR-3 cells. After a second screening for reactivity to control nonmelanoma cell lines, 46 hybrids were discarded, 8 from the Me43 fusions and 38 from the IGR-3 fusions. The reactivity spectrum of the 9 remaining hybridomas showed that the hybrid products could be classified into three groups: antibodies binding to melanomas only, antibodies binding to melanomas and gliomas, and antibodies directed against HLA-DR antigens. Antibodies from clones Me1-5, Me1-14, and Me3-TB7 displayed a broad reactivity with the majority of the melanoma lines tested, suggesting that they recognize antigenic structures widely expressed on melanoma cells. The hybridoma product from clone Me1-7 bound only to a proportion of melanoma cell lines, suggesting the existence of a more restricted melanoma antigen. Among the various control cell lines tested, antibodies from clones Me1-5, Me1-14, and Me3-TB7 showed some reactivity for 5 of the 13 glioma lines tested. Antibodies from clone Me3-NE4 were found to react with some melanomas, some gliomas, and B-cell lines, suggesting a reactivity for HLA-DR antigens known to be present on some melanoma cell lines (Wilson et al., 1979; Winchester et al., 1978). Further investigations confirmed the anti-Ia specificity of these antibodies. None of the selected 9 hybridoma products was directed against fibronectin, even though this protein seems to represent a major antigen expressed by the two melanoma cell lines, Me43 and IGR-3, that were used for immunization. When the 9 hybridoma products were analyzed for their cytolytic activity, in the presence of rabbit complement, it appeared that only 3 of 9 antibodies were able to lyse the melanoma cells. The lack of lytic activity for Me1-5 antibodies can be explained easily, since isotype analysis showed that these antibodies belong to the non-complement-binding class of immunoglobulins, IgG_1. However, IgM antibodies from clone Me1-7 and IgG_2 antibodies from clone Me1-14 were also noncytolytic even though these immunoglobulins are complement-binding. The reasons for this behavior are unknown. One might envisage that the antigens detected by these two monoclonal antibodies are expressed on the cell surface in a configuration or a density that does not allow complement-dependent lysis. Preliminary experiments using antibody-dependent cell-mediated cytotoxicity with either human PBL or mouse cells as effector killer cells gave the same negative result. The melanoma specificity of the three antibodies, Me1-5, Me1-14, and Me3-TB7, directed against one or more putative common melanoma-associated antigens was confirmed by a series of quantitative absorption experiments. These studies showed that pretreatment with melanoma cells Me1-67, Me1-57, and IGR-3 removed the binding activity of these three monoclonal antibodies for melanoma target cells, whereas up to 80 times more colon-carcinoma cells Co-115 or endometrial-carcinoma cells END-1 could not reduce the reactivity of the respective culture fluids. In addition, we could demonstrate by reciprocal binding-inhibition experiments that antibodies from clones Me1-5, Me1-14, and Me3-TB7 were directed against different antigenic determinants expressed on the membrane of melanoma cells.

The reactivity of Me1-5, Me1-14, and Me3-TB7 antibodies for glioblastoma cell lines suggests the existence of common antigens for cells of a common origin, since it is generally accepted that both cell types, melanocytes and glial cells, originate from the neural crest. The close relationship between melanocytes and glial cells has recently been confirmed by Gaynor et al. (1980), who demonstrated the presence of S100 protein in melanocytes, this protein being a typical marker for glial cells. Antibodies that displayed a cross-reactivity for cells of common origin have already been reported by Kennett and Gilbert (1978). These authors raised a monoclonal antineuroblastoma antibody that cross-reacted with glioblastoma. Since the antimelanoma antibodies described in this paper did not bind to the neuroblastoma cells tested, it seems unlikely that the antineuroblastoma antibody of Kennett and Gilbert (1978) detects similar antigenic determinants. Schnegg et al. (1981) produced three monoclonal antiglioblastoma antibodies, one of which, Gli1-C6, secreted antibodies cross-reacting with melanomas. The reactivity spectrum for 13 different glioblastoma lines (see Table X) suggests that the antigenic determinant recognized by Gli1-C6 is different from the determinants recognized by the antimelanoma antibodies, since Gli1-C6 bound to glioma lines not detected by the antimelanoma antibodies, Mel-5, Mel-14, and Me3-TB7. The reactivity spectrum of these three antimelanoma antibodies for gliomas further suggests that the antigenic determinants detected by these antibodies are not located on the same molecule, since they were not concomitantly expressed on all glioma lines tested. Further immunochemical studies are in progress to characterize, at the molecular level, the various antigens recognized by the different monoclonal antimelanoma antibodies and to develop sensitive assays for each of them, which we believe will help to determine the degree of tumor specificity of melanoma-associated antigens.

ACKNOWLEDGMENTS. The authors wish to thank Drs. N. de Tribolet, A.-C. Diserens, and J.-F. Schnegg from the Neurological Department of the University Hospital (CHUV), Lausanne, Switzerland, for providing us with glioma cell lines, and express their gratitude for expert technical assistance to Mrs. S. Salvi and E. Duruz.

References

Accolla, R. S., Carrel, S., and Mach, J.-P., 1980, Monoclonal antibodies specific for carcinoembryonic antigen (CEA) produced by hybrid cell lines, Proc. Natl. Acad. Sci. U.S.A. 77:563–566.

Aubert, C., Lagrange, C., Rorsman, H., and Rosengren, E., 1976, Catecholes in primary and metastatic human malignant melanoma cells in monolayer culture, Eur. J. Cancer 12:441–445.

Brunner, K. T., Mauel, J., Cerottini, J.-C., and Chappuis, B., 1968, Quantitative assay of the lytic action of immune lymphoid cells on ^{51}Cr labeled allogenic target cells in vitro: Inhibition by isoantibody and drugs, Immunology 14:181–196.

Bystryn, J.-C., 1977, Release of cell-curface tumor-associated antigens by viable melanoma cells from humans, J. Natl. Cancer Inst. 59:325–328.

Carey, T. E., Takahashi, T., Resnick, L. A., Oettgen, H. F., and Old, L. J., 1976, Cell surface antigens of human malignant melanoma: Mixed hemadsorption assay for humoral immunity to cultured autologous melanoma cells, Proc. Natl. Acad. Sci. U.S.A. 73:3278–3282.

Carrel, S., Delisle, M.-C., and Mach, J.-P., 1977, Antibody dependent cell-mediated cytolysis of human colon carcinoma cells induced by specific antisera against carcinoembryonic antigen, Cancer Res. 36:2644–2650.

Carrel, S., Gross, N., Heumann, D., and Mach, J.-P., 1979, Expression of "Ia-like" antigens on cells from a human endometrial carcinoma cell line End-1, Transplantation 27:431–433.

Carrel, S., Dent, P. B., and Liao, S. K., 1980a, Demonstration of the specificity of a monkey antiserum against human melanoma: Evidence that the cytotoxic antibodies from the specific antiserum belong to the IgM class, Cancer Immunol. Immunother. 8:192–203.

Carrel, S., Accolla, R. S., Carmagnola, A. L., and Mach, J.-P., 1980b, Common human melanoma associated antigen(s) detected by monoclonal antibodies, Cancer Res. 40:2523–2428.

Carrel, S., Accolla, R. S., Carmagnola, A. L., and Mach, J.-P., 1980c, Demonstration of human melanoma associated antigen(s) by monoclonal antibodies, in: *Protides of Biological Fluids,* Vol. 27 (H. Peeters, ed.,), Pergamon Press, Oxford (in press).

Carrel, S., Tosi, R., Gross, N., Tanigaki, N., Carmagnola, A. L., and Accolla, R. S., 1981, Subsets of human Ia-like molecules defined by monaclonal antibodies *Mol. Immunol.* **18**:403–411.

Cornain, S., De Vries, J. E., Collard, J., Vennegoor, C., van Wingarden, I., and Rumke, P., 1975, Antibodies and antigen expression in human melanoma detected by the immune adherence test, *Int. J. Cancer* **16**:981–997.

Cowan, N. J., Secher, D. S., and Milstein, C., 1974, Intracellular immunoglobulin chain synthesis in non-secreting variants of a mouse myeloma: Detection of inactive light chain messenger RNA, *J. Mol. Biol.* **90**:697–701.

Ferrone, S., and Pellegrino, M. A., 1977, Cytotoxic antibodies to cultured melanoma cells in the sera of melanoma patients, *J. Natl. Cancer Inst.* **58**:1201–1204.

Fritze, D., Kern, D. H., Drogemuller, C. R., and Pilch, Y. H., 1976, Production of antisera with specificity for malignant melanoma, *Cancer Res.* **36**:458–466.

Gaynor, R., Irie, R., Morton, D., and Herschman, H. R., 1980, S100 protein is present in cultured human malignant melanomas, *Nature (London)* **286**:400–401.

Gupta, R. K., and Morton, D. L., 1975, Suggestive evidence for *in vivo* binding of specific antitumor antibodies of human melanomas, *Cancer Res.* **35**:58–62.

Herlyn, M., Steplewski, Z., Herlyn, D., and Koprowski, H., 1979, Colorectal carcinoma-specific antigen: Detection by means of monoclonal antibodies, *Proc. Natl. Acad. Sci. U.S.A.* **76**:1438–1442.

Hersey, P., Honeyman, M., Edwards, A., Adams, E., and McCarthy, W. H., 1976, Antigens on melanoma cells detected by leukocyte dependent antibody assay of human melanoma antisera, *Int. J. Cancer* **18**:546–573.

Kennett, R. H., and Gilbert, F., 1979, Hybrid myelomas producing antibodies against a human neuroblastoma antigen present on fetal brain, *Science* **203**:1120–1121.

Klinman, N. R., 1972, The mechanism of antigenic stimulation of primary and secondary clonal precursor cells, *J. Exp. Med.* **136**:241–260.

Köhler, G., and Milstein, C., 1975, Continuous cultures of fused cells secreting antibody of predefined specificity, *Nature (London)* **256**:495–497.

Köhler, G., Howe, S. C., and Milstein, C., 1976, Fusion between immunoglobulin secreting and non-secreting myeloma cell lines, *Eur. J. Immunol.* **6**:292–295.

Koprowski, H., Steplewski, Z., Herlyn, D., and Herlyn, M., 1978, Study of antibodies against human melanoma produced by somatic cell hybrids *Proc. Natl. Acad. Sci. U.S.A.* **75**:3405–3409.

Lewis, M. G., Ikonopisov, R. L., Nairn, R. C., Phillips, T. M., Fairley, G. H., Bodenham, D. C., and Alexander, P., 1969, Tumour specific antibodies in human malignant melanoma and their relationship to the extent of the disease, *Br. Med. J.* **3**:547–552.

Liao, S. K., Leong, S. P. L., Sutherland, C. M., Dent, P. B., Kwong, P. C., and Krementz, E. T., 1978, Common human melanoma membrane antigens detected by mixed hemadsorption microassay with serum from a patient undergoing immunotherapy with autologous tumor cells, *Cancer Res.* **38**:4394–4399.

Liao, S. K., Kwong, P. C., Thompson, J. C., and Dent, P. B., 1979, Spectrum of melanoma antigens on cultured human malignant melanoma cells as detected by monkey antibodies, *Cancer Res.* **39**:183–192.

Lozzio, C. B., and Lozzio, B. B., 1975, Human chronic meylogenous leukemia cell line with positive Philadelphia chromosome, *Blood* **45**:324–334.

McCabe, R. P., Ferrone, S., Pellegrino, M. A., Kern, D. H., Holmes, E. C., and Reisfeld, R. A., 1978, Purification and immunological evaluation of human melanoma-associated antigens, *J. Natl. Cancer Inst.* **60**:773–777.

Metzgar, R. S., Bergoc, P. M., Moreno, M. Y., and Seigler, H. F., 1973, Melanoma-specific antibodies produced in monkey by immunization with human melanoma cell lines, *J. Natl. Cancer Inst.* **50**:1065–1068.

Morton, D. L., Malmgreen, R. A., Holmes, E. C., and Ketcham, A. S., 1968, Demonstration of antibodies against human malignant melanoma by immunofluorescence, *Surgery* **64**:233–240.

Muna, N. M., Marcus, S., and Smart, C., 1969, Detection by immunofluorescence of antibodies specific for human malignant melanoma cells, *Cancer* **23**:88–95.

Pontecorvo, G., 1975, Production of mammalian somatic cell hybrids by means of polyethylene-glycol treatment, *Somatic Cell Genet.* **1**:397–400.

Schmidt-Ulrich, R., Ferber, E., Kneufermann, H., Fischer, H., and Hoelzl-Wallach, D. F., 1974, Analysis of the proteins in thymocyte plasma membrane and smooth endoplasmic reticulum by sodium dodecyl-sulfate gel electrophoresis, *Biochim. Biophys. Acta* **332**:175-191.

Schnegg, J. F., Diserens, A. C., Carrel, S., and de Tribolet, N., 1981, Human glioma-associated antigens detected by monoclonal antibodies, *Cancer Res.* **41**:1209.

Shiku, H., Takahashi, T., Oettgen, H. F., and Old, L. J., 1976, *J. Exp. Med.* **144**:873-881.

Shiku, H., Takahashi, T., Oettgen, H. F., and Old, L. J., 1977, Cell surface antigens of human malignant melanoma. III. Recognition of auto-antibodies with unusual characteristics, *J. Exp. Med.* **145**:784-789.

Sorg, C., Brüggen, J., Seibert, E., and Macher, E., 1978, Membrane-associated antigens of human malignant melanoma. IV. Changes in expression of antigens on cultured melanoma cells, *Cancer Immunol. Immunother.* **3**:259-271.

Steplewski, Z., Herlyn, M., Herlyn, D., Clark, W., and Koprowski, H., 1979, Reactivity of monoclonal anti-melanoma antibodies with melanoma cells freshly isolated from primary and metastatic melanoma, *Eur. J. Immunol.* **9**:94-96.

Stuhlmiller, G. M., and Seigler, H. F., 1975, Characterization of a chimpanzee anti-human melanoma anti-serum, *Cancer Res.* **35**:2132-2137.

Viza, D., and Phillips, J., 1975, Identification of an antigen associated with malignant melanoma, *Int. J. Cancer* **16**:312-317.

Williams, A. F., 1977, Differentiation antigens of the lymphocyte cell surface, in: *Contemporary Topics in Molecular Immunology,* Vol. 6 (G. L. Ada and R. R. Porter, eds.), pp. 93-116, Plenum Press, New York.

Wilson, B. S., Indiveri, F., Pellegrino, M. A., and Ferrone, S., 1979, DR. (Ia-like) antigens on human melanoma cells: Serological detection and immunochemical characterization, *J. Exp. Med.* **149**:658-668.

Winchester, R. J., Wang, C., Gibofsky, A., Kunkel, H. G., Lloyd, K. O., and Old, L. J., 1978, Expression of Ia-like antigens on cultured human malignant melanoma cells lines, *Proc. Natl. Acad. Sci. U.S.A.* **75**:6235-6239.

Woodbury, R. G., Brown, J. P., Yeh, M. X., Hellström, I., and Hellström, K. G., 1980, Identification of a cell surface protein, P97, in human melanomas and certain other neoplasms, *Proc. Natl. Acad. Sci. U.S.A.* **77**:2183-2187.

Yeh, M. Y., Hellström, I., Brown, J. P., Warner, G. A., Hansen, J. A., and Hellström, K. E., 1979, Cell surface antigens of human melanoma identified by monoclonal antibody, *Proc. Natl. Acad. Sci. U.S.A.* **76**:2927-2931.

Zardi, L., Carnemolla, B., Siri, A., Santi, L., and Accolla, R. S., 1980, Somatic cell hybrids producing antibodies specific to human fibronectin, *Int. J. Cancer* **25**:325-328.

5

Tumor-Directed Cellular Immunity in Malignant Melanoma and the Antigens That Evoke It

ALISTAIR J. COCHRAN

1. Introduction

The stimulus to study host responses in patients with malignant melanoma is provided by the observation that the clinical course of this neoplasm is not as uniformly bad as was previously believed by the medical profession and the informed laity (Solzhenitsyn, 1968). In favorable groups of patients with small superficial tumors [< 0.76 mm by micrometric measurement (Breslow, 1970)], the cure rate may considerably exceed 50%. Even in patients with disease in the regional lymph nodes, between 20 and 36% (Cochran, 1969a; Callery *et al.*, 1982) will remain tumor-free 5 years after therapeutic lymphadenectomy. Prognosis can be, in fact, quite accurately quantified prospectively (Cochran, 1968; MacKie *et al.*, 1972; Callery *et al.*, 1982). Some of the variability in prognosis is undoubtedly due to biological characteristics of the primary tumor such as thickness (Breslow, 1970) (which probably correlates with tumor volume and thus tumor-cell number), depth of invasion relative to anatomical landmarks of the skin (Clark, 1967; Cochran, 1969b), histogenetic pattern, mitotic rate, blood vascular or lymphatic invasion (McGovern *et al.*, 1973), and number of regional nodes replaced by tumor (Callery *et al.*, 1982; Cochran, 1969a). It is highly probable that the manner in which the patient reacts to the developing tumor is also very relevant.

Clinical evidence for human responses to spontaneous tumors is strong, if diverse. I have reviewed this evidence recently (Cochran, 1978) and will merely summarize the situation here. The concept that a well-functioning immunological system protects against the

ALISTAIR J. COCHRAN • Division of Surgical Oncology and Departments of Surgery and Pathology, UCLA School of Medicine, University of California, Los Angeles, California 90024.

development of malignant disease has been widely canvassed (Thomas, 1959; Burnet, 1967). There is support for this theory from observations that individuals with inherited deficiencies of immunological function and those receiving immunosuppressive therapy with or without an associated allograft have an increased incidence of malignant disease. However, the increased frequency of tumors in the immunologically abnormal does not reflect the incidence of tumor types seen in the general population. The theory of general immune surveillance is thus difficult to sustain. The key role of T-lymphocyte-mediated immunity in immune surveillance has also been challenged, the current candidate for the central role in this function being the natural killer (NK) cell (Herberman and Holden, 1979). A decline in immunological efficiency with *age* has been considered important for understanding the increased incidence of cancer in the elderly. Some such decline does occur, but is limited and small when compared to that associated with tumor progression (Todd *et al.,* 1980). Spontaneous regression of primary and, rarely, of metastatic cancer does occur (Everson and Cole, 1966). In malignant melanoma, partial or total regression of a primary tumor is not uncommon and may be associated with a better-than-average prognosis for some patients (Cochran *et al.,* 1970). Certainly not all regressive phenomena are immunologically based. Variations in the rate of tumor progression and in the period during which tumor cells may lie dormant indicate biologically "negotiable" relationships between host and tumor. The investigation of such phenomena presents many difficulties, but the potential insights that such studies may yield suggests that they deserve more determined attention.

The common association of immunocytes and macrophages with tumors, particularly with early invasive tumors or carcinoma-*in-situ,* suggests an immunological reaction similar in morphology to immunological reactions seen in the tissues affected by organ-specific autoimmune disease. Attempts to demonstrate tumor-specific sensitization *in vitro* or tumoricidal capacities for these peritumoral or tumor-infiltrating lymphocytes have so far been inconclusive. The application of newer techniques permitting expansion of tumor-infiltrating lymphocyte subpopulations *in vitro* may finally settle the role and biological significance of these cells.

The role of immunological factors in families with a high incidence of cancer and in single individuals with multiple malignancies remains speculative. New knowledge of immonogenetics should greatly assist in elucidating such problems.

The nature of host factors that may influence tumor growth, whether it grows progressively, develops metastatic capacities, and eventually kills the tumor-bearing host, remains obscure. While multiple and diverse systems are undoubtedly involved in the host–tumor relationship, it is highly probable that the immune system plays some role. The extent and significance of that role are of critical interest to all tumor immunologists. The degree of immune-system involvement is probably widely variable from one tumor system to another. The extent to which molecules not usually present on normal adult cells are present on tumor cells will vary according to the nature of the inducing carcinogen(s), the dose and kinetics of carcinogenic exposure, the route of administration of the carcinogens, and the concurrent exposure to cocarcinogens and anticarcinogens. The species and/or strain of the carcinogen-exposed animal is also relevant, since it can reflect genetic susceptibility to the agent employed.

A major problem that the diversity of tumor antigenicity and host responsiveness poses is the limited extent to which the findings may be extrapolated from one carcinogen–species combination to others. In particular, there is concern that the findings from experiments with small, inbred experimental animals exposed to high doses of strong, rapid-acting carcinogens may not be directly applicable to genetically heterogeneous man, in whom most tumors probably arise following long-continued conditioning by many different weak carcinogens. Therefore, in my view, it is a mistake to rigidly seek to obtain experimental findings in man that are identical to those previously found in animals. Conversely, we should not be surprised to find that human tumor-associated antigens (TAAs) are expressed differently from those of animals and that men react to such antigens in a manner quite different from that found in experimental animals. The pressures to study the diseases of man in man are thus considerable.

The goals of the immunologist studying human tumors are simple and may be expressed as a series of questions:

1. Are there molecules expressed in or on tumor cells that are not expressed on the normal cells from which the tumor derives?
2. Are these molecules recognizably foreign to the autochthonous host? If they are, can we detect evidence of humoral or cellular immunity to these molecules in tumor-bearing individuals?
3. If tumor-directed immunity does exist, does it have a significant biological effect *in vivo,* reducing or augmenting tumor growth locally or affecting its capacity to metastasize?
4. If tumor-directed immunity does develop spontaneously, why do cancers progress so lethally in many patients?
5. If tumor immunity does exist spontaneously but is incapable of inhibiting tumor growth and spread in its natural form, can we modify it to the patient's benefit?
6. If tumor immunity does not develop naturally, can we bring it into being with a beneficial result for the patients?

The latter two questions cover the central problems for those who would develop strategies for thus far elusive immunotherapy.

With the aforestated questions and aims as our motivation, I and various colleagues have conducted numerous studies over the past decade on animal and human tumors, including malignant melanoma, lymphocytic leukemia, Burkitt's lymphoma, breast cancer, colon cancer, and neuroblastoma. The remainder of this chapter summarizes our findings, concentrating on malignant melanoma in view of the central theme of this book.

2. Studies Employing the Direct One-Stage Capillary Leukocyte-Migration-Inhibition Technique

The direct leukocyte-migration-inhibition technique (DLMT) described by Søborg and Bendixen in 1967 was developed from Vaughan (1962). Blood leukocytes are mixed with tumor cells or tumor-cell extracts, and the production of leukocyte-inhibitory activity is assessed. In this one-stage assay, the mixed leukocyte population acts as both the source of the inhibitory materials and the indicator system. The DLMT was first applied to human malignant disease in a study of women with breast cancer (Andersen *et al.,* 1970). Numerous reports have since established its usefulness and limitations. In our

experience, the technique is relatively simple, and the necessary equipment is uncompli-
cated and inexpensive. There is evidence that the effect is due to release of soluble mediators
from sensitized lymphocytes (Ross *et al.*, 1979). Whether the mediators act exclusively
against macrophages (monocytes) or against granulocytes as well, or whether separate lymphokines act on different cell populations, has been the subject of debate. There is recent
evidence for separate leukocyte- and macrophage-inhibitory lymphokines (see below).

There is little unanimity as to what constitutes the best antigenic preparation for use
in DLMTs. Sources of antigen that we have investigated include whole and fractionated
fluids from cystic melanoma metastases (Cochran *et al.*, 1973; Jackson *et al.*, 1978), the
centrifuged supernatants of homogenized melanomas and other tumors (Cochran *et al.*,
1972a), and formalin-fixed single-cell suspensions from melanomas, other tumors, and normal tissues (Ross *et al.*, 1975). The exact nature of the antigens being detected on tumors
and the role of fetal antigens remains to be elucidated.

The migration technique was employed as follows: A 20-ml aliquot of heparinized
venous blood (10 IU preservative-free heparin/ml blood) was sedimented for 1–2 hr at
37°C. The white-cell-rich plasma was removed and spun at $100g$ for 10 min at 22°C. The
white-cell pellet was then washed twice ($70g$ for 5 min) in phosphate-buffered saline (PBS)
(pH 7.4) and resuspended in Eagle's Minimal Essential Medium (EMEM) containing
10% fetal calf serum (FCS), to a concentration of 10^8 cells/ml. This concentration gave a
cell button 2–3 mm long when spun in a 50-μl capillary tube. Samples of suspension, 200
μl, were placed in 10 × 60 mm plastic test tubes. The appropriate amount of antigen was
added [usually a range of 50–200 μg/ml leukocyte suspension or formalinized cells (FC)
at ratios of from 50 : 1 to 200 : 1 leukocytes/FC]. The tubes were stoppered tightly to
reduce evaporation and incubated for 1 hr at 37°C. Control tubes contained leukocytes and
medium alone or leukocytes with antigens from sources other than melanoma. The test
tubes were then agitated before four 50-μl aliquots were drawn into capillary tubes (Gel-
man-Hawksley Ltd., Sussex, England) that were sealed at one end with inert clay. The
capillary tubes were centrifuged at $50g$ for 5 min before the tubes were cut with a diamond
at the cell–fluid interface. The cell-containing portions of the capillaries were mounted on
a spot of silicone grease (Edwards, London, U.K.) in disposable tissue-culture plates [19
mm diameter planchette (Univers. Mekaniska Verkstad AB, Enskede, Sweden)]. EMEM
with 10% FCS was added to fill the plates, which were then closed with coverslips held in
place by silicone grease.

The completed plates were incubated in air at 37°C for 18–24 hr. Areas of migration
were drawn by means of a drawing tube attached to a light microscope. The areas were
measured by planimetry.

The migration areas of cells preexposed to antigen were compared with those of the
same cells exposed only to medium with FCS. The ratio of the mean of quadruplicate tubes
with and without antigen, or the *migration index*, was calculated.

Results obtained with quadruplicate samples of the same leukocytes in the presence
and absence of antigen were compared by the Mann–Whitney–Wilcoxon U test of ranking. Significance was assessed at the 5% level. This is, in our view, a more satisfactory
method of assessing a positive result than employing an arbitrary cutoff at, say, 20%
inhibition.

The reaction frequencies of different subpopulations with the various tumor-cell suspensions and other tumor-derived materials were compared by the χ^2 technique, applying
Yates correction where appropriate. Significance was assessed where p was less than 0.05.

2.1. Reactions of Melanoma Patients' Leukocytes with Autologous Melanoma-Derived Materials (Table I)

The migration of melanoma patients' leukocytes was significantly inhibited by autologous formalinized melanoma cells (FMC) in 18 of 23 instances (78%) and by supernatants (SN) of homogenized autologous melanoma cells in 8 of 10 experiments (80%). That melanoma patients' leukocytes react with cells or materials *derived from their own tumors* in a test known to be an *in vitro* correlate of delayed cutaneous hypersensitivity *in vivo* is in keeping with the existence of autoimmunogenic melanoma-associated antigens.

2.2. Reactions of Melanoma Patients' Leukocytes with Autologous and Allogeneic Melanoma-Derived Materials and of Control Donors' Leukocytes with Allogeneic Melanoma-Derived Materials (Table I)

The reaction frequencies of melanoma patients' leukocytes with allogeneic and autologous melanoma-derived materials were similar regardless of whether the antigen was FMC [190 of 225 (84%) and 18 of 23 (78%), respectively; $p > 0.05$]. These reaction frequencies were significantly greater ($p < 0.001$ and < 0.01, respectively) than those observed when (necessarily allogeneic) control donor leukocytes were exposed to the same

TABLE I

Reaction Frequency of Melanoma Patients' and Control Donors' Leukocytes against Different Preparations of Tumor- and Tissue-Associated Antigen in a One-Stage Leukocyte-Migration Assay

| | | Source of leukocytes | | | | |
| | | Melanoma patients | | Control donors | | |
Antigenic material	Technique	$+/T^a$	%	$+/T^a$	%	p^b
Melanoma-derived						
1. Fluid from cystic melanoma	DLMT	22/37	60	3/34	9	<0.01
2. Low-molecular-weight Sephadex # of (1)	DLMT	16/40	40	2/32	6	<0.05
3. Supernate tumor homogenate						
Autologous and allogeneic	DLMT	41/65	63			
Autologous only	DLMT	8/10	80			
Allogeneic only	DLMT	33/55	60	10/74	14	<0.01
4. Formalinized tumor cells						
Autologous and allogeneic	DLMT	208/248	84			
Autologous only	DLMT	18/23	79			
Allogeneic only	DLMT	190/225	84	76/250	30	<0.001
Control-tissue-derived						
6. Supernatant of homogenate	DLMT	5/52	10	37/157	24	NS
7. Formalinized cells	DLMT	19/68	22	42/146	29	NS

^{a}Number positive/total number tested.
^{b}The p value A-B was assessed by the χ^2 technique with Yates correction where appropriate. (NS) Not significant ($p > 0.05$).

FMC [76 of 250 (30%)] and SN [10 of 74 (14%)] in parallel experiments. Significant selective activity was also observed in comparisons of the reaction frequency of melanoma patients' and control donors' leukocytes in experiments employing whole fluid ($p < 0.01$) and fractionated fluid ($p < 0.05$) from cystic metastatic melanomas.

The reaction of melanoma patients' leukocytes with materials from autologous and allogeneic melanomas at a similar frequency suggests that antigens of at least closely similar structure occur on different melanomas.

2.3. Reaction of Melanoma Patients' and Control Donors' Leukocytes with Allogeneic Materials Derived from Tumors Other Than Melanoma and from Normal Tissues (Table I)

Melanoma patients' leukocytes were reactive with materials from melanomas significantly more often than with control tissues. This was observed with FMC (208 of 248 vs. 19 of 68, $p < 0.001$) and with SN (41 of 65 vs. 5 of 52, $p < 0.01$). By contrast, control donors' leukocytes were inhibited to a similar extent by melanoma-derived and control materials, whether FMC (76 of 250 vs. 42 of 146 $p > 0.05$) or SN (10 of 74 vs. 37 of 157, $p > 0.05$).

Melanoma patient reactivity with materials from other tumors and from normal tissues was low, indicating that the reactivity to FMC or SN antigens was to a degree melanocyte- and tumor-specific.

3. Clinical Stage and Tumor-Directed Cellular Immunity (Table II)

While a stage relationship of the frequency of reaction to tumor and recall antigens is clear, the major difference in response is between patients with limited disease (Stages I and II), 56–84% reactive, and patients with disseminated disease (Stage III), 0–50% reactive for both melanoma and breast-cancer patients. That the loss of reactivity is not tumor-antigen-specific is indicated by a comparable loss of response to tuberculoprotein as a "recall" antigen (Todd et al., 1980).

The mechanisms of stage-related reduction in detectable sensitization to tumor antigens and "recall" antigens are incompletely understood. It is not absolute or irreversible, as shown by the (re)development of cytotoxic lymphocytes after immunization with autologous irradiated tumor cells in patients with advanced malignancy (Currie et al., 1971). Furthermore, when patients with advanced melanoma receive systemic or intralesional bacillus Calmette Guérin (BCG) (with or without autologous irradiated or formalinized tumor cells), the frequency of detectable DLMT reactions is approximately the same as that of patients with localized disease. If immune paralysis exists in the patient with advanced malignancy, it is only partial and is remediable. High-zone tolerance cannot be excluded as cause for the decline in reactivity, because tumor cells administered in the "unnatural" form of a suspension could break the tolerance. The administration of tumor cells with or without an adjuvant may also stimulate concomitant immunity (Gershon, 1974).

TABLE II

Frequency of Leukocyte-Migration Inhibition Related to Clinical Stage

Cancer type and stage[a]	Leukocyte-migration-inhibited/total tested					
	SN antigens[b]		FMC antigens[b]		BCG[c]	
	Number	%	Number	%	Number	%
Malignant melanoma						
Stage I	24/37	65	16/19	84	14/17	82
Stage II	7/15	47	21/21	100	12/24	50
Stage III	0/6	0	12/24	50	11/30	37
Stage III, immunotherapy			35/37	95	25/36	69
Tumor-free under 2 years	13/16	81	23/25	92		
Tumor-free for over 2 years	3/12	25	22/38	58		
Breast carcinoma						
Stage I	32/57	56				
Stage II	20/31	65				
Stage III	6/22	27				
Local recurrence	6/10	60				

[a]Stage I: primary tumor only; Stage II: primary tumor + ipsilateral draining lymph nodes involved; Stage III: spread to internal viscera or remote lymph nodes.
[b]SN antigens are centrifuged supernatants of homogenized tumors; FMC antigens are formalinized single-cell suspensions of tumors.
[c]Data from Todd *et al.* (1980) and unpublished UCLA studies.

Another possibility is that large volumes of tumor may sequester active committed lymphocytes from the peripheral blood. Against this possibility is the observation that lymphocytic infiltration is characteristic of early rather than advanced tumors, although a limited number of lymphocytes might appear sparse if spread through extensive tumor. Changes may occur in tumor cells rendering them less immunogenic, and in the absence of continued stimulation, the immune response may wane, resulting in fewer detectable sensitized cells and lesser quantities of antitumor antibodies. The memory-cell population would remain, as witnessed by the prompt response to immunization with tumor cells. Reduced immunogenicity could result from population evolution, from antigenic alteration by modulation or selection, or from masking of antigens by immunologically inert materials such as sialic acid.

The stage-related decline of antitumor and other immunity is probably the end result of complex interactions of some or all of the aforementioned factors, acting simultaneously or sequentially. Recent studies have highlighted the role of free tumor antigen and antigen–antibody complexes in immune suppression.

Tumor-directed cellular immunity persists in patients who remain tumor-free 2 years after surgical excision. Beyond this point, the reaction frequency declines as the period of tumor freedom increases (Table II), on observations made previously in patients with bladder cancer (O'Toole *et al.*, 1972). The decline in reactivity most likely reflects a reduced level of immune response in the absence of continued antigenic stimulation. Serial studies are necessary to define the kinetics of this situation and relate them more precisely to clinical events.

TABLE III

Humoral and Cellular Immunity in Children with Stage IVS
Neuroblastoma before, during, and after Tumor Regression[a]

	Technique			
	Leukocyte-migration assay		Immunofluorescence	
Subjects	+/T[b]	Positive (%)	+/T[b]	Positive (%)
Stage IVS NB patients				
Before regression	4/8	50	1/6	17
During regression	0/8	0	0/8	0
After regression	4/19	21	2/4	50
Control donors	24/76	31	6/40	15

[a]Based on studies of two Stage IVS NB patients.   [b]Tests positive/total tests.

4. Tumor-Directed Immunity during Tumor Regression (Table III)

We have not systematically studied tumor-directed immunity in melanoma patients during regression. Lindsay Morrison, working in my laboratories in Glasgow, examined this in neuroblastoma (NB) patients, and since her as yet unpublished findings are of interest, I will summarize them. Dr. Morrison serially examined two young children who had spontaneous regression of prognostically favorable Stage IVS NB (for the definition, see D'Angio *et al.*, 1971) for tumor-directed cellular immunity (one-stage leukocyte-migration assay) and humoral immunity (indirect membrane immunofluorescence) before, during, and after the regression.

The children were respectively 14 and 16 weeks at presentation with overt tumor and elevated urinary vanillylmandellic acid (VMA) levels. After partial resection of tumor, both had complete regression of detectable tumor, and their VMA levels returned to normal. Prior to and following regression, both showed positive leukocyte-migration inhibition by NB extracts, and one had IgG antibody reactive with cultured NB. *During remission, neither humoral nor cellular tumor-directed immunity was detected in either child in repeated tests.*

That the patients were reactive before or after regression suggests that the absent reactivity during regression either is due to immunological incompetence or reflects transient immune suppression associated with the regression. The tumor extracts and NB cultures employed had shown selective reactivity with the cells and sera of these and other NB patients previously (Morrison *et al.*, 1982) and thus bear TAAs. Treatment-related immunosuppression can be excluded, since neither patient had radiotherapy or chemotherapy and their surgery predated regression by several weeks.

Two disparate theories may be used to explain the absence of detectable immunity during regression. Immune factors may be critically important to regression and the involvement of tumor-directed immunocytes and antibodies in the area of the regressing tumor so complete that they are totally removed from the peripheral blood. Alternatively, it is possible that regression may proceed in the absence of detectable tumor immunity and be induced by endocrine or maturative mechanisms.

5. Effects of Treatment on Tumor-Directed Immunity

Two main questions have to be answered: (1) Is there evidence that conventional cancer therapy increases or diminishes the activity of the immune system to an extent that can be reflected by clinical events such as increased or slowed tumor progression or spread or increased susceptibility to infection? (2) Can we identify techniques that will increase general and (tumor)-specific immunity, and if we can, are such manipulations associated with improved prognosis?

5.1. Surgery

Surgical operations induce complex alterations in the patient's physiology and biochemistry, alterations akin to those associated with severe trauma. That the immunological system is also affected is indicated by reports of transient postoperative depression of (T)-lymphocyte transformation by phytohemagglutinin (PHA) and purified protein derivative (PPD) and reduced leukocyte-migration inhibition by PPD.

In a study of postsurgical immunodepression, we investigated 13 breast-cancer patients and 12 melanoma patients serially over the operative period by the leukocyte migration-inhibition assay for evidence of a decline of tumor-directed cell-mediated immunity (Cochran *et al.*, 1972a). We found that patients who reacted positively preoperatively were nonreactive for a period of 3–22 days following the operation, after which reactivity returned to preoperative levels (Table IV). This finding has since been confirmed by McCoy *et al.* (1975), using the leukocyte-migration-inhibition assay, and by Vose and Moudgil (1975, 1976), using lymphocytotoxicity and antibody-dependent cell-mediated cytotoxicity assays. All studies suggest that the reduction of tumor-directed immunity is merely part of general postoperative immune depression that varies with the degree of

TABLE IV

Postoperative Reduction of Tumor-Antigen-Induced Leukocyte-Migration Inhibition

Tumor type	Postoperative abolition of MI[a]	Subsequent recovery of MI[a]	Time to return of MI (days)	
			Mean	Range
Melanoma	12/12	11/12	11	6–22
Breast cancer	13/13	7/7	7	3–10
All	25/25	18/19	10	3–22

[a](MI) Leukocyte-migration by tumor antigen.

operative trauma. The effect appears to be cumulative, and a patient who has three surgical operations within three successive weeks—for example, a biopsy, a radical excision, followed by a skin graft procedure—will remain immunologically nonreactive for a total of 28–40 days.

Studies of the mechanisms of this effect have been inconclusive. The intraoperative release of steroids from the adrenal cortex has been considered potentially important, although the kinetics of corticosteroid release and depressed (tumor-specific) immunity are quite different. Posttraumatic immune depression does occur in adrenalectomized animals (Munster *et al.*, 1972). Anesthetic agents can depress lymphocyte function *in vitro*, but the significance of this *in vivo* remains doubtful. In our own study, we could not relate immune depression to particular anesthetic agents or to their routes or duration of administration. Immunosuppressive materials that have been extracted from traumatized tissues and identified in the serum of trauma patients are also potential mediators of immune depression. Activation of T suppressor cells may be involved in minimizing autoimmune reactions to antigens exposed after injury.

The clinical significance of these observations is unknown. It remains of interest that tumor-directed cell-mediated immunity, including effector cells with the capacity to kill tumor cells *in vitro*, is eclipsed at a time when small numbers of tumor cells may have been dislodged and disseminated by operative manipulations. It is certainly possible that this "window" in the host defense may permit tumor cells to establish themselves in areas remote from the operation site and that such cells may be the basis of latent metastases. It is perhaps relevant that rats show increased acceptance of tumor grafts after a surgical operation (Buinauskas *et al.*, 1965).

5.2. Radiation Therapy

Radiation therapy depresses lymphocyte numbers and some lymphocyte activities to a considerable extent for extended periods. That these alterations are associated with clinically significant immune deficiency in most patients is far from certain. Opportunistic infection, an excellent marker of significantly reduced host defenses, is certainly less common in patients treated with radiotherapy than in those treated by chemotherapy.

We have found leukocyte-migration inhibition by tumor-associated and other antigens to be abolished or severely reduced after radiotherapy, and this reduction may persist for many months (Cochran, 1978).

While the clinical significance of postradiation alterations of immunological activity remains unproved, there is little doubt that irradiated tissues have a reduced capacity to resist infection, indicated by the development of herpes zoster in irradiated patients with Hodgkin's disease. Radiated tissues also show a susceptibility to tumor growth, as, for example, the growth of recurrent breast carcinoma in areas of irradiated skin. Whether this increased susceptibility to infection and tumor growth has a purely immunological basis remains to be ascertained.

Radiant energy is certainly capable of causing cancer. In man, it has been incriminated in the etiology of skin cancers, thryoid cancer, and leukemia. While direct mutagenesis is undoubtedly the main mechanism of such carcinogenesis, it is of interest to speculate whether immune suppression may have some relevance.

5.3. Chemotherapy

Most agents used in the chemotherapy of cancer cause identifiable alterations in lymphocyte and macrophage numbers and affect their function *in vitro* and *in vivo,* as indicated by opportunistic infections. The literature on the effects of single cytotoxic agents, and their endless combinations, on the immunological system is vast, and a review is beyond the scope of this chapter. Our comparatively limited experience of the effects of these agents on laboratory tests of lymphocyte function confirms the view that the severity and duration of the effect induced vary with the agents used and the dose, rhythm, and duration of treatment. In contrast to the major prolonged alterations of lymphocyte populations and function seen after radiotherapy, the effects of chemotherapy measured *in vitro* in this way seem less severe and distinctly transient (Cochran *et al.,* 1979). Immunological rebound or overshoot 10–20 days after cessation of therapy is a common occurrence.

5.4. Immunotherapy

Table V gives a summary of the alterations seen in various laboratory tests including the leukocyte-migration assay during BCG immune stimulation (for therapeutic and technical details, see Cochran *et al.,* 1977). Conversion of a negative reaction to positive in the autologous situation was seen in 8 of 12 patients (67%) so tested, but positive conversion in the homologous situation was less frequent [19 of 37 (51%)]. Other patients maintained an initially positive reaction against advancing disease, but reactions became negative terminally in 2 of the 37 patients.

The results of the other techniques are included for comparison purposes. PHA-induced transformation was increased in almost all patients. PPD transformation also

TABLE V

Variations in Results in Various Tests of Immunological Function in Patients Receiving Immunotherapy

Technique	Variation in test results			
	Negative to positive or increased value	No change	Positive to negative or decreased value	Inconstant
Leukocyte-migration test				
Autologous	8/12 (67%)	4/12 (33%)	—	—
Allogeneic	19/37 (51%)	16/37 (44%)	2/37 (5%)	—
Effect of autologous serum on leukocyte migration	10/25 (40%)	9/25 (36%)	6/25 (24%)	—
PHA transformation	13/14 (93%)	—	3/14 (21%)	1/14 (7%)
PDP transformation	5/11 (46%)	3/11 (27%)	—	3/11 (27%)
Indirect membrane immunofluorescence	7/11 (64%)	3/11 (27%)	1/11 (9%)	—
Lymphocytotoxicity	6/12 (50%)	3/12 (25%)	3/12 (25%)	—
Mantoux test	13/23 (56%)	10/23 (44%)	—	—
Other recall skin tests	1/11 (9%)	10/11 (91%)	—	—

increased in some patients, but such an increase was not observed in all patients who converted from Mantoux negativity to positivity during BCG administration.

Membrane reactive antibodies developed in 7 of 11 patients tested during BCG stimulation, and lymphocytes cytotoxic for cultured melanoma cells were detected in 6 of 12 previously nonreactive patients at this time. Mantoux conversion was the rule. Anamnestic conversion of reactions to other recall skin tests (*Candida, T. rubrum*, mumps, Streptokinase-Streptodornase) was seldom seen.

Autologous serum became inhibitory to leukocyte migration in 10 of 25 patients (40%), but inhibitory activity was lost in 6 of 25 individuals (24%) (Cochran *et al.*, 1976).

The administration of BCG to patients thus alters many specific and nonspecific tests of immunological function including tumor-mediated leukocyte-migration inhibition. Unfortunately, in the small group of patients studied to date, these changes do not correlate with clinical status, and in our view, such patients are best monitored for clinical effects and apparent complications of therapy by clinical examination.

6. Correlation of Tumor-Directed Immunity and Histology

Certain histological and cytological characteristics of tumors may be associated with a relatively favorable prognosis. This approach has been well developed in the case of melanoma (McGovern *et al.*, 1973). Favorable outcome could be due to tumor-cell characteristics, but might also result in part from a host reaction, which seems likely to have an immunological component. We studied this by relating the occurrence of tumor-directed cell-mediated immunity in patients with localized melanoma to prognostically relevant histological features of their primary tumors (MacKie *et al.*, 1973) including cross-sectional profile, ulceration, histogenetic pattern, vascular invasion, mitotic activity, peritumoral lymphoid-cell aggregation, cytology, and extent and distribution of melanin. Cell-mediated reactivity correlated significantly only with mitotic rate and the presence of tumor cells in vascular channels. The first finding may indicate that tumor-associated antigens are relatively more expressed on actively growing tumors and the second that critical amounts of tumor cells or their antigens must have access to lymph nodes to permit the development of a detectable response. Nairn *et al.* (1971) found a correlation between antitumor immunity and peritumoral reaction, but we were unable to demonstrate this.

This potentially productive approach has been surprisingly little exploited.

7. Formalinized Cell Suspensions as "Antigen" in One- and Two-Stage Leukocyte-Migration Assays

We investigated FMC suspensions from 50 melanomas: 45 from surgically excised tumor tissue, 3 from metastatic tumors from autopsies, and 2 from tissue cultures. The surgical materials comprised tissue from 9 primary tumors, 20 lymph-node metastases, 9 local recurrences, and 6 cutaneous deposits from patients with blood-spread disease.

A total of 22 suspensions were prepared from tissues other than melanoma: primary breast cancer (14), fibrosarcoma (1), renal carcinoma (1), neuroblastoma (1), testicular seminoma (1), colon cancer (1), normal liver (1), normal breast (1), and normal testis (1) (Table VI).

Lymph nodes replaced by tumor provided most cells, from 12 to 240 $\times$ 10^6 with an average of 116 $\times$ 10^6. The average cell yield from primary tumors, local cutaneous recurrences, and subcutaneous hematogenous metastases was similar (62 $\times$ 10^6).

FMC preparations are stable at 4°C and show no tendency to aggregate. The reaction frequency of a typical preparation was quite steady for up to 2 years.

Different FMC preparations vary widely in the frequency with which they inhibit melanoma patients' leukocytes (22–96%) and control donors' leukocytes (0–100%). The majority of melanoma FMC inhibit a high proportion of melanoma patients' leukocytes and a low proportion of control donors' leukocytes. The mean figure for inhibition of melanoma patients' leukocytes by FMC was 60% and that for control donors' leukocytes was 27% ($p < 0.001$). Formalinized control-cell (FCC) preparations showed a similar range of reaction frequencies against melanoma patients' leukocytes (0–45%, mean 20%) and control donors' leukocytes (0–36%, mean 22%).

FMC from nodal metastases and local cutaneous recurrences were most active against melanoma patients' leukocytes [367 of 567 (65%) and 116 of 180 (64%), respectively], followed by those from primary tumors [144 of 244 (59%)], with suspensions from hematogenous deposits least active [74 of 149 (50%)]. The frequency of reaction of control donor leukocytes with FMC was similar regardless of the stage of melanoma from which the FMC was derived.

A total of 43 FMC preparations were tested against a sufficient number of patients' and donors' leukocytes to permit a statistical comparison. Of these 43 preparations, 24 inhibited patients' leukocytes significantly more frequently than control donor leukocytes. This selectivity was most frequent with FMC from lymph nodes [13 of 17 (77%)], from primary tumors [5 of 8 (63%)] and local cutaneous recurrences [4 of 8 (50%)], and least with FMC from autopsy tissues [1 of 3 (33%)] and cutaneous metastases from patients with advanced disease [1 of 5 (20%)]. FMC from tissue-culture lines showed no selective inhibitory activity against patients' leukocytes. Nonmelanomatous cell suspensions showed no selective activity for melanoma leukocytes.

TABLE VI

Frequency of Reactions Induced by Melanoma-Cell Suspensions from Different Stages of the Disease and by Nonmelanoma-Cell Suspensions

Source of formalinized cells	Melanoma patients			Control donors		
	Number[a]	Number[b]	Positive %	Number[a]	Number[b]	Positive %
All melanoma	1157	712	62	770	216	28
Primary melanoma	244	144	59	164	43	26
Local recurrence	180	116	64	132	41	31
Nodal metastases	567	367	65	340	96	28
Hematogenous metastases[c]	149	74	50	126	31	25
Nonmelanoma cells[d]	98	25	26	154	43	28

[a]Total tests with this type of cell suspension.   [b]Total positive tests.
[c]Subcutaneous deposits and visceral metastases.   [d]See text for source of these cells.

Tumors from which FMC were prepared were examined for tumor-cell morphology, frequency of mitoses, lymphocytic infiltration, the presence and extent of necrosis, and melanin content. Although tumors producing FMC specifically reactive with melanoma leukocytes showed more cytological pleomorphism, more mitotic figures, and less necrosis, the differences between such tumors and those yielding nonselectively active FMC were not statistically significant.

We compared the proportion of individuals producing FMC with and without selective activity against melanoma leukocytes who reacted positively with autologous and/or allogeneic FMC preparations in the 3 months *prior to removal of tissue* for FMC preparation. In both groups, a majority reacted with autologous FMC preparations, while reactions with allogeneic FMC were less frequent.

Thus FMC preferentially inhibit melanoma patients' leukocytes, whereas FCC do not. Not all FMC are preferentially active for melanoma patients' leukocytes. Each new preparation must be tested against leukocytes from a preliminary panel of at least 10 melanoma patients and 10 control donors and titrated over a wide range of ratios of leukocytes to tumor cells before using it routinely. Maximum discrimination is usually obtained with preferentially active FMC in the range of 100 : 1 to 200 : 1 (leukocytes to tumor cells).

The factors governing whether an individual FMC preparation will or will not be specifically inhibitory for melanoma patients' leukocytes are not entirely clear. The best sources of specific preparations were primary tumors, local recurrences, and nodal metastases. Hematogenous metastases were less satisfactory, autopsy tissues were inactive, and cultured cells were nonspecifically inhibitory for leukocytes, regardless of their source. We could not identify histological features that could predict whether the FMC derived from a tissue would preferentially inhibit melanoma patients' leukocytes. Neither could such a prediction be based on the reaction of the tissue donor with autologous or allogeneic FMC at or shortly before surgery to obtain the tissue.

Formalinized tumor and control cells are not the ideal method of presenting TAAs for *in vitro* testing, mainly because they induce fairly frequent "false-positive" reactions with control donors' leukocytes. Nonetheless, much may be learned from the use of carefully categorized FC in leukocyte-migration inhibition and allied tests.

8. Reaction of Melanoma Patients' and Control Donors' Leukocytes with Fetal Materials (Table VII)

Melanoma patients' leukocytes reacted significantly more frequently [51 of 169 (30%)] with SN from first-trimester fetuses than did control leukocytes [58 of 339 (17%)], $p < 0.02$). No significant difference in reaction frequency was observed when melanoma patients' and control leukocytes were exposed to SN from second-trimester fetuses or placental tissues (regardless of placental age) (Cochran *et al.*, 1982).

These findings are consistent with published evidence that some TAAs are molecules that, while not expressed on normal adult cells, are expressed transiently during embryogenesis (Coggin and Anderson, 1974; Avis and Lewis, 1973; Irie *et al.*, 1976, 1979; Baldwin and Price, 1976). We found materials from first-trimester fetuses to selectively inhibit

TABLE VII

TABLE VII

Reaction of Melanoma Patients' and Control Donors' Leukocytes against Melanoma and Fetal Extracts in a One-Stage Leukocyte-Migration Assay

	Source of leukocytes				
	Melanoma patients		Control donors		
Source of tissue extract	(A) $+/T^a$	%	(B) $+/T^a$	%	p^b
Supernatant homogenate of:					
Malignant melanoma	56/97	58	62/317	20	< 0.01
Fetus					
First-trimester	51/169	30	58/339	17	< 0.02
Second-trimester	24/104	23	63/252	25	NS[3]
Placental tissues	10/51	20	27/134	20	NS

[a]Number positive/total tested.
[b]The p value A-B was assessed by the χ^2 test with Yates correction where appropriate. (NS) Not significant ($p > 0.05$).

melanoma patients' leukocytes relative to those of normal donors (including 142 pregnant women, of differing parity and at different stages of pregnancy). Materials from older fetuses and from placental tissues showed no selective activity for melanoma patients' leukocytes. This suggests that antigens cross-reactive with melanoma-associated antigens are expressed transiently during early embryogenesis and that a (possibly minor) component of the TAAs detected by our studies is oncofetal in type.

9. Reactions of Melanoma Patients' and Control Donors' Leukocytes with Materials from Nevi, Perimelanomatous Skin, Skin Involved by Lentigo Maligna, and Normal Skin (Table VIII)

Melanoma patients' leukocytes were selectively reactive with SN from nevocytic nevi [melanoma patients, 16 of 50 (32%); control donors, 14 of 98 (14%); $p < 0.02$], perimelanomatous skin containing hyperplastic and dysplastic melanocytes [melanoma patients, 28 of 45 (62%); control donors, 4 of 30 (13%); $p < 0.001$], and skin involved by lentigo maligna [melanoma patients, 20 of 35 (57%); control donors, 5 of 22 (23%); $p < 0.05$]. No significant difference in reaction frequency was observed in a comparison of melanoma patients' leukocytes and control donors' leukocytes exposed to SN from clinically and histologically normal skin (Wilson *et al.*, 1979). The possibility that the TAAs of melanoma cells are specific for the malignantly transformed melanocyte is largely discounted, since melanoma patients' leukocytes are selectively reactive with materials from tissues containing abnormal but not malignant melanocytes. This includes the nevocytes of benign tumors,

TABLE VIII

Reaction Frequency of Melanoma Patients' and Control Donors' Leukocytes against Extracts of Melanoma, Nevi, and Normal and Abnormal Skin in a One-Stage Leukocyte-Migration Assay

	Source of leukocytes				
	Melanoma patients		Control donors		
Antigenic material	(A)+/T^a	%	(B) +/T^a	%	p^b
Supernatant homogenate of:					
Melanoma, malignant	33/57	61	10/64	16	< 0.001
Nevocytic nevi	16/50	32	14/98	14	< 0.02
Skin	28/45	62	4/30	13	< 0.001
Lentigo melanoma	20/35	57	5/22	23	< 0.05
Normal melanocytes	4/20	20	1/20	5	NS

^{a}Number of positive reactors/total tested.
^{b}The p value A-B was assessed by the χ^2 test with Yates correction where appropriate. (NS) Not significant ($p > 0.05$).

melanocytes in the epidermis around primary malignant melanomas showing hyperplastic and dysplastic changes, and partially transformed intraepidermal melanocytes of *melanoma-in-situ* (lentigo maligna). Extracts of skin containing normal melanocytes showed no selective activity for melanoma patients' leukocytes. Thus, a variety of pathological processes other than malignant transformation in which the morphological and behavioral characteristics of melanocytes are modified are associated with the expression of molecules that selectively inhibit melanoma patients' leukocytes. It is likely that these antigens are similar to those on the cells of malignant melanomas, antigens against which melanoma patients are autoimmunized.

Are the antigens detected on melanomas, nevi, fetal tissues, and other tumorous and normal tissues blood-group-related or transplantation antigens? We believe not, on the basis of the similar frequency of autologous and allogeneic reactions with melanoma patients' leukocytes and the low frequency of control donor reactions. There was no excess of alloimmunizing situations, such as multiple blood transfusions, multiple pregnancies (reactivity to melanoma materials is just as selective in male patients), and organ transplantations in our melanoma patients.

10. Indirect Leukocyte-Migration Assays

Although we have obtained extensive results with the one-stage capillary leukocyte-migration technique, we remain dissatisfied with this technique on the grounds of an unacceptable high frequency of apparently false-positive and false-negative results, the fact that the technique is cumbersome, and the requirement for relatively large quantities of reagents, which limits the range of experimental and control studies possible on a blood sample of reasonable size. It is also unsatisfactory to use a single mixed-cell population to generate migration-inhibiting materials and to act as the indicator of the effect of any such materials produced.

We therefore examined a two-stage assay based on that of Thor *et al.* (1968). A relatively pure population of lymphoid cells is exposed to antigens to which it is putatively sensitized, and the supernatant from this coculture is assayed for migration-inhibitory activity against normal human peripheral-blood leukocytes (Morrison *et al.*, 1979).

10.1. Responder and Indicator Leukocyte Donors

Responder lymphocyte donors were 72 patients with histologically proven malignant melanoma and 75 individuals without malignant melanoma, the latter group comprising normal individuals, 29 patients with nonmalignant diseases, and 10 patients with solid tumors other than malignant melanoma. *Indicator* leukocyte donors were 72 normal adults.

10.2. Antigen Source

Formalin-fixed tumor and normal cell suspensions were prepared by the technique of Ross *et al.* (1975).

10.3. Preparation of Mononuclear-Cell Suspensions

Between 25 and 30 ml heparinized blood (10 IU preservative-free heparin/ml blood) was obtained. A 10-ml aliquot of blood was carefully layered onto 10 ml Ficoll-Hypaque (FH) solution, taking special care not to mix the blood with the FH, and spun at $400g$ for 20 min at 22°C. The upper layer was pipetted off carefully and the mononuclear layer at the FH–blood interface transferred to a nonsiliconized tube and diluted at least 1 : 3 in PBS at pH 7.4. The mononuclear cells were thoroughly resuspended and spun at $100g$ for 10 min. The supernatant was pipetted off and the resulting cell pellet washed twice in PBS ($100\,g$ for 5 min). This cell suspension consisted of approximately 90% lymphocytes and monocytes, 5% erythrocytes, and 5% granulocytes. These were resuspended in Eagle's minimal essential medium (EMEM) with 10% FCS to a concentration of 2.5×10^6 cells/ml.

10.4. Preparation of Indicator Leukocytes

These were prepared by gravity sedimentation and washing as described previously (Cochran *et al.*, 1972a).

10.5. Indirect Leukocyte Migration-Inhibition Test

Stage I. Cultures were established in 2 ml EMEM supplemented with 10% FCS. The cultures contained 5×10^6 FH-separated mononuclear cells and formalinized cells (melanoma or control cells) at ratios of 100:1 or 50:1 (mononuclear cells/fixed cells). Simultaneous control cultures consisted of medium plus mononuclear cells alone, medium plus formalin-fixed cells alone, and medium alone.

Stage II. After 18–24 hr at 37°C, the culture tubes were spun at $70g$ for 5 min, and the cell-free SN was pipetted off and its pH adjusted to approximately 7.4 by gassing with 5% CO_2 in air. Indicator leukocytes were placed in capillaries and the cell-containing capillary stumps mounted in tissue-culture dishes (Cochran *et al.*, 1972a), four for each experimental and control situation. The appropriate SN was added and the plates closed with a coverslip and incubated at 37°C for 18–24 hr.

Migration areas were drawn using a drawing tube attached to a standard light microscope and measured by planimetry. A *migration index* was calculated by dividing the mean area of migration of indicator leukocytes in SN of cultures of mononuclear cells cultivated with formalinized tumor or control cells by the mean area of migration of indicator leukocytes from the same donor in the SN of cultures of mononuclear cells alone, or in the presence of formalinized, unrelated tumor cells or formalinized normal cells. Significance was assessed at the 5% level by comparing the migration areas of four replicate capillaries from the relevant test and control situations using the Mann–Whitney–Wilcoxon U test of ranking. Variation in migration between the replicate capillaries was seldom greater than 1%.

10.6. Reactions Observed on Combining the Leukocytes of Melanoma Patients or Control Donors with Formalinized Cells of Melanomas or Control Tissues (Table IX)

Leukocytes from 65 melanoma patients tested against FMC generated an inhibitory SN in 31 cases (48%), a reaction frequency very significantly higher than that observed when control leukocytes were tested against FMC [5 of 38 (13%), $p < 0.001$]. The reaction frequency of melanoma patients' leukocytes with FMC was significantly higher than that with FCC [6 of 35 (17%) $p < 0.01$]. The reaction frequencies of control donor leukocytes with FMC [5 of 38 (13%)] and FCC [5 of 31 (16%)] were not significantly different, nor was there a significant difference between the reaction frequency of melanoma patients' and control donors' leukocytes with FCC (Morrison *et al.*, 1979).

10.7. Reaction Frequency Related to Clinical Stage of the Melanoma Patients (Table IX)

Stage II patients [7 of 26 (65%)] were significantly more often reactive than were Stage I patients [9 of 22 (41%), $p < 0.05$] and Stage III patients [5 of 17 (29%), $p < 0.05$]. A similar order of reaction frequency was observed when the melanoma patients

TABLE IX

Reactions Observed on Combining Leukocytes
from Melanoma Patients or Control Donors with
Formalinized Cells from Melanomas or Control
Tissues in an Indirect Leukocyte-Migration-
Inhibition Test

Leukocyte source	Formalinized melanoma cells[a]	Formalinized control cells[a]
Melanoma patients	31/65 (48%)	6/35 (17%)
Melanoma		
Stage I	9/22 (41%)	2/12 (17%)
Stage II	17/26 (65%)	4/11 (36%)
Stage III	5/17 (29%)	0/12 (0%)
Control donors	5/38 (13%)	5/31 (16%)

[a]Results are individuals giving a positive reaction with at least one preparation of formalinized cells/total number of individuals tested. The figures in parentheses are the percentages of positive results.

were tested against FCC. Four of 11 Stage II patients (36%), two of 12 Stage I patients (17%), and none of 12 Stage III patients reacted with FCC. The difference in reaction frequency of Stage II and Stage III with FCC patients was statistically significant ($p < 0.05$).

10.8. Reaction Frequency Related to Presence or Absence of Clinically Detectable Tumor in Leukocyte Donors (Table X)

A comparison of patients with and without clinically detectable tumor (regardless of clinical stage) showed an identical reaction frequency.

Stage I patients with clinically detectable tumor were more frequently reactive with FMC [7 of 12 (58%)] than were those clinically tumor-free after surgery [2 of 10 (20%)] ($0.10 > p > 0.05$)]. There was a similar frequency of reactions with leukocytes from Stage II patients with detectable tumor [7 of 11 (63%)] and those ostensibly tumor-free [10 of 15 (67%)].

10.9. Reactivity Related to the Number of Formalinized-Cell Preparations Tested

The likelihood that a melanoma patient's leukocytes would yield an inhibitory SN increased directly with the number of different FMC preparations against which they were tested. Patients' leukocytes tested against one FMC preparation reacted in 13 of 35 instances (37%); against two and three FMC preparations, in 11 of 20 instances (55%);

TABLE X

*Reaction Frequency of Melanoma Patients with
and without Clinically Detectable Tumor*

Leukocyte-donor status	Formalinized melanoma cells	
	$+/T^a$	Positive (%)
All stages		
Tumor present	19/40	48
Tumor absent	12/25	48
Stage I		
Tumor present	7/12	58
Tumor absent	2/10	20
Stage II		
Tumor present	7/11	63
Tumor absent	10/15	67

[a]Individuals giving a positive reaction with at least one
preparation of FMC/total number of individuals
tested.

and against four or more FMC preparations, in 7 of 10 instances (70%). The difference between the first and last reaction frequencies was statistically significant ($p < 0.05$). A similar though less steep increase was seen when control leukocytes were exposed to increasing numbers of FMC: with one FMC preparation, no reactions (0/16); with two or three preparations, 2 reactions from 11 donors (18%); and with four or more preparations, 8 reactions from 15 donors (53%). Again, the difference between the first and the last figures was statistically significant ($p < 0.05$). No comparable increase was seen when melanoma patients' or control donors' leukocytes were combined with FCC.

The reaction frequency of melanoma leukocytes with FMC was significantly greater than with FCC, regardless of the number of FMC tested ($p < 0.05$ in each case). The reaction frequency of melanoma leukocytes with FMC was significantly higher than that of control leukocytes when up to three FMC preparations were employed ($p < 0.05$).

10.10. Reactions Induced by Formalinized Melanoma Cells from Primary and Metastatic Tumors

Reactivity of control donors' leukocytes with FMC was low regardless of whether they were derived from primary or secondary tumors. Melanoma patients' leukocytes reacted most frequently with FMC from primary melanomas [11 of 26 (42%)], less frequently with those from metastases [Stage III, 3 of 9 (33%); Stage II, 28 of 93 (30%)]. FMC from all clinical stages effectively discriminated between melanoma-patient and control-donor populations. Differences between reaction frequencies were statistically significant (Stage I and III antigens, $p < 0.05$; Stage II antigens, $p < 0.01$).

11. Concordance of Indirect and Direct Leukocyte-Migration Assays

Concordance of positivity or negativity was observed in 31 of 52 experiments in which direct and indirect leukocyte-migration assays were performed simultaneously with the same FMC or FCC and leukocytes. Concordance was significantly more frequent than discordance ($p < 0.01$).

12. Mechanism of Tumor-Cell-Induced Inhibition of Human Leukocyte Migration (Ross *et al.*, 1979)

We investigated the mechanism of leukocyte-migration inhibition by formalin-fixed tumor cells. Peripheral-blood leukocytes were separated into the component populations, granulocytes, lymphocytes, lymphocyte subpopulations, and monocytes, and incubated for 24 hr with FMC or FCC. The SN of these cultures were tested for their capacity to inhibit the migration of normal peripheral-blood leukocytes. Inhibitory activity was generated by cocultures of FMC with populations containing a substantial proportion of melanoma patients' lymphocytes. Studies with enriched populations indicated that T cells generated the inhibitory activity; our inability to totally purify the T cells meant that a cooperative role for Fc-receptor-bearing lymphocytes including B cells could not be excluded.

The indirect assay thus confirms the results obtained with the one-stage assay and is clearly a more malleable technique. While we remain interested in the former technique as a means of analysis of the mechanisms of lymphokine production in tumor immunity systems, it will remain unwieldy as long as the detection of lymphokines requires a migrating cell population. The provision of a suitable indicator-cell population remains a problem. "Normal" leukocyte populations, even from a single individual, may vary widely in their constitution and responsiveness from day to day. The situation would be much improved if an alternative to human leukocytes could be used or if physical or chemical techniques could be devised for the detection of lymphokines.

13. Tissue-Cultured Lymphoblastoid Cells as Indicators of Lymphokine Generation (Culbert *et al.*, 1982)

As indicated above, human leukocytes are far from ideal as indicators of lymphokine activity. Leukocytes from different individuals may vary widely in their responsiveness to leukocyte-inhibition factor (LIF). Leukocytes obtained sequentially from a single individual may also vary in LIF responsiveness due to changes in health and in the general immunological status of the donor. Sequential assays are therefore difficult to compare and evaluate. There is also a practical logistic problem in obtaining a regular supply of appropriate leukocytes.

Suspension-cultured lymphoid tumor cells actively migrate from capillary tubes, a process that is inhibited by immunoglobulin and by immune complexes (Cochran, 1971; Cochran et al., 1972b). As part of an effort to identify a stable and responsive indicator cell for the second stage of the two-stage assay, we investigated the migration characteristics and lymphokine responsiveness of five continuous human lymphoblastoid cell lines, QIMR-WIL, NAMALWA, BJAB, RAJ16HAT, and 8 AdHDI. Only two, QIMR-WIL and NAMALWA, were actively migratory, a process that was metabolically active, being abolished at 4°C and reduced by inhibitors of anaerobic glycolysis (iodoacetate), oxidative phosphorylation (dinitrophenol), and RNA synthesis (actinomycin D).

To assess the effect of leukocyte-migration-inhibitory lymphokines on QIMR-WIL and NAMALWA migration, we exposed them to the SN of mouse spleen cells pulsed with PHA or cocultured with histoincompatible mouse spleen cells, situations known to generate migration-inhibitory lymphokines. In such experiments, the migration of QIMR-WIL and of mouse spleen cells was inhibited, the degree of inhibition varying with the period of exposure of the mouse spleen cells to PHA or incompatible cells. Characterization of the inhibitory material showed it to be nondialyzable, relatively heat-stable (57°C for 30 min), unaffected by α-L-fucose, and neutralized by the serine esterase inhibitor phenylmethly sulphonyl fluoride, and to have a molecular size similar to that of albumin, characteristics similar to those of human LIF but unlike those of macrophage migration-inhibition factor (Rocklin, 1972). The migration of NAMALWA was completely unaffected by the lymphokine-containing supernatants.

At this point, it was clear that QIMR-WIL was responsive to a lymphokine that was the murine equivalent of human LIF. The question was whether it would also respond to human LIF.

We therefore set up experiments in which peripheral lymphocytes from melanoma patients or normal individuals were exposed to FMC in simultaneous direct leukocyte-migration assays, indirect assays using allogeneic normal human peripheral-blood leukocytes as indicator cells, and indirect assays using QIMR-WIL cells as indicators (Table XI). There was a higher frequency of reactions with melanoma patients' lymphocytes in all three tests, but only with QIMR-WIL as indicator was the difference between patients and controls significant (12 of 20 vs. 5 of 20, $p < 0.01$). We feel that this is a useful

TABLE XI

Comparison of the Reaction Frequencies of Melanoma Patients and Control Donors against Formalinized Melanoma Cells Using Direct and Indirect Leukocyte-Migration Assays

	Melanoma patients		Control donors		
Indicator cell	Number of tests	Positive[a]	Number of tests	Positive	p value[b]
Human leukocytes					
Direct LMT	20	8 (40%)	20	5 (25%)	> 0.05
Indirect LMT	20	6 (30%)	20	5 (25%)	> 0.05
QIMR-WIL	20	12 (60%)	20	5 (25%)	< 0.05

[a]Significant difference in test and control migration at 5% level by Mann–Whitney–Wilcoxon U test of ranking.
[b]Comparison of reaction frequencies of patients and control (χ^2).

approach to the detection of cell-mediated immunity in man that may permit standardization of serial results from a single patient and among different patients and different laboratories.

Much remains to be learned about the nature and biological significance of melanoma-associated molecules. It is likely that further advances will derive from serological investigations employing new technology and reagents such as monoclonal antibodies. In the enthusiasm for the new, it would be unfortunate if attempts to refine longer-established approaches were totally abandoned.

ACKNOWLEDGMENTS. The studies described in this chapter were undertaken in collaboration with colleagues in Stockholm (George Klein, Jan Stjernswärd, Volker Diehl, Ulrich Jehn, and Balwant Gothoskar), Glasgow (Rona Mackie, Alan Jackson, Geoffrey Clements, Robert Grant, Kate Ross, Lindsay Morrison, Deidre Hoyle, Gaye Todd, Eric Culbert, and Ian McGregor), Manchester (Brent Vose), and Los Angeles (Duan-Ren Wen and Annice Burdeos). Financial support was provided by the Peel Medical Research Trust, London; the Swedish Cancer Society; The Secretary of State for Scotland; The McMillan Research Funds of the University of Glasgow; The Cancer Research Campaign, London: The World Health Organization Cancer Unit; and USPHS Grant CA 09010 from the U.S. National Institutes of Health.

References

Andersen, V., Bjerrum, O., and Bendixen, G., 1970, Effect of autologous mammary tumour extracts on human leukocyte migration *in vitro, Int. J. Cancer* 5:357.

Avis, P., and Lewis, M. E., 1973, Brief communication: Tumor-associated fetal antigens in human tumors, *J. Natl. Cancer Inst.* 51:1063.

Baldwin, R. W., and Price, M. R., 1976, Nature and expression of tumor antigens associated with experimental animal and human tumors, *Ann. Clin. Biochem.* 13(5):488.

Breslow, A., 1970, Thickness, cross-sectional area and depth of invasion in the prognosis of cutaneous melanoma, *Ann. Surg.* 172:902.

Buinauskas, P., Brown E. R., andCole, W. H., 1965, Inhibiting and enhancing effect of various chemical agents on rat's resistance to inoculated Walker 25 tumor cells, *J. Surg. Res.* 5:538.

Burnet, F. M., 1967, Immunological aspects of malignant disease, *Lancet* 1:1171.

Callery, C., Roe, D., Cochran, A. J., and Morton, D. L., 1982, Natural history of Stage II melanoma, *Ann. Surg* (in press).

Clark, W. H., 1967, A classification of malignant melanoma in man correlated with histogenesis and biological behavior, in: *Advances in Biology of the Skin,* Vol. 8 (W. Montagna and F. Hu, eds.), pp. 621, Pergamon Press, Oxford.

Cochran, A. J., 1968, Method for assessment of prognosis in malignant melanoma, *Lancet* 2:1062.

Cochran, A. J., 1969a, Malignant melanoma: A review of 10 years' experience in Glasgow, Scotland, *Cancer* 23:1190.

Cochran, A. J., 1969b, Histology and prognosis in malignant melanoma, *J. Pathol.* 97:459.

Cochran, A. J., 1971, Tumor cell migration, *Eur. J. Clin. Biol. Res.* 16:44.

Cochran, A. J., 1978, *Man, Cancer and Immunity,* Academic Press, London, New York, San Francisco.

Cochran, A. J., Diehl, V., and Stjernswärd, J., 1970, Regression of primary malignant melanoma associated with a good prognosis despite metastasis to lymph nodes, *Rev. Eur. Etud. Clin. Biol.* 15:969.

Cochran, A. J., Spilg, W. G. S., Mackie, R. M., and Thomas, C. E., 1972a, Postoperative depression of tumor-directed cell mediated immunity in patients with malignant disease, *Br. Med. J.* 3:67.

Cochran, A. J., Klein, E., and Kiessling, R., 1972b, The effect of immune factors on the motility of lymphoma cells, *J. Natl. Cancer Inst.* **48**:1657.

Cochran, A. J., Jehn, U. W., and Gothaskar, B. P., 1973, Cell-mediated immunity to malignant melanoma, *Pigment Cell* **1**:360.

Cochran, A. J., Mackie, R. M., Ross, C. E., Ogg, L. J., and Jackson, A. M., 1976, Leukocyte migration inhibition by sera from melanoma patients, *Int. J. Cancer* **18**:274.

Cochran, A. J., Mackie, R. M., Jackson, A. M. Ogg., L. J., and Ross, C. E., 1977, Immunological changes in cancer patients receiving BCG, *Dev. Biol. Standard* **38**:441.

Cochran, A. J., Mackie, R. M., Morrison, L. J. A., Jackson, A. M., and Todd, G., 1979, Laboratory studies in the early detection of metastatic malignant melanoma, in: *Proceedings of the XII International Cancer Congress*, (S. Kumar, ed.), pp. 113–120, Pergamon Press, Oxford.

Cochran, A. J., Todd., G., Hart, D. M., Morrison, L. H. A., and MacKie, R. M., 1982, Patterns of reaction of melanoma patients and control donors, including pregnant women, with melanoma and fetus-derived materials, *Int. J. Cancer* (in press).

Coggin, J. H., and Anderson, N. G., 1974, Cancer, differentiation and embryonic antigens: Some central problems, *Adv. Cancer Res.* **19**:105.

Culbert, E. J., Cochran, A. J., and Clements, G. B., 1982, Tissue cultured lymphoblastoid cells as indicators of lymphokine generation, *Scand. J. Immunol.* (in press).

Currie, G. A., Lejeune, F., and Fairley, G. H., 1971, Immunization with irradiated tumor cells and specific cytotoxicity in malignant melanoma, *Br. Med. J.* **2**:305.

D'Angio, G. L., Evans, A., and Everett Koop, C., 1971, Special patterns of widespread neuroblastomas with a favorable prognosis, *Lancet* **2**:1046.

Everson, T. C., and Cole, W. H., 1966, *Spontaneous Regression of Cancer,* W. B. Saunders, Philadelphia.

George, M., and Vaughan, J. H., 1962, *In vitro* cell migration as a model for delayed hypersensitivity, *Proc. Soc. Exp. Biol. Med.* **111**:514.

Gershon, R. K., 1974, Regulation of concomitant immunity activation of suppressor cells by tumor excision, in: *Immunological Parameters of Host–Tumor Relationships,* Vol. III (D. Weiss, ed.), pp. 198–209, Academic Press, New York and London.

Herberman, R. B., and Holden, H. T., 1979, Natural killer cells as anti-tumor effector cells, *J. Natl. Cancer Inst.* **62**:441.

Irie, R. F., Irie, K., and Morton, D. L., 1976, A membrane antigen common to human cancer and fetal brain tissue, *Cancer Res.* **36**:3510.

Irie, R. F., Guiliano, A. E., and Morton, D. L., 1979, Oncofetal antigen (OFA): A tumor-associated fetal antigen immunogenic in man, *J. Natl. Cancer Inst.* **63**:367.

Jackson, A. M., Vose, B. M., and Cochran, A. J., 1978, Tumor-associated antigens in cystic melanomas, *Eur. J. Cancer* **14**:543.

MacKie, R. M., Carfrae, D. C., and Cochran, A. J., 1972, The assessment of prognosis in patients with malignant melanoma, *Lancet* **2**:455.

MacKie, R. M., Spilg, W. G. S., Thomas, C. E., Cameron-Mowat, D. E., Grant, R. M., and Cochran, A. J., 1973, A comparison of tumor-directed cell mediated immunity and tumor histology in melanoma patients, *Rev. Inst. Pasteur Lyon* **6**:281.

McCoy, J. L., Jerome, L. F., Dean, J. H., Perlin, E., Oldham, R. K., Char, D. H., Cohen, M. H., Felix, E. L., and Herberman, R. B., 1975, Inhibition of leukocyte migration by tumor-associated antigens in soluble extracts of human malignant melanoma, *J. Natl. Cancer Inst.* **55**:19.

McGovern, V. J., Mihm, M. C., Bailly, C., Booth, J. C., Clark, W. H., Cochran, A. J., Hardy, E. G., Hicks, J. D., Levene, A., Lewis, M. G., Little, J. H., and Milton, G. W., 1973, The classification of malignant melanoma and its histologic reporting, *Cancer* **32**:1446.

Morrison, L. J. A., Cochran, A. J., MacKie, R. M., Ross, C. E., Todd, G., and Garland, C. G., 1979, Indirect leukocyte migration assay in patients with malignant melanoma, *Int. J. Cancer* **24**:11.

Morrison, L. J. A., Cochran, A. J., Baird, G. M., Campbell, A. M., and Willoughby, M. L. N., 1982, Tumor-directed immunity in human neuroblastoma, *Am. J. Pediatr. Hematol. Oncol.* (in press).

Munster, A. M., Eurenius, K., Mortensen, R. F., and Mason, A. D., 1972, Ability of splenic lymphocytes from injured rats to induce a graft versus host reaction, *Transplantation* **14**:106.

Nairn, R. C., Guli, E. P. G., Nind, A. P. D., Miller, H. K., Rolland, J. M., and Minty, G. C., 1971, Specific immune response in human skin carcinoma, *Br. Med. J.* **4**:701.

O'Toole, C., Perlmann, P., Unsgaard, B., Moberger, G., and Edsmyr, F., 1972, Cellular immunity to human urinary bladder cancer. II. Effect of surgery and preoperative irradiation, *Int. J. Cancer* **10**:92.

Rocklin, R. E., Remold, H. G., and David, J. R., 1972, Characterization of human migration inhibitory factor (MIF) from antigen-stimulated lymphocytes, *Cell. Immunol.* **5**:436.

Ross, C. E., Cochran, A. J., Hoyle, D. E., Grant, R. M., and Mackie, R. M., 1975, Formalin-fixed tumour cells in the leukocyte migration test, *Clin. Exp. Immunol.* **22**:126.

Ross, C. E., Cochran, A. J., Jackson, A. M., Mackie, R. M., and Ogg, L. J., 1979, The mechanism of tumor cell induced inhibition of human leukocyte migration, *Eur. J. Cancer* **15**:995.

Søborg, M., and Bendixen, G., 1967, Human lymphocyte migration as a parameter of hypersensitivity, *Acta Med. Scand.* **181**:247.

Solzhenitsyn, A. I., 1968, *Cancer Ward,* Bodley Head, London.

Thomas, L., 1959, Mechanisms involved in tissue damage by the endotoxins of gram-negative bacteria, in:*Cellular and Humoral Aspects of the Hypersensitivity State* (H. S. Lawrence, ed.),   451–468, Hoeber, New York.

Thor, D. E., Jureziz, R. E., Veach, S. R., Miller, E., and Drays, S., 1968, Cell migration inhibition factor released by antigen from human peripheral lymphocytes, *Nature (London)* **219**:755.

Todd, G., Chan, C. W., Cochran, A. J., Kennedy, R., MacKie, R. M., and Morrison, L. J. A., 1980, *In vitro* reaction of cancer patients and others to bacillus Calmette Guérin, *Int. J. Cancer* **26**:285.

Vose, B. M., and Moudgil, G. C., 1975, Effect of surgery on tumour-directed leukocyte responses, *Br. Med. J.* **1**:56.

Vose, B. M., and Moudgil, G. C., 1976, Postoperative depression of antibody-dependent lymphocyte cytotoxicity following minor surgery and anesthesia, *Immunology* **30**:123.

Wilson, N. I. L., Ross, C. E., MacKie, R. M., and Cochran, A. J., 1979, A study of the immunology of nonmalignant melanocytic lesions, *Cancer Immunol. Immunother.* **6**:27.

6

Heterogeneity of Human Melanoma-Associated Antigens Revealed by Alloantisera and Xenoantisera

PETER B. DENT AND SHUEN-KUEI LIAO

1. Introduction

As repeatedly stressed by other authors in this volume, human malignant melanoma is a good model for the study of tumor immunology. A number of fundamental questions have been raised in this model, and reliable answers may now be emerging. These questions include the following: (1) Do human tumor-specific antigens that function as rejection antigens exist? (2) Are these antigens immunogenic in man, and if they are, how should they be measured? (3) Are there antigens on melanoma cells that are recognized only by heterologous species, and if there are, might they be of any use in immunodiagnosis and therapy?

   In this review, we will outline our experience in attempting to answer some of these questions. We refer throughout to melanoma-associated antigens (MAAs) rather than melanoma-specific antigens, since the former designation is more accurate in light of the available data. We will begin by reviewing some methodological considerations that we feel are essential for an appreciation of the relationship of our work to that of others and also for the definition of the limitations that they impose on our results. We have restricted our work to serology not because we do not appreciate the potential importance of antigens recognized by cell-mediated immune reactions, but rather because to define entities that are unknown, or in fact may not even exist, serology is a more reproducible, quantifiable, and sensitive approach. We will outline our results with human sera using different techniques

PETER B. DENT AND SHUEN-KUEI LIAO • Departments of Pediatrics and Pathology, McMaster University; The Ontario Cancer Treatment & Research Foundation (Hamilton Clinic), Hamilton, Ontario, L8N 3Z5 Canada.

and then summarize our studies with heteroantisera raised in nonhuman primates and rabbits as well as our preliminary work with the hybridoma technique. We will review factors that affect the expression of antigens by melanoma cells in culture, such as interferon and theophylline. We will present our findings that indicate similarity between histocompatibility antigens and MAAs defined by heteroantisera. Finally, we will comment briefly on the potential clinical implications of studies of melanoma antigens. This review concentrates largely on the work done in our laboratory and is not meant to be a comprehensive review of the literature relevant to each of the areas under discussion. While we have referred to the work of others where appropriate, we recognize that we have been selective in this regard.

2. Methodological Considerations

Before we discuss the results of our work on the serological definition of human MAAs, it is important to briefly point out some of the methodological features of our work. We have relied in large part on cultured cell lines of tumor tissue as a substrate for our studies. Cell lines have the advantage of relative uniformity for repetitive studies and ready availability. We have also used short-term cultures and fresh tissue homogenates to complement our work with cell lines and to verify the fact that antigens described *in vitro* are also found on tumor cells *in vivo*.

We have made great efforts to fully characterize the melanoma cell lines with which we work, to ensure that the cells are truly melanoma. We have studied their properties *in vitro* in terms of morphology and growth characteristics and have been able to identify three different morphological types (Liao *et al.*, 1975). Seven of the most frequently used cell lines have undergone extensive cytogenetic analysis, and it has been possible to identify specific marker chromosomes for each (McCulloch *et al.*, 1976). In addition, the cytohistochemical properties and heterotransplantability in the hamster cheek pouch and in nude mice have been described (Qizilbash *et al.*, 1977; Liao *et al.*, 1977, 1979a). To date, we have made few clinicopathological correlations, but with the development of our knowledge of MAAs, we expect that such correlations may be forthcoming. We have been able to correlate malignant potential in nude mice with saturation density *in vitro* using clonal sublines derived from a pigmented melanoma cell line (Liao *et al.*, 1979a). We have also studied the primary outgrowth of fresh melanoma tissues and have suggestive evidence for a correlation of favorable prognosis with a homogeneous triangular dendritic cellular morphology (Liao *et al.*, 1976). We are currently maintaining and using 26 melanoma cell lines and have over 40 different nonmelanoma lines including various carcinomas, sarcomas, normal and malignant lymphoblastoid cell lines, and fibroblasts for these studies. The importance of such a large panel of target cells is illustrated in the discussion of the specificity of monoclonal antibodies (see Section 6). The use of continuous cell lines is not without significant technological problems. The possibility of contamination of one cell line with another is always present (Nelson-Rees and Flandermeyer, 1976), though not widely appreciated. The contamination of cell lines by mycoplasma is also a serious hazard, since such contamination has been shown to alter the reactivity of such cells in both cellular (Aldridge *et al.*, 1977; Brooks *et al.*, 1979) and antibody-dependent (Bloom, 1973) immunological reactions. We observed a profound inhibitory effect in mixed-lymphocyte tumor-interaction experiments of tumor lines containing "noncultivatable" mycoplasma organisms (Lui et al., 1977). As a result, we have maintained a strict mycoplasma surveillance and prevention protocol that has successfully eliminated this organism from our cell lines (Dent et al., 1980a).

An additional factor that interferes with the analysis of specificity of immunological reactions against cultured cell lines is the absorption and/or incorporation of components of calf serum in the medium supplements into the target-cell membranes (Hamburger et al., 1963). Most sera contain antibodies to these components if sensitive enough detection methods are used, and of course antisera derived from animals or from patients immunized against cultured cell lines will have high titers of reactivity against calf serum antigens (Irie et al., 1974; Liao et al., 1979b; Houghton et al., 1980). This problem can be controlled by growing cells in human serum (Irie et al., 1974) or chemically defined medium (Liao et al., 1979b) or by absorbing the test serum with insolubilized calf serum or with a nonmelanoma cell line grown in calf serum (Liao et al., 1979b).

An additional problem in the use of cell lines for immunological studies is that of antigen deletion. It is well known that certain antigens are expressed to a different degree among cell lines such as the oncofetal antigen (OFA) described by Irie et al. (1976) or the carcinoembryonic antigen (CEA)-like antigen on melanoma cells (Dent et al., 1980b). The loss or decline of MAAs with prolonged passage has been previously described (Irie et al., 1976; Stuhlmiller and Seigler, 1977). We have not observed this phenomenon in our work; however, we do not subject our cell lines to prolonged in vitro passage, but rather go back to early frozen stocks at regular intervals.

Finally, much of the confusion in the serology of human malignant melanoma is due to the large number of antibody-detection methods used. Some of the problems with the use of immunofluorescent-antibody techniques are described below. Despite evolving improvements in technology, the continued lack of methodological standardization continues to stand in the way of comparison of the results of different investigators. We have concentrated our work on the mixed hemadsorption assay (MHA) technique, and we have been able to miniaturize it so that very small volumes of serum (5–10 μl) and very few target cells (100/well) are required (Liao et al., 1980a). It is possible to measure antibodies of different isotypes with this assay, and it is highly suitable for antigen quantitation using classic quantitative absorption methods.

3. Human Antibodies to Melanoma

Malignant melanoma in man has provided a strong stimulus for the study of tumor immunity because of the belief that host factors may account for its occasional unpredictable behavior, particularly for the high incidence of spontaneous regression. The serology of human melanoma took its beginning from the work of Martin Lewis (1967), whose perceptive analysis of the natural history of melanoma in Africa attracted him to the study of antitumor immunity in patients with this disease. These studies led to the serological definition of individually specific cell-surface antigens, while common cross-reacting antigens could be demonstrated in the cytoplasm of melanoma cells (Lewis et al., 1969). Patients with limited disease or recently resected tumor had antibody to autologous membrane antigens as well as to the cross-reacting cytoplasmic antigens. With disease progression, antibody tended to disappear. Donald Morton (Morton *et al.,* 1968) reported similar results with respect to the presence of a common cytoplasmic melanoma antigen detectable by immunofluorescence techniques. He was also able to demonstrate reactivity against melanoma surface antigens; however, unlike Lewis, he felt that the surface antigens detected by sera from melanoma patients were not individually specific, but rather common to all melanomas tested.

Encouraged by the evidence from these two laboratories and the additional indications from the work of the Hellströms (Hellström *et al.,* 1968) that patients with melanoma were responding immunologically to their tumors, in 1972 we initiated our own studies of antitumor immunity in melanoma. We first sought to confirm the existence of common cytoplasmic antigens in melanoma cells using sera from patients with melanoma and acetone-fixed cultured melanoma cell lines as substrate in the indirect immunofluorescent-antibody technique as described by Lewis *et al.* (1969). We found that all cell lines tested, both melanoma and nonmelanoma, gave high background fluorescence so that it was very difficult to score the reactions. We found no discernible differences in the reactivity of sera from melanoma patients, nonmelanoma cancer patients, and normal controls.

Because these technical difficulties were being experienced by other investigators in the field, a workshop on fluorescent-antibody studies in malignant melanoma was held in Lewis's laboratory at McGill University in March 1975, sponsored by the National Cancer Institute of Canada. The conclusions of the workshop were that there were considerable technical problems with this antibody-detection system. Both cultured cells and fresh tumor imprints gave a high degree of background fluorescence, and the quality of these substrates was highly variable. It was possible to define criteria of positivity. While it was not the purpose of the workshop to evaluate the ability of the test to detect melanoma-specific reactions, sufficiently large numbers of control sera and nonmelanoma tumor tissues were included to indicate that unequivocally positive reactions were not melanoma-specific. This lack of specificity of the reaction of melanoma sera against the common cytoplasmic antigen in melanoma cells has since been confirmed by a number of other investigators (Dore *et al.,* 1973; Wood and Barth 1974; Peter *et al.,* 1975).

We also examined the reactivity of sera from melanoma patients against surface antigens on melanoma cell lines by indirect membrane immunofluorescence and found an increased incidence of reactivity of sera from melanoma patients (33.7%) compared to other cancer patients (24.2%) or normal controls (22.2%) (Dent *et al.,* 1978). Patients with more advanced disease were less reactive against melanoma target cells than patients with limited disease, although the reactivity against nonmelanoma targets was identical. While the differences observed were statistically significant, they were small differences, and the clinical or biological significance was not clear. The nature of the specificities involved in this reactivity was also not clear, although tissue-culture artifacts such as fetal calf serum and blood group as well as heterophile antigens were excluded as possible targets of the patients' antibody.

The fluorescent-antibody technique proved unsatisfactory for these studies because of lack of sensitivity and specificity, as well as its unsuitability for screening and titrating large numbers of sera. We therefore adapted and miniaturized the well-established antiglobulin antibody-detection technique, the MHA, for these studies (Liao *et al.*, 1980a). Using this technique, we have examined further the specificity of the antimelanoma reactivity of sera from patients with melanoma (Dent *et al.*, 1982). To exclude weak or equivocal reactivity, sera were screened at a dilution of 1 : 20 against nine different melanoma cell lines. Of 48 patients, 9 showed reactivity against one or more of these lines; 7 of the 9 patients were also reactive against at least one of four nonmelanoma cell lines and 4 of the 9 had cytotoxic antibodies against two or more normal lymphocyte preparations obtained from a panel of at least 30 different donors. After absorption with platelets from a pool of 200 different donors or with nonmelanoma tumor cells or both, no patient had residual melanoma reactivity, indicating that the antimelanoma reactions observed were not against antigens found exclusively on melanoma cells. It is of interest that all the reactive patients were parous females, indicating that the target antigens may be either fetal in origin or paternal alloantigens.

The number of patients studied was too small to make meaningful clinical correlations; however, patients with limited but evident disease had the strongest antimelanoma reactivity, and among the same group of patients there was a suggestive survival benefit for those with antibody against cultured melanoma cells. Because it is well known that females with melanoma carry a better prognosis (Shaw *et al.*, 1980) and because of the possible role of fetal antigens in protective immunity in animal systems (Coggin and Anderson, 1974), further examination of the nature of the reactivity observed in our study may be of importance.

The studies referred to above utilized sera from patients who we postulated might have become spontaneously immunized by their own tumors. The conclusion that we have drawn is that under these circumstances, no antibodies were formed that recognized melanoma-specific surface antigens common to the patient's own tumor and to the cultured allogeneic cells used as targets in the assay. There are at least three features of these studies that must be borne in mind that prevent us from making categorical pronouncements about the absence of melanoma-specific antibodies in patients with melanoma. The first is the observation that melanoma patients make antibodies that are reactive only with their own tumor cells (Lewis *et al.*, 1969; Bodurtha *et al.*, 1975; Shiku *et al.*, 1976; Carey *et al.*, 1976). The frequency and clinical correlates of such reactivity are not yet fully appreciated.

The second is the fact that in our studies, only antibodies of the immunoglobulin G (IgG) isotype are being detected. Studies of antitumor antibody in animal (Lando *et al.*, 1977, 1980; Carrel *et al.*, 1980a) and human systems (Thiry *et al.*, 1977; Sofen and O'Toole, 1978; Houghton *et al.*, 1980) indicate that IgM antibodies may be the predominant or most important isotype. In terms of melanoma specificity, Seibert *et al.* (1977) have used the immune-adherence assay, which readily detects IgM antibody, and have concluded that most of the observed reactivity is not melanoma-specific. Absorption with human erythrocytes, platelets, fetal calf serum, and homogenized fetal tissues virtually eliminated the activity of melanoma patients' sera against melanoma target cells. Irie *et al.* (1976) have described an antifetal antibody in melanoma patients that recognizes an antigen on various cultured tumor cells and is also found on fetal brain cells and that they have called OFA. This antibody is predominantly of the IgM isotype (Sidell *et al.*, 1979). Houghton *et al.* (1980) have recently described IgM antibodies in the serum of a small number of normal males that react with antigens shared by some melanoma cell lines and astrocytoma lines, a specificity that is identical to their previously described class II antigens. Thus, it is unlikely that more extensive study of antibodies of the IgM isotype will reveal reactivity that is truly restricted to melanoma antigens.

Finally, none of the patients in our studies was deliberately immunized with vaccines composed of melanoma tissues or extracts. This may be significant with respect to the question of whether patients with melanoma can ever recognize tumor-specific allogeneic surface structures and, as a corollary, whether such structures do exist. Ikonopisov et al. (1970) first reported that immunotherapy with autologous tumor cells could stimulate production of antibodies against melanoma cells. Leong et al. (1977) have presented evidence that allogeneic as well as autologous melanoma cell immunotherapy can induce production of antibody against shared melanoma surface antigens detectable by the fluorescent-antibody technique. We have studied one of Leong's autoimmunized patients using the MHA and have shown that after extensive absorption with normal tissues and a cultured nonmelanoma cancer line, high titers of apparently melanoma-specific antibody could be revealed (Liao et al., 1978). We are unable to draw any general conclusions from the study of this one serum and are therefore currently analyzing a large number of sera from patients with melanoma undergoing adjuvant allogeneic tumor-vaccine immunotherapy. Preliminary results indicate that almost all such immunized patients make high titers of antibody not only against melanoma cells but also, as expected, against other nonmelanoma antigens. Absorption analysis is under way to determine the specificity of such reactivity and whether there are any correlations with clinical outcome. It is of interest that very few immunotherapy studies have attempted to correlate clinical effectiveness of therapy with antibody responses to tumor antigens (Ikonopisov et al., 1970; Shibata et al., 1976). Irie et al. (1979) have recently reported that allogeneic tumor-vaccine immunotherapy stimulated the production of antibody against fetal antigen not specific for melanoma, but had very little effect on the development of specific antimelanoma antibody.

4. Nonhuman Primate Antibodies to Melanoma

Because of their close phylogenetic relationship to man, nonhuman primates would seem to be ideal for the production of antisera against antigens that might be less readily recognized by lower species. Metzgar et al. (1973) first showed that monkey antisera raised against cultured melanoma cells after absorption with human erythrocytes, peripheral-blood leukocytes, and cultured nonmelanoma cells were reactive with fresh and cultured melanoma cells, one of four nonmelanoma cell lines, and not with fibroblasts or lymphoid cells. Subsequently, Stuhlmiller and Seigler (1975) found that a chimpanzee antiserum against fresh melanoma tissue after absorption with erythrocytes and peripheral-blood cells derived from the same individual as the tumor reacted with 14 of 14 cultured melanoma cell lines, but not with any of the 8 nonmelanoma lines. There was a reduction but not elimination of melanoma reactivity following absorption with fetal tissues, leading them to conclude that monkey antisera to melanoma cells could identify both common MAAs and distinct fetal MAAs.

We have raised antisera in African green monkeys against cultured melanoma cell lines that after absorption with human erythrocytes, leukocytes, normal adult liver homogenate, and cultured oral carcinoma cells (KB) can be shown to react against most if not all cultured melanoma cell lines (Liao *et al.,* 1979c). These antisera failed to react with a variety of carcinoma cell lines, fibroblasts, xenogeneic melanomas, normal skin, bacillus Calmette Guérin (BCG), or sheep red blood cells (SRBC). They also react with fresh, noncultured melanoma tissues. However, while the large variety of nonmelanoma cell lines and tissues listed above were nonreactive with the absorbed monkey antisera by quantitative-absorption analysis, we found that some tumor cell lines of neuroectodermal origin were reactive. The antiserum against melanoma line CaCL 73-36 was reactive against one of three retinoblastoma lines and four of four glioblastomas, and the antiserum against CaCL 78-4 melanoma cell line was reactive against one of four glioblastomas (Liao *et al.,* unpublished data). An example of the spectrum of reactivity revealed by one monkey antiserum against melanoma cells is seen in Table I.

TABLE I

Spectrum of Reactivity of Monkey Antiserum[a] Raised against
Melanoma Cell Line CaCL 73-36

Reactive tissues	Nonreactive tissues
Melanoma cell lines	Neuroblastoma cell lines
CaCL 73-36	SK-N-MC
CaCL 74-36	IMR 6
CaCL 78-1	NMB 7
CaCL 78-4	Carcinoma cell lines
CaCL 79-3	HeLa (cervix)
RPMI 4445	Hep 2 (larynx)
RPMI 5966	A-427 (lung)
RPMI 8322	CaLu (lung)
RPMI 8342	HT 29 (colon)
RPMI 7932	Normal epithelial lines
M40	HH (heart)
LeCa Str 19-4	HAE/70
UCLA-SO-M14	Normal fibroblasts
SK-Mel-1	RAM
Melanoma fresh cells	A6
4/5	A2
Retinoblastoma cell line	XXX35
Y-79	J004-42
Glioblastoma cell lines	Lymphoid cell lines
LN 18	Raji
LN 40	Daudi
LN 140	Leukemic cell lines
LN 229	K562
	CCL 119
	Xenogeneic cells
	SRBC
	Pig melanoma
	Mouse melanoma
	BCG

[a]Antiserum absorbed with human erythrocytes, leukocytes, liver homogenate, and oral carcinoma cells (KB) (Liao *et al.,* 1979c).

With respect to the involvement of fetal antigens in the observed reactivity of the monkey antisera, we found that antimelanoma reactivity was reduced but not eliminated after repetitive absorption with tissues of 9 of 13 fetuses (Liao *et al.*, 1979c). A lack of reduction of melanoma reactivity after absorption with two different colon-carcinoma cell lines known to express CEA (Liao *et al.*, unpublished data) indicates that the anti-MAA reactivity was not directed against CEA or the related cross-reacting antigen that is also found on melanoma cells (Dent *et al.*, 1980b).

In more extensive analyses with five different monkey antisera including the three antisera previously reported, two of five have been shown to recognize common MAAs, i.e., MAAs shared by all the cell lines tested. The remaining three antisera reacted against melanomas in a more restricted fashion, i.e., with some but not all melanomas tested. In none of the antisera studied to date were we able to detect any individually specific (melanoma) antigens (Vennegoor *et al.*, 1978), since one or more melanoma lines other than the immunizing line were able to remove reactivity against the latter completely.

Our results are in agreement with the previously referred to data of Metzgar *et al.* (1973) and Stuhlmiller and Seigler (1975), in that common MAAs in addition to fetal specificities were recognized. We also obtained evidence for the existence of shared neuroectodermal antigens that may be similar to those identified by hybridoma antibodies (see below). In addition, monkey antisera recognize antigens that are not shared by all melanomas, indicating a heterogeneity of MAAs similar to that suggested by Brüggen *et al.* (1978) and Vennegoor *et al.* (1978) in their studies with nonhuman primate antimelanoma antisera.

Since our technique measures antibody only on the basis of its ability to bind to the target, we wished to determine whether the same melanoma specificity could be detected with respect to the ability of the antibody to mediate complement-dependent cytotoxicity (CDC) (Carrel *et al.*, 1980a). We found that one such antiserum (anti-CaCL 73-36) was active in CDC and that melanoma specificity was evident after absorption with 4×10^8 T and B lymphoid cells/ml antiserum. This is in contrast to the much more extensive absorption required to remove nonmelanoma specificity for the MHA. A surprising observation that remains unexplained was that even without absorption, the monkey antiserum that was strongly positive in both CDC and the MHA failed to react in antibody-dependent cell-mediated cytotoxicity (ADCC) using either human or monkey effector cells. To determine whether the failure to react in ADCC was due to an imbalance in antibody isotype or to the presence of immune complexes, the unabsorbed serum was fractionated on a Sephadex G200 column, and the IgM, IgG, and albumin fractions were tested separately before and after lymphoid-cell absorption. There was no ADCC reactivity against melanoma cells in any fraction before or after absorption. Before absorption, cytotoxic antibody was present in both IgG and IgM fractions, but after removal of reactivity against nonmelanoma targets, only the IgM fraction was active against melanoma cell lines. Four additional specific monkey antimelanoma sera (obtained from Dr. G. Stuhlmiller, Duke University, and Dr. C. Sorg, Münster, Germany) were fractionated, and all four showed melanoma-specific cytotoxic antibody in the IgM fraction, while only one of four had specific IgG antibody. The explanation for the predominance of cytotoxic antibody activity in the IgM isotype may reflect the greater efficiency of this antibody in cytolytic reactions. It may also be related to the biochemical nature of the antigen on the melanoma-cell surface. These studies indicate that the melanoma specificity of monkey antibodies can be demonstrated by two different techniques. The more sensitive MHA reveals reactivity against nonmelanoma cells in sera that appear to be specific for melanoma by CDC tests. This undetected non-specific reactivity could cause difficulties if such sera were used in binding studies for antigen analysis or purification.

In anticipation of the possible use of specific active immunotherapy in patients with regionally recurrent melanoma, we wished to determine the immunogenicity of various tumor vaccine preparations. To facilitate multiinstitutional trials, a stable inactivated vaccine would be desirable. We carried out in monkeys a small-scale preclinical comparison of vaccines comprised of fresh melanoma cells, freshly irradiated cells, stored lyophilized cells, and stored glutaraldehyde-treated cells (Dent et al., unpublished data). The response was assessed only in terms of antibody production, and the preliminary results indicate that significantly reduced antibody levels are obtained with any of the three inactivated vaccines, the glutaraldehyde-treated cells giving the lowest responses. Peak titers are obtained after 2–4 months of continuous monthly immunization, but by 7–9 months, melanoma-specific antibodies are virtually undetectable with all four vaccine preparations. These results suggest that melanoma-specific antigens are less readily recognized by xenogeneic hosts than nonspecific xenoantigens, which may overwhelm the immune response of the animal. In this respect, MAAs may be similar to histocompatibility antigens in that xenogeneic antisera are rarely capable of recognizing true allospecificities (Sanderson, 1977).

5. Rabbit Antibodies to Melanoma

There have been a number of reports of melanoma antisera prepared in rabbits that demonstrated sufficient specificity to be useful in clinical detection of melanoma antigen in tissue sections (Goodwin et al., 1972), serum (Viza and Phillips, 1975), or urine (Carrel and Theilkaes, 1973). These reports have not yet been followed by more definitive descriptions of the antigens involved. Nevertheless, they appeared to show sufficient promise for our laboratory to proceed along similar lines to prepare melanoma antisera in rabbits. We felt that working with nonhuman primates was costly and possibly that additional antigenic specificities might be revealed by rabbit antisera.

We have raised antisera against antigens present on intact cells freshly derived from biopsies or from cultured cell lines, against antigens derived by protease treatment and by sonication, and against antigens recovered from spent culture medium of melanoma cell lines (Rahman et al., 1979; Dent et al., unpublished data). The most highly reactive and specific antisera were obtained from rabbits immunized with fresh melanoma homogenates, cultured cells, or spent culture medium. We have obtained one antiserum that appears to be melanoma-specific, reacting with six of seven lines tested, three of six fresh melanoma tumors, and with none of six nonmelanoma tumor lines (see Table II). The remaining antisera react strongly with some melanoma lines, weakly with some, and not at all with others. They also react weakly with some nonmelanoma lines, most notably with some neuroblastoma and lung-carcinoma lines. This "preferential" melanoma reactivity is similar to that observed by other investigators using rabbit antisera against melanoma (Bystryn and Smalley, 1977; McCabe et al., 1979; Imai and Ferrone, 1980). These antisera are currently being used for molecular characterization of melanoma cell-surface antigens.

TABLE II

Spectrum of Reactivity of Rabbit Antiserum[a] Raised against Crude Homogenate of Melanoma Tissue

Reactive tissues	Nonreactive tissues
Melanoma cell lines	Melanoma cell lines
RPMI-8322	CaCL 73-36
LeCa Str 19-4	Nonmelanoma cell lines
RPMI-8252	CaLu (lung carcinoma)
CaCL 78-4	HeLa (cervic carcinoma)
CaCL 78-1	HT29 (colon carcinoma)
SK-Mel-26	SK-N-MC (neuroblastoma)
Fresh melanoma homogenates	NMB7 (neuroblastoma)
GAR I	IMR6 (neuroblastoma)
DON	Y-79 (retinoblastoma)
MCD	WERI-RB1 (retinoblastoma)
Nude mouse xenograft homogenates	LN-18 (glioma)
Melanoma	LN-40 (glioma)
RPMI 83	LN-140 (glioma)
CaCL 78-4	LN-229 (glioma)
	HAE/70 (human amnion)
	Raji (Burkitt's lymphoblastoid)
	Fresh melanoma homogenates
	GAR II
	HEA
	LAB
	Nude mouse xenograft homogenates
	Melanoma
	CaCL 73-36
	RPMI 8252
	Nonmelanoma
	HT29
	SK-N-MC
	NMB7
	IMR6
	Xenogeneic tissues
	Mouse liver
	Mouse kidney

[a]Antiserum absorbed with human erythrocytes, leukocytes, liver homogenate, and oral carcinoma cells (KB).

Most are obviously not specific for melanoma cells and are also not of very high titer. The relevance of melanoma specificity remains to be determined, since true tumor specificity as detected serologically may not exist. It therefore seems reasonable to proceed with antigen characterization with impure ("nonspecific") antisera or to use these antisera to select antigens for the development of more potent second-generation reagents.

6. Monoclonal Antibodies to Melanoma

The new and powerful technique of monoclonal-antibody production developed by Köhler and Milstein (1975) may provide the ultimate tool for defining the spectrum of cell-surface antigens on melanoma. By careful selection of antibody-producing clones derived from hybrids of murine myeloma cells and splenocytes from mice immunized with human tumor cells, it will be possible to generate large volumes of highly specific antisera for use in serological and immunochemical studies. Although the method has certain limitations that cannot be discussed here, several groups have already put it to use in the melanoma system (Koprowski *et al.*, 1978; Steplewski *et al.*, 1979; Yeh *et al.*, 1979; Woodbury *et al.*, 1980; Carrel *et al.*, 1980b; Herlyn *et al.*, 1980).

Our own experience with this technique is still limited, although we have studied in detail two antibodies that seemed initially to be melanoma-specific but that on further testing were detecting antigens common to several other tissues of neuroectodermal origin and to fetal brain tissue (Liao *et al.*, 1981)(Table III). The antibodies were derived from fused splenocytes taken from a mouse immunized with a cultured melanoma cell line (CaCL 78-1). They were found to react with ten of ten and nine of ten melanoma lines, respectively,

TABLE III

Spectrum of Reactivity of Two Hybridoma Antibodies (7.51 and 7.60) Raised against Melanoma Cell Line CaCL 78-1[a]

Tissues	7.51	7.60	Tissues	7.51	7.60
Melanomas			Glioblastomas		
CaCL 78-1	+	+	LN-18	−	+
CaCL 73-36	+	+	LN-40	+	+
CaCL 78-4	+	+	LN-135	+	+
CaCL 79-3	+	+	LN-140	+	+
UCLA-SO-M14	+	+	LN-229	+	+
RPMI-4445	+	+	Carcinomas		
RPMI-8252	+	+	KB	−	−
RPMI-8322	+	+	HeLa	−	−
RPMI-5966	+	+	CaLu	−	−
RPMI-7932	+	+	HT29	−	−
Fresh tumors (3)	+	+	MCF-7	−	−
Neuroblastomas			A549	−	−
SK-N-MC	+	+	LN (lung, fresh)	−	−
SHSY-5Y	+	+	NP (hypernephroma, fresh)	−	−
1MR6	+	+	Lymphoid cell lines		
1MR7	+	+	Daudi	−	−
Retinoblastomas			Raji	−	−
WERI-Rb1	+	+	Leukemias		
Y-79	+	+	CCL 119	−	−
RB267	+	+	K562	−	−
RB302A	+	+	Fibroblasts		
RB369E	−	+	C003	−	−
RB385 (fresh)	+	+	A23	−	−
			Fetal brain (fresh)		
			FT (20 weeks)	+	+
			BJ (26 weeks)	+	+
			Adult brain		
			ME	−	−
			SA	−	−

[a] Reactivity was determined by quantitative absorption followed by testing against immunizing cell line according to the method of Liao *et al.* (1979c)

but with none of four carcinoma lines and none of five nonmalignant cell lines. They did, however, react with two neuroblastoma lines, and on further testing they were reactive with one additional neuroblastoma line, six retinoblastomas, and five glioma lines. No reactivity was seen with a variety of carcinoma lines, leukemias, lymphoid-cell lines, or fibroblasts. The two antibodies did react with cell suspensions prepared from three fresh melanomas, two retinoblastomas, and two fetal brains, but not with adult brain, lung-carcinoma, or hypernephroma tissue. We have concluded that these antibodies are defining fetal neuroectodermal antigens that are present on melanoma cells (Carrel and Theilkaes, 1973; Pfreundschuh et al., 1978; Liao et al., 1979c). Kennett and Gilbert (1979) produced a monoclonal antibody against neuroblastoma cells that reacted with six neuroblastoma lines, one of two retinoblastomas, one of one glioblastoma, and fetal but not adult brain. They did not look for reactivity with melanoma cells. Several laboratories have reported the detection of common melanoma antigens using monoclonal antibodies, and in at least three of these reports, melanoma specificity was implied (Steplewski et al., 1979; Yeh et al., 1979; Carrel et al., 1980b). However, no other neuroectodermally derived tissues were examined. Carrel et al. (1980b) utilized a large panel of both malignant and nonmelanoma targets to demonstrate convincingly the melanoma specificity of three different monoclonal antibodies. The panel included only one glioblastoma cell line that was not reactive with any of the three antibodies by direct testing. Recently, Herlyn et al. (1980), extending the previous reports of Koprowski et al. (1978) and Steplewski et al. (1979), have defined the specificity of their monoclonal antibodies. They found that two antibodies that cross-react widely with melanoma cell lines also react with brain-tumor lines and have suggested that a neuroectodermal antigen may be involved. Two of their other antibodies appear to identify immune-associated (Ia)-like antigens. In our own work, we did not find complete melanoma cross-reactivity of one of our antibodies by direct tests, but absorption studies did demonstrate complete cross-reactivity among all the melanoma lines with two antibodies. Furthermore, even by absorption, one of the antibodies failed to react with one of five gliomas and one of six retinoblastomas, suggesting the existence of more than one type of neuroectodermal antigen.

7. Factors That Affect Expression of Melanoma-Associated Antigens

One of the advantages of our standard assay is that it involves the direct observation of the target cells for evaluation, and this has revealed that there are quantitative variations in antigen expression on the melanoma cells. We have also observed a small and variable proportion of cells that are totally nonreactive while the majority are strongly reactive. Whether we are dealing with stable antigen-deficient variants or whether these cells represent a stage in the normal replicative cycle of cells in culture is not known. We have observed no differences in MAA expression (defined by nonhuman primate antisera) during exponential and stationary phases of growth. We have recently examined the effect of two growth-inhibitory factors, interferon (IF) (Liao et al., 1980b) and theophylline (Th) (Liao et al., 1980c), which also have immunomodulating and differentiation-inducing properties, on the surface-antigen expression of cultured melanoma cells.

Exposure of melanoma cells to human leukocyte IF for 64 hr resulted in a dose-dependent inhibition of growth with a 46% reduction in cell number at 10^3 U/ml and 74% reduction at 10^5 U/ml. The expression of MAAs and β_2-microglobulin (β_2m) was enhanced 2- to 5-fold and 5- to 12-fold, respectively, while no change in Ia-like antigenic expression was seen by IF treatment. Enhancement of antigen expression was evident as early as 16 hr after addition of IF to the cultures, with a maximum increase occurring at 96 hr. The effect was reversible on removal of IF from the culture medium. Enhancement of antigen expression did not appear to be related to the inhibitory effect of IF on cell proliferation.

Th, a potent phosophodiesterase inhibitor that causes increased intracellular cyclic AMP levels, is known to promote the maturation of mouse melanoma cells (Kreider et al., 1975; Steinberg and Whittaker, 1976, 1978; Lotan and Lotan, 1980). We have shown that Th causes a dose-dependent inhibition of melanoma-cell growth with a 64% reduction in plating efficiency and a 50% reduction in saturation density at a concentration of 1 mM (Liao et al., 1980c). In contrast to IF, which did not induce any visible changes in the cultured cells, Th induced marked morphological differentiation characterized by elongation and increased complexity of dendritic processes and loss of close and diffuse contact of plasma membranes. Th also augmented MAA and β_2m expression, 4- and 12-fold respectively, while the expression of Ia-like antigen was decreased on the same cells. We are at present attempting to elucidate the mechanism of action of IF and Th in antigen enhancement. Since IF in particular (Borden, 1979; Krim, 1980), but also Th (DeWys and Bathina, 1980), are thought to have therapeutic potential, it is intriguing to speculate that enhanced antigenicity may be a contributing factor in this situation.

While the variability in antigen expression referred to above is not of sufficient magnitude to interfere with serological studies, we wished to determine whether fixation of the target cells with glutaraldehyde (GA) might proivde us with a large amount of stable, uniform substrate for long-term studies (Liao and Dent, 1979). We observed that GA fixation of the target melanoma cells *in situ* interfered with the MHA directly, probably because of the need for movement of surface antigens within the lipid bilayer to permit indicator-red-cell adherence (Dierich and Reisfeld, 1975). We went on to show by quantitative-absorption studies with monkey anti-MAA that treatment of melanoma cells for 15 min at room temperature at concentrations of GA greater than 0.0025% resulted in significant loss of antigenicity. GA also impaired reactivity with human alloantisera against histocompatibility antigens and with the rabbit antiserum against β_2m. Treatment of colon cancer cells (HT29) with up to 2.5% GA failed to alter their reactivity with antisera against CEA or blood group A antigen.

8. Characterization of Melanoma-Associated Antigens

The definition of tumor-associated antigen in man continues to be an elusive goal. The original, and for some the only interesting, tumor-associated antigen is one that acts as a rejection antigen and hence has a role to play in host control of neoplasia. It is clear that even if such antigens do exist in human tumors, it will, for ethical reasons, be difficult to obtain conclusive proof of their existence. Nonetheless, from among the myriad of surface structures that may be recognized immunologically by man or lower species on the surface of human melanoma cells, there are undoubtedly some that may be important in immunodiagnosis if not in therapy. However, before this can occur, the molecules involved will have to be isolated and purified, and it is safe to say that as yet, no such molecules have been described, although candidate molecules are evolving in different laboratories. The lack of standardization of sources of antibody, serological assays, and antigenic substrate makes comparison of the properties of MAAs as defined by different laboratories difficult. We have begun to characterize the MAAs that we defined by monkey and rabbit antisera and will discuss our preliminary findings briefly.

The structural and functional similarities of histocompatibility antigens and tumor-associated antigens have been recently reviewed (Poulik, 1978; Parmiani *et al.*, 1979). The constant association of β_2m with histocompatibility antigens was the basis of experiments reported by Thomson *et al.* (1976, 1978), in which it was shown that papain-solubilized tumor-specific antigens from a number of human tumors, including malignant melanoma, are associated with β_2m in a manner that permits their specific binding to an anti-β_2m immunoabsorbent. Malley *et al.* (1979) subsequently showed that MAAs reactive *in vivo* and in *in vitro* tests of cell-mediated immunity are enriched 10-fold in material bound to an anti-β_2m immunoabsorbent. At variance with these findings, structural association of β_2m with MAAs was not found in spent medium from melanoma cultures (McCabe *et al.*, 1978) or in a papain digest of a cultured melanoma cell line (Carey *et al.*, 1979). We have found that MAA activity concentrated from melanoma-culture supernatants was enriched at least 10-fold in material that bound to an anti-β_2m affinity column compared to the unbound material (Khosravi *et al.*, unpublished data). Human leukocyte antigen (HLA) activity was also enriched in the bound fraction, while there was no binding of Ia antigen to anti-β_2m column. The binding of MAAs to the affinity column could be blocked competely by pretreating the column with purified β_2m. These data indicate either that MAAs are linked to β_2m as are HLA antigens or that they are in close spatial proximity in the cell membrane such that they are shed together from the cell surface. Further immunochemical studies will be necessary to elucidate the nature of the association and to reconcile the difference between our results and those of other investigators (McCabe *et al.*, 1978; Carey *et al.*, 1979). The latter however, may be due to differences in MAAs in each of the three studies.

We have obtained similar discrepant results in attempts to dissociate MAAs from classic histocompatibility antigens using physical–chemical techniques. McCabe *et al.* (1978) and Malley *et al.* (1979) found that histocompatibility antigens can be recovered separately from MAAs using KBr ultracentrifugal flotation. They found that HLA activity was present in the upper fraction and MAAs were concentrated in the bottom fraction as determined by skin testing in patients or leucocyte-adherence-inhibition tests. Stuhlmiller *et al.* (1978), using column-chromatographic techniques, were able to dissociate HLA activity from MAAs as assessed by monkey anti-MAA in a pronase digest of a fresh melanoma. Carey *et al.* (1979) obtained similar separation of HLA and MAAs (defined by an autologous human antibody) in papain extracts of a cultured melanoma cell line.

We have followed the approach of McCabe *et al.* (1978) using KBr flotation of MAAs derived from spent culture medium and found, as they did, HLA in the top fraction (Khosravi *et al.*, unpublished data). However, MAAs defined by our monkey antisera were also recovered in the top fraction. MAAs were enriched over 10-fold, while HLA-A10 activity was enriched over 15-fold. MAAs defined by rabbit antisera were also enriched in the top fraction. We have sent, under code, aliquots of top and bottom KBr fractions derived from melanoma as well as colon-carcinoma culture supernatants to Dr. D. M. P. Thomson, McGill University. He has identified MAA activity only in the top fraction of the melanoma-derived material using the leucocyte-adherence-inhibition technique as previously described in his laboratory (Thomson *et al.*, 1978, 1980). We conclude that the similarity of serologically defined MAAs and HLA in terms of flotation on KBr gradients implies certain common physical and chemical features indicating that these antigens are members of the same class of cell-surface structures.

In addition to the reports referred to above, there have been numerous other reports of the use of various extracts and partially purified melanoma materials in immunological surveys of patients with melanoma. These are not directly related to our findings and are too numerous to review here. Some recent studies have shed light on the biochemical and molecular nature of MAAs defined by human (Gupta *et al.*, 1979; Hersey *et al.*, 1979; Embelton *et al.*, 1980) and rabbit antisera (Imai and Ferrone, 1980).

9. Clinical Implications of Melanoma Immunology

One of the goals of tumor immunology research is to determine whether there are tumor-specific antigens on human cancer that can be utilized for the benefit of patients with cancer. With respect to melanoma, which is probably the best-studied human tumor, it is apparent that we have not yet defined the full antigenic spectrum nor do we know whether there are antigens that are truly restricted to melanoma tumor cells. It follows that any measurement of antitumor immune responses is limited by the lack of precise definition of the target of such responses. Nevertheless, despite this great deficiency in our knowledge base, a few studies have documented a relationship between the quantitative and/or qualitative aspects of immune reactions to MAAs and the clinical status of the patient.

The majority of investigators have documented a decline in antitumor immunity with advancing disease (Morton *et al.*, 1968; Lewis *et al.*, 1969; Currie and Basham, 1972; DeVries *et al.*, 1972; Canevari *et al.*, 1975; Hersey *et al.*, 1978). We also found that among patients with visceral metastases, there was a decreased incidence of antibody against melanoma target cells, while no decrease in reactivity against nonmelanoma target cells was observed using the immunofluorescence technique (Dent *et al.*, 1978). Our findings implied that the decrease in antibody reactivity was specific for melanoma cells and not simply a manifestation of general immunological incompetence that is seen with advanced disease in cancer patients (Lui *et al.*, 1975). It may be that with advancing disease, serum blocking factors appear that interfere with anti-MAA reactivity (Hellström *et al.*, 1973; Cochran *et al.*, 1976; Grosser and Thomson, 1976). It has been suggested that these blocking factors could be immune complexes (Jerry *et al.*, 1976; Murray *et al.*, 1977). The intriguing possibility would be if the complexes did contain melanoma antigens (Theofilopoulos *et al.*, 1977). The correlation of circulating antigen levels with tumor extent has already been demonstrated for other tumor products, such as CEA and α-fetoprotein. Characterization and isolation of MAAs may provide the means for a more specific test for the assessment of disease extent and response to therapy and for early diagnosis of recurrence in patients with melanoma. Viza and Phillips (1975) have detected circulating melanoma antigen in the sera of 28 of 150 patients with melanoma using a rabbit antibody against melanoma membranes. They were unable to make any correlations between the presence of antigen and the clinical status of the patient. Carrel and Theilkaes (1973) have described similar findings of antigen in the urine of melanoma patients using a rabbit antiserum. These early reports have not been confirmed or extended, probably because of difficulties relating to the definition of antigen specificity.

Stuhlmiller *et al.* (1977) have reported the usefulness of a monkey antimelanoma antiserum in the immunohistochemical verification of a difficult pathological diagnosis in three cases of melanoma metastases to lymph nodes. Brüggen *et al.* (1978) have suggested that melanoma cells may be classified on the basis of reactivity with certain monkey anti-MAA antisera and that the classification defines different malignant phenotypes. Similarly, Werkmeister *et al.* (1980) have found that the presence of certain antigens on melanoma tumors, as defined by patient sera, may have predictive value regarding prognosis. It is thus not inconceivable that as the spectrum of antigens on melanomas becomes better defined, we may be able to use immunological tumor-typing to assist in determining prognosis and designing specific therapy.

10. Summary

In our studies of the serology of human melanoma, we have come to a better appreciation of the extent of the antigenic diversity in this tumor. This has been sharply focused by the hybridoma technique, which has confirmed some of the suggestions of antigenic complexity revealed in studies using classic heteroantisera and alloantisera. The spectrum of antigens already uncovered by this technique is summarized in idealized form in Table IV. In addition to the private, common cross-reactive, and partially cross-reactive melanoma antigens, we should expect to see monoclonal antibodies against growth factors (Fabricant *et al.*, 1977), hormone receptors (Fisher *et al.*, 1976), and a variety of other membrane molecules. It is our feeling that much more information is still needed to serologically and biochemically define the antigens on melanoma cells. The use of human allo- and autoantisera as well as the use of classic heteroantisera should not be abandoned in favor of the monoclonal antibody technique; rather, all three methods should be studied in parallel, since the ideal approach to melanoma serology has yet to be determined. The next decade will see the characterization of specific antigens by individual laboratories and, it is to be hoped, the standardization of serological techniques to permit the exchange and comparison of reagents and results. It is also clear that a modified view will emerge of what tumor antigens are in man, and from this may come truly useful advances in tumor diagnosis and treatment.

ACKNOWLEDGMENTS. The research carried out in our laboratories has been supported primarily by grants from the Ontario Cancer Treatment & Research Foundation and the Medical Research Council of Canada. The authors wish to acknowledge the contributions of a number of students and laboratory personnel without whose diligent work these studies could never have reached fruition. In addition, the support and interest of our clinical col-

TABLE IV

Antigenic Heterogeneity of Melanoma Cell Surface as Revealed by Monoclonal Antibodies (Idealized)

Serological reactivity against different target-cell lines

Specificity designation	Melanoma						Carcinoma						Neuroblastoma	Retinoblastoma	Glioblastoma	Lymphoid	Fibroblast	References
	1	2	3	4	5	6	1	2	3	4	5	6						
Melanoma																		
Private	+	−	−	−	−	−	−	−	−	−	−	−	−	−	−	−	−	—
Common	+	+	+	+	+	+	−	−	−	−	−	−	−	−	−	−	−	Carrel et al. (1980b)
Shared	+	+	−	−	+	+	−	−	−	−	−	−	−	−	−	−	−	Liao et al. (unpublished), Carrel et al. (1980b), Koprowski et al. (1978)
Neuroectodermal	+	+	+	+	+	+	−	−	−	−	−	−	+	+	+	−	−	Liao et al. (1981), Herlyn et al. (1980)
CEA-like antigen	+	+	+	+	+	+	+	+	+	+	+	+	−	−	−	−	−	Liao et al. (unpublished)
Transformed or neoplastic cells	+	+	+	+	+	+	+	+	+	+	+	+	+	+	+	−	−	Woodbury et al. (1980), Herlyn et al. (1980), Liao et al. (unpublished)
Ia-like antigen	+	+	+	+	+	+	−	−	−	−	+	+	−	−	+	+	−	Herlyn et al. (1980)

leagues, in particular Dr. Peter B. McCulloch, our associates in the laboratory, and the nursing staff of the Hamilton Clinic of the Ontario Cancer Foundation is gratefully acknowledged. Finally, the patience, skill, and cheerfulness of Mrs. J. Giles have made the preparation of this manuscript a bearable exercise.

References

Aldridge, K. E., Cole, B. S., and Ward, J. R., 1977, Mycoplasma-dependent activation of normal lymphocytes: Induction of a lymphocyte-mediated cytotoxicity for allogeneic and syngeneic mouse target cells, *Infect. Immunol.* **18**:377.

Bloom, E. T., 1973, Microcytotoxicity tests on human cells in culture: Effect of contamination with mycoplasma, *Proc. Soc. Exp. Biol. Med.* **143**:244.

Bodurtha, A. J., Chee, D. O., Laucius, J. F., Mastrangelo, M. J., and Prehn, R. T., 1975, Clinical and immunological significance of human melanoma cytotoxic antibody, *Cancer Res.* **35**:189.

Borden, E. C., 1979, Interferons: Rationale for clinical trials in neoplastic disease, *Ann. Intern. Med.* **91**:472.

Brooks, C. G., Rees, R. C., and Leach, R. H., 1979, High nonspecific reactivity of normal lymphocytes against mycoplasma infected target cells in cytotoxicity assays, *Eur. J. Immunol.* **9**:159.

Brüggen, J., Sorg, C., and Macher, E., 1978, Membrane associated antigens of human malignant melanoma. V. Serological typing of cell lines using antisera from nonhuman primates, *Cancer Immunol. Immunother.* **5**:53.

Bystryn, J. C. and Smalley, J. R., 1977, Identification and solubilization of iodinated cell surface human melanoma associated antigens, *Int. J. Cancer* **20**:165.

Canevari, S., Fossati, G., DellaPorta, G., and Balzarini, G. P., 1975, Humoral cytotoxicity in melanoma patients and its correlation with the extent and course of the disease, *Int. J. Cancer* **16**:722.

Carey, T. E., Takahashi, T., Resnick, L. A., Oettgen, H. F., and Old, L. J., 1976, Cell surface antigens of human malignant melanoma. I. Mixed hemadsorption assays for humoral immunity to cultured autologous melanoma cells, *Proc. Natl. Acad. Sci. U.S.A.* **73**:3278.

Carey, T. E., Lloyd, K. O., Takahashi, T., Travassos, L. R., and Old, L. J., 1979, Solubilization and partial characterization of the AU cell surface antigen of human malignant melanoma, *Proc. Natl. Acad. Sci. U.S.A.* **76**:2898.

Carrel, S., and Theilkaes, L., 1973, Evidence for a tumor-associated antigen in human malignant melanoma, *Nature (London)* **242**:609.

Carrel, S., Dent, P. B., and Liao, S. K., 1980a, Demonstration of the specificity of a monkey antiserum against human melanoma: Evidence that the cytotoxic antibodies from the specific antiserum belong to the IgM class, *Cancer Immunol. Immunother.* **8**:197.

Carrel, S., Accolla, R. S., Carmagnola, A. L., and Mach, J. -P., 1980b, Common human melanoma antigen(s). 1. Detection by monoclonal antibodies, *Cancer Res.* **40**:2523.

Cochran, A. J., Mackie, R. M., Ross, C. E., Ogg, L. J., and Jackson, A. M., 1976, Leukocyte migration inhibition by cancer patients' sera, *Int. J. Cancer* **18**:274.

Coggin, J. H., Jr., and Anderson, N. G., 1974, Cancer, differentiation and embryonic antigens: Some central problems, *Adv. Cancer Res.* **19**:105.

Currie, G. A., and Basham, C., 1972, Serum mediated inhibition of the immunological reactions of the patient to his own tumor: A possible role for circulating antigen, *Br. J. Cancer* **26**:427.

Dent, P. B., Liao, S. K., McCulloch, P. B., Blajchman, M. A., and MacNamara, J., 1978, Characterization of human melanoma cell lines. III. Membrane immunofluorescence reactivity with sera from patients with melanoma, *Cancer Immunol. Immunother.* **3**:239.

Dent, P. B., Cleland, G., and Liao, S. K., 1980a, Detection and control of occult mycoplasma contamination in human tumor cell lines, *Cancer Immunol. Immunother.* **8**:27–32.

Dent, P. B., Carrel, S., and Mach, J. -P., 1980b, Detection of new crossreacting carcinoembryonic antigen(s) on cultured tumor cells by mixed hemadsorption assay, *J. Natl. Cancer Inst.* **64**:309.

Dent, P. B., Liao, S. K., McCulloch, P. B., Stone, B. R., and Singal, D. P., 1982, Absence of melanoma specificity in the reactivity of melanoma patients' sera with cultured allogeneic melanoma cell lines, *Cancer* (in press).

DeVries, J. E., Rümke, P., and Bernheim, J. L., 1972, Cytotoxic lymphocytes in melanoma patients, *Int. J. Cancer* 9:567.

DeWys, W. D., and Bathina, S. H., 1980, Synergistic anti-leukemic effect of theophylline and 1,3-bis(2-chloroethyl)-1-nitrosourea, *Cancer Res.* 40:2202.

Dierich, M. P., and Reisfeld, R. A., 1975, C_3-mediated cytoadherence. Formation of C_3 receptor aggregates as prerequisites for cell attachment. *J. Exp. Med.* 142:242.

Dore, J. F., Bourgoin, J. J., Gulbout, C., and Diatloff, C., 1973, Recherche d'anticorps reagissant avec les cellules des melanomes malins dans le serum des malades porteurs de tumours cutanées, *Rev. Inst. Pasteur Lyon* 6:307.

Embleton, M. J., Price, M. R., and Baldwin, R. W., 1980, Demonstration and partial purification of common melanoma-associated antigen(s), *Eur. J. Cancer* 16:575.

Fabricant, R. N., Delarco, J. E., and Todaro, G. J., 1977, Nerve growth factor receptors on human melanoma cells in culture, *Proc. Natl. Acad. Sci. U.S.A.* 74:565.

Fisher, R. I., Neifeld, J. P., and Lippman, M. E., 1976, Oestrogen receptors in human malignant melanoma, *Lancet* 2:337.

Goodwin, D. P., Hornung, M. O., Leong, S. P. L., and Krementz, E. T., 1972, Immune responses induced by human malignant melanoma in the rabbit, *Surgery* 72:737.

Grosser, N., and Thomson, D. M. P., 1976, Tube leukocyte (monocyte) adherence inhibition assay for the detection of anti-tumor immunity. III. "Blockade" of monocyte reactivity by excess free antigen and immune complexes in advanced cancer patients, *Int. J. Cancer* 18:58.

Gupta, R. K., Irie, R. F., Chee, D. O., Kern, D. H., and Morton, D. L., 1979, Demonstration of two distinct antigens in spent tissue culture medium of a human malignant melanoma cell line, *J. Natl. Cancer Inst.* 63:347.

Hamburger, R. N., Pious, D. A., and Milles, S. E., 1963, Antigenic specificities acquired from growth medium by cells in tissue culture, *Immunology* 6:439.

Hellström, I., Hellström, K. E., Pierce, G. E., and Yang, J. P. S., 1968, Cellular and humoral immunity to different types of human neoplasms, *Nature (London)* 320:1352.

Hellström, I., Warner, G., Hellström, K. E., and Sjögren, H. O., 1973, Sequential studies on cell-mediated tumor immunity and blocking serum activity in ten patients with malignant melanoma, *Int. J. Cancer* 11:280.

Herlyn, M., Clark, W. H., Jr., Mastrangelo, M. J., Guerry, D., IV., Elder, D. E., LaRossa, D., Hamilton, R., Bondi, E., Tuthill, R., Steplewski, Z., and Koprowski, H., 1980, Specific immunoreactivity of hybridoma-secreted monoclonal anti-melanoma antibodies to cultured cells and freshly derived human cells, *Cancer Res.* 40:3602.

Hersey, P., Edwards, A., Milton, G. W., and McCarthy, W. H., 1978, Relationship of cell mediated cytotoxicity against melanoma cells to prognosis in melanoma patients, *Br. J. Cancer* 37:505.

Hersey, P., Murray, E., Werkmeister, J., and McCarthy, W. H., 1979, Detection of a low-molecular-weight antigen on melanoma cells by a human antiserum in leukocyte-dependent antibody assays, *Br. J. Cancer* 40:615.

Houghton, A. N., Taormina, M. C., Ikeda, H., Watanabe, T., Oettgen, H. F., and Old, L. J. 1980, Serological survey of normal humans for natural antibody to cell surface antigens of melanoma, *Proc. Natl. Acad. Sci. U.S.A.* 77:4260.

Ikonopisov, R. L., Lewis, M. G., Hunter-Craig, I. D., Bodenham, D. C., Phillips, T. R., Cooling, I. C., Proctor, J. W., Hamilton-Fairley, G., and Alexander, P., 1970, Autoimmunization with irradiated tumor cells in malignant melanoma, *Br. Med. J.* 2:752–754.

Imai, K., and Ferrone, S., 1980, Indirect rosette microassay to characterize human melanoma-associated antigens recognized by operationally specific xenoantisera, *Cancer Res.* 40:2252.

Irie, R. F., Irie, K., and Morton, D. L., 1974, Natural antibody in human serum to a neoantigen in human cultured cells grown in fetal bovine serum, *J. Natl. Cancer Inst.* 52:1051.

Irie, R. F., Irie, K., and Morton, D. L., 1976, A membrane antigen common to human cancer and fetal brain, *Cancer Res.* 36:3510.

Irie, R. F., Giuliano, A. E., and Morton, D. L., 1979, Oncofetal antigen: A tumor-associated fetal antigen immunogeneic in man, *J. Natl. Cancer Inst.* 63:367.

Jerry, L. M., Rowden, G., Cano, P. O., Phillips, T. M., Deutsch, G. F., Capek, A., Hartmann, D., and Lewis, M. G., 1976, Immune complexes in human melanoma, a consequence of deranged immune regulation, *Scand. J. Immunol.* 5:845.

Kennett, R., and Gilbert, F., 1979, Hybrid myelomas producing antibodies against a human neuroblastoma antigen present on fetal brain, *Science* **203**:1120.

Köhler, G., and Milstein, C., 1975, Continuous culture of fused cells secreting antibody of predefined specificity, *Nature (London)* **256**:495.

Koprowski, H., Steplewski, Z., Herlyn, D., and Herlyn, M., 1978, Studies of antibodies against human melanoma produced by somatic cell hybrids, *Proc. Natl. Acad. Sci. U.S.A.* **75**:3405.

Kreider, J. W., Wade, D. R., Rosenthal, M., and Densley, T., 1975, Maturation and differentiation of B16 melanoma cells induced by theophylline treatment, *J. Natl. Cancer Inst.* **54**:1457.

Krim, M., 1980, Towards tumor therapy with interferons. II. Interferons: *In vivo* effects, *Blood* **55**:875.

Lando, P., Gabriel, J., Berzins, K., and Perlmann, P., 1980, Determination of the immunoglobulin class of complement-dependent cytotoxic antibodies in serum of D23 hepatoma-bearing rats, *Scand. J. Immunol.* **11**:253.

Lando, P., Blomberg, F., Raftell, M., Berzins, K., and Perlmann, P., 1977, Complement-dependent cytotoxicity against hepatoma cells mediated by IgM antibodies in serum from tumor bearing rats, *Scand. J. Immunol.* **6**:1081.

Leong, S. P. L., Sutherland, C. M., and Krementz, E. T. 1977, Immunofluorescent detection of common melanoma membrane antigens by sera of melanoma patients immunized against autologous or allogeneic cultured melanoma cells, *Cancer Res.* **37**:4035.

Lewis, M. G., 1967, Possible immunological host factors in human malignant melanoma, *Lancet* **2**:921.

Lewis, M. G., Ikonopisov, R. L., Nairn, R. C., Phillips, T. M., Hamilton Fairley, G., Bodenham, D. C., and Alexander, P., 1969, Tumor specific antibodies in human malignant melanoma and their relationship to the extent of the disease, *Br. Med. J.* **2**:547.

Liao, S. K., and Dent, P. B., 1979, Preservation of melanoma-associated antigens on human malignant melanoma cells by glutaraldehyde fixation, *Proc. Am. Assoc. Cancer Res.* **20**:270.

Liao, S. K., Dent, P. B., and McCulloch, P. B., 1975, Characterization of human malignant melanoma cell lines. I. Morphology and growth characteristics in culture, *J. Natl. Cancer Inst.* **54**:1037.

Liao, S. K., Dent, P. B., and McCulloch, P. B., 1976, Cellular morphology of human malignant melanoma in primary culture, *In Vitro* **12**:654.

Liao, S. K., Dent, P. B., and Qizilbash, A., 1977, Characterization of human malignant melanoma cell lines: Heterotransplantation in the hamster cheek pouch, *Z. Krebsforsch.* **88**:121.

Liao, S. K., Leong, S. P. L., Sutherland, C. M., Dent, P. B., Kwong, P. C., and Krementz, G. T., 1978, Common human melanoma membrane antigens detected by mixed hemadsorption microassay with serum from a patient undergoing immunotherapy with autologous tumor cells, *Cancer Res.* **38**:4395.

Liao, S. K., Dent, P. B., and McCulloch, P. B., 1979a, Relationship of malignant potential to *in vitro* saturation density of human melanoma cell clones, *Pigment Cell* **5**:235.

Liao, S. K., Rahman, A. F. R., Kwong, P. C., and Dent, P. B., 1979b, A simple microassay for detection of antibodies to fetal calf serum and related antigens and its application to the serological definition of human tumor antigens, *J. Immunol. Methods* **17**:111.

Liao, S. K., Kwong, P. C., Thompson, J. C., and Dent, P. B., 1979c, Spectrum of melanoma antigens on cultured human malignant melanoma cells as detected by monkey antibodies, *Cancer Res.* **39**:183.

Liao, S. K., Khosravi, M., Kwong, P. C., Singal, D. P., and Dent, P. B., 1980a, Miniaturization makes mixed hemadsorption assays more sensitive, reliable and economic, *Immunol. Lett.* **2**:123.

Liao, S. K., Kwong, P. C., and Dent, P. B., 1980b, Interferon enhances the expression of melanoma-associated antigens and β-2 microglobulin on cultured human melanoma cell, *Proc. Am. Assoc. Cancer Res.* **21**:205.

Liao, S. K., Kwong, P. C., and Dent, P. B., 1980c, Effect of theophylline on the growth and expression of different surface antigens of cultured human melanoma cells, *Yale J. Biol. Med.* **53**:416.

Liao, S. K., Clarke, B. J., Kwong, P. C., Brickenden, A., Gallig, B. L., and Dent, P. B., 1981, Common neuroectodermal antigens of human melanoma, neuroblastoma, retinoblastoma, glioblastoma and fetal brain revealed by hybridoma antibodies raised against melanoma cells, *Eur. J. Immunol.* **11**:450.

Lotan, R., and Lotan, D., 1980, Stimulation of melanogenesis in a human melanoma, *Cancer Res.* **40**:3345.

Lui, V. K., Karpuchas, J., Dent, P. B., McCulloch, P. B., and Blajchman, M. A., 1975, Cellular immunocompetence in melanoma: Effect of extent of disease and immunotherapy, *Br. J. Cancer* **32**:323.

Lui, V. K., Dent, P. B., and Liao, S. K., 1977, Characterication of human malignant melanoma cell lines. VI. Inhibition of ^{3}H-thymidine uptake by normal stimulated lymphocytes, *Oncology* **34**:251.

Malley, A., Burger, D. R., Vandenbark, A. A., Frikke, M., Finke, P., Begley, D., Acott, K., Black, J., and

Vetto, R. M., 1979, Association of melanoma tumor antigen activity with β2-microglobulin, *Cancer Res.* **39**:619.

McCabe, R. P., Ferrone, S., Pellegrino, M. A., Kern, D. H., Holmes, E. C., and Reisfeld, R. A., 1978, Purification and immunologic evaluation of human melanoma associated antigens, *J. Natl. Cancer Inst.* **60**:773.

McCabe, R. P., Quaranta, V., Frugis, L., Ferrone, S., and Reisfeld, R. A., 1979, A radioimmunometric antibody-binding assay for evaluation of xenoantisera to melanoma associated antigens, *J. Natl. Cancer Inst.* **62**:455.

McCulloch, P. B., Dent, P. B., Hayes, P. R., and Liao, S. K., 1976, Common and individually specific chromosomal characteristics of cultured human melanoma, *Cancer Res.* **36**:398.

Metzgar, R. S., Bergoc, P. M., Moreno, M. A., and Seigler, H. F., 1973, Melanoma specific antibodies produced in monkeys by immunization with human melanoma cell lines, *J. Natl. Cancer Inst.* **50**:1065.

Morton, D. L., Malmgren, R. A., Holmes, E. C., and Ketcham, A. S., 1968, Demonstration of antibodies against human malignant melanoma by immunofluorescence, *Surgery* **64**:233.

Murray, E., McCarthy, W. H., and Hersey, P., 1977, Blocking of factors against leucocyte-dependent melanoma antibody in the sera of melanoma patients, *Br. J. Cancer* **36**:7.

Nelson-Rees, W. A., and Flandermeyer, R. R., 1976, HeLa cultures defined, *Science* **191**:96.

Parmiani, G., Carbone, G., Invernizzi, G., Pierotti, M. A., Sensi, M. L., Rogers, M. J., and Appella, E., 1979, Alien histocompatibility antigens on tumor cells, *Immunogenetics* **9**:1.

Peter, H. -H., Kalden, J. R., Seeland, P., Diehl, V., and Eckert, G., 1975, Humoral and cellular immune reactions "in vitro" against allogeneic and autologous human melanoma cells, *Clin. Exp. Immunol.* **20**:193.

Pfreundschuh, M., Shiku, H., Takahashi, T., Veda, C., Ransohoff, J., Oettgen, H. F., and Old, L. J., 1978, Serological analysis of cell surface antigens of malignant human brain tumors, *Proc. Natl. Acad. Sci. U.S.A.* **75**:5122.

Poulik, M. D., 1978, Structure of tumor antigens related to transplantation antigens, *Scand. J. Immunol.* **7**(Suppl. 6,):63.

Qizilbash, A. H., Liao, S. K., and Dent, P. B., 1977, Characterization of human malignant melanoma cell lines. IV. Cytological and histochemical characteristics, *Acta Cytol.* **21**:147.

Rahman, A. F. R., Liao, S. K., and Dent, P. B., 1979, Common surface antigens of human melanoma cell lines detected by rabbit xenoantisera, *Proc. Am. Assoc. Cancer Res.* **10**:237.

Sanderson, A. R., 1977, HLA "help" for human β2 microglobulin across species barriers, *Nature (London)* **269**:414.

Seibert, E., Sorg, C., Happle, R., and Macher, E., 1977, Membrane associated antigens of human malignant melanoma. III. Specificity of human sera reacting with cultured melanoma cells, *Int. J. Cancer* **19**:172.

Shaw, H. M., McGovern, V. J., Milton, G. W., Farago, G. A., and McCarthy, W. H., 1980, Histologic features of tumors and the female superiority in survival from malignant melanoma, *Cancer* **45**:7.

Shibata, H. R., Jerry, L. M., Lewis, M. G., Mansell, P. W. A., Capek, A., and Marquis, G., 1976, Immunotherapy of human malignant melanoma with irradiated human cells, oral bacillus Calmette-Guérin, and levamisole, *Ann. N.Y. Acad. Sci.* **277**:355.

Shiku, H., Takahashi, T., Oettgen, H. F., and Old, L. J., 1976, Cell surface antigens of human malignant melanoma. II. Serological typing with immune adherence assays and definition of two new surface antigens, *J. Exp. Med.* **144**:873.

Sidell, N., Irie, R. F., and Morton, D. L., 1979, Immune cytolysis of human malignant melanoma by antibody to oncofetal antigen I (OFA-I). I. Complement-dependent cytotoxicity, *Cancer Immunol. Immunother.* **7**:151.

Sofen, H., and O'Toole, C., 1978, Antisquamous tumor antibodies in patients with squamous cell carcinoma, *Cancer Res.* **38**:199.

Steinberg, M. L., and Whittaker, J. R., 1976, Stimulation of melanotic expression in a melanoma cell line by theophylline, *J. Cell Physiol.* **87**:265.

Steinberg, M. L., and Whittaker, J. R., 1978, Theophylline incorporation into the nucleic acids of theophylline stimulated melanoma cells. *J. Invest. Dermatol.* **71**:250.

Steplewski, Z., Herlyn, M., Herlyn, D., Clark, W. H., and Koprowski, H., 1979, Reactivity of monoclonal antimelanoma antibodies with melanoma cells freshly isolated from primary and metastatic melanoma, *Eur. J. Immunol.* **9**:94.

Stuhlmiller, G. M., and Seigler, H. F., 1975, Characterization of a chimpanzee antihuman melanoma antiserum, *Cancer Res.* **35**:2132.

Stuhlmiller, G. M., and Seigler, H. F., 1977, Enzyme susceptibility and spontaneous release of human melanoma tumor-associated antigens, *J. Natl. Cancer Inst.* **58**:215.

Stuhlmiller, G. M., Boylston, J. A., Seigler, H. F., and Fetter, B. F., 1977, Immunodiagnosis of melanoma
using chimpanzee antihuman melanoma antiserum, *Am. J. Clin. Pathol.* **67**:573.

Stuhlmiller, G. M., Green, R. W., and Seigler, H. F., 1978, Solubilization and partial isolation of human
melanoma tumor-associated antigens, *J. Natl. Cancer Inst.* **61**:61.

Theofilopoulos, A. N., Andrews, B. S., Urist, M. M., Morton, D. L., and Dixon, F. J., 1977, The nature of
immune complexes in human cancer sera, *J. Immunol.* **119**:657.

Thiry, L., Sprecher-Goldberger, S., Hannecart-Pokorni, E., Gould, I., and Bossens, M., 1977, Specific non-
immunoglobulin G antibodies and cell-mediated response to herpes simplex virus antigens in women with
cervical carcinoma, *Cancer Res.* **37**:1301.

Thomson, D. M. P., Gold, P., Freedman, S. O., and Shuster, J., 1976, The isolation and characterization of
tumor-specific antigens of rodent and human tumors, *Cancer Res.* **36**:3518.

Thomson, D. M. P., Rauch, J. E., Weatherhead, J. C., Friedlander, P., O'Connor, R., Grosser, N., Shuster,
J., and Gold, P., 1978, Isolation of human tumor specific antigens associated with β2 microglobulin, *Br.
J. Cancer* **37**:753.

Thomson, D. M. P., Tataryn, D. N., Weatherhead, J. C., Friedlander, P., Rauch, J., Schwartz, R., Gold, P.,
and Shuster, J., 1980, A human colon tumor antigen associated with β2-microglobulin and isolated from
solid tumor, serum and urine is unrelated to carcinoembryonic antigen, *Eur. J. Cancer* **16**:539.

Vennegoor, C., Jonker, A., Van Smeerdi, D., Van Es, J. K. A., and Rümke, P., 1978, Specificity of a monkey
antiserum for a melanoma cell line IPC-48, in: *Protides of the Biological Fluids* (H. Peeters, ed.), p. 731,
Pergamon Press, Oxford and New York.

Viza, D., and Phillips, J., 1975, Identification of an antigen associated with malignant melanoma, *Int. J. Cancer*
16:312.

Werkmeister, J., Edwards, A., McCarthy, W., and Hersey, D., 1980, Prognostic significance of expression of
antigens on melanoma cells, *Cancer Immunol. Immunother.* **9**:233.

Wood, G. W., and Barth, R. F., 1974, Immunofluorescent studies of the serologic reactivity of patients with
malignant melanoma against tumor-associated cytoplasmic antigens, *J. Natl. Cancer Inst.* **53**:309.

Woodbury, R. G., Brown, J. P., Yeh, M.-Y., Hellströom, I., and Hellström, K. E., 1980, Identification of a
cell surface protein p97 in human melanomas and certain other neoplasms, *Proc. Natl. Acad. Sci. U.S.A.*
77:2183.

Yeh, M.-Y., Hellström, I., Brown, J. P., Warner, G. A., Hansen, J. A., and Hellström, K. E., 1979, Cell
surface antigens of human melanoma identified by monoclonal antibody, *Proc. Natl. Acad. Sci. U.S.A.*
76:2927.

7

Protein Antigens of Mouse Melanomas

DOUGLAS M. GERSTEN AND JOHN J. MARCHALONIS

1. Introduction

Two lines of evidence suggest that B16 melanoma cells express immunological determinants. The first is that syngeneic C57BL/6 mice may be immunized outright to B16 preparations—either whole-cell (Fidler *et al.,* 1977) or extract (Bystryn, 1978). The second is that cultured cells, when injected into B16-sensitized hosts, exhibit *in vivo* behavior different from that observed following administration into naïve hosts (Fidler *et al.,* 1977; Gersten, 1980). It follows, then that B16 cells should possess unique molecules that are both absent from other C57BL/6 cells and immunogenic.

We have approached the search for and identification of these molecules as shown schematically in Fig. 1. The xenogeneic serological approach to the isolation of tumor antigens has been hampered in the past by the failure to produce antisera that withstand analysis by rigorous criteria. Consequently, experimental design and interpretation of results must be performed with caution. We shall endeavor to point out and discuss areas where such ambiguities may exist.

DOUGLAS M. GERSTEN • Department of Pathology and National Biomedical Research Foundation, Georgetown University, Washington, D.C. 20007.   JOHN J. MARCHALONIS • Department of Biochemistry, Medical University of South Carolina, Charleston, South Carolina 29403.

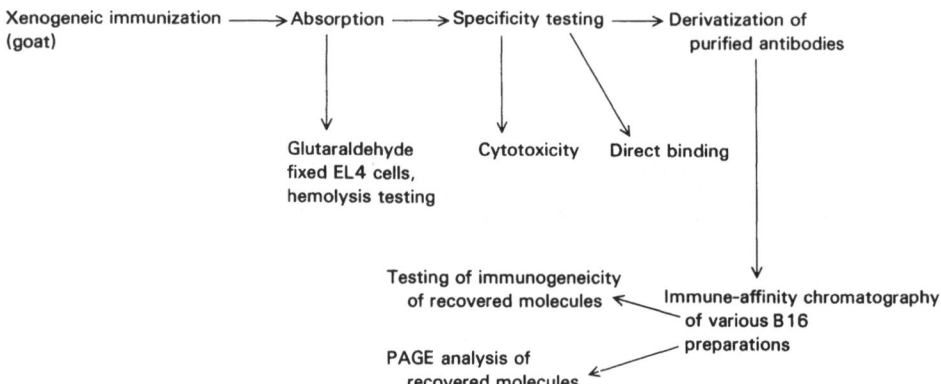

Figure 1. Flow chart of approach to identification of melanoma antigens.

2. Xenogeneic Immunization

B16 melanoma and UV-112 fibrosarcoma were obtained from Dr. I. J. Fidler, who injected the goats. Both B16 and UV-112 (syngeneic to C57BL/6 mice) were inoculated subcutaneously into syngeneic hosts and allowed to grow until the tumors reached a size of 1.5–2.5 cm. At this time, they were removed aseptically, minced in cold Hanks' solution, and dispersed mechanically to prepare single-cell suspensions. Cell viability as measured by Trypan blue exclusion ranged from 25 to 35%. The cell suspension was mixed with complete Freund's adjuvant (CFA) at 4 : 1 ratio. Each goat was injected intradermally at four different sites with 0.5 ml of cell–CFA mixture. A total of 2×10^7 viable cells were injected per goat. Two weeks later, the injection of 2×10^7 viable cells/goat was repeated without CFA. Seven days thereafter, each goat was injected intravenously (i.v.) with 1×10^6 viable cells and bled 2 weeks later. Thereafter, goats were given a booster i.v. injection of 1×10^6 viable cells and were bled on alternate weeks (total of three bleedings). The serum was passed through a 0.22-μm Millipore filter and frozen in liquid nitrogen until absorption. This method is similar to that reported for production of goat anti-mouse macrophage serum (Peterson et al., 1977).

3. Absorption

Whenever mixtures of antigens such as whole cells are used to immunize xenogeneic species, the host animals produce antibodies to many determinants in the mixture. It was necessary, therefore, to absorb out the irrelevant antibodies. These, in the case of murine tumor cells, include antibodies to histocompatibility antigens, viral gycoproteins, and the so-called mouse-specific xenoantigens. An appropriate cell line to use as an absorbant is EL4 lymphoma, since it is syngeneic to C57BL/6 and expresses several viral antigens.

3.1. Growth and Fixation of EL4 Lymphoma Cells

EL4 lymphoma cells were grown at 37°C in 10 liters spinner culture to early stationary phase. The medium was Roswell Park Memorial Institute (RPMI) 1640, supplemented with 10% fetal calf serum (FCS) (Flow Labs, Rockville, Maryland), 1% (vol./vol.) sodium pyruvate, 1% nonessential amino acids, 1% penicillin–streptomycin, 1% glutamine, and 2% Minimal Essential Medium vitamins (GIBCO, Grand Island, New York). The cells were harvested by centrifugation at 350g and washed three times in phosphate-buffered saline [(PBS), 0.145 M NaCl, 0.02 M Na$_2$HPO$_4$, pH 7.4]. The cells were then fixed with 0.5% (wt./vol.) glutaraldehyde in PBS for 1 hr at 4°C. Following the fixation, the cells were washed three times in PBS and 1 mg/ml bovine serum albumin (BSA) as above and stored until use in PBS + 1.0 mg/ml NaN$_3$ at 4°C.

3.2. Absorption of Sera

A pellet of 1 × 10^9 glutaraldehyde-fixed EL4 cells was prepared by washing three times in a solution of 1 mg/ml fraction V BSA (Sigma Chemical Co., St. Louis, Missouri). A 5-ml quantity of goat anti-B16 melanoma or goat anti-UV-112 fibrosarcoma was diluted with 20 ml PBS and added to the EL4 pellet. The suspensions were incubated for 1 hr at 37°C, then 2 hr at 4°C, centrifuged at 500 g, and the supernatants tested for reactivity against C57BL/6 erythrocytes by complement-mediated hemolysis. Hemolysis was assessed by optical measurement of hemoglobin released into the supernatant (OD at 410 μm). Routinely, two to four cycles of absorption were necessary before hemolysis approached background levels. The results, shown in Fig. 2, indicate that reactivity to C57BL/6 erythrocytes could be completely abolished for both the goat-anti B16 (Fig. 2A) and the goat-anti UV-112 (Fig. 2B) sera.

At this juncture, it became necessary to establish that the decrease in reactivity to C57BL/6 erythrocytes was, in fact, attributable to specific absorption, rather than to nonspecific events. We therefore eluted the anti-B16 serum adsorbed to the glutaraldehyde-fixed EL4 cells with elution buffer (0.145 M NaCl + 0.01 M CH$_3$COOH, pH 2.9) and compared the hemolytic activity of the eluate to that of fully absorbed anti-B16 serum, partially absorbed anti-B16 serum, and normal goat serum. Figure 3 indicates the expected specificity of the absorption. On an equal protein basis, the eluate had the strongest complement-mediated hemolytic activity. Normal goat serum and fully absorbed anti-B16 serum had no appreciable hemolytic activity, while the activity of partially absorbed serum was intermediate.

4. Specificity Testing

Having established that the goat anti-B16 serum had no residual activity against C57BL/6 erythrocytes, and that this was due to specific absorption, we could then proceed to assess the specificity of the absorbed serum. The activity of the absorbed anti-B16 serum was titered against cultured B16 cells and then assessed, at appropriate concentrations against various targets.

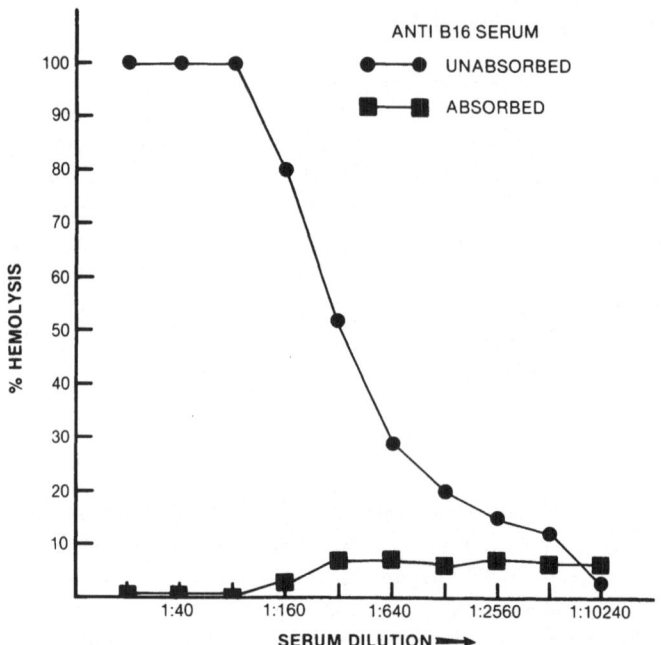

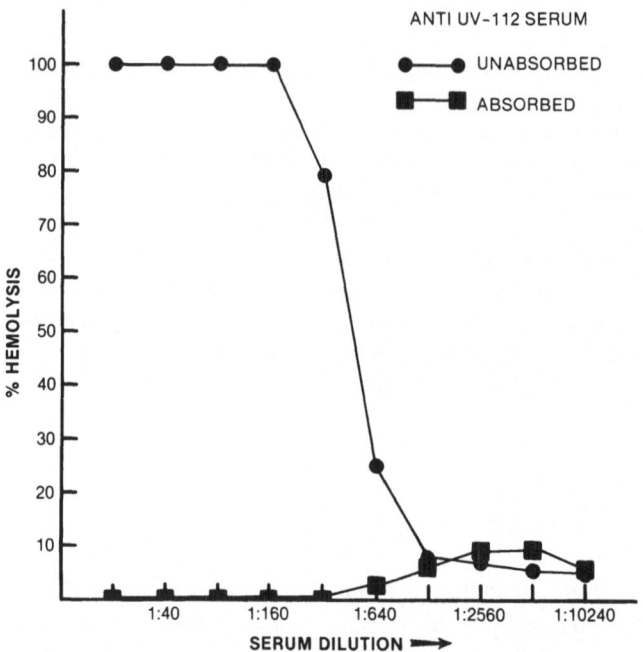

FIGURE 2. Complement-dependent hemolytic activity of goat antisera against C57BL/6 erythrocytes. (A) Goat anti-B16 serum; (B) goat anti UV-112 serum.

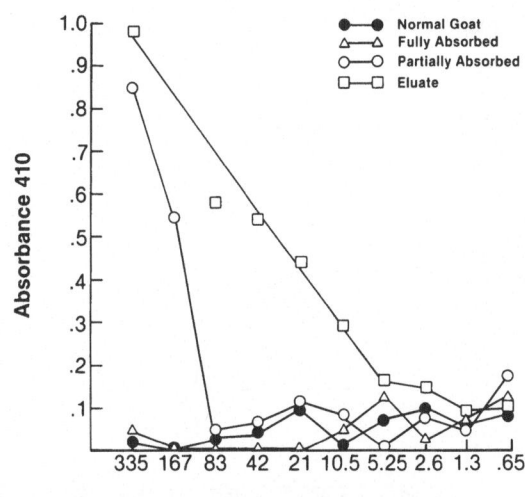

FIGURE 3. Complement-dependent hemolytic activity of normal goat serum and goat anti-B16 melanoma serum against C57BL/6 erythrocytes.

4.1. Titration

Complement-dependent cytotoxicity was assessed by serial dilution against cultured B16 melanoma and UV-112 fibrosarcoma cells by the method of Gately and Mayer (1974).

B16-subline F10 or UV-112 target cells were harvested from the monolayer by brief trypsinization, washed twice in Hanks' solution, and resuspended in Hanks' to a concentration of approximately 1×10^6/ml. A 0.1-ml aliquot of cell suspension was mixed with 0.1 ml antiserum appropriately diluted in PBS and incubated at 37°C in a 12 × 75 mm polypropylene culture tube. The suspension was agitated at 10-min intervals to prevent the cells from plating out on the walls of the tube. After 30 min, 0.02 ml freshly thawed guinea pig complement was added, and the incubation was continued for an additional 45 min. The interaction was terminated by moving the cells to an ice bath while maintaining the agitation at intervals. The cells were washed from the incubation tubes with 10 ml "Isoton" counting electrolyte (Coulter Electronics, Hialeah, Florida), and the cell numbers were determined. The number of intact cells remaining at the end of the incubation was determined by counting the target-cell suspension in a Coulter Counter (Model ZB_1) fitted with a 100-μm aperture tube. The setting of the lower threshold discriminator was adjusted according to the target cell used. The data represent the means of duplicate determinations of at least two separate experiments. The percentage cytotoxicity was calculated by subtracting the number of intact cells remaining in the incubation tube following antiserum treatment from the number of cells in the PBS blank divided by the number of cells in the PBS blank.

Figure 4 indicates that the absorbed goat anti-B16 serum had strong lytic activity against B16 line F10 target cells, but there was no appreciable lysis of UV-112. The background lysis of UV-112 did not vary with antibody concentration and therefore was nonspecific.

It was important to establish that UV-112 was an appropriate negative control in these studies, since the possibility existed that goats are incapable of producing antiserum that recognizes UV-112. Consequently, the goat anti-UV-112 serum was tested for speci-

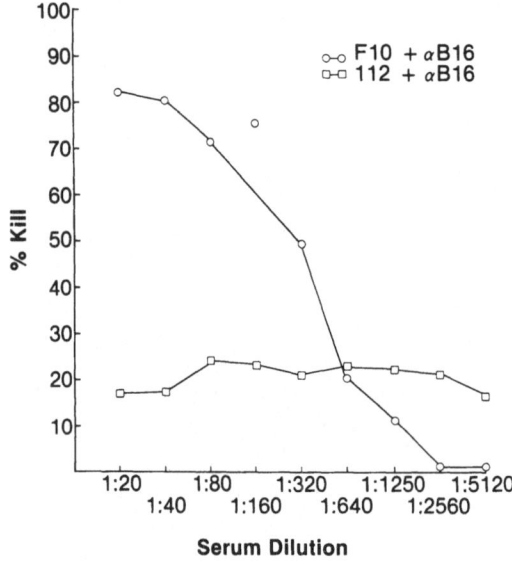

FIGURE 4. Titration curve of absorbed goat anti-B16 serum (complement-dependent lysis) against B16-F10 melanoma and UV-112 fibrosarcoma.

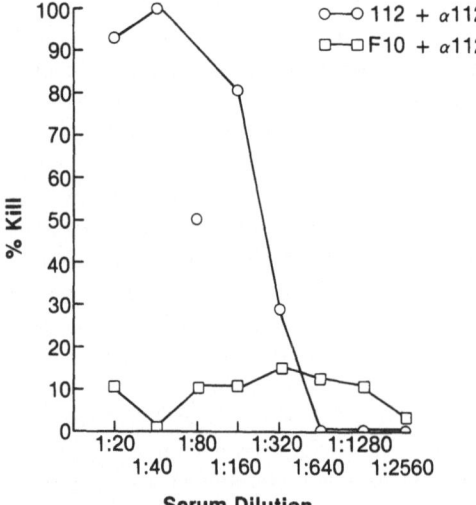

FIGURE 5. Titration curve of absorbed goat anti-UV-112 serum (complement-dependent lysis) against B16-F10 melanoma and UV-112 fibrosarcoma.

ficity. It can be seen in Fig. 5 that absorbed goat anti-UV-112 serum was indeed highly specific for UV-112. Less than 15% lysis of B16-F10 was observed at any serum concentration.

4.2. Specificity Assessment

Based on the titration curve shown in Fig. 4, a serum dilution of 1 : 100 was used for the assessment of specificity against various target-cell lines. Complement-mediated cytotoxicity was measured as above. This dilution gave approximately 60% cytotoxicity of B16-F10.

One of the major problems with the serological approach to isolation of tumor antigens is the definition of the specificity of those antibodies remaining after absorption. Since the number of possible antibody specificities produced by immunization of the goat is undefined, the question of unspecified reactivities cannot be unequivocally answered. Nevertheless, we have been able to rule out the most likely candidates for residual, extraneous activity using the battery of targets listed in Table I.

Table I indicates that the only appreciable complement-mediated cytotoxicity of the absorbed goat anti-B16 melanoma serum is against B16-F10 and B16-F10^{Lr-6} mouse melanoma. At this serum dilution, activity against UV-112 was 11%. This is insignificant, since Fig. 4 indicates a constant background of approximately 15% for this cell line. Since both B16 melanoma and UV-112 fibrosarcoma have the same strain of origin, the absorbed antiserum is not directed against the major histocompatibility complex of the C57BL/6 mouse. The serum recognizes neither UV-112 or UV-112 infected with a C-type virus of C57BL/6 origin. This suggests that whatever antibodies might have been directed against viral glycoproteins were removed by the EL4 absorption. Similarly, the absence of cytotoxicity against AKR low-passage fibroblasts and AKR-Tu argues against viral glycoproteins. Three different strains of mice, C57BL/6, C₃H, and AKR, were tested. On this basis, mouse-specific xenoantigens may be ruled out.

TABLE I

Complement-Mediated Cytotoxicity of Absorbed Goat Anti-B16 Melanoma Serum against Various Targets

Target-cell description	Description	Host of origin	C-type virus[a]	Cytotoxicity (%)[b]	References[c]
B16-F10	Melanoma	C57BL/6 mouse	Positive	57 ± 6	Fidler (1973)
B16-F10^{Lr-6}	Melanoma	C57BL/6 mouse	Positive	32 ± 3	Fidler *et al.* (1976)
UV-112	Fibrosarcoma	C57BL/6 mouse	Negative	11 ± 2	Kripke (1977)
UV-112[d]	Fibrosarcoma	C75BL/6 mouse	Positive	0 ± 0	Kripke (1977)
UV-2237	Fibrosarcoma	C₃H mouse	Negative	3 ± 1	Kripke (1977)
AKR low-passage	Fibroblast	AKR mouse	Negative	4 ± 1	Fidler (1978)
AKR-Tu	Adenocarcinoma	AKR mouse	Positive	0 ± 0	Fidler (1978)
DMBA-II	Fibrosarcoma	F344 rat	Negative	5 ± 1	Fidler (1978)

[a]The presence of endogenous C-type virus (MuLV) was determined by radioimmune precipitation (Fidler, 1978).
[b]Data are the means ± S.E.M. of data pooled from two experiments each representing two observations of each of three separate determinations.
[c]Reference for characterization of tumor lines.
[d]Produced by deliberate infection of UV-112 virus negative cell line.

4.3. Antibody Binding

The assessment of antibody specificity by complement-mediated cytotoxicity may be performed by many different assays. Each is subject to its own particular limitations. The most severe problem of the Coulter Counter assay used above is the requirement that the tumor cells, which normally grow in culture as monolayers, must be trypsinized to yield single-cell suspensions. We sought, therefore, to verify and further quantitate the binding of antibody by a technique that utilized native rather than trypsinized cell surfaces.

Goat immunoglobulin G (IgG) was purified from the absorbed serum by affinity chromatography on a column of protein A–Sepharose (Pharmacia Fine Chemicals, Piscataway, New Jersey) as described previously (Marchalonis *et al.*, 1978). Tumor cells were inoculated into a 96-well microtest plate (Falcon Plastics, Oxnard, Canada) at a concentration of $1–10 \times 10^3$ cells/0.2 ml well and allowed to grow to confluence. The wells were washed twice with PBS and the monolayers fixed to the plastic with glutaraldehyde according to the method of Segal and Klinman (1976). The fixation solution was 0.1 M potassium phosphate buffer, pH 7.0, to which glutaraldehyde was added to a final concentration of 0.15 (wt./vol.). After 5-min incubation at room temperature, the wells were washed twice with a solution of fraction V BSA, 1.0 ml/ml, containing 1 mg/ml NaN_3. The plates were stored at 4°C until use.

Immediately prior to use, the plates were warmed to room temperature and the wells were washed twice with PBS to remove residual BSA and NaN_3. Appropriately diluted IgG, 50 µl, was overlaid on the monolayer and incubated for 2 hr at room temperature. The wells were washed twice more with PBS and overlaid with 100 µl protein A from *Staphylococcus aureus* that had been prelabeled with ^{125}I by the chloramine T method (Greenwood *et al.*, 1963). Although goat IgG does not bind protein A as well as IgG antibodies of other species, we and others (Langone, 1980) have found that effective assays can be developed using goat antibodies and protein A. The protein A solution contained 100–200 ng protein A/ml in 1 mg/ml BSA. Following overnight incubation of the plates at 4°C, unbound radioactivity was removed by two washes in PBS. The monolayers were harvested and counted for radioactivity.

In Fig. 6, a serial dilution is depicted in which the binding of goat anti-B16 melanoma IgG antibodies is quantitated. As in Fig. 4, the antibody shows strong reactivity to B16-

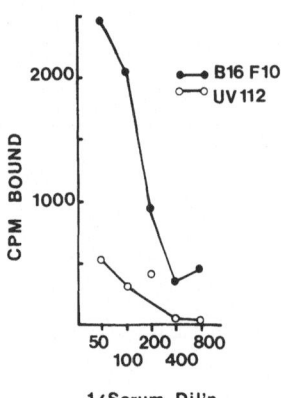

Figure 6. Quantitation of binding of absorbed goat anti-B16 melanoma antibodies to B16-F10 melanoma monolayers and UV-112 fibrosarcoma monolayers.

F10 in the absence of binding to UV-112 fibrosarcoma. Serial dilution experiments were also performed using the absorbed goat-anti B16 melanoma serum against another mouse melanoma, 1735-Mel 8 (Kripke, 1979). This melanoma is syngeneic to C_3H mice. Therefore, the negative control used was UV-2237, also of C_3H origin. The antiserum has been shown in Table I to have no reactivity toward UV-2237. This serial dilution (Fig. 7) indicates that mouse melanoma 1735-Mel 8 has serological cross-reactivity to B16-F10, albeit at a lower level, while being unreactive to UV-2237.

A 1 : 100 dilution of purified goat anti-B16 melanoma IgG was used to quantitate binding to various melanoma derivatives and nonmelanoma controls. The data (Table II) represent the means ± S.E.M. of three observations in at least two separate experiments. Counts per minute bound refers to the amount of [^{125}I] protein A remaining in the microtest wells following antibody binding and washing. Five derivatives (kindly provided by I. J. Fidler) of B16 melanoma were tested. All the B16 sublines bound antiserum, but quantitative variation was observed, and the following rank order was established: F10 = $F10^{Lr-6}$ > FO > FO-U_1 = FO-U_2. On this basis, it is unlikely that the antiserum is directed against melanin. FO-U_1 and FO-U_2 are paired pigmented and nonpigmented isolates and show equal reactivity. F10 and FO presumably contain equal amounts of melanin, yet bind

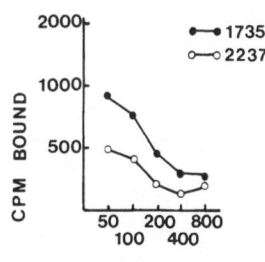

FIGURE 7. Quantitation of binding of absorbed goat anti-B16 melanoma antibodies to 1735-Mel 8 melanoma monolayers and 2237 fibrosarcoma monolayers.

TABLE II

Goat Anti-B16 Melanoma Antiserum Binding to Surface of Fixed Murine Melanoma Cells[a]

Target-cell designation	Strain of origin	Description	Counts per minute bound[b]
B16-FO	C57BL/6	Parent tumor to which antiserum was raised; pigmented; low metastasis	1620 ± 40
B16-FO-U_1	C57BL/6	Pigmented variant; low metastasis	1360 ± 130
B16-FO-U_2	C57BL/6	Nonpigmented variant; low metastasis	1220 ± 130
B16-F10	C57BL/6	Selected *in vivo;* pigmented; high metastasis	2050 ± 180
B16-$F10^{Lr-6}$	C57BL/6	Selected *in vitro;* pigmented; resistant to lysis by syngeneic lymphocytes; low metastasis	1960 ± 180
UV-112	C57BL/6	Fibrosarcoma syngeneic to C57BL/6 mouse	330 ± 18
1735-Mel 8	C_3H	Melanoma syngeneic to C_3H mouse	1460 ± 170
UV-2237	C_3H	Fibrosarcoma syngeneic to C_3H mouse	405 ± 20

[a]Reprinted from Gersten and Marchalonis (1979) with permission from Academic Press.
[b]Data are the means ± S.E.M. of three observations in at least two separate experiments.

different amounts of antibody. The C_3H melanoma 1735 bound an average of 1460 cpm, while the C_3H fibrosarcoma bound only 405 cpm.

To summarize the results of the specificity studies, the purified goat anti-B16 melanoma serum recognizes all mouse melanoma tumor lines tested but none of the others. Both the complement-dependent cytotoxicity studies and the direct binding studies agree. The antiserum does not appear to react with histocompatibility antigens, mouse-specific or rat-specific xenoantigens, C-type viral glycoproteins, or melanin. We have therefore considered the antiserum to be purified to apparent specificity. We recognize the limitations of this consideration.

5. Derivatization

In considering the methods available for covalent linkage of IgG antibodies to solid-phase matrices, it was apparent that these tend to be low-efficiency procedures. The reason is that there are numerous sites on the IgG molecule that can be coupled to the activated matrix. Thus, the orientation of the IgG molecule relative to the matrix is often such that the combining site participates in the linkage or is sterically blocked. We have used the method of Gersten and Marchalonis (1978) in which IgG antibodies are adsorbed via their constant fragment (Fc) portions to protein A–Sepharose. Cross-linking is then performed using the bifunctional reagent dimethyl-suberimidate. Thus, the antibody is attached in a high-efficiency orientation by its Fc portion and uses both the Fc portion and the protein A as spacers from the Sepharose bead.

6. Immune-Affinity Chromatography

Having purified the goat anti-B16 melanoma serum to apparent specificity, demonstrated that it recognizes melanoma-associated surface components, and derivatized the antibodies to a solid-phase matrix, we could proceed to recover the antigen(s) from cell-culture preparations. In the initial experiments, B16-F10 and UV-112 monolayer cultures were washed free of conditioned medium and allowed to "shed" components into serumless medium. The released material was exhaustively dialyzed against distilled water, lyophilized, and radioiodinated. The radioiodinated material was allowed to adsorb, in batch, to matrices of goat anti-B16–protein A–Sepharose or normal goat IgG–protein A–Sepharose. The results indicated specific binding of the B16 shed material but not the UV-112 shed material (Table III). The affinity-purified material was eluted from the matrix using "elution buffer" as described in Section 3.2. Portions of these iodinated, shed, specifically bound preparations were analyzed by sodium dodecyl sulfate–polyacrylamide gel electrophoresis (SDS-PAGE) as described in Section 7.

Two other types of preparation were subjected to immune-affinity column chromatography: Triton X-100 extracts of whole-cell preparations of B16-F10 and Triton X-100 extracts of metabolically labeled whole-cell preparations.

TABLE III
Immune-Affinity Binding of ¹²⁵I-Labeled Shed Material[a]

	Preparation	
Matrix	UV-112 shed material	B16-F10 shed material
Normal goat IgG–protein A–Sepharose	1300	11,600
Anti B16 IgG–protein A–Sepharose	830	44,700

[a]Reprinted from Gersten and Marchalonis (1979) with permission from Academic Press.

7. Sodium Dodecyl Sulfate–Polyacrylamide Gel Electrophoresis

Several different preparations of "shed" and cell-extract material, purified by immune-affinity chromatography, were analyzed by SDS-PAGE. The method was essentially that of Laemmli and Favre (1973) using conditions and standards described previously (Atwell and Marchalonis, 1975).

The first preparations analyzed were the shed materials of B16-F10 melanoma and UV-112 fibrosarcoma described in Section 6, since this has been reported to be a rich source of B16 melanoma antigens (Bystryn, 1978). The results, shown in Fig. 8A, indicate that affinity-purified material from B16-F10 melanoma consists of a major peak of approxi-

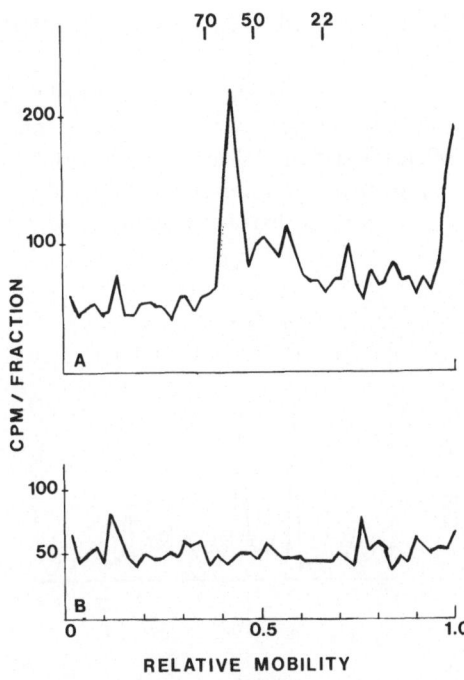

FIGURE 8. SDS-PAGE of ¹²⁵I-labeled "shed" material recovered by immune-affinity chromatography in 10% SDS-polyacrylamide gels. (A) Material shed by B16-F10 melanoma monolayers; (B) Material shed by UV-112 fibrosarcoma monolayers.

mately 65,000, a second peak of approximately 50,000, and a minor peak of 15,000–20,000. The presence of the 15,000–20,000 peak was variable with culture conditions. The corresponding UV-112 shed prepartion, purified by immune-affinity chromatography, was similarly analyzed and is shown in Fig. 8B. It can be seen that no specific peaks are present in the UV-112 preparation. This is consistent with the titration data indicating a low, constant background (see Figs. 4 and 6 and Table III).

Due to the 65,000-dalton nature of the primary protein, it became necessary to ensure that this was not an albumin artifact of the culture technique. We therefore grew a B16-F10 melanoma culture to mid-log phase and replaced the medium after washing with leucineless RPMI 1640 medium supplemented with 2% FCS and [^{3}H]leucine. A Triton X-100 extract was prepared from the metabolically labeled cells, and the antigens were purified and analyzed by SDS-PAGE. All labeled, high-molecular-weight material must therefore be a product of cellular metabolism and cannot be an artifact of the culturing process. Figure 9 indicates that the 65,000, 50,000, and 15,000 peaks are again obtained, although the proportions are slightly different—probably the result of different culture conditions.

The next preparation analyzed was a bulk-affinity isolation from a 0.1% Triton X-100 extract of whole B16-F10 cells, grown to subconfluence in culture. In this preparation, the primary peak of 65,000 is again recovered when the analysis is run under reducing conditions (Fig. 10). A preliminary experiment indicates that under nonreducing conditions, the antigens remain near the origin of the gel, suggesting an aggregate molecular weight of over 150,000.

8. Testing of Recovered Molecules

To ensure that the affinity-purified fraction in fact contained specific B16-melanoma-associated antigens, two rabbits were immunized with the putative antigen preparation isolated from material released into serum-free medium. The fraction was eluted from the immunoadsorbent using elution buffer, dialyzed against PBS, and passed through a column of protein A–Sepharose to remove any IgG that might have eluted from the matrix. Two

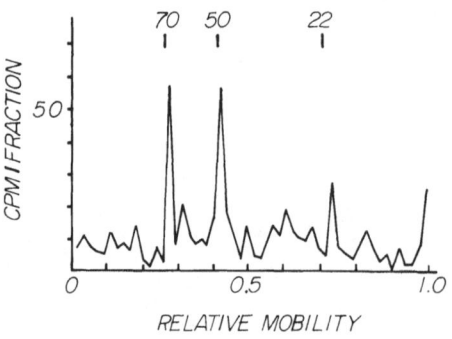

FIGURE 9. SDS-PAGE of ^{3}H-metabolically labeled cell extracts, recovered by immune-affinity chromatography. 10% SDS–polyacrylamide gels.

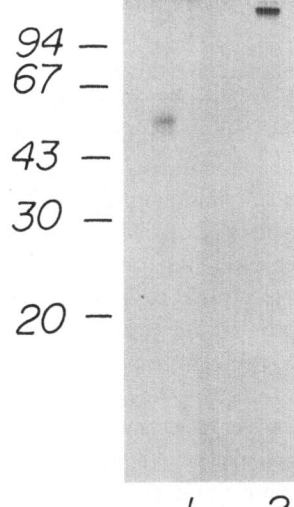

FIGURE 10. SDS-PAGE of unlabeled cell extracts, recovered by immune-affinity chromatography. 10% SDS–polyacrylamide gels. (1) Sample reduced with mercaptoethanol; (2) sample not reduced with mercaptoethanol.

FIGURE 11. Binding to B16-F10 melanoma and UV-112 fibrosarcoma target cells of rabbit antisera produced against the melanoma-associated xenoantigen preparation isolated using goat antibodies.(●) Antiserum tested on B16 cells; (■) antiserum tested on UV-112 cells; (○) preimmunization serum tested on B16 cells. Reprinted from Gersten and Marchalonis (1979) with permission from Academic Press.

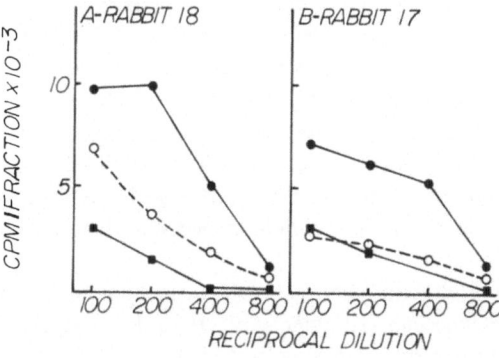

rabbits were each given two injections consisting of 200 μg (Lowry) of purified antigen preparation. The first injection was given in CFA; the second was given 3 weeks later using incomplete FA. Serum was obtained 2 weeks following the second injection. In addition, serum samples were obtained from the same rabbits prior to the immunization, to serve as a control for naturally occurring antibodies. Both preimmune and immune sera were absorbed with EL4 cells to remove antimouse activity. The binding to monolayers of B16-F10 melanoma and UV-112 fibrosarcoma was then assessed as described in Section 4.3.

Immunization with the specifically purified antigen preparation induced the rabbits to produce antibodies that recognized components of the cell surface of B16 melanoma cells but not UV-112 cells (Fig. 11). One rabbit (No. 18) demonstrated some activity against B16 cell-surface components prior to immunization, but binding to B16 was substantially increased by the immunization.

9. Discussion

We have raised a xenogeneic antiserum in goats to the murine B16 melanoma. After exhaustive absorption, the antiserum has been purified to apparent specificity. The reactivity of the purified antiserum appears to be directed against protein determinants unique to the immunizing tumor, B16 melanoma, and to the allogeneic melanoma, 1735-Mel 8. A solid-phase immune absorbant was made by derivatizing the purified IgG antibodies to a matrix of protein A–Sepharose using the bifunctional cross-linking agent dimethylsuberimidate. Preparations of Triton X-100 extracts of cultured B16 cells and of material shed from cultured cells into serumless medium were purified by immune-affinity chromatography and analyzed by SDS-PAGE. Injection of the affinity-purified material into rabbits induced them to produce IgG antibodies that specifically recognized moieties resident on the surface of the B16 melanoma cells.

The major antigen recovered has a molecular weight of approximately 65,000. A less prominent band of 50,000 and minor peak at 15,000–20,000 are also seen when the SDS gels are run under reducing conditions. The relative proportions of the antigens recovered by this approach appear to vary with culture conditions (see Figs. 8–10), an observation that has been made previously for B16 antigens (Poskitt et al., 1976) and for other B16 properties as well (Bosmann et al., 1973; Gersten and Bosmann, 1975; Satoh et al., 1974).

In previous attempts to isolate B16 melanoma antigens (Bystryn et al., 1974; Bystryn, 1976), a glycoprotein of 150,000–200,000 was prepared by gel filtration on Sephadex G200. This glycoprotein was reactive to their antibody (Bystryn et al., 1974) and conferred partial protection, against a tumor challenge, to mice preimmunized with that preparation (Bystryn, 1978). We demonstrated (Fig. 10) that the nonreduced molecular weight of the primary (65,000) band is in the 150,000–200,000 range. The nature and number of molecular species in the broad G200 peak have yet to be determined (Smalley, personal communication). This would be necessary before identity could be established between the two preparations.

Protein patterns of B16 melanoma have been compared to those of C57BL/6 normal melanocytes (Klingler et al., 1976; Hearing and Nicholson, 1979). In an elegant series of experiments, Hearing and Nicholson (1979) have studied the major protein of normal (C700) and B16 (B700) melanosomes. They have suggested, on the basis of N-terminal analysis, C-terminal analysis, amino acid analysis, and fingerprint analysis, that B700 is a deletion variant of C700, possibly the result of intragenic spacers and defective splicing. They have further demonstrated that B700 but not C700 gives a positive response when tested for antigenicity in a syngeneic system (Hearing et al., 1978; Kerney et al., 1977). The molecular weight of B700 is 68,000. Since the reduced molecular weight of the primary peak in Figs. 8A, 9, and 10 is approximately 65,000, it would be attractive to speculate on their identity. Experiments to determine this are currently in progress.

Finally, proteins similar to B700 have been found in Cloudman melanoma and in the serum and urine of human melanoma patients (Tomecki et al., 1980). These observations support the idea of structural similarity among proteins of similar tumors from different species. It should be remembered, of course, that structural similarity, as in the case of B700 and C700 above, does not necessitate antigeneic cross-reactivity. Nevertheless, it may be possible to demonstrate such cross-reactivity using xenogeneic antisera such as the one described herein. It is likely that such sera will be capable of recognizing distinct alternate sites on the antigeneic molecules. Studies directed toward determining precisely the antigenic sites of B16 antigens will be aided materially by the production of monoclonal antibodies against the purified proteins reactive with the specific xenoantisera described herein.

References

Atwell, J. L., and Marchalonis, J. J., 1975, Phylogenetic emergence of immunoglobulin classes distinct from IgM, *J. Immunogenet.* **1**:367.

Bosmann, H. B., Bieber, G. F., Brown, A. E., Case, K. R., Gersten, D. M., Kimmerer, T. W., and Lione, A., 1973, Biochemical parameters correlated with tumour cell implantation, *Nature (London)* **246**:487.

Bystryn, J. C., 1976, Release of tumor associated antigens by murine melanoma cells, *J. Immunol.* **116**:1302.

Bystryn, J. C., 1978, Antibody response and tumor growth in syngeneic mice immunized to partially purified B16 melanoma associated antigens, *J. Immunol.* **120**:96.

Bystryn, J. C., Shenkein, I., Baur, S., and Uhr, J. W., 1974, Partial isolation and characterization of antigen(s) associated with murine melanoma, *J. Natl. Cancer Inst.* **52**:1263.

Fidler, I. J., 1973, Selection of successive tumor lines for metastasis, *Nature (London) New Biol.* **242**:148.

Fidler, I. J., 1978, Recognition and destruction of target cells by tumoricidal macrophages, *Isr. J. Med, Sci.* **14**:177.

Fidler, I. J., Gersten, D. M., and Budmen, M. B., 1976, Characterization *in vivo* and *in vitro* of tumor cells selected for resistance to syngeneic lymphocyte-mediated cytotoxicity, *Cancer Res.* **36**:3160.

Fidler, I. J., Gersten, D. M., and Riggs, C. W., 1977, Relationship of host immune status to tumor cell arrest, distribution and survival in experimental metastasis, *Cancer* **40**:46.

Gately, M. K., and Mayer, M. M., 1974, The molecular dimensions of guinea pig lymphotoxin, *J. Immunol.* **112**:168.

Gersten, D. M., 1980, Control of growth and vascularity of B16 melanoma by syngeneic lymphocytes, *Cell Biol. Int. Rep.* **4**:407.

Gersten, D. M., and Bosmann, H. B., 1975, Surface properties of plasma membranes following ionizing radiation exposure, *Exp. Cell Res.* **96**:215.

Gersten, D. M., and Marchalonis, J. J., 1978, A rapid, novel method for the solid phase derivatization of IgG antibodies for immune-affinity chromatography, *J. Immunol. Methods* **24**:305.

Gersten, D. M., and Marchalonis, J. J., 1979, Demonstration and isolation of murine melanoma-associated antigenic surface proteins, *Biochem. Biophys. Res. Comm.* **90**:1015.

Greenwood, F. C., Hunter, W. M., and Glover, J. S., 1963, The preparation of ^{131}I-labelled human growth hormone of high specific activity, *Biochem. J.* **89**:114.

Hearing, V. J., and Nicholson, J. M., 1979, Abnormal protein synthesis in malignant melanoma cells, *Cancer Biochem. Biophys.* **4**:59.

Hearing, V. J., Kerney, S. E., Montague, P. M., Ekel, T. M., and Nicholson, J. M., 1978, Characterization of the intracellular location of tumor associated antigens in B16 murine malignant melanoma, *Pigment Cell* **5**:148.

Kerney, S. E., Montague, P. M., Cretien, P. B., Nicholson, J. M., Ekel, T. M., and Hearing, V. J., 1977, Intracellular localization of tumor associated antigens in murine and human malignant melanoma, *Cancer Res.* **37**:1519.

Klingler, W. G., Montague, P. M., and Hearing, V. J., 1976, Unique melanosomal proteins in murine melanomas, *Pigment Cell* **2**:1.

Kripke, M. L., 1977, Latency, histology and antigenicity of tumors induced by ultraviolet light in three inbred mouse strains, *Cancer Res.* **37**:1395.

Kripke, M. L., 1979, Speculation on the role of ultraviolet radiation in the development of malignant melanoma, *J. Natl. Cancer Inst.* **63**:541.

Laemmli, U. K., and Favre, M., 1973, Maturation of the head of bacteriophage T4. I. DNA packaging events, *J. Mol. Biol.* **80**:575.

Langone, J. J., 1980, ^{125}I labeled protein as a general tracer in immunoassay: Suitability of goat and sheep antibodies, *J. Immunol. Methods* **34**:93.

Marchalonis, J. J., Atwell, J. L., and Goding, J. W., 1978, Immunoglobulins of a monotreme, the echidna *Tachyglossus aculeatus:* Two distinct isotypes which bind a protein of *Staphylococcus aureus, Immunology* **34**:97.

Peterson, P. E., Bucana, C. D., Fidler, I. J., 1977, Immunologic specificity and reactivity of goat anti-guinea pig and goat anti-mouse macrophage sera, *J. Reticuloendothel. Soc.* **21**:119.

Poskitt, P. F., Poskitt, T. R., and Wallace, J. H., 1976, Release into culture medium of membrane associated, tumor specific antigen by B16 melanoma cells, *Proc. Soc. Exp. Biol. Med.* **152**:76.

Satoh, C., Banks, J., Horst, P., Kreider, J. W., and Davidson, E. A., 1974, Polysaccharide production by cultured B16 mouse melanoma cells, *Biochemistry* **13**:1233.

Segal, G. P., and Klinman, N. R., 1976, Defining the heterogeneity of anti-tumor antibody responses, *J. Immunol.* **116**:1539.

Tomecki, K. J., Montague, P. M., and Hearing, V. J., 1980, Serum and urine protein differences in patients with malignant melanoma, *J. Natl. Cancer Inst.* **64**:29.

8

Clinical Significance of Tumor-Associated Antigens and Antitumor Antibodies in Human Malignant Melanoma

RISHAB K. GUPTA AND DONALD L. MORTON

1. Introduction

The concept that an immune response similar to that of infectious diseases is elicited in patients suffering from malignancy is well established. This concept was first developed during the early 1900s when it was observed that transplantable neoplasms in randomly bred laboratory mice could induce a strong immunity. On the basis of these observations, it was hypothesized that immune defense could play an important role in controlling the growth of cancer in man. This hypothesis was supported by the following findings: (1) spontaneous regression of established tumor (Everson and Cole, 1966); (2) delayed recurrence of rapidly progressive disease after successful treatment of the primary tumor (Lewis and Kiryabwire, 1968); (3) association of lymphocyte and other cellular infiltration into tumor with an improved prognosis (Black *et al.*, 1956); (4) presence of tumor cells in lymphatics, peripheral blood, pleural cavity, and operative wounds of patients without subsequent development of metastases (Griffiths, *et al.*, 1973; Roberts *et al.*, 1967); and (5) inhibition of tumor autotransplants when mixed with autologous leukocytes or plasma in almost half the patients studied (Southam *et al.*, 1966).

RISHAB K. GUPTA AND DONALD L. MORTON • Division of Oncology, Department of Surgery, UCLA School of Medicine, University of California, Los Angeles, California 90024; and Surgical Service, V. A. Medical Center, Sepulveda, California 91343.

2. Immune Response vs. Development of Malignancy

The importance of immune response of the host in controlling the development and progression of the malignancy is evident from various clinical observations. Human beings with congenital immunological deficiency disorders, i.e., ataxia–telangiectasia and Wiscott–Aldrich syndrome, have a high incidence of spontaneous neoplasms (Gatti and Good, 1971; Peterson et al., 1964). Immunosuppressive therapy has been reported to be associated with increased incidence of development of malignancy (Gatti and Good, 1971; McKhann, 1969; Penn et al., 1969; Penn, 1970). Various forms of immunotherapy of cancer patients have been shown to cause regression of the disease (Eilber et al., 1976; Morton et al., 1975; Nathanson, 1974; Oettgen et al., 1976; Pilch et al., 1976; Pinsky et al., 1972; Seigler et al., 1972). Impaired cell-mediated immune response appeared to correlate with poor prognosis of clinical course of the malignant disease (Eilber and Morton, 1970; Morton et al., 1971b).

3. Recognition of Tumor-Associated Antigens Expressed by Human Melanoma

Numerous attempts have been made to detect tumor-associated antigens (TAAs) in human malignant melanoma by a variety of in vitro and in vivo cellular reactions and by in vitro serological tests. In the latter instance, both sera from cancer patients and antisera produced in xenogeneic hosts have been used as the source of antibody.

3.1. In Vivo Cellular Reactions

Delayed cutaneous hypersensitivity reaction (DCHR) in cancer patients has been used to recognize TAAs in extracts of cultured and biopsy melanoma cells (Bluming et al., 1972; Char et al., 1974; Della Porta et al., 1979; Fass et al., 1970; Hollinshead et al., 1974; Roth et al., 1976; Stewart, 1969). Hollinshead et al. (1974) and Char et al., (1974) have been successful in eliciting DCHR using partially purified antigen from low-frequency sonic extracts of melanoma cells. Roth et al. (1976) used 3 M KCl extracts (Reisfeld et al., 1971) of melanoma specimens to purify the antigenic component. Though DCHR reflects cellular immune reaction, it is a relatively complex reaction, and precise quantitation of different antigenic components is difficult. It has been pointed out by Ristow and McKhann (1977) that the ideal conditions of testing the extracts in the patient who provided the tumor were generally not met, thus raising the possibility of false-positive or false-negative reactions. Furthermore, the skin is capable of a limited range of responses and inflammation may occur following injection of many materials. Oren and Herberman (1971) have reported that use of too much material, even of control, might result in false-positive reactions.

3.2. *In Vitro* Cellular Reactions

Specific cytotoxicity against human malignant melanoma has been documented by a number of investigators (Fossati *et al.*, 1971; DeVries *et al.*, 1972; I. Hellström *et al.*, 1973b; Heppner *et al.*, 1973; Peter *et al.*, 1975; Canevari *et al.*, 1976; Steel *et al.*, 1976) using lymphcoytes from cancer patients. In these assays, it is believed that the lymphocytes are cytotoxic because of sensitization to TAAs expressed by the melanoma cells. However, nonspecific reactions have also been observed (Tagasuki *et al.*, 1973; I. Hellström *et al.*, 1973a; Rosenberg *et al.*, 1974). Despite the nonspecificity and technical problems associated with *in vitro* cellular assays, the presence of TAAs in tumor-cell extracts and patients' sera has been demonstrated by inhibition studies (Currie and Basham, 1972; Embleton and Price, 1975; K. E. Hellström and I. Hellström, 1974).

3.3. Serological Reactions

Detection and definition of TAAs in melanoma cells has been achieved by autologous and allogeneic antibody (sera from melanoma patients) as well as by xenoantibody (antisera raised in heterospecies).

3.3.1. Xenoantibody

Despite a great deal of effort to produce specific antisera in heterospecies for TAAs expressed by human melanoma cells, there has been little success. The antisera that were initially thought to be specific for melanoma TAAs were later found to react with normal antigens as well (Ting and Herberman, 1976). Only in recent years have xenoantisera that possess some degree of specificity been developed (Seigler *et al.*, 1975a; Stuhlmiller and Seigler, 1975; Ghose *et al.*, 1975; Viza and Phillips, 1975; McCabe *et al.*, 1978a, 1979; Gupta *et al.*, 1980; Ax *et al.*, 1976; Bystryn and Smalley, 1977).

Stuhlmiller and Seigler (1975) produced antisera in a chimpanzee that contained antibodies to melanoma TAAs and fetal antigens. Ghose *et al.*, (1975) were successful in developing antisera in rabbits and goats that reacted, after absorptions, with melanoma cells and not with normal counterparts. The TTAs were expressed in cytoplasm as well as on the surface of melanoma cells. Partially purified membrane extracts of melanoma have been used by Viza and Phillips (1975) to produce antisera in rabbits. Recently, McCabe *et al.*, (1978a, 1979) and Gupta *et al.* (1980) have been able to raise antibodies to melanoma TAAs by immunizing rabbits with antigens isolated from spent culture medium of melanoma cells.

More recently, melanoma TAAs have been recognized by the use of monoclonal antibodies (Koprowski *et al.*, 1978; Yeh *et al.*, 1979; I. Hellström *et al.*, 1980). Carrel *et al.* (1980) have defined common melanoma-associated antigen(s) that were expressed by at least 15 different melanoma cell lines. These investigators used two monoclonal antibodies directed against different common antigenic determinants. Gallaway *et al.* (1980) have been successful in isolation and characterization of melanoma TAAs with the use of monoclonal antibody. However, it remains to be determined, as with other xenoantibody, whether or not these melanoma TAAs are also recognized by the antibody elicited in melanoma patients in response to their disease.

3.3.2. Sera from Melanoma Patients

There is a wealth of data in the literature that provides evidence regarding the expression of certain components by malignant melanoma cells that are immunogenic in autologous and allogeneic hosts. Though the biological and biochemical characteristics of these antigens are not fully understood, they are recognized as TAAs. A variety of serological techniques, listed in Table I, have been used to demonstrate the immunological reactivity between these antigens and sera from melanoma patients.

4. Types of Tumor-Associated Antigens Expressed by Melanoma Cells

On the basis of humoral cross-reactivity and absorption studies, melanoma TAAs, detected by the use of patients' antibody, can be grouped into four categories: (1) fetal antigens (Seibert et al., 1977; Romsdahl and Cox, 1970; Irie et al., 1976); (2) common melanoma-associated antigens (Morton et al., 1968; Romsdahl and Cox, 1970; Cornain et al., 1975); (3) group-specific antigens—antigens that are expressed by a few but not all melanomas (Shiku et al., 1976); and (4) individually specific antigens (Nairn et al., 1972; Bodurtha et al., 1975; Lewis and Phillips, 1972; Shiku et al., 1976; Carey et al., 1976; The et al., 1975).

TABLE I

In Vitro Serological Assays Used for Detection of Melanoma Tumor-Associated Antigens or Antibodies in Sera from Melanoma Patients

Serological technique	References
Antibody-mediated cytotoxicity	Lewis et al. (1969), Gray et al. (1971), Bodurtha et al (1975), Romsdhal and Cox (1973), Hersey et al. (1976), Ferrone and Pellegrino (1977)
Immune adherence	Cornain et al. (1975), Macher et al. (1975), Irie et al. (1976), Shiku et al. (1976)
Immunofluorescence	Morton et al. (1968), Oettgen et al. (1968), Lewis et al. (1969, 1971, 1973), Muna et al. (1969), Morton (1971), Lewis and Phillips (1972), Nairn et al (1972), Elliott et al. (1973), Mukherji et al. (1973), Wood and Barth (1974)
Mixed hemadsorption	Carey et al. (1976), Seibert et al. (1977), Liao et al. (1978)
Complement fixation	Morton et al. (1970, 1971a), Gupta and Morton (1975a), Gupta et al. (1978a, 1979c,d)
Radioimmunoassay	Gupta (1980), Gupta and Morton (1979c)

Some of the melanoma TAAs have been localized on the cell surface (Bodurtha *et al.*, 1975; Lewis and Phillips, 1972; Gray *et al.*, 1971; Romsdahl and Cox, 1970; Morton *et al.*, 1968), others in the cytoplasm (Wood and Barth, 1974; Bourgoin and Bourgoin, 1973; Lewis and Phillips, 1972). McBride *et al.* (1972) detected the presence of antinucleolar antibodies in the sera of patients with malignant melanoma. The nucleolar antigen, apparently a ribonucleoprotein, is not melanoma-specific; however, its presence in tumor cells correlates directly with the clinical status of the patient and represents a poor prognosis for the disease (Bowen *et al.*, 1976).

Of the two groups of antigens, one individually specific and the other common to most melanomas, identified by the immunofluorescence technique by Morton *et al.* (1968), Muna *et al* (1969), and Lewis *et al.* (1969), the first group was associated with the cell surface and the second with the cytoplasm. Localization of the common group of melanoma TAAs defined by the complement-fixation assay was not possible because disrupted melanoma cells were used as the target antigens (Morton, 1971).

The membrane-rich fraction of an autopsied melanoma showed a wide cross-reactivity against sera from patients with malignancies of various histological types in complement fixation (Gupta, 1975). Extracts of sarcoma and carcinoma tissues were also widely cross-reactive. Absorption of the sera with fetal tissue homogenates revealed that the cross-reactivity was probably due to antigens of fetal origin (Gupta and Morton, 1977). Similar wide cross-reactivity was observed by Grimm *et al.* (1976) when partially purified spent culture medium of a melanoma cell line was used. A membrane antigen common to both human cancer cells and fetal brain tissue has been reported by Irie *et al.* (1976). This antigen has been termed the oncofetal antigen (OFA). OFA has been shown to be immunogenic in man by its ability to elicit humoral antibody in patients with cancer (Irie *et al.*, 1976).

From the foregoing reports, it is obvious that the antigenic composition of human malignant melanoma is quite diverse. Of course, this antigenic diversity could be due to the use of different serological assays, patients' sera, and target antigens. Since the conditions of *in vitro* culture are not similar to those of *in vivo* tumor growth, the selective pressure of culture conditions may lead to changes in antigenic expression on or in the melanoma cells. Human melanoma TAAs have been shown to fluctuate markedly in their expression on the cell surface with passage from one generation to another (Sorg *et al.*, 1978; Carey *et al.*, 1976; Cornain *et al.*, 1975). Incorporation of exogenous components from growth medium into membranes of cultured cells has been reported by several investigators (Irie *et al.*, 1974a; Laine and Kakorman, 1973; Hamburger *et al.*, 1963; Coombs *et al.*, 1961). Thus, results of many serological assays may be influenced by the presence of these heteroantigens on cultured melanoma cells. The stage of the disease of melanoma patients from whom the sera were drawn could also have influenced the results of serological assays. Many investigators (Bodurtha *et al.*, 1975; Canevari *et al.*, 1975; Cochran *et al.*, 1976; Lewis *et al.*, 1969; Morton, 1971; Dent *et al.*, 1978) have documented that the incidence and level of antibodies in melanoma patients were higher when the disease was localized than when the disease was disseminated. Surgery and/or immunotherapy with bacillus Calmette Guérin (BCG), and autologous and allogenic tumor-cell vaccine, have been shown to increase the circulating antibody levels in melanoma patients (Cornain *et al.*, 1975; deKernion *et al.*, 1975; Minden *et al.*, 1976; Seigler *et al.*, 1975b; Shibata *et al.*, 1976). With the recent advent of hybridoma technology, however, monoclonal antibodies have been developed that recognize TAAs expressed only on autologous melanoma cells

(Yeh *et al.*, 1979), expressed on some melanomas (Koprowski *et al.*, 1978), expressed on almost all melanomas (Carrel *et al.*, 1980), and expressed on melanomas and on tumors of other histological types (Kasai *et al.*, 1981). Thus, despite the use of varied serological assays and unstandardized reagents by various investigators, it is obvious that the four groups of TAAs on melanoma cells recognized by allogeneic antibody were real.

5. Significance of Melanoma Tumor-Associated Antigens Recognized by Allogeneic Antibody

In many reports, antibodies elicited in melanoma patients in response to TAAs of their tumors have been shown to be complement-fixing and to participate in antibody-dependent cellular cytotoxicity. Such antibodies may play a role in blocking or augmenting cell-mediated immunity, or they may be directly cytotoxic to the tumor cells *in vivo* (I. Hellström *et al.*, 1973b; Sjögren *et al.*, 1971, 1972). Attempts have been made by various investigators to utilize immunological parameters for diagnostic and prognostic purposes. However, as stressed by Ferrone and Pellegrino (1979), the information concerning the kinetics of the antibody response to melanoma TAAs is at present too fragmentary to draw any definite conclusions. This lack of information on kinetic studies was, perhaps, largely due to the use of crude reagents, especially the TAAs. Such preparations, as we know, are complex antigenically.

Though a number of melanoma TAAs have been recognized by the use of autologous and allogeneic antibody, progress in solubilization, purification, and physicochemical characterization of these antigens has been slow. Some of these antigens have been solubilized and partially purified by 3 M KCl extraction (Holmes *et al.*, 1975; Roth *et al.*, 1976), by sonication of cell membranes (Hollinshead *et al.*, 1974), by treatment with nonionic detergents (Bystryn and Smalley, 1977), by phenol–water extraction (Suter *et al.*, 1978), and by isolation from spent culture medium (Grimm *et al.*, 1976). Most of these soluble antigenic fractions have been immunologically characterized by *in vivo* and *in vitro* cell-mediated immune reactions. The advancement in the characterization of the soluble antigens by the serological assays has been hampered by the unavailability of continued supply of antigen and/or allogeneic antibody sources. Without availability of melanoma TAAs that are immunogenic in the host, it may be difficult to fully appreciate the importance of such antigens in terms of immunobiology, diagnosis, and prognosis of human melanoma.

6. Antibodies Bound *in Vivo* to Melanoma Cells

It is conceivable that the serological reactions observed *in vitro* between sera from melanoma patients and their tumor cells could also occur *in vivo*. The presence of tumor-bound immunoglobulins on biopsy specimens supports this hypothesis (Ran *et al.*, 1976). It has been shown that tumor cells may contain constant-fragment (Fc) receptors for immunoglobulin G (IgG). These Fc receptors may be on tumor-infiltrating host mononu-

TABLE II

Antigenic Activity of Human Melanoma before and after Elution of Tumor-Bound Immunoglobulins by Complement Fixation

	Antigen titer against	
Melanoma tumor	Autologous serum	Eluted antibody
Before elution	1 : 8	< 1 : 2
After elution with 15% NaCl	1 : 512	1 : 64
After elution with low pH (2.6)	1 : 256	1 : 32

clear cells (Wesenberg, 1978). Tonder *et al.* (1976) reported that tumor-associated immunoglobulins were associated with Fc receptors. Our studies reported earlier (Gupta and Morton, 1975a) suggest that although a proportion of tumor (melanoma)-bound immunoglobulins could be due to Fc receptors, the antigenic activity of a melanoma to autologous serum increased by 32 to 64-fold after elution of the immunoglobulins (Table II). The eluted immunoglobulins contained IgG and IgM.

7. Isolation of Antitumor Antibodies by Affinity Chromatography

Sera from melanoma patients may contain antibodies to a spectrum of antigens, including bacterial, viral, and alloantigens. Mere isolation of immunoglobulins by conventional biochemical techniques will be of no value in terms of specificity. Therefore, we adopted an immunoaffinity chromatographic approach using a melanoma-cell-membrane immunoadsorbent column to isolate and characterize antitumor antibodies from sera of melanoma patients.

7.1. Membrane Fractions

The membrane-rich fractions were prepared from biopsied melanoma cells obtained from a patient with blood group O by two methods: (1) hypotonic cell lysis as described by Oren and Herberman (1971) and (2) homogenization and differential centrifugation followed by discontinuous sucrose-gradient centrifugation (Gupta *et al.*, 1980). The specific activity of a membrane marker enzyme, 5′-nucleotidase, was 4–12 times higher in the extracted fractions than in the initial cell homogenate, suggesting that biochemically these fractions were rich in plasma membranes. The membranes extracted by the homogenization and differential centrifugation method were slightly more antigenic than those obtained by the hypotonic cell-lysis method (Table III). The complement-fixation assay as described by Gupta *et al.* (1978a) was used to assess the antigenic activity.

TABLE III

Immunoreactivity of Melanoma-Cell Membranes
against Sera from Melanoma Patients by
Complement Fixation

Serum source[a] (Patient No.)	Antigen titer of membrane prepared by:	
	Differential centrifugation method	Hypotonic cell-lysis method
1	1 : 64	1 : 64
2	1 : 64	1 : 64
3	1 : 128	1 : 256
4	1 : 32	1 : 32
5	1 : 8	1 : 16
6	1 : 16	1 : 32

[a]Sera were used as source of antibody at a dilution of 1 : 8.

7.2. Affinity Chromatography

The melanoma membranes were covalently linked to cyanogen-bromide-activated Sepharose 4B by the method of Parikh *et al.* (1974). The immobilized membranes were packed into a small column and washed four times alternately with 0.1 M acetate buffer (pH 4) and 0.1 M borate buffer (pH 8.5). The final wash was given with 0.01 M borate buffer (pH 8.5). A 4-ml serum sample diluted to 20 ml with the borate buffer was circulated through the column for 16 hr at 4°C. The column was flushed with the buffer until absorbency of the eluent was less than 0.025 OD_{280}. The unwashable proteins retained by the column were eluted with 2.5 M $MgCl_2$ at pH 6.5.

A significant amount of 280 nm absorbing material was eluted when the immunoadsorbent column was treated with sera from autologous or allogeneic melanoma patients. Similar treatments of the column with a randomly selected human normal serum resulted in elution of negligible amounts of 280 nm absorbing material. When an immunoadsorbent column prepared from a human normal liver membrane was used with a serum from melanoma patient, the elution of 280 nm absorbing material was again negligible. These results suggested that isolation of antibodies from melanoma serum by immunoadsorbent chromatography was successful.

7.3. Immunochemical Analysis

Qualitative analysis of the 280 nm absorbing materials isolated from cancer sera by melanoma-membrane affinity chromatography revealed that they contained mainly immunoglobulins (IgG in most and IgM in some) and traces of albumin (Table IV). The material isolated from human normal serum by melanoma-membrane immunoadsorbent or from melanoma serum by human normal liver-membrane column was devoid of IgG or IgM.

To determine the proportions of immunologically active IgG and IgM antibodies, the isolated immunoglobulins were subjected to absorption with immobilized rabbit anti-human IgG and rabbit anti-human IgM. The absorbed antibodies were then tested in complement fixation using melanoma-cell membranes as the target. Absorption of the isolated antibodies with rabbit anti-human IgG completely removed the complement-fixing antibody activity in the allogeneic system and reduced the activity by 4-fold in the autologous system (Fig. 1). This suggested that isolated immunoglobulins from allogeneic serum contained IgG antibodies only, whereas similar preparations from autologous serum contained both IgG and IgM antibodies. This observation was confirmed by quantitative absorption with rabbit anti-human IgM, which resulted in partial removal of antibody activity in the autologous system and no effect in the allogenic system.

7.3.1. Purification of IgG and IgM

To separate the IgG and IgM antibodies from isolated immunoglobulins, the preparations were radioiodinated with ^{125}I and subjected to sequential absorption with rabbit anti-human IgG and IgM immunobeads. The ^{125}I-labeled IgG and IgM antibodies were recovered from the respective immunobeads by elution with 2.5 M $MgCl_2$ at pH 6.5 and dialyzed against 0.025 M phosphate-buffered saline (PBS). The recovery of ^{125}I activity from the immunobeads was about 75%. The homogeneity of the affinity-purified IgG and IgM was confirmed by polyacrylamide gel electrophoresis.

The immunoreactivity of the purified IgG and IgM was determined by mixing them with the antigen solubilized from the autologous melanoma-cell membranes by freeze–thaw and sonication. The mixture was incubated at 37°C for 1 hr. The mixture of IgG and IgM fractions untreated with the soluble antigen was included as control. The control and the

TABLE IV

Immunodiffusion and Immunoelectrophoretic Analysis of 280 nm Absorbing Material Isolated from Melanoma and Normal Sera by Immunoadsorbent Column Chromatography

Serum source	Diagnosis	Affinity column	Immunodiffusion[a]		Immunoelectrophoresis[a]	
			IgG	IgM	IgG	IgM
J.G.	Melanoma	Melanoma membrane	+	+	+	+
J.R.	Melanoma	Melanoma membrane	+	−	+	−
N.B.	Normal	Melanoma membrane	±	−	−	−
J.G.	Melanoma	Human normal liver-cell membrane	−	−	−	−

[a] (+) Present; (−) absent; (±) questionable.

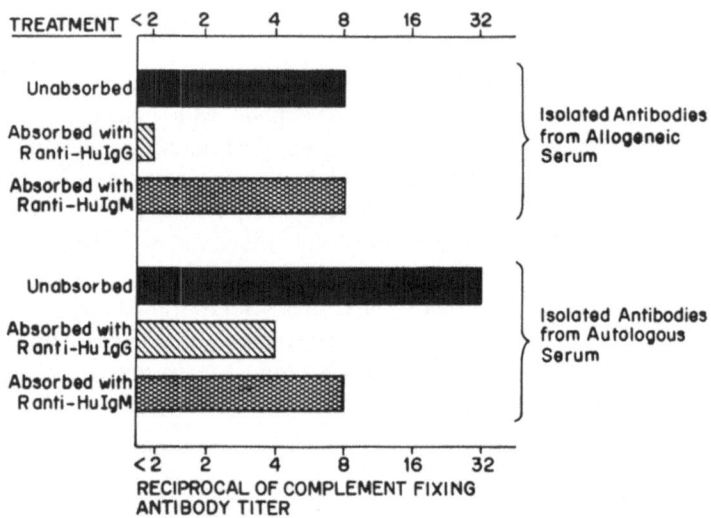

FIGURE 1. Effect of absorption with rabbit anti-human IgG (R anti-HuIgG) and rabbit anti-human IgM (R anti-HuIgM) of isolated immunoglobulins (Ig) isolated from autologous and allogeneic melanoma sera by melanoma-membrane affinity chromatography. The rabbit anti-human IgG and IgM were covalently linked to CNBr-activated Sepharose 4B, mixed with the isolated Ig, incubated at 37°C for 30 min, and centrifuged at 2000g for 10 min. The supernatants were analyzed for antibody activity by complement fixation against melanoma-cell membranes as the target. This figure illustrates the point that isolated antibodies from allogeneic serum contained immunoreactive IgG only, whereas isolated antibodies from autologous serum contained both IgG and IgM.

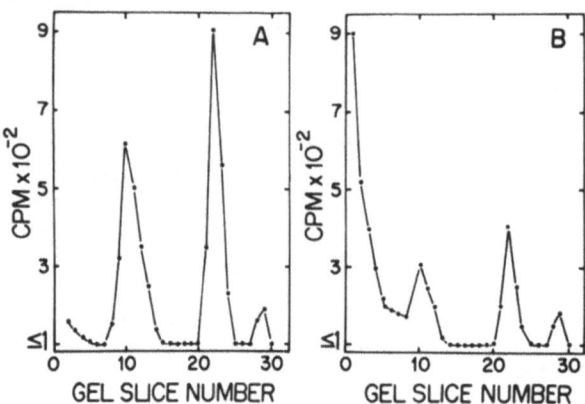

FIGURE 2. Comparison of profiles of ^{125}I activity in 0.5% agarose–2.5% polyacrylamide gels when a mixture of ^{125}I-labeled IgG and IgM purified from melanoma serum by autologous tumor-cell-membrane affinity chromatography was electrophoresed before and after treatment with melanoma TAAs. (A) Mixture of ^{125}I-labeled IgG and IgM without any treatment; (B) mixture of ^{125}I-labeled IgG and IgM after incubation with solubilized antigen (TAAs) from melanoma-cell membrane.

mixture of antibodies and antigen were electrophoresed in 0.5% agarose–2.5% acrylamide gels under nondissociating conditions (Peacock and Dingman, 1968). Under the experimental conditions, $[^{125}I]$-IgG migrated to a distance of about 5.4 cm and $[^{125}I]$-IgM to about 2.0 cm (Fig. 2A). The treatment of the IgG and IgM mixture with the soluble antigen reduced the amount of radioactivity that migrated to the 2.0- and 5.4-cm regions. Also, it caused an increase in radioactivity that remained within the top 1-cm region (Fig. 2B).

7.3.2. Specificity of Isolated Immunoglobulins

The specificity of immunoreactivity of the isolated immunoglobulins initially was determined by complement fixation. A number of melanoma, sarcoma, and normal tissues were used as target antigens (Table V). No histological type specificity for reactivity of the isolated antibodies was observed. This was possibly due to expression of fetal antigens by melanoma cells used in this study. Expression of OFA has been shown to occur on tumors of various histological types (Irie, 1980).

The isolated immunoglobulins from autologous serum (serum taken from a patient whose melanoma-tumor-cell membranes were used in affinity chromatography) were absorbed with the following allogeneic cultured cells: melanoma-UCLA-SO-M14 (M14), sarcoma-UCLA-SO-S1 (S1), and a lymphoblastoid cell line established from the M14 donor (ML14). The absorbed and unabsorbed preparations were tested against autologous melanoma membrane, M14, and S1. Both M14 and S1 were known to express OFA (Irie et al., 1976; Saxton et al., 1978). ML14 cells were ineffective in removing any antibody activity. Absorption with sarcoma (S1) cells completely removed the antibody activity against S1; however, this activity against autologous melanoma membrane or M14 cells was reduced but was not eliminated completely even after three consecutive absorptions. Absorption with M14 cells, either directly or after absorption with S1, of the isolated immunoglobulins completely abolished the reactivity against all target antigens (Table VI). The fact that the isolated immunoglobulins were not directed against blood group antigens or heterophile antigens was determined by their inability to react with erythrocyte membranes of human (blood groups A, B, and O), sheep, and cattle.

These results suggest that the immunoglobulins isolated from melanoma serum by autologous tumor-cell-membrane affinity chromatography contained antibodies of at least two specificities: (1) anti-OFA and (2) anti-melanoma-associated antigen. Therefore, it was concluded that plasma membranes of melanoma cells obtained at biopsy contain antigenic

TABLE V

Immunoreactivity of Isolated Immunoglobulins from Melanoma Sera by Autologous Melanoma-Membrane Affinity Chromatography in the Complement-Fixation Assay

Target antigen	Antibody titer of affinity-purified Ig from melanoma serum	
	JG	JR
JG-melanoma	1:32	1:8
JR-melanoma	1:8	1:8
RC-melanoma	1:16	1:16
JV-melanoma	1:32	1:16
Si-sarcoma	1:16	1:8
PA-sarcoma	1:16	1:8
Normal fibroblasts	1:2	1:2
Normal lung	< 1:2	< 1:2
Normal liver	1:2	< 1:2

Table VI

Effect of Absorption[a] of Isolated Immunoglobulins with Melanoma Cells (M14), Lymphoblastoid Cells (ML14), and Sarcoma (S1) Cells on Immunoreactivity against Melanoma Membranes, Melanoma Cells, Sarcoma Cells, and Normal Fibroblast Cells, by Complement Fixation

	Complement-fixing antibody titer against:		
Absorbed with:	Melanoma membrane (autologous)	Melanoma cells (M14) (allogeneic)	Sarcoma cells (S1)
None (control)	1 : 32	1 : 32	1 : 16
ML14 cells (2×)	1 : 32	1 : 32	1 : 8–1 : 16
S1 cells (3×)	1 : 8	1 : 8	< 1 : 2
M14 cells (2×)	< 1 : 2	< 1 : 2	< 1 : 2

[a] Each absorption was performed by mixing 100 μl of the isolated immunoglobulins with 100 μl packed cell volume, incubating at 37°C for 1.0 hr, and centrifuging at 2000 rpm for 15 min.

components that are immunogenic in the host. Some of these antigenic components are shared in common with melanoma and tumors of other histological types, whereas others are possessed by melanomas only.

8. Melanoma Tumor-Associated Antigens in Spent Culture Medium

It has been our and others' experience that spent culture medium of M14 cells reacts with sera from cancer patients (Grimm *et al.*, 1976; Leong *et al.*, 1978a). Biopsy specimens provide only a limited supply of material to warrant any extensive antigen purification and characterization procedures. Since certain antigenic components of plasma membrane of biopsy melanoma cells showed immunological cross-reactivity with cultured M14 cells, we initiated our studies to purify melanoma TAAs from spent culture medium of the M14 cell line.

Approximately 50% of serum samples from humans contain antibodies to fetal calf serum (FCS) components (Irie *et al.*, 1974a; Gupta *et al.*, 1978a). Cells in culture are known to incorporate macromolecules from the medium supplements, e.g., FCS (Irie *et al.*, 1974b; Smith and Jacobs, 1979). Since our sources of antibody were allogeneic sera from melanoma patients, the M14 cells were adapted to grow in chemically defined serum-free medium (Chee *et al.*, 1976). This was done to avoid confusions that could arise during antigen purification by the presence of FCS components to which sera from melanoma patients might have antibodies.

The spent culture medium of M14 cells that were adapted to grow in the chemically defined medium for several months was harvested biweekly and was processed as follows:

The pooled M14 spent medium was concentrated by 5000-molecular-weight exclusion-limit hollow-fiber concentrator. The concentrate was ultrafiltered through a 100,000-molecular-weight exclusion-limit membrane. The material retained on the membrane was chromatographed on a Sepharose 6B column. The antigenic fractions were pooled and concentrated to the original volume by vacuum dialysis. Three allogeneic sera from melanoma patients containing antibodies to OFA and melanoma TAAs were employed as the source of antibody to monitor the antigenic activity of the fractions by complement fixation during the antigen-purification procedures (Gupta *et al.*, 1979c). One serum contained antibodies to OFA and melanoma TAAs, the second serum contained antibodies to OFA only, and the third serum contained antibodies to TAAs only.

8.1. Separation of Oncofetal Antigen and Melanoma Tumor-Associated Antigens

The antigenic fraction of the spent culture medium contained both OFA and melanoma TAAs. These two antigenic components could not be separated by conventional physical and chemical techniques, i.e., ultrafiltration, gel filtration and ion-exchange chromatography, ultracentrifugation and ammonium sulfate precipitation. Therefore, efforts were made to separate these antigenic components (OFA and TAAs) by heat treatment, Sepharose–concanavalin A beads, proteolytic enzymes, or solvent extraction. Extraction with chloroform–methanol (C : M) resulted in separation of OFA and TAAs into C : M-insoluble and C : M-soluble fractions, respectively (Fig. 3). The precipitate formed during the extraction procedure did not react against any of the three typing sera. Also, as illustrated in Fig. 3, no detectable OFA activity could be observed in the C : M-soluble fraction and no TAA activity in the C : M-insoluble fraction.

When tested by complement fixation, 82% (74 of 90) sera from melanoma patients reacted against the crude M14 spent medium. In contrast, only 40% (36 of 90) and 29% (26 of 90) of these sera were reactive to the C : M-insoluble (OFA) and C : M-soluble (TAA) fractions, respectively. Absorption of the 90 sera with cultured lymphoblastoid cells from the M14 donor reduced the positive incidence against crude M14 spent medium to 58% (52 of 90), whereas reactions against C : M fractions were virtually unaffected. Of the 90 absorbed sera, 21% reacted against the C : M-insoluble (OFA) fraction and not against the C : M-soluble (TAA) fraction. Conversely, only 10% of sera reacted against TAAs and not against OFA. About 19% of sera contained antibodies to both antigens. The incidence of antibody to melanoma TAAs (C : M-soluble fraction) in sera from sarcoma, carcinoma, and normal donors ranged from 6 to 8%. Thus, the incidence of antibody to melanoma TAAs in sera from melanoma patients was significantly higher than the other groups of sera ($P < 0.05$).

8.2. Absence of M14-Associated Human Leukocyte Antigen in Chloroform–Methanol Fractions

Serum samples that contained significant levels of anti-human leukocyte antigen (HLA) antibodies (HLA specifically expressed by M14 cells) and virtually no antibodies

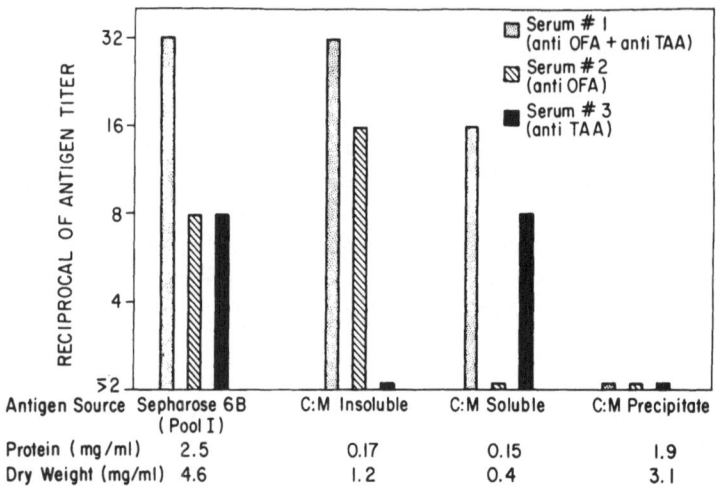

FIGURE 3. Comparison of reactivity of chloroform–methanol-extracted fractions of spent culture medium of a melanoma cell line against three typing sera from melanoma patients in the complement-fixation assay. Serum-free spent culture medium of a melanoma cell line was concentrated 200-fold by a hollow-fiber concentrator and chromatographed on a Sepharose 6B column (1.6 × 100 cm) after fractionation by ultrafiltration on a 100,000-molecular-weight exclusion-limit membrane. The antigenic fraction from the column that had both TAA and OFA activities was extracted with a mixture of chloroform (2 parts) and methanol (1 part). One part of the antigenic fraction (2.5 mg protein/ml) was mixed with 8.5 parts of the organic solvent. After continuous shaking at room temperature for 15 min, the organic and inorganic phases and the precipitate formed were collected. The solvent from each fraction was evaporated under vacuum. The residues were dissolved in 0.025 M PBS and tested for antigenic activity. Though pool I of crude spent culture medium from the Sepharose 6B column contained both TAA and OFA activities, the C : M-insoluble fraction reacted against anti-OFA (Serum No. 2) and not against anti-TAA (Serum No. 3), whereas the C : M-soluble fraction reacted against anti-TAA (Serum No. 3) and not against anti-OFA (Serum No. 2). The precipitate formed during the extraction procedure did not react against any of the three sera.

to OFA and TAAs did not react with either C : M-soluble or C : M-insoluble fractions by complement fixation. The absence of anti-OFA and anti-TAA in these sera was determined by absorption with M14 cells. These absorbed sera were unreactive to M14 cells.

8.3. Immunological Dissimilarity between Melanoma Tumor-Associated Antigens and Bacillus Calmette Guérin

Using xenoantisera, Minden *et al.* (1976) and Bucana and Hanna (1974) have demonstrated that certain antigenic components are shared by BCG and human melanoma cells. Inasmuch as most melanoma donors in our investigation received immunotherapy with BCG and tumor-cell vaccine, it was investigated whether a part of the reactivity against melanoma TAAs was due to antigenic determinants cross-reactive with BCG. In fact, several of the sera from melanoma patients were positive in complement fixation when BCG was used as the target antigen. Therefore, seven sera that were positive to BCG and melanoma TAAs were randomly selected and absorbed quantitatively with BCG and tested against both BCG and melanoma TAAs. All seven sera remained positive to melanoma TAAs, but became negative to BCG. Thus, it appeared that BCG was not a major component in reactivity of sera from melanoma patients to melanoma TAAs.

9. Development of Radioimmunoassay

The TAAs isolated from serum-free spent culture medium of M14 cell lines appeared to be rather specific for the melanoma system. However, the incidence of antibodies in sera of melanoma patients was low (26%). This could have been due to the use of the complement-fixation assay, which is less sensitive and the results of which are affected by the anticomplementary activity of the samples. Therefore, attempts were made to develop a radioimmunoassay (RIA).

9.1. Radioiodination and Further Purification of Melanoma Tumor-Associated Antigens

The TAA fraction was radiolabeled by the vapor-phase chloramine T method as outlined in Fig. 4 (Gupta and Morton, 1979a). The ^{125}I-labeled TAA was further purified by Sephacryl S-200 column (0.9 × 25 cm) chromatography (Fig. 5). Individual tubes obtained from the fractionation procedure were analyzed for binding of [^{125}I]-TAA to a constant amount of allogeneic anti-TAA. Tubes collected under the areas of minor first peak were found to show significant bindings with the anti-TAA.

9.2. Radioimmunoassay Procedure

The RIA procedure used in these studies is briefly outlined in Fig. 6 and described in detail elsewhere (Gupta and Morton, 1980). Borate buffer (boric acid, 6 g/liter, and

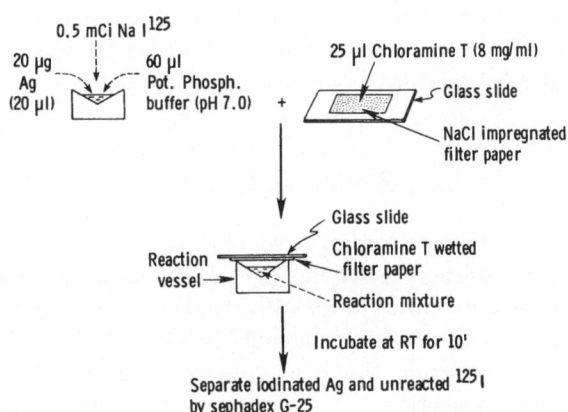

FIGURE 4. Outline of vapor-phase chloramine T method of radioiodination of melanoma TAA (Ag). Potassium phosphate buffer (1 M, pH 7.0) was added to the reaction mixture to neutralize the Na^{125}I.

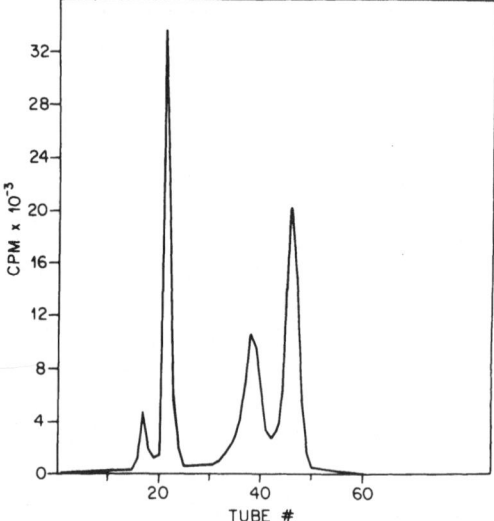

FIGURE 5. Elution profile of chloroform-methanol-extracted TAA after radioiodination from a Sephacryl S-200 column. Borate buffer at pH 8.2 supplemented with 0.15 M NaCl, 0.01 M EDTA, and 0.5% Triton X-100 was used as the eluent. The antigenic activity against anti-TAA as detected by RIA was associated with the first peak only.

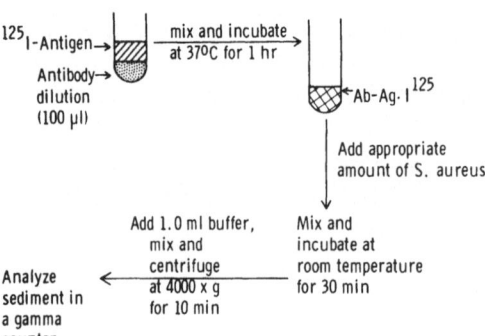

FIGURE 6. Outline of RIA procedure using protein-A-bearing *Staphylococcus aureus* cells. A 200-μl aliquot of a 10% suspension of formalin-fixed and heat-killed *S. aureus* was used to separate the bound and free [^{125}I]-TAA. For competitive inhibition, the limiting amount of anti-TAA (100 μl) was mixed with the test sample (100 μl) and incubated at 37°C for 1 hr, followed by addition of [^{125}I]-TAA (7500 cpm in 100 μl). The remaining steps were similar to those outlined in the figure.

sodium tetraborate, 9.5 g/liter) at pH 8.2 supplemented with 0.15 M NaCl, 0.01 Methylenediamine tetraacetic acid (EDTA), and 0.5% Triton X-100 was used as diluent of reagents in the assay. A 10% suspension of protein-A-bearing *Staphylococcus aureus* (200 μl/tube) was used to separate bound and free labeled antigen.

9.3. Primary Binding in Radioimmunoassay

A primary binding curve of [^{125}I]-TAA vs. various dilutions of serum from a melanoma patient is shown in Fig. 7. The antibody titer was defined as the highest dilution of the serum showing at least 10% binding (a base line well above nonspecific binding). The unabsorbed serum had an antibody titer of 1 : 1200. This titer remained almost the same when the serum sample was absorbed with lymphoblastoid cells of the M14 donor or human fetal brain cells. Absorption of the serum with M14 cells decreased the titer to 1:15.

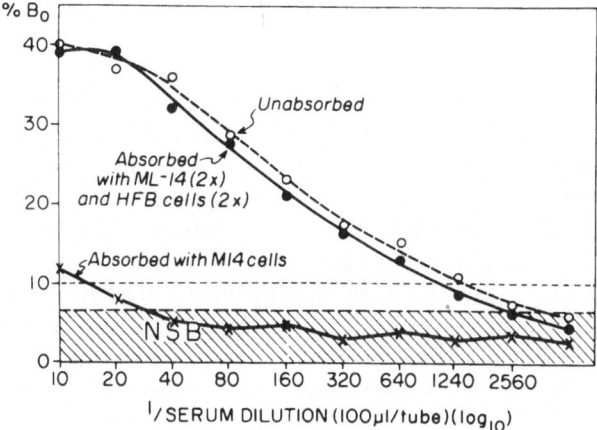

FIGURE 7. Primary binding of [^{125}I]-TAA by various dilutions of a melanoma serum in RIA. The serum was used before and after absorption with lymphoblastoid cells (LM14) autologous to the TAA source, human fetal brain (HFB) cells, and M14 cells (source of [^{125}I]-TAA). (NSB) Nonspecific binding.

These results suggested that the antigen immunologically similar to [^{125}I]-TAA was present on M14 cells and not on human fetal brain or lymphoblastoid cells of the M14 donor.

9.4. Distribution of Anti-Tumor-Associated Antigen Antibody in Various Human Sera

A number of serum samples from melanoma, sarcoma, carcinoma, and normal donors were analyzed in RIA for their extent of reactivity to [^{125}I]-TAA. Both incidence and mean antibody titers of sera from melanoma patients were significantly higher than those from other groups (Fig. 8). A serum with antibody titer of higher than 1 : 100 was considered positive.

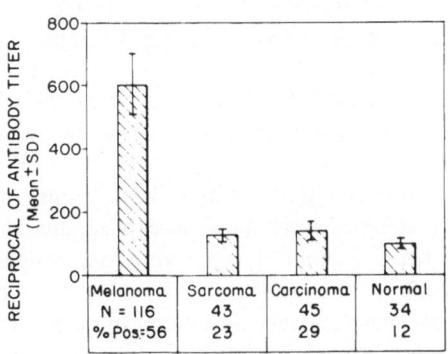

FIGURE 8. Distribution and mean titer of anti-TAA antibody in serum samples taken from melanoma, sarcoma, and carcinoma patients, and normal volunteers, by RIA. A serum was considered anti-TAA- antibody-positive when the titer was higher than 1 : 100. The mean antibody titer (1 : 609 ± 98) was significantly higher ($p < 0.005$) compared to other groups by student's t test.

9.5. Distribution of Melanoma Tumor-Associated Antigens in Various Cell Lines and Tumor Tissues

To determine the presence or absence of immunologically similar melanoma TAAs in a given sample, a competitive-inhibition RIA was developed. In this assay, the limiting amount of antibody was preincubated with the test sample. The binding of [^{125}I]-TAA to this treated antibody was compared with binding to the untreated antibody. Analysis of crude spent media of various cell lines by the competitive-inhibition RIA revealed that spent media of sarcoma, colon carcinoma, and breast carcinoma did not result in any significant inhibition even at protein concentrations of greater than 300 μg per tube, whereas 50% inhibition of binding occurred by melanoma spent media at protein concentrations of less than 100 μg. Similar competitive inhibition was observed when M14 cells cultured in chemically defined medium or FCS were used as the inhibitor. Using M14 cells grown in FCS as the standard inhibitor, the percentage of cross-reactivity between these cells and other histological types of cancer cells was determined by calculating the ratio of number of cells required to bring about 50% inhibition and multiplying the ratio by 100. A cell line was considered antigen-positive when the cross-reactivity was greater than 5%. By this criterion, 11 of 17 (65%) melanoma cell lines were positive for the TAA. On the contrary, 0 of 3 sarcoma, 0 of 1 renal carcinoma, 1 of 3 breast carcinoma and 0 of 1 cultured fetal fibroblast were positive. Similar results were observed when extracts or minced-cell suspensions of biopsy specimens were used as the inhibitor. Of 23 melanomas, 15 (61%) were positive. Among carcinoma, 12% (2 of 17) exhibited cross-reactivity. Nine sarcoma, 7 human fetal tissues (brain, skin, muscle), 4 human placenta, 24 human normal tissues, 4 human viral antigens (simian virus 40, herpes, adeno, cytomegalovirus) and 15 different bacterial antigens so far tested were not inhibitory in the competitive RIA. These results suggest that melanoma TAAs are expressed by a majority of human melanomas and by only a very limited number of neoplasms of other histological types. It should be pointed out that the nonmelanoma tumors that showed inhibition in RIA were breast, ovarian, and teratocarcinomas. The degree of cross-reactivity exhibited by these carcinomas ranged from 8 to 14%, whereas melanoma tumors consistently showed cross-reactivity of greater than 20%. Thus, the melanoma TAAs purified from spent culture medium of M14 cell line may be melanoma-specific.

9.6. Detection of Free Circulating Melanoma Tumor-Associated Antigens in Sera from Cancer Patients by Radioimmunoassay

RIA is considered to be sensitive enough to detect minute quantities of antigen. During the screening of sera from melanoma patients for the presence of anti-TAA antibodies, a number of sera were found to be negative. This could be due either to lack of expression of immunologically similar TAA by the tumors of these hosts (only about 65% of melanomas tested were found to express this antigen) or to lack of circulating free antibody. Therefore, antibody-negative serum samples were analyzed in competitive RIA to determine whether these sera contained detectable levels of free antigen. Sera from sarcoma and carcinoma patients and normal volunteers were included as controls. The mean competitive inhibition in RIA by 100 μl serum from melanoma patients was 16.7 $\pm$ 26.1% compared to 2.3 ± 5.9% by sarcoma, 6.4 ± 16.4% by carcinoma, and 1.0 ± 4.4% by normals. Considering a serum with greater than 10% inhibition (normal mean ± 2 S.D.) as positive, 35% (49 of 139) sera from melanoma, 3% (1 of 40) sera from sarcoma, 9% (3 of 35) sera from carcinoma, and 0% (0 of 25) sera from normals were positive for melanoma-TAA-like activity. At present, we do not have an explanation for the ability of sarcoma and carcinoma sera to exhibit occasional inhibition in RIA developed with the melanoma system. This may simply be due to rare expression of cross-reactive antigen by tumors of these individuals. However, none of the normals was positive for melanoma-TAA-like activity, and the extent of inhibition by these sera was negligible.

10. Presence of Tumor-Associated Antigens in Urine of Melanoma Patients

Excretion of antigens into urine from tumors originating outside the genitourinary tract has been observed by various investigators. Jehn *et al.* (1970) reported a case in which an antigen excreted into the urine of a melanoma patient was mitrogenic for lymphocytes from another patient. The antigen reacted with rabbit antibody prepared against cystic fluid of tumor. The urinary antigen was identical with that extracted from the cystic fluid by immunodiffusion using rabbit antimelanoma antibody (Jehn *et al.*, 1970). A common melanoma antigen has been detected in the urine of a high percentage of patients with melanotic and amelanotic tumors (Carrel and Theilkaes, 1973; Bennett *et al.*, 1978; Volkers *et al.*, 1978). Excretion of TAAs into urine is not restricted to melanoma only, such excretion of antigens into urine having been reported in sarcoma (Gupta and Morton, 1975b, 1979b; Huth *et al.*, 1979), breast carcinoma (Lopez and Thomson, 1977; Thomson and Lopez, 1978), and other types of carcinomas (Gupta and Morton, 1976; Rote *et al.*, 1978, 1980a, b). Importance of sequential analyses of urinary TAAs to monitor the clinical course and to assess the *in vivo* effectiveness of tumoricidal chemotherapy and radiation therapy of cancer patients has been reported by Gupta and Morton (1975b), Huth *et al.* (1979, 1981a, b), and Copeman (1979).

10.1. Detection by Complement Fixation

In the complement-fixation assay using serum (antibody) from a source autologous with the source of urine (antigen), 91.3% (21 of 23) melanoma patients were positive for urinary TAAs, while only 6.9% (2 of 29) normal controls were positive. When the serum from an allogeneic source was used, the incidence of positivity for urinary TAAs remained the same (91.3%) for melanoma patients, whereas it increased to 35.1% (13 of 37) for normal controls. No correlation was observed between the presence of carcinoembryonic antigen (CEA) and reactivity of urine samples against autologous ($\gamma = 0.22$) and allogeneic ($\gamma = 0.02$) sera. Therefore, the reactivity observed in the urine samples could not have been due to CEA or like material (Rote *et al.*, 1980a).

There are two reasons to believe that the antigenic activity detected in urine of melanoma patients could be tumor-associated: (1) The reactivity between urine and autologous serum was abolished only after absorption of the serum with tumor cells and not by the normal tissues. (2) The presence of antigenic activity depended on the presence of tumor in the host. Patients who underwent curative surgery became urinary-antigen-negative.

10.2. Detection by Radioimmunoassay

Excretion of antigenic components into the urine of cancer patients may represent a spectrum of antigens (TAAs) associated with tumor cells. Since we have been able to isolate melanoma TAAs and have developed an RIA, we analyze urine samples from melanoma patients and normal volunteers for their ability to exhibit competitive inhibition. Results presented in Table VII denote that, on an average, normal urine samples did not competitively inhibit binding between [^{125}I]-TAA and allogeneic antibody, whereas a significant level of inhibition was caused by urine samples from melanoma patients. The urine samples from both melanoma patients and normal volunteers were processed immediately after reception and in an identical manner. None of the normal urines showed inhibition greater than 20%, whereas 7 of 12 melanoma urines caused greater than 40% inhibition. These studies confirmed the earlier observations that TAAs expressed by tumor cells may be excreted into the urine of cancer patients. Such urine may be utilized as a source of TAAs for molecular and chemical characterization and for immunoprognosis.

10.3. Detection by Enzyme Immunoassay

By RIA, we could detect the presence of melanoma TAAs in the urine of patients with malignant melanoma. However, a urine may contain a spectrum of antigens similar to those associated with melanoma cells. We have observed a disparity between the results of complement fixation and RIA. Some of the antigens present in melanoma urine were found to be heat-stable and were apparently different from the melanoma TAAs (Cheng et al., 1981). Thus, to fully realize the presence of TAAs in the urine of cancer patients, another sensitive assay, enzyme immunoassay (EIA), was developed (Huth et al., 1981a).

TABLE VII

Comparison of Competitive Inhibition in Radioimmunoassay Caused by Urine Samples from Melanoma Patients and Normal Donors[a]

Urine Donors[b]	Number	Protein (mg/ml) (Mean ± S.D.)	Inhibition (%) in RIA[c] (mean ± S.D.)
Melanoma patients	12	9.1 ±8.2	39.9 ±40.8
Normal volunteers	12	12.3 ±9.8	−1.8 ±12.2

[a] Serum from a Melanoma Patient with known Anti-TAA activity and [^{125}I]melanoma TAA were used in the assay.

[b] Urine samples (24-hr) were concentrated 100-fold by ultrafiltration (5000-molecular-weight exclusion limit) and dialyzed against 0.025 M phosphate buffer supplemented with 0.15 M NaCl.

[c] 100-µl aliquot of each sample was used for competitive inhibition in RIA.

The EIA was performed according to the procedures described by Voller *et al.* (1976) and Engvall and Perlmann (1971). The antigen used as target in the EIA was partially purified from the urine of a melanoma patient by heat treatment and Sephacryl S-200 gel-filtration chromatography. Autologous serum was used as the standard antibody. Of 18 patients with clinicial Stage I melanoma, 8 were positive for urinary TAAs by competitive inhibition in RIA. In 5 patients studied serially, the urinary TAA activity became negative following excision of the primary tumor. Of 14 patients with Stage II melanoma, 10 were positive for urinary TAAs following lymphadenectomy. Of these 10 urinary-TAA-positive patients, 9 developed recurrent disease. Of 29 patients with Stage III melanoma, 26 were positive for urinary TAAs. Thus, urinary TAAs appear to be a promising marker for subclinical residual disease (Huth, Gupta, and Morton, unpublished data).

11. Relationship of Serum Tumor-Associated Antigens and Immune Complexes with Inhibition of Lymphocyte Blastogenesis

In vivo and *in vitro* manifestations of defects in cell-mediated immune function in patients with malignant melanoma have been reported by several investigators (Catalona *et al.*, 1973; Butterworth *et al.*, 1974; Golub *et al.*, 1974; Eilber *et al.*, 1975; Lee *et al.*, 1975). Factors capable of inhibiting normal lymphocyte function are demonstrable in the sera of cancer patients (Glasgow *et al.*, 1974; I. Hellström *et al.*, 1971, 1973b; Heppner *et al.*, 1973; Nelson and Gatti, 1976), which may contribute to the immunosuppression associated with malignant disease. Some of these blocking factors have been tentatively identified as free tumor-associated antigens (Baldwin *et al.*, 1973; Currie, 1973; Thomson *et al.*, 1973) and/or antigen–antibody immune complexes (Sjögren *et al.*, 1972; Jose and Seshadri, 1974; Baldwin *et al.*, 1973; Baldwin and Robins, 1976), and their means of functioning has been postulated (K. E. Hellström and I. Hellström, 1977; Theofilopoulos and Dixon, 1978).

In our studies on immunocompetence in melanoma patients, we demonstrated that their lymphoproliferative capacity was nearly normal (Golub *et al.*, 1977), but many of these patients' sera inhibited mitogen-induced blastogenesis of lymphocytes from normal donors (Guiliano *et al.*, 1977; Rangel *et al.*, 1977). We also observed that many serum samples from melanoma patients were anticomplementary and that the incidence depended on body burden of tumor (Gupta *et al.*, 1979a). The anticomplementary activity in selected melanoma sera was documented to be due to circulating immune complexes (CICs) composed of tumor (melanoma)-associated antigen(s) and antibodies directed against them (Gupta *et al.*, 1979e). Therefore, an investigation was undertaken to answer the following questions: (1) Does the presence of CICs in melanoma patients correlate with the ability of their serum samples to inhibit mitogen-induced normal lymphocyte blastogenesis? (2) Is the ability of CIC-positive melanoma sera to inhibit the lymphocyte blastogenesis influenced by the concurrent presence of free antigen or antibody?

The lymphocyte blastogenesis–inhibition assay was performed as described by Rangel *et al.* (1977). Normal lymphocytes were stimulated with 0.5% phytohemagglutinin (PHA)

for 72 hr. [^{3}H]-Thymidine incorporated during the last 18 hr of culture was used to estimate the stimulation or inhibition of PHA-induced blastogenesis by the following equation:

$$\Delta cpm = cpm \text{ with reference serum} - cpm \text{ with test serum}$$

A positive Δcpm value denoted inhibition of lymphocyte blastogenesis and a negative Δcpm
value denoted stimulation by the test serum. The reference serum was a pool of normal
sera from blood-group-AB-positive donors. Antibody activity in the test serum samples was
measured using the melanoma UCLA-SO-M21 (M21) cell line as the target, and xenoantiserum raised against human melanoma extract (Gupta *et al.*, 1978b) was used to determine the presence or absence of antigen by complement fixation. The CIC activity was
measured by the complement-consumption method (Gupta *et al.*, 1979b).

The presence of antibody alone in melanoma sera did not correlate with inhibition of
lymphocyte blastogenesis, and in fact was associated with slightly higher than normal
responses to PHA. Antigen-positive sera ($N = 29$) were significantly ($P < 0.01$) more
inhibitory in the lymphocyte-blastogenesis assay (mean cpm $\pm$ S.E. $= 6941 \pm 1848$) than
antigen-negative sera ($N = 69$) (mean cpm $= 826 \pm 1399$). Likewise, CIC-positive sera
were significantly ($P < 0.01$) more inhibitory than CIC-negative sera (Table VIII). CIC-
and antigen-positive sera ($N = 18$) exhibited greater inhibition in the lymphocyte-blastogenesis assay (mean cpm $= 10,606 \pm 3707$) than CIC-positive but antigen-negative sera
($N = 25$) (mean cpm $= 4215 \pm 2602$). CIC- and antigen-negative sera ($N = 44$) or
CIC-negative but antigen-positive sera ($N = 11$) were not inhibitory (mean cpm $=$
-1098 ± 1572 and 942 ± 3485, respectively). These results suggested that inhibition of
PHA-induced lymphocyte blastogenesis by melanoma sera was independent of antibody
activity, but closely correlated with their CIC activity. The inhibition caused by CICs was
potentiated by the concomitant presence of antigen and diminished by the presence of
antibody.

Serum samples from melanoma patients with no evidence of disease were not inhibitory in lymphocyte blastogenesis, whereas sera from patients with minimal and large tumor
burden showed moderate to significant inhibition (Fig. 9). CIC-positive sera were more
inhibitory than CIC-negative sera at each level of tumor burden. Thus, presence of CICs
and inhibition of lymphocyte blastogenesis appeared to be related to tumor burden.

A number of possible mechanisms for nonspecific inhibition of cellular immune
responses by immune complexes (ICs) can be visualized. It is possible that ICs themselves

TABLE VIII
Inhibition of Phytohemagglutinin-Induced Blastogenesis of Normal
Lymphocytes by Sera from Melanoma patients with and without
Circulating Immune Complexes

CIC activity	Number tested	Lymphocyte-blastogenesis inhibition (mean cpm $\pm$ S.E.)
Positive	43	6889 ± 2194
Negative	55	-690 ± 1427

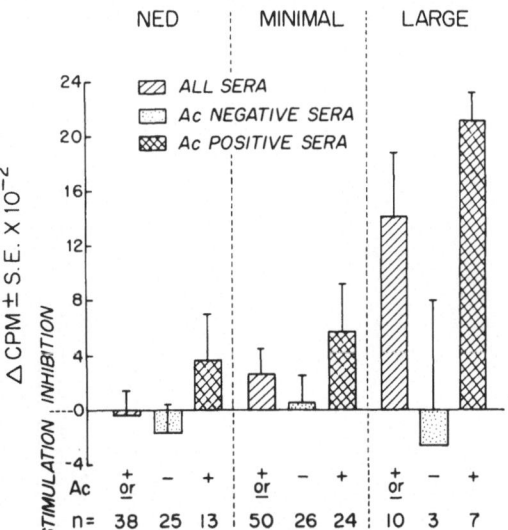

FIGURE 9. Comparison of mean inhibition of PHA-induced lymphocyte blastogenesis caused by CIC-positive [denoted by activity (Ac)] sera from melanoma patients with no evidence of disease (NED), with MINIMAL tumor burden (localized disease), and with LARGE tumor burden (disseminated disease). Inhibition or stimulation of the lymphocyte blastogenesis was expressed as mean difference (Δ) $\pm$ S.E. cpm of [³H]thymidine incorporation between pooled normal human serum and the test serum.

have no inhibitory activity, but that certain clinical situations lead to the presence of both ICs and a higher level of some other factor. Thus it is certainly possible that the presence of CICs and inhibitory activity of serum may be coincidental. However, in some preliminary studies, we have observed that in some sera from cancer patients that were both inhibitory to PHA-induced lymphocyte blastogenesis and positive for ICs, both activities could be removed by absorption of the serum with *S. aureus* Cowan strain I. Since protein A from this bacterium binds to immunoglobulins and can remove ICs that are inhibitory in other systems (Steel *et al.*, 1974), it may be that ICs themselves are the inhibitory factor, or as suggested by Kilburn *et al.* (1976), ICs may interact with other serum components that in turn may exhibit inhibitory activity. It is also possible that the ICs interact with the cells bearing Fc receptors and that these cells are either directly inhibitory or have an indirect suppressor function. Suppressor activity of cells with receptors for the Fc fragment of IgG has been reported in human systems (Moretta *et al.*, 1977).

12. Conclusions

As mentioned earlier, a wide variety of serological techniques have been used to demonstrate the existence of TAAs in human malignant melanoma. These antigens were recognized by both allogeneic antibody (patient's serum) and xenogeneic antibody. On the basis of these observations, a number of clinical trials in immunotherapy have been tried—some unsuccessfully and some with moderate success. The reason may be, in part, that the techniques used to study the antigens expressed by human melanoma were relatively crude. Despite several years of continuous efforts by numerous investigators, we are in an early stage of understanding the host response to these antigens. Indeed, the problem of tumor–host interactions is extremely complex. The key to our complete understanding of

TABLE IX

Partial List of Reports on Solubilization and Isolation of Tumor Antigens Associated with Human Malignant Melanoma

Investigators	Source of TAA	Isolation procedures[a]	Approximate molecular weight of TAA ($\times$1000)	Probable chemical nature of TAA
Carrel and Theilkaes (1973)	Urine	Gel-filtration chromatography and Pevikon block electrophoresis	40 and 60	—
Hollinshead et al. (1974)	Autologous and allogeneic tumors	Low-frequency sonication, gel-filtration chromatography, and PAGE	—	—
Malley et al. (1976)	Tumor tissue	3 M CCl extraction and gel-filtration chromatography	—	—
Roth et al. (1976)	Tissue-culture cells	3 M KCl extraction and gel-filtration chromatography, and PAGE	—	—
Bystryn and Smalley (1977)	Tissue-culture cells	Nonionic detergent and gel-filtration chromatography	160	—
Reisfeld et al. (1977), McCabe et al. (1978b)	Tissue-culture cells and spent culture medium	3 M KCl extraction, KBr gradient, CMC, and lectin affinity chromatography	50	Glycoprotein
Bystryn and Smalley (1978)	Spent media of ^{125}I-labeled cells	Gel filtration and Con A affinity chromatography	120	Glycoprotein

Reference	Source	Method	Molecular weight	Nature
Hersey et al. (1978)	Sera from melanoma patients	Gel filtration, Con A affinity chromatography, and PAGE	300 and < 60	Glycoprotein
Leong et al. (1978b)	Spent culture medium	Gel filtration and CMC chromatography	< 200	—
Stuhlmiller et al. (1978)	Tissue-culture cells	Pronase digestion and gel-filtration chromatography	48–17	—
Carey et al. (1979)	Tissue-culture cells	Papain digestion and LcH lectin	20–50	Glycoproteins
Gallaway et al. (1979)	Spent culture medium	Indirect immunoprecipitation and lectin affinity chromatography	160 and 94	Glycoproteins
Hersey et al. (1979)	^{125}I-labeled melanoma cells	Urea–acetate extraction, gel-filtration and Con A chromatography, and preparative IEF	15	Glycoprotein
Gupta (1980)	Spent culture medium	Chloroform–methanol extraction and gel-filtration chromatography	180	Lipoprotein
Cheng et al. (1981)	Urine	Gel-filtration and lectin affinity chromatography	300	Glycoprotein
Gallaway et al. (1981)	Spent culture medium	Indirect immune precipitation	240 and 94	Glycoproteins

a(CMC) Carboxymethyl cellulose; (Con A) Concanavalin A; (IEF) isoelectric focusing; (LcH) Lens culinaris hemagglutinin (lentil lectin); (PAGE) polyacrylamide gel electrophoresis.

the problem is to work toward a more refined approach to the study of the human melanoma antigens and the response of the host of these antigens.

The antigens with individual host specificity, though important from an academic point of view, may not be of practical value in terms of diagnosis, prognosis, or therapy. In this regard, TAAs that are specific for a particular histological type of malignancy, e.g., melanoma, or that are broadly cross-reactive, e.g., OFAs, would be important. However, with regard to their use in active immunotherapy, it must be pointed out that OFAs are components of normal embryonic cells. It is possible that residual embryonic cells may exist in the adult and perform important functions, e.g., repair and regeneration of damaged tissues, or that adult cells may express subthreshold levels of OFAs below the sensitivity of current *in vitro* assays. Therefore, active immunization with OFAs may induce an autoimmune response. Furthermore, successful immunization against cancer with OFAs may not be possible because the species in its evolutionary history of phylogeny and ontogeny has developed a fail-safe homeostatic system for its survival against such an event (Chee and Gupta, 1980). Perhaps the greatest utilitarian value of OFAs could be their use in diagnosis or prognosis of cancer in its early stage of development.

During recent years, progress made in isolation and characterization of melanoma-associated antigens obviously points toward a diverse nature of such antigens. Table IX gives a partial list of reports that deal with solubilization and isolation of antigens associated with human malignant melanoma. By and large, these antigens are comprised of glycoproteins that are molecules generally present in plasma membrane and inside the cell. However, the molecular size has ranged from 14,000 to 300,000. Though the solubilization and extraction procedures might be responsible for such a heterogeneity in molecular size, it is hard to conceptualize that these represent subspecies of the same melanoma-associated antigen or fetal antigens. One direct way to resolve this would be to exchange the reagents (antigen isolated and the antibody utilized to recognize the detected antigen). We have begun to do so. No immunological cross-reactivity was seen when melanoma TAA recognized by the patient's antibody and isolated by chloroform–methanol extraction (Gupta, 1980) was tested in RIA using xenoantisera developed and made specific for melanoma-associated antigen by Bystryn and Smalley (1978). A partial immunological cross-reactivity has been observed by Morgan and Reisfeld (unpublished results) between an antigen isolated from the urine of a melanoma patient recognized by the patient's antibody (Gupta *et al.*, unpublished data) and monoclonal antibody to 94K antigen (Gallaway *et al.*, 1981). Nevertheless, it is clear that a number of antigens are expressed by human melanoma cells. Some of the antigens recognized by xeno- or monoclonal antibody may not be necessarily immunogenic in patients.

We believe that to understand the immunobiology of tumor–host interaction, it is necessary to isolate and purify melanoma TAAs that are recognized by the patient's antibody. Such reagents are important to identify and immunochemically characterize the immune complexes detected in sera from melanoma patients. We realize that continuous use of patient's antibody may not be feasible because these reagents are in limited supply.

Since the availability of hybridoma technology, a number of antigens associated with human melanoma have been identified using either whole cells or their crude extracts. However, it remains to be determined what proportion of these antigens are recognized by the host (patient). It is possible that production of hybridoma may provide greater success in obtaining monoclonal antibodies that are specific for these antigens. These antibodies, in turn, can be used for the development of sensitive assays, e.g., RIA and EIA, to detect and quantitate the TAAs in serum and urine of melanoma patients, to localize the subclinical tumor nodule(s) *in vivo*, and as a vehicle to carry and retain therapeutic agent(s) at the tumor site. Immunochemists can utilize these monoclonal antibodies for immunoaffinity purification of the TAAs to obtain quantities sufficient for molecular and structural characterization.

ACKNOWLEDGMENTS. These investigations were supported by Grants ROl CA30019 and CA 12582 awarded by the National Cancer Institute (DHEW) and by the Medical Research Service of the Veterans Administration.

References

Ax, W., Sedlacek, H. H., and Johennsen, R., 1976, Antigenic specificities of human melanoma cells *in vitro*: Detection by xenogeneic antisera and HLA isoantisera, *Behring Inst. Mitt.* **59**:71.

Baldwin, R. W., and Robins, R. A., 1976, Interference with immunological rejection of tumors, *Br. Med. Bull.* **32**:118.

Baldwin, R. W., Bowen, J. G., and Price, M. R., 1973, Detection of circulating hepatoma D23 antigen and immune complexes in tumor bearer serum, *Br. J. Cancer* **28**:16.

Bennett, C., Cooke, K. B., and Geck, p., 1978, Protein insolubilization as an aid to the detection of melanoma antigen in human urine, *Protides Biol. Fluids Proc. College* **24**:667.

Black, M. M., Opler, S. R., and Speer, F. D., 1956, Structural representations of tumor–host relationship in gastric carcinoma, *Surg. Gynecol. Obstet.* **102**:599.

Bluming, A. Z., Vogel, C. L., Ziegler, J. L., and Kiryabwire, J. W. M., 1972, Delayed cutaneous sensitivity reaction to extracts of autologous malignant melanoma: A second look, *J. Natl. Cancer Inst.* **48**:17.

Bodurtha, H. J., Chee, D. O., and Lancius, J. F., 1975, Clinical and immunological significance of human melanoma cytotoxic antibody, *Cancer Res.* **35**:189.

Bourgoin, J., Jr., and Bourgoin, A., 1973, Cytoplasmic antigens in human malignant melanoma cells, in: *Pigment Cell Mechanisms in Pigmentation* (V. G. McGovern and P. Russell Sidney (eds.). *Int. Pigm. Cell. Conf.*, Vol. 1, pp. 366–371, S. Karger, Basel.

Bowen, J. M., McBride, C. M., Miller, M. F., and Dmochowski, L., 1976, The relationship of nucleolar antigens in malignant melanoma cells to disease prognosis, *Pigm. Cell* **2**:174.

Bucana, C., and Hanna, H. M., 1974, Immunoelectron microscopic analysis of surface antigens common to *Mycobacterium bovis* (BCG) and tumor cells, *J. Natl. Cancer Inst.* **53**:1313.

Butterworth, C., Oon, C. T., Westburg, G., and Hobbs, J. R., 1974, T-lymphocyte responses in patients with malignant melanoma, *Eur. J. Cancer* **10**:639.

Bystryn, J.-C., and Smalley, J. R., 1977, Identification and solubilizaton of iodinated cell surface human melanoma associated antigens, *Int. J. Cancer* **20**:165.

Bystryn, J.-C., and Smalley, J. R., 1978, Purification of a cell-surface human melanoma associated antigen (MAA), *Clin. Res.* **26**:432A.

Canevari, S., Fossati, G., Della Porta, G., and Balzanni, G. P. 1975, Humoral cytotoxicity in melanoma patients and its correlation with the extent and the course of the disease, *Int. J. Cancer* **16**:722.

Canevari, S., Fossati, G., and Della Porta, G., 1976, Cellular immune reaction to human malignant melanoma and breast carcinoma cells, *J. Natl. Cancer Inst.* **56**:705.

Carey, T., Takahashi, T., Resnick, L. A., Oettgen, H. F., and Old, L. J., 1976, Cell surface antigen to human malignant melanoma. I. Mixed hemadsorption assays for humoral immunity to cultured autologous melanoma cells, *Proc. Natl. Acad. Sci. U.S.A.* **73**:3278.

Carey, T. E., Lloyd, K. O., Takahashi, T., Travassos, L. R., and Old, L. J., 1979, AU cell-surface antigen of human malignant melanoma: Solubilization and partial characterization, *Proc. Natl. Acad. Sci. U.S.A.* **76**:2898.

Carrel, S., and Theilkaes, L., 1973, Evidence for tumor-associated antigen in human malignant melanoma, *Nature (London)* **242**:609.

Carrel, S., Accolla, R. S., Carmgnola, A. L., and Mach, J. P. 1980, Common human melanoma-associated antigen(s) detected by monoclonal antibodies, *Cancer Res.* **40**:2523.

Catalona, W. L., Sample, W. F., and Chretien, P. B., 1973, Lymphocyte reactivity in cancer patients: Correlation with tumor histology and clinical stage, *Cancer* **31**:65.

Char, D. M., Hollinshead, A., Cogan, D. G., Ballintine, E. J., Hogan, M. J., and Herberman, R. B., 1974, Cutaneous delayed hypersensitivity reactions to soluble melanoma antigen in patients with ocular malignant melanoma, *N. Engl. J. Med.* **291**:274.

Chee, D. O., and Gupta, R. K., 1980, Tumor immunology and chemical carcinogenesis, in: *Genetic Differences in Chemical Carcinogenesis* (R. E. Kouri, ed.), pp. 151–184, CRC Press, Boca Raton, Florida.

Chee, D. O., Boddie, A. W., Jr., Roth, J. A., Holmes, E. C., and Morton, D. L., 1976, Production of melanoma-associated antigen by a human malignant melanoma cell strain grown in chemically defined medium, *Cancer Res.* **36**:1505.

Cheng, L. Y., Gupta, R. K., Huth, J. F., and Morton, D. L., 1981, Characterization of urinary antigen detected in melanoma patients by autologous and allogeneic antibody, *Proc. Am. Assoc. Cancer Res.* **22**:292.

Cochran, A. J., Mackie, R. M., Grant, R. M., Ross, C. E., Connell, M. D., Sandilands, G., Whaley, K., Hoyle, D. E., and Jackson, A. M., 1976, An examination of cancer patients, *Int. J. Cancer* **18**:298.

Coombs, R. R. A., Daniel, M. R., Gurner, B. W., and Kelus, A., 1961. Recognition of the species of cell origin in culture by mixed agglutination. II. Use of heterophile (anti-Forssman) sera, *Int. Arch. Allergy* **19**:210.

Copeman, P. W., 1979, Significance of melanoma antigen (melanoma specific protein) in the urine, *J. R., Soc. Med.* **72**:95.

Cornain, S., deVries, J. E., Collard, J., Vennegoor, C., Wingerden, I. V., and Rumke, P., 1975, Antibodies and antigen expression in human melanoma detected by the immune adherence test, *Int. J. Cancer* **16**:981.

Currie, A., 1973, Circulating antigen as an inhibitor of tumor immunity in man, *Br. J. Cancer* **28**(1):153.

Currie, G., and Basham, C., 1972, Serum mediated inhibition of the immunologic reactions of the patients to his own tumor: A possible role for circulating antigen, *Br. Med. J.* **26**:427.

DeKernion, J. B., Golub, S. H., Gupta, R. K., Silverstein, M. J., and Morton, D. L., 1975, Successful transurethral intralesional BCG therapy of a bladder melanoma, *Cancer* **36**:1661.

Della Porta, G., Calvari, S., Della Torre, G., Fossati, G., Pierotti, M. A., Vezzoni, P., and Vaglini, M., 1979, Skin test for delayed hypersensitivity to cancer extracts in cancer patients, in: *Current Trends in Tumor Immunology* (S. Ferrone, S. Gorini, R. B. Herberman, and R. A. Reisfeld, eds.), pp. 85–92, Garland STM Press, New York.

Dent, P. B., Liao, S. K., McCulloch, P. B., Blajchman, M. A., and Macnamera, J., 1978, Characterization of human malignant melanoma cell lines. III. Membrane immunofluorescence reactivity with sera from patients with melanoma, *Cancer Immunol. Immunother.* **3**:239.

DeVries, J. E., Rumke, P., and Berneheim, J. L., 1972, Cytotoxic lymphocytes in melanoma patients, *Int. J. Cancer* **9**:567.

Eilber, F. R., and Morton, D. L., 1970, Impaired immunologic reactivity and recurrence following cancer surgery, *Cancer* **25**:362.

Eilber, F. R., Nizze, J. A., and Morton, D. L., 1975, Sequential evaluation of general immune competence in cancer patients: Correlation with clinical course, *Cancer* **35**:660.

Eilber, F. R., Morton, D. L., Holmes, E. C., Sparks, F. C., and Ramming, K. P., 1976, Adjuvant immunotherapy with BCG in treatment of regional lymph node metastases from malignant melanoma, *N. Engl. J. Med.* **294**:237.

Elliott, P. G., Turlow, B., Needham, P. R. G., and Lewis, M. G., 1973, The specificity of cytoplasmic antigen in human malignant melanoma, *Eur. J. Cancer* **9**:606.

Embleton, M. J., and Price, M. R., 1975, Inhibition of *in vitro* lymphotoxic reactions against tumor cell by melanoma membrane extracts, *Behring Inst. Mitt.* **56**:157.

Engvall, E., and Perlmann, P., 1971, Enzyme linked immusorbent assay (ELISA): Quantitative assay of IgG, *Immunochemistry* **8**:871.

Everson, T. C., and Cole, W. H., 1966, *Spontaneous Regression of Cancer*, W. B. Saunders, Philadelphia.

Fass, L., Herberman, R. B., Ziegler, J. L., and Kiryabwire, J. W. M., 1970. Cutaneous hypersensitivity reactions to autologous extracts of malignant melanoma cells, *Lancet* **1**:116.

Ferrone, S., and Pellegrino, M. A., 1977, Cytotoxic antibodies to cultured melanoma cells in sera of melanoma patients, *J. Natl. Cancer Inst.* **58**:1201.

Ferrone, S., and Pellegrino, M. A., 1979, Serological detection of human melanoma associated antigens, in: *Immunodiagnosis of Cancer* (R. B. Herberman and K. R. McIntire, eds.), pp. 588–632, Marcell Dekker, New York.

Fossati, G., Colnaghi, M. I., and Della Porta, G., 1971, Cellular and humoral immunity against human malignant melanoma, *Int. J. Cancer* 8:344.

Gallaway, D. R., McCabe, R. P., Pellegrino, M. A. Ferrone, S., and Reisfeld, R. A., 1979, Molecular profile of human melanoma-associated antigens purified from spent culture medium, *Fed Proc. Fed. Am. Soc. Exp. Biol.* 38:1105.

Gallaway, D. R., Walker, L. E., and Ferrone, S., 1980, Isolation and characterization of human tumor-associated antigens with monoclonal antibody, *Proc. Am. Assoc. Cancer Res.* 21:25.

Gallaway, D. R., McCabe, R. P., Pellegrino, M. A., Ferrone, S., and Reisfeld, R. A., 1981, Tumor-associated antigens in spent culture medium of human melanoma cells: Immunochemical characterization with xenoantisera, *J. Immunol.* 126:62.

Gatti, R. A., and Good, R. A., 1971, Occurrence of malignancy in immunodeficiency diseases, *Cancer* 28:89.

Ghose, T., Norvell, S. T., Guclu, A., and McDonald, A. S., 1975, Immunochemotherapy of human malignant melanoma with chlorambucil-carrying antibody, *Eur. J. Cancer* 11:321.

Glasgow, A. H., Nimberg, R. B., Menzoian, J. O., Sporaschetz, I., Cooperband, S. R., Schmidt, K., and Mannik, J. A., 1974, Association of energy with an immunosuppressive peptide fraction in serum of patients with cancer, *N. Engl. J. Med.* 291:1263.

Golub, S. H., O'Connell, T. X., and Morton, D. L., 1974, Correlation of *in vivo* and *in vitro* assays of immunocompetence in cancer patients, *Cancer Res.* 34:1833.

Golub, S. H., Rangel, D. M., and Morton, D. L., 1977, *In vitro* assessment of immunocompetence in patients with malignant melanoma, *Int. J. Cancer* 20:873.

Gray, B. R., Mehigan, J. T., and Morton, D. L., 1971, Demonstration of antibodies in melanoma patients cytotoxic to human melanoma cells, *Proc. Am. Assoc. Cancer Res.* 12:79.

Griffith, J. D., McKinna, J. A., Rowbatham, H. D., Tsolakidis, P., and Salsbury, A. J., 1973, Carcinoma of the colon and rectum: Circulating malignant cells and five-year survival, *Cancer* 31:226.

Grimm, E. A., Silver, H. K. B., Roth, J. A., Chee, D. O., Gupta, R. K., and Morton, D. L., 1976, Detection of tumor associated antigen in human melanoma cell line supernatants, *Int. J. Cancer* 17:559.

Giuliano, A. E., Rangel, D. M., Holmes, E. C., Golub, S. H., and Morton, D. L., 1977, Serum-mediated immunosuppression in cancer, *Surg. Forum* 28:163.

Gupta, R. K., 1975, Common cancer associated antigen(s) in human neoplasms, *Proc. Am. Assoc. Cancer Res.* 15:262.

Gupta, R. K., 1980, Antigenic complexity in human malignant melanoma tumors detected by allogeneic antibody, in: *Serologic Analysis of Human Cancer Antigens* (S. A. Rosenberg, ed.), pp. 339–380, Academic Press, New York.

Gupta, R. K., and Morton, D. L., 1975a, Suggestive evidence for *in vivo* binding of specific antitumor antibodies of human melanomas, *Cancer Res.* 35:58.

Gupta, R. K., and Morton, D. L., 1975b, Presence of tumor-associated antigens in urine of patients with cancer, *Surg. Forum* 26:158.

Gupta, R. K., and Morton, D. L., 1976, Tumor-associated antigens in urine of cancer patients, *Proc. Am. Assoc. Cancer Res.* 17:92.

Gupta, R. K., and Morton, D. L., 1977, Distribution of antibodies to common tumor-associated antigen(s) in cancer and non-cancer sera, *Proc. Am. Assoc. Cancer Res.* 18:184.

Gupta, R. K., and Morton, D. L., 1979a, Double antibody method and the protein-A bearing *Staphylococcus aureus* cells method compared for separating bound and free antigen in radioimmunoassay, *Clin. Chem.* 25:752.

Gupta, R. K., and Morton, D. L., 1979b, Detection of cancer-associated antigens in urine of sarcoma patients, *J. Surg. Oncol.* 11:65.

Gupta, R. K., and Morton, D. L., 1979c, Specificity by radioimmunoassay of tumor-associated antigen isolated from spent culture medium of a human melanoma cell line, *Fed. Proc. Fed. Am. Soc. Exp. Biol.* 39:1144.

Gupta, R. K., and Morton, D. L., 1980, Radioimmunoassay for the analysis of tumor associated antigens with allogeneic antibody, in: *Serologic Analysis of Human Cancer Antigens* (S. A. Rosenberg, ed.), pp. 645–650, Academic Press, New York.

Gupta, R. K., Irie, R. F., and Morton, D. L., 1978a, Antigens on human tumor cells assayed by complement fixation with allogeneic antisera, *Cancer Res.* **38**:2573.

Gupta, R. K., Silver, H. K. B., and Morton, D. L., 1978b, Reactivity of human tumor extracts to xenogeneic antisera raised against human melanoma extracts, *Proc. Am. Assoc. Cancer Res.* **19**:360.

Gupta, R. K., Golub, S. H., and Morton, D. L., 1979a, Correlation between tumor burden and anticomplementary activity in sera from cancer patients, *Cancer Immunol. Immunother.* **6**:63.

Gupta, R. K., Golub, S. H., Rangel, D. M., and Morton, D. L., 1979b, Inhibition of mitogen-induced lymphocyte proliferation correlated to anticomplementary activity in sera from melanoma patients, *Cancer Immunol. Immunother.* **5**:221.

Gupta, R. K., Irie, R. F., Chee, D. O., Kern, D. H., and Morton, D. L., 1979c, Demonstration of two distinct antigens in spent tissue culture medium of a human malignant melanoma cell line, *J. Natl. Cancer Inst.* **63**:347.

Gupta, R. K., Silver, H. K. B., Reisfeld, R. A., and Morton, D. L., 1979d, Isolation and immunochemical characterization of antibodies from cancer patients' sera reactive against human melanoma cell membranes by affinity chromatography, *Cancer Res.* **39**:1683.

Gupta, R. K., Theofilopoulos, A. N., Dixon, F. J., and Morton, D. L., 1979e, Circulating immune complexes as possible cause for anticomplementary activity in humans with maligant melanoma, *Cancer Immunol. Immunother.* **6**:211.

Gupta, R. K., Silver, H. K. B., and Morton, D. L., 1980, Production and characterization of xenogeneic antisera to tumor-associated antigen(s), *J. Surg. Oncol.* **13**:75.

Hamburger, R. N., Pioris, D. A., and Milles, S. E., 1963, Antigenic specificities acquired from the growth medium by cells in tissue culture, *Immunology* **6**:439.

Hellström, I., Sjögren, H. O., Warner, G. A., and Hellström, K. E., 1971, Blocking of cell mediated tumor immunity by sera from patients with growing neoplasms, *Int. J. Cancer* **7**:226.

Hellström, I., Hellström, K. E., Sjögren, H. O., and Warner, G. A., 1973a, Destruction of cultivated melanoma cells by lymphocytes from healthy black (North American Negro) donors, *Int. J. Cancer* **11**:116.

Hellström, I., Warner, G. A., Hellström, K. E., and Sjögren, H. O., 1973b, Sequential studies on cell-mediated tumor immunity and blocking serum activity in ten patients with malignant melanoma, *Int. J. Cancer* **11**:280.

Hellström, I., Brown, J. P., Woodbury, R., Yen, Y. M., Nishiyama, K., and Hellström, K. E., 1980, Monoclonal antibodies to tumor-associated antigens in human melanoma, *Proc. Am. Assoc. Cancer Res.* **21**:221.

Hellström, K. E., and Hellström, I., 1974, Lymphocyte-mediated cytotoxicity and blocking serum activity to tumor antigens, *Adv. Immunol.* **18**:209.

Hellström, K. E., and Hellström, I., 1977, Immunologic enhancement of tumor growth, in: *Mechanisms of Tumor Immunity* (I. Green, S. Cohen, and R. T. McCluskey, eds.). pp. 147–191, Wiley, New York.

Heppner, G. H., Stolbach, L., Byrne, M., Cummings, F. J., McDonough, E., and Calabrest, E., 1973, Cell-mediated reactivity to tumor antigens in patients with malignant melanoma, *Int. J. Cancer* **11**:245.

Hersey, P., Honeyman, M., Edwards, A., Adams, E., and McCarthy, W. H., 1976, Antigens on melanoma cells detected by leukocyte dependent antibody assays of human melanoma antisera, *Int. J. Cancer* **18**:564.

Hersey, P., Murray, E., and Ruygrok, S., 1978, Characterization of melanoma antigens in sera of melanoma patients and in supernatants of melanoma cell cultures, *Fed. Proc. Fed. Am. Soc. Exp. Biol.* **37**:1595.

Hersey, P., Murray, E., Werkmeister, J., and McCarthy, W. H., 1979, Detection of a low molecular weight antigen on melanoma cells by a human antiserum in leukocyte-dependent antibody assay, *Br. J. Cancer* **40**:615.

Hollinshead, A. C., Herberman, R. B., Jaffurs, W. J., Alpert, L. K., Minten, J. P., and Harris, J. E., 1974, Soluble membrane antigens of human maligant melanoma cells, *Cancer* **34**:1235.

Holmes, E. C., Roth, J. A., and Morton, D. L., 1975, Delayed cutaneous hypersensitivity reactions to autologous extracts of malignant melanoma cells, *Surgery* **78**:160.

Huth, J. F., Gupta, R. K., and Morton, D. L., 1979, Sequential analysis of urinary antigens in sarcoma patients, *Surg. Forum* **30**:150.

Huth, J. F., Gupta, R. K., and Morton, D. L., 1981a, Development of an enzyme immunoassay to detect and quantitate tumor-associated antigens in the urine of sarcoma patients, *Cancer* **47**:28–56.

Huth, J. F., Gupta, R. K., and Morton, D. L., 1981b, Assessment of the *in vivo* effectiveness of tumoricidal chemotherapy and radiation therapy by serial analysis of tumor-associated urinary antigen titers in sarcoma patients, *Cancer Treatment Rep.* (in press).

Irie, R. F., 1980, Oncofetal antigen (OFA-I): A human tumor associated fetal antigen immunogenic in man, in: *Serologic Analysis of Human Cancer Antigens* (S. A. Rosenberg, ed.), pp. 493–513, Academic Press, New York.

Irie, R. F., Irie, K., and Morton, D. L., 1974a, Natural antibody in human serum to a neoantigen in human cultured cells grown in fetal bovine serum, *J. Natl. Cancer Inst.* **52**:1051.

Irie, R. F., Irie, K., and Morton, D. L., 1974b, Characteristics of heterologous membrane antigen on cultured human cells, *J. Natl. Cancer Inst.* **53**:1545.

Irie, R. F., Irie, K., and Morton, D. L., 1976, A membrane antigen common to human cancer and fetal brain tissues, *Cancer Res.* **36**:3510.

Jehn, V. W., Nathanson, L., Schwartz, R. S., and Skinner, M., 1970, *In vitro* lymphocyte stimulation of a soluble antigen from malignant melanoma, *N. Engl. J. Med.* **283**:329.

Jose, D. G., and Seshadri, R., 1974, Circulating immune complexes in human neuroblastoma: Direct assay and role in blocking specific cellular immunity, *Int. J. Cancer* **13**:824.

Kasai, M., Saxton, R. E., Holmes, E. C., Burk, W. M., and Morton, D. L., 1981, Membrane antigens detected on human lung carcinoma cells by hybridoma monoclonal antibody, *J. Surg. Res.* **30**:403.

Kilburn, D. G., Fairhurst, M., Levey, J. G., and Whitney, R. B., 1976, Synergism between immune complexes and serum from tumor-bearing mice in the suppression of mitogen responses, *J. Immunol.* **117**:1612.

Koprowski, H., Steplewski, Z., Herlyn, D., and Herlyn, M., 1978, Studies of antibodies against human melanoma produced by somatic cell hybrid, *Proc. Natl. Acad. Sci U.S.A.* **75**:3405.

Laine, R. A., and Kakorman, A., 1973, Incorporation of exogenous glycosphingolipid in plasma membranes of cultured hamster cells and concurrent change of growth behavior, *Biochim. Biophys. Acta* **54**:1039.

Lee, Y. T. N., Sparks, F. C., Eilber, F. R., and Morton, D. L., 1975, Delayed cutaneous hypersensitivity and peripheral lymphocyte counts in patients with advanced cancer, *Cancer* **35**:748.

Leong, S. P., Cooperband, S. R., Sutherland, C. M., Krementz, E. T., and Deckers, P. J., 1978a, Detection of human melanoma antigens in cell-free supernatants, *Biochem. Med.* **24**:245.

Leong, S. P., Cooperband, S. R., Deckers, P. J., Sutherland, C. M., and Krementz, E. T., 1978b, Isolation of human melanoma membrane antigens, *Clin. Res.* **26**:224A.

Lewis, M G., and Kiryabwire, J. W. M., 1968, Aspects of behavior and natural history of malignant melanoma in Uganda, *Cancer* **21**:876.

Lewis, M G., and Phillips, T. M., 1972, Specificity of surface membrane immunofluorescence in human malignant melanoma, *Int. J. Cancer* **10**:105.

Lewis, M G., Ikonopisov, R. L., Nairn, R. C., Phillips, T. M., Hamilton-Fairley, G., Bodenham, D. C., and Alexander, P., 1969, Tumour specific antibodies in human malignant melanoma and their relationship to the extent of the disease, *Br. Med. J.* **3**:547.

Lewis, M.G., Phillips, T. M., Cook, K. B., and Blake, J., 1971, Possible explanation for loss of detectable antibody in patients with disseminated malignant melanoma, *Nature (London)* **232**:52.

Lewis, M. G., Avis, P. J. G., Phillips, T. M., and Sheikh, K. M. A., 1973, Tumor-associated antigens in human malignant melanoma, *Yale J. Biol. Med.* **46**:661.

Liao, S. K., Leong, S. P. L., Sutherland, C. M., Dent, P. B., Kwong, D. C., and Krementz, E. T., 1978, Common human melanoma membrane antigens detected by mixed hemadsorption assay with sera from a patient undergoing immunotherapy with autologous tumor cells, *Cancer Res.* **38**:4394.

Lopez, M J., and Thomson, D. M. P., 1977, Isolation of breast tumor antigen from serum and urine, *Int. J. Cancer* **20**:834.

Macher, E., Muller, C., Sorg, G., Gassen, A., and Sorg, C., 1975, Evidence for cross-reacting membrane-associated specific melanoma antigens as detected by immunofluorescence and immune adherence, *Behring Inst. Mitt* **56**:86.

Malley, A., Frikke, M. J., Burger, D. R., Black, J. A., and Vandenbark, A. A., 1976, Fractionation of human melanoma tumor antigens, *Fed. Proc. Fed. Am. Soc. Exp. Biol.* **35**:547.

McBride, C. M., Bowen, J. M., and Dmochowski, L. L., 1972, Anti-nucleolar antibodies in the sera of patients with malignant melanoma, *Surg. Forum* **23**:92.

McCabe, R. P., Ferrone, S., Pellegrino, M. A., Kern, D. H., Homes, E. C., and Reisfeld, R. A., 1978a, Purification and immunological evaluation of human melanoma associated antigens, *J. Natl. Cancer Inst.* **60**:773.

McCabe, R. P., Frugis, L., Ferrone, S., Kern, D., and Reisfeld, R. A., 1978b, Detection and purification of human melanoma-associated cell surface antigens, *Proc. Am. Assoc. Cancer Res.* **19**:206.

McCabe, R. P., Quaranta, V., Frugis, L., Ferrone, S., and Reisfeld, R. A., 1979, A radioimmunometric antibody binding assay for the evaluation of xenoantisera to melanoma associated antigens, *J. Natl. Cancer Inst.* **62**:455.

McKhann, C. F., 1969, Primary malignancy in patients undergoing immunosuppression for renal transplantation, *Transplantation* **8**:209.

Minden, P., Sharpton, T. R., and McClatchy, J. K., 1976, Shared antigens between human malignant melanoma cells and *Mycobacterium bovis* (BCG), *J. Immunol.* **116**:1407.

Moretta, L., Webb, S. R., Girossi, C. E., Lydyard, T. M., and Cooper, M D., 1977, Functional analysis of two human T-cell subpopulations: Help and supression of B-cell responses by T-cell bearing receptors for IgM and IgG, *J. Exp. Med.* **146**:184.

Morton, D. L., 1971, Immunologic studies with human neoplasms, *J. Reticuloendothel. Soc.* **10**:137.

Morton, D. L., Malmgren, R. A., Holmes, E. C., and Ketcham, A. S., 1968, Demonstration of antibodies against human malignant melanoma by immunofluorescence, *Surgery* **64**:233.

Morton, D. L., Eilber, F. R., Malmgren, R. A., and Wood, W. C., 1970, Immunologic factors which influence response to immunotherapy in malignant melanoma, *Surgery* **68**:158.

Morton, D. L., Eilber, F. R., and Malmgren, R. A., 1971a, Immune factors in human cancer: Malignant melanomas, skeletal and soft tissue sarcomas, *Prog. Exp. Tumor Res.* **14**:25.

Morton, D. L., Holmes, E. C., Eilber, F. R., and Wood, W. C., 1971b, Immunologic aspects of neoplasia: A rational basis for immunotherapy, *Ann. Intern. Med.* **74**:587.

Morton, D. L., Golub, S. H., Sulit, H. L., Gupta, R. K., Eilber, F. R., Holmes, E. C., and Sparks, F. C., 1975, Immunologic and clinical responses to active immunotherapy of malignant melanoma, in: *Fundamental Aspects of Neoplasia* (A. A. Gottlieb, O. J. Plescia, and D. H. L. Bishop, eds.), pp. 181–201, Springer-Verlag, New York.

Mukherji, B., Nathanson, L., and Clark, D. A., 1973, Studies of humoral and cell-mediated immunity in human melanoma, *Yale J. Biol. Med.* **46**:681.

Muna, N. M., Marcus, S., and Smart, C., 1969, Dectection by immunofluorescence of antibodies specific for human malignant melanoma cells, *Cancer* **23**:88.

Nairn, R. C., Nind, A. P., Guli, E. P., Davies, K. J., Little, J. H., Davies, N. C., and Whitehead, R. H., 1972, Anti-tumor immunoreactivity in patients with malignant melanoma, *Med. J. Aust.* **1**:397.

Nathanson, L., 1974, Use of BCG in the treatment of human neoplasms: A review, *Semin. Oncol.* **1**:337.

Nelson, D. S., and Gatti, R. A., 1976, Humoral factors influencing lymphocyte transformation, *Prog. Allergy* **21**:261.

Oettgen, H. F., Aoki, T., Old, L. J., Boys, E. A., deHarven, E., and Mills, G. M., 1968, Suspension culture of a pigment-producing cell line derived from a human malignant melanoma, *J. Natl. Cancer Inst.* **41**:827.

Oettgen, H. F., Pinsky, C. M., and Delmonte, L., 1976, Treatment of cancer with immunomodulators: *Corynebacterium parvum* and Levamisole, *Med. Clin. North Am.* **60**:511.

Oren, M. E., and Herberman, R. B., 1971, Delayed cutaneous hypersensitivity reactions to membrane extracts of human tumor cells, *Clin. Exp. Immunol.* **9**:45.

Parikh, I., March, S., and Cuatrecasas, P., 1974, Topics in the methodology of substitution reactions with agarose, in: *Methods in Enzymology*, Vol. 34 (Part B) (W. B. Jakoby and M. Wilchek, eds.), pp. 77–102, Academic Press, New York.

Peacock, A. C., and Dingman, C. W., 1968, Molecular weight estimation and separation of ribonucleic acid by electrophoresis in agarose–acrylamide composite gels, *Biochemistry* **7**:668.

Penn, I., 1970, Chemical immunosuppression and human cancer, *Cancer* **34**:1474.

Penn, I., Hammond, W., Brettschmeider, L., and Sturzl, T. E., 1969, Malignant lymphomas in transplantation patients, *Transplant. Proc.* **1**:106.

Peter, H. H., Pavie-Fischer, J., Fridman, W., Aubert, C., Cesarini, J. P., Roubin, R., and Kounilsky, F., 1975, Cell-mediated cytoxicity *in vitro* of human lymphocytes against a tissue culture melanoma cell line (1GR3), *J. Immunol.* **115**:539.

Peterson, R. D. A., Kelly, W. D., and Good, R. A., 1964, Ataxia telangiectasia: Its association with defective thymus, immunological-deficiency diseases and malignancy, *Lancet* **1**:1189.

Pilch, Y. H., Fritze, D., and Kern, D. H., 1976, Immune RNA in the immunotherapy of cancer, *Med. Clin. North Am.* **60**:567.

Pinsky, C., Hirshaut, Y., and Oettgen, H., 1972, Treatment of malignant melanoma by intratumoral injection of BCG, *Proc. Am. Assoc. Cancer Res.* **13**:21.

Ran, M., Klein, G., and Witz, I. P., 1976, Tumor bound immunoglobulins: Evidence for the *in vivo* coating of tumor cells by potentially cytotoxic anti-tumor antibodies, *Int. J. Cancer* **17**:90.

Rangel, D. M., Golub, S. H., and Morton, D. L., 1977, Demonstration of lymphocyte blastogenesis-inhibiting factors in sera of melanoma patients, *Surgery* **82**:224.

Reisfeld, R. A., Pellegrino, M. A., and Kahan, B. D., 1971, Salt extraction of soluble HL-A antigens, *Science* **172**:1134.

Reisfeld, R. A., McCabe, R. P., Ferrone, S., Pellegrino, M. A., and Holmes, E. C., 1977, Characterization of melanoma associated antigens isolated from cultured melanoma cells, *Proc. Am. Assoc. Cancer Res.* **18**:205.

Ristow, S., and McKhann, C. F., 1977, Tumor-associated antigens, in: *Mechanisms of Tumor Immunity* (I. Green, S. Cohen, and R. T. McClusky, eds.), pp. 109–145, John Wiley, New York.

Roberts, S. S., Hengesh, J. W. McGrath, R. G., Valaitis, J., McGrew, E. A., and Cole, W. H., 1967, Prognostic significance of cancer cells in circulating blood: A ten year evaluation, *Am. J. Surg.* **113**:757.

Romsdahl, M. M., and Cox, I. S., 1970, Human malignant melanoma antibodies demonstrated by immunofluorescence, *Arch. Surg.* **100**:491.

Romsdhal, M. M., and Cox, I. S., 1973, Immunological studies on malignant melanomas of man, *Yale J. Biol. Med.* **46**:693.

Rosenberg, E. B. McCoy, J. L., Green, S. S., Donnelly, F. C., Siwarski, D. F., Levine, P. H., and Herberman, R. B., 1974, Destruction of human lymphoid tissue-culture cell line by human peripheral blood lymphocytes in ⁵¹Cr-release cellular cytotoxicity assays, *J. Natl. Cancer Inst.* **52**:345.

Rote, N. S., Gupta, R. K., and Morton, D. L., 1978, Detection of tumor-associated antigens in the urine of sarcoma patients *Proc. Am. Assoc. Cancer Res.* **19**:134.

Rote, N. S., Gupta, R. K., and Morton, D. L., 1980a, Determination of incidence of tumor-associated antigens found in the urine of patients bearing solid tumors, *Int. J. Cancer* **26**:203

Rote, N. S., Gupta, R. K., and Morton, D. L., 1980b, Tumor-associated antigens detected by autologous sera in urine of patients with solid neoplasms, *J. Surg. Res.* **29**:18.

Roth, J. A., Slocum, H.K., Pellegrino, M A., Holmes, E. C., and Reisfeld, R. A., 1976, purification of soluble melanoma-associated antigens, *Cancer Res.* **36**:2360.

Saxton, R. E., Golub, S. H., and Morton, D. L., 1978, Specificity of antibody induced in sarcoma patients immunized with allogeneic sarcoma cells, *Proc. Am. Assoc. Cancer Res.* **19**:135.

Seibert, E., Sorg, C., Happle, R., and Macher, E., 1977, Membrane associated antigens of human malignant melanoma. III. Specificity of human sera reacting with cultured melanoma cells, *Int. J. Cancer* **19**:172.

Seigler, H. F. Shingleton, W. W., Metzgar, R. D., Buckley, C. E., Bergoc, C. M., Miller, D. S., Fatter, B. F., and Phaup, M. B., 1972, Non-specific and specific immunotherapy in patients with melanoma, *Surgery* **72**:162.

Seigler, H. F., Metzgar, R. S., Mohankumar, T., and Stuhlmiller, G. M., 1975a, Human melanoma and leukemia-associated antigens defined by non-human primate antisera, *Fed. Proc. Fed. Am. Soc. Exp. Biol.* **34**:1642.

Seigler, H. F., Shingleton, W. W., Horne, B. J., and Pickness, K. L., 1975b, The use of BCG, adoptive transfer, and neuraminidase treated cells in the management of melanoma, *Behring Inst. Mitt.* **56**:214.

Shibata, H. R., Jerry, L. M., Lewis, M. G., Manself, P. W. A., Capek, C., and Marquis, G., 1976, Immunotherapy of malignant melanoma with irradiated tumor cells, oral bacillus Calmette-Guérin and levamisole, *Ann. N.Y. Acad. Sci.* **277**:355.

Shiku, H., Takahashi, T., Oettgen, H. F., and Old, L. J., 1976, Cell surface antigen of human malignant melanoma. II. Serologic typing with immune adherence assays and definition of two new surface antigens, *J. Exp. Med.* **144**:873.

Sjögren, H. O., Hellström, I., Bansal, S. C., and Hellström, K. E., 1971, Suggestive evidence that "blocking antibodies" of tumor bearing individuals may be antigen antibody complexes, *Proc. Natl. Acad. Sci. U.S.A.* **68**:1372.

Sjögren, H. O., Hellström, I., Bansal, S. C., Warner, G. A., and Hellström, K. E., 1972, Elution of blocking factors from human tumors capable of abrogating tumor-cell destruction by specifically immune lymphocytes, *Int. J. Cancer* **9**:274.

Smith, W. J., and Jacobs, B. B., 1979, Modification of melanoma antigen expression *in vitro*, *Fed. Proc. Fed. Am. Soc. Exp. Biol.* **38**:1105.

Sorg, C., Brüggen, J., Seibert, E., and Macher, E., 1978, Membrane associated antigens of human malignant melanoma. IV. Changes in expression of antigens on cultured melanoma cells, *Cancer Immunol. Immunother.* **3**:259.

Southam, C. M., Brunschwig, W., Levin, A. G., and Dixon, Q. S., 1966, The effect of leukocytes on transplantability of human cancer, *Cancer* **19**:1743.

Steel, G., Jr., Ankerst, J., and Sjögren, H. O., 1974, Alteration of *in vitro* anti-tumor activity of tumor-bearer sera by absorption with *Staphylococcus aureus*, Cowan I., *Int. J. Cancer* **14**:83.

Steel, G., Jr. Sjögren, H. O., and Stradenberg, I., 1976, *In vitro* cell-mediated immune reactions of melanoma and colorectal carcinoma patients demonstrated by long-term ^{51}Cr assay, *Int. J. Cancer* **17**:27.

Stewart, T. H. M., 1969, The presence of delayed hypersensitivity reactions in patients toward cellular extracts of their malignant tumors, *Cancer* **23**:1368.

Stuhlmiller, G. M., and Seigler, H. F., 1975, Characterization of a chimpanzee anti-human melanoma antiserum, *Cancer Res.* **35**:2132.

Stuhlmiller, G. M., Green, R. W., and Seigler, H. F., 1978, Solubilization and partial isolation of human melanoma tumor-associated antigens, *J. Natl. Cancer Inst.* **61**:61.

Suter, L., Tilkorn, H., and Kovary, P. M., 1978, Human malignant melanoma antigenic properties of phenol water extracts, *Arch. Dermatol. Res.* **264**:37.

Tagasuki, M., Mickey, M. R., and Terasaki, P. I., 1973, Reactivity of lymphocytes from normal persons on cultured tumor cells, *Cancer Res.* **33**:2898.

The, T. H., Huiges, H. A., Koops, H. S., Lambarts, H. B., and Niewg, H. O., 1975, Surface antigens on cultured malignant melanoma cells as detected by membrane immunofluorescence method with human sera: Lack of tumor specific reaction on melanoma cell lines, *Ann. N. Y. Acad. Sci.* **254**:528.

Theofilopoulos, A. N., and Dixon, F. J., 1978, Immune complexes associated with neoplasia, in: *Immunodiagnosis of Cancer*, Part 2 (R. B. Herberman, ed.), pp. 896–937, Marcel Dekker, New York.

Thomson, D. M. P., and Lopez, M. J., 1978, Isolation of human tumor antigen from serum and urine, *Proc. Am. Assoc. Cancer Res.* **19**:171.

Thomson, D. M. P., Steel, K., and Alexander, P., 1973, The presence of tumorspecific membrane antigen of a chemically induced sarcomata, *Br. J. Cancer* **27**:27.

Ting, C. C., and Herberman, R. B., 1976, Humoral host defense mechanisms against tumors, *Int. Rev. Exp. Pathol.* **15**:93.

Tonder, O., Krishnan, E. C., Jewell, W. R., Morse, P. A., and Humphrey, L. J., 1976, Tumor Fc receptors and tumor-associated immunoglobulins, *Acta Pathol. Microbiol. Scand.* **84**:105.

Viza, D., and Phillips, J., 1975, Identification of an antigen associated with malignant melanoma, *Int. J. Cancer* **16**:312.

Volkers, C., Cooke, B., Bennett, C., Byrom, N., Campbell, M., Elliott, P., and Whitfield, P., 1978, The significance of urinary melanoma antigen excretion and the ability of thymosin to raise the level of depleted lymphocytes *in vitro* in malignant melanoma, *Aust. N. Z. J. Surg.* **48**:32.

Voller, A., Bidwell, D. E., and Bartlett, A., 1976, Microplate enzyme immunoassay for immunodiagnosis of virus infections, in: *Manual of Clinical Immunology* (N. R. Rose and H. Friedman, eds), pp. 506–512, American Society for Microbiology, Washington, D.C.

Wesenberg, F., 1978, Fc receptors and IgG associated with human malignant tumors *Acta Pathol. Microbiol. Scand.* **86**:259.

Wood, G. W., and Barth, R. F., 1974, Immunofluorescent studies of the serologic reactivity of patients with malignant melanoma against tumor-associated cytoplasmic antigens, *J. Natl. Cancer Inst.* **53**:309.

Yeh, M.-Y., Hellström, I., Brown, J. P., Warner, G. A., Hansen, J. A., and Hellström, K. E., 1979, Cell surface antigens of human melanoma identified by monoclonal antibody, *Proc. Natl. Acad. Sci. U.S.A.* **76**:2927.

9

Specificity of Cell-Mediated Immunoreactivity in Melanoma and Comments on the Nature of Serum Blocking Factors

W. J. HALLIDAY

1. Introduction

Malignant melanoma is, from the immunological viewpoint, one of the most extensively studied of all cancers. It is sometimes stated that the reason lies in the tendency of melanoma to undergo spontaneous regression. The assumption is made that regression necessarily has an immunological basis and furthermore that host immunity should thus be more readily demonstrable in melanoma than in other cancers. These concepts are simplistic: tumor regression might have many different mechanisms, and identifiable criteria of immuno-reactivity in melanoma patients are typical of many cancers. Nevertheless, there are good practical reasons for choosing to study melanoma as a model of tumor immunity. In Queensland, melanoma is not uncommon; the incidence is the highest in the world at over 30 per 100,000, and clinical material is thus relatively abundant. The visibility of the cutaneous tumor, and intensive health education, combine to ensure that many melanomas are detected at an early stage, identified by experienced clinicians and histopathologists, and removed successfully by adequate surgery (Smith, 1979).

As recounted previously (Halliday, 1979), studies of melanoma have played an important part in the development of leukocyte-adherence inhibition (LAI). Most of this chapter will deal with the influence of LAI on ideas concerning cell-mediated immunity (CMI) in cancer and its regulation by serum factors.

W. J. HALLIDAY • Department of Microbiology, University of Queensland, Brisbane, Australia 4067.

2. Techniques of Cell-Mediated Immunity *in Vitro*

Specific adaptive CMI may be defined, somewhat inconsistently, as immunity dependent on reactions of T lymphocytes. Other cells, particularly mononuclear phagocytes
(monocytes and macrophages), are involved not only in nonspecific innate cellular immunity, but also as accessory cells or effector cells in specific CMI. The *in vivo* manifestations
of CMI (tumor rejection, delayed hypersensitivity) are difficult to observe, quantitate, and
analyze. Hence, there has been a great attraction to *in vitro* reactions as a means of investigating the host response to tumor antigens.

In vitro reactions of CMI fall broadly into two classes, those that involve antigens on
cells and that that involve soluble antigens.

2.1. Reactions That Require Intact Target Cells

Fresh or cultivated melanoma cells form suitable targets for the cytotoxic activities of
sensitized lymphocytes from melanoma patients (I. Hellström *et al.*, 1968; I. Hellström
and K. E. Hellström, 1973). Antigens on the target-cell surface and receptors on the lymphocyte surface are demonstrated by this reaction of lymphocyte cytotoxicity.

The current status of lymphocyte cytotoxicity reactions in melanoma is fully covered
in Chapter 11. The original observations (I. Hellström *et al.*, 1968) of specificity related
to tumor type have been clouded by the discovery of widespread reactivity in normal
subjects and patients with other cancers. Nevertheless, the concept of an underlying
tumor specificity is an important one, which reappears in connection with other reactions and is elaborated in Sections 2.2, 2.3, and 3.1.

A characteristic property of lymphocytotoxicity is its ability to be "blocked" by factors
in certain sera (I. Hellström *et al.*, 1973). This phenomenon is dealt with more fully in
Section 5.

2.2. Reactions with Soluble Antigens

When soluble antigens from tumors or other sources are recognized by sensitized lymphocytes, a cytotoxic reaction in a target cell obviously cannot result. The lymphocyte is
activated in alternative ways, resulting in DNA synthesis (lymphocyte transformation,
stimulation, or blastogenesis) and in the production of lymphokines. These phenomena may
also be triggered by antigens on intact tumor cells, but this mode of presentation is not
essential. Usually, accessory cells are required, in the form of macrophages or monocytes,
in order that lymphocytes and soluble antigens will interact effectively.

Leukocyte-migration inhibition (LMI) is the most familiar example of a lymphokine-
mediated reaction involving soluble tumor antigens. Several different techniques have been
developed to demonstrate the interaction between melanoma patients' blood leucocytes and
allogeneic extracts or other crude preparations of melanoma antigens, resulting in migration inhibition (see Chapter 5). The data appear to reflect reactivity related to common
antigens in melanomas from different sources and the ability of many patients to respond

immunologically to their own tumor antigens. The proportion of false-negative reactions in some studies is disturbingly high. It is not clear whether this unreliability is a consequence of lack of sensitivity in the technique, unresponsiveness in the patient, heterogeneity of melanoma antigens, or more subtle factors. A possible additional cause of spurious non-reactivity is a phenomenon reported by McCoy *et al.* (1980), namely, that certain individuals' polymorphonuclear leukocytes are poorly susceptible to the lymphokine involved in LMI and therefore cannot function as indicator cells in the reaction. To avoid this source of error, it is recommended that LMI reactions be conducted as indirect or two-stage tests; the patient's leukocytes are reacted with the tumor extract in the first stage, then the cell-free supernatant is tested on normal polymorphs of known susceptibility in the second stage.

Modern forms of the LMI technique (McCoy *et al.*, 1980) have improved on the conventional capillary-tube method, which was slow and tedious and required large numbers of cells. In an effort to obviate these disadvantages of LMI, the reaction of LAI was developed (Halliday and Miller, 1972). Although LAI has a mechanism quite different from lymphocyte cytotoxicity, these reactions have remarkable similarities as indicators of antitumor CMI and of serum blocking factors.

2.3. Leukocyte-Adherence Inhibition

LAI is an immunological reaction first demonstrated with murine tumor antigens. It is now established for use with a variety of soluble antigens in man and several animal species. A recent workshop (Goldrosen and Howell, 1979) summarized the status of the technique in cancer.

When suitable leukocytes (from blood, spleen, or peritoneal cavity of a subject previously sensitized to a certain antigen) are exposed to antigen *in vitro*, they rapidly become less likely to adhere to solid surfaces. This simple outline of LAI conceals many complexities. One must immediately ask: Which cells in the leukocyte population are antigen-reactive? Are these cells the ones the adherence of which is inhibited, or are other cells affected and how? Does antigen concentration affect the outcome, and what is the time–course of the reaction? What controls are employed to establish normal adherence? How is cell adherence quantitated? Is LAI directly related to antitumor immunoreactivity? These and many other questions present themselves, and complete answers to all of them are not yet available. Nevertheless, a picture is emerging, and a brief summary can be attempted.

2.3.1. Hemocytometer Leukocyte-Adherence Inhibition

Our first observations of LAI in the mouse (Halliday and Miller, 1972) and in man (Halliday *et al.*, 1974b) involved tumor antigens, and only this aspect will be pursued here. LAI with other antigens is described elsewhere (Holt *et al.*, 1975; Powell *et al.*, 1978; Koppi *et al.*, 1979; Dunn and Halliday, 1980; Noonan and Halliday, 1980). Murine peritoneal cells or human blood leukocytes from tumor-bearing subjects were mixed with appropriate tumor extracts in a serum-rich medium and introduced into hemocytometer chambers. During a 1-hr incubation period, most of the cells adhered to the glass surface of the slide, with varying degrees of affinity. The total numbers of cells were then counted in predetermined areas, the less adherent cells were removed by a standard manual washing procedure, and the remaining adherent cells were counted. The percentage adherence was calculated. Statistical comparisons were made between adherences with and without tumor extract (antigen). The raw data and calculations pertaining to an actual LAI assay by this "hemocytometer method" have been published (Maluish and Halliday, 1979); these were obtained during a blind trial of LAI in human cancer, including melanoma.

The specifically reactive cells in human LAI are T lymphocytes (Powell *et al.*, 1978; Koppi *et al.*, 1979). In the mouse, they have the Thy.1 and Ly.1 markers and require macrophages as accessory cells (Koppi and Halliday, unpublished data). The lymphocytes are stimulated by antigen to produce leukocyte-adherence-inhibition factor (LAIF), a lymphokine that reduces the glass-adherence of a range of indicator leukocytes, including those from other animal species (Noonan *et al.*, 1977; Koppi *et al.*, 1979). Hemocytometer LAI has been shown to have tumor specificity of a type reminiscent of that found in other assays, namely, related to individual chemically induced tumors in mice (Halliday and Miller, 1972; Halliday *et al.*, 1974c) and to tumor type in man (Halliday *et al.*, 1974a,b; Powell *et al.*, 1975). Further details of the mechanism are available from studies with nontumor antigens (Creemers, 1977; Powell *et al.*, 1978; Dunn and Halliday, 1980).

Relatively few of the laboratories reporting LAI investigations in cancer have employed the original method. Hemocytometer LAI is a technically demanding technique, and many adaptations have been introduced in attempts to make the assay more suitable for routine use. The two most prominent of these adaptations employ different adherence vessels, namely, glass or plastic test tubes and plastic microplates.

2.3.2. Test-Tube Leukocyte-Adherence Inhibition

When leukocyte–antigen mixtures are incubated in test tubes lying horizontally, cell adherence occurs and the nonadherent cells are readily counted (Holáň *et al.*, 1974; Grosser and Thomson, 1975). The proportion of nonadherent cells increases when there is specific interaction between the leukocytes of cancer patients and a tumor extract of the same type of cancer, compared with mixtures containing a different tumor type as control. Media poor in serum have generally been used. Many of the recent LAI investigations in human melanoma have employed the tube technique (I. Hellström *et al.*, 1977; Vandenbark *et al.*, 1979; Winter *et al.*, 1980).

An extraordinary and unexpected consequence of the introduction of this variant procedure has been the discovery of a different mechanism of LAI. In both human and animal experiments, antigen appears to reduce the glass-adherence of monocytes or macrophages in a direct fashion, with no soluble mediator (Holáň *et al.*, 1974). The tumor antigen has been shown to react with cytophilic antitumor antibody on human blood monocytes (Marti *et al.*, 1976), so that test-tube LAI is not a reaction of specific CMI in the strict sense. Only in tumor-type specificity does this variant assay closely resemble the prototype. On further reflection, even this appears strange, since antibody-mediated and cell-mediated antitumor immune reactions often have different specificities, as though different antigens were involved (see Sections 3.1 and 5.4).

Changes in LAI reactivity and in specific serum effects in relation to tumor progression are different in hemocytometer and test-tube LAI. These distinctions are confusing but assume some importance in interpretation of laboratory data.

2.3.3. Microplate Leukocyte-Adherence Inhibition

In this variation, leukocytes are incubated with antigens in the 60-well microtest plates; the nonadherent cells are washed away, and adherent cells are stained and counted. The potential for automation of all steps is most appealing. Many independent replicate mixtures can be counted, and great economy of reagents is achieved. Microplate LAI was first introduced in studies of CMI in mice (Holt *et al.*, 1975); these early observations established the existence of LAIF and its dependence on T lymphocytes. More recently, the technique was applied by the Goldrosen group (Russo *et al.*, 1978) to human cancer, especially pancreatic carcinoma.

The cellular mechanism of microplate LAI in human cancer is not well established. B lymphocytes have been implicated (Goldrosen *et al.*, 1979). Current work in this laboratory (J. J. Harper and W. J. Halliday, unpublished data) has demonstrated a soluble mediator that is not species-restricted, so that assays are conveniently done in two stages with mouse leukocytes as the final indicator cells.

3. Specificity of Leukocyte-Adherence Inhibition in Melanoma

The content of this section derives mainly from our own studies using hemocytometer LAI, in which the indispensable collaboration of Dr. Annette Maluish, Dr. Frances Noonan, and Mrs. Thelma Koppi is gratefully acknowledged. Other aspects of LAI in melanoma, especially as related to test-tube LAI, are discussed in Chapter 21.

The term *specificity* is used in several different ways in tumor immunology, reflecting some of the special attributes of this area. In the strict academic sense, specificity should be related to the nature of the antigenic determinants involved. However, three special meanings of the word have emerged. With *in vitro* reactions, if one tests a cancer patient's cells against several antigens from different types of tumors and observes a selective recognition of one type, this is taken as evidence of tumor-type specificity. Conversely, if even a single antigen preparation is tested with cells from several subjects (including healthy normals) and there are few false-positive reactions, one claims specificity in the diagnostic sense. Finally, if an antigen is found only in tumor cells and not in normal cells of any kind, it is said to have tumor specificity in the most restricted sense of the term.

3.1. Specificity with Regard to Tumor Type

Reactions of CMI related to murine virus-induced tumors exhibit pronounced cross-reactivity between individual tumors caused by the same virus. This extends to *in vitro* correlates such as LAI (Creemers, 1977; Mortensen, 1979; Koppi and Halliday, 1981). On the other hand, individual chemically induced tumors cross-react weakly or not at all, so that mice sensitized to one methylcholanthrene-induced tumor do not readily recognize another separately derived tumor. This statement holds for LAI *in vitro* (Halliday and Miller, 1972; Halliday *et al.*, 1974c; Leveson *et al.*, 1979). Serological studies with chemically induced tumors show no such clear-cut differences in individual antigenic specificity;

the antibodies produced by tumor-bearing mice are numerous and cross-reacting, partly because they recognize adventitious viral antigens expressed on tumor cells. For some obscure reason, CMI displays a much more restricted perspective. LAI has strong affinities with the other reactions of CMI, rather than with antibody-mediated reactions.

In all of the aforementioned assays—excluding tumor challenge, where the opportunities for experimentation are limited—spontaneous human tumors resemble virus-induced tumors of animals. Tumors of the same histological type and tissue of origin cross-react (I. Hellström et al., 1968). For example, antigens of melanoma cells are recognized preferentially by melanoma-sensitized allogeneic lymphocytes (I. Hellström and K. E. Hellström, 1973). In other words, the antigens taking part in these reactions are common to the type of tumor and are absent from other types. Melanoma patients' leukocytes reacted specifically in LAI with melanoma extracts, rather than with colorectal or breast-carcinoma extracts, with a high frequency (Halliday et al., 1975, 1980).

The basis for antigenic cross-reactivity in melanomas is not known. Attempts to identify a common virus have not been successful, and even the reports of specific immunoreactivity in healthy contacts of melanoma patients (Vandenbark et al., 1979) do not necessarily prove the existence of an infectious agent. The antigen or antigens may be differentiation antigens characteristic of the tissue of origin. Little is known of the chemical structure of melanoma antigens (see Chapters 10 and 22). Studies in this area lag behind the work in breast cancer, from which a peptide has been isolated, identified, and synthesized; it is claimed to be a specific antigenic determinant common to that neoplasm (R. H. Reid, unpublished data).

These remarks are not meant to exclude the possibility of antigens common to all cancers, but absent from normal adult cells. Common cancer antigens appear to be relatively inactive in the extracts normally used for LMI and LAI, otherwise the observed tumor-type specificity would be obscured; this point is mentioned again in Section 3.2.

An important further consequence of the observed widespread cross-reactivity within tumor types is concerned with human leukocyte antigen compatibility. Since a single tumor extract can react in LAI with lymphocytes of many different allogeneic donors, there can be no stringent requirement for matching of HLA type. A similar lack of restriction has been observed in LAI with murine virus-induced tumors in allogeneic strains (Mortensen and Elson, 1980; Koppi and Halliday, 1981).

3.2. Specificity with Regard to False-Positive Reactions

A shadow has been cast over lymphocytotoxicity techniques in human cancer by the discovery that most individuals have cells capable of killing tumor cells *in vitro* (Herberman and Holden, 1979). These natural killer (NK) cells are thus nonspecific, in the sense that they give rise to widespread reactivity unrelated to tumor type or even to presence of cancer. If one is anticipating specific tumor-related reactivity, such phenomena are called "false-positives." The underlying specificity is then difficult to discern. NK cells are an important natural phenomenon, possibly contributing to surveillance against cancer *in vivo*, but they confuse diagnostic applications of lymphocytotoxicity. Fortunately, analogous cells with reactivity against soluble tumor antigens do not appear to interfere with LMI and LAI. This may be because NK cells cannot produce lymphokines.

LAI reactions in melanoma are relatively free of nonspecific reactions. Normal subjects rarely exhibit false-positive LAI with melanoma extracts (Halliday *et al.*, 1975, 1980). There appears to be a slight excess of reactivity in other cancer patients, compared with normal subjects; this may be reactivity to a common cancer antigen.

Two special situations complicate the discussion of false-positive reactions. These situations are found in benign and premalignant conditions related to melanoma and in close contacts of melanoma patients.

3.2.1. Benign and Premalignant Conditions

These have not been studied extensively in melanoma with respect to LAI, but there is considerable evidence from LMI studies that some nevi and other lesions induce melanoma-related reactivity (Chapter 5). In relation to breast carcinoma (Halliday *et al.*, 1980; O'Connor *et al.*, 1978), some patients with relevant benign pathological conditions exhibited positive LAI reactivity. It is difficult to be sure whether this reflects an early stage of developing malignancy or alternately the existence of common organ-specific antigens in benign and malignant tumors. The latter explanation seems to be the more likely in mammary dysplasia, where false-positive reactions occur frequently as determined by a variety of techniques (Avis *et al.*, 1976).

3.2.2. Patient Contacts

The idea that healthy contacts of cancer patients may exhibit increased cell-mediated reactivity to tumor antigens stems from the Hellström school (I. Hellström *et al.*, 1970) and is supported by many *in vitro* observations. The phenomenon has been studied extensively in melanoma by Burger and co-workers using tube LAI (Burger *et al.*, 1977; Vandenbark *et al.*, 1979). Family members and other unrelated close contacts of patients often reacted immunologically to melanoma extracts. The mechanism of sensitization is unknown; it is perhaps more likely to be the ingestion of tumor antigens, rather than infection with a tumor virus. Close contacts constitute an unusual group in that they may have specific antitumor immunoreactivity in the absence of tumor growth. There is a tendency to use such persons as a convenient source of substances of possible therapeutic benefit, for example, transfer factor. In many instances, the donors are assumed to be specifically immunoreactive without any form of testing, simply because they are close contacts of cancer patients of the appropriate type. A further unsubstantiated assumption is that the "immunity" of donors is related to antigens involved in protection or tumor rejection. Almost all cancer patients already have "immunity" demonstrable by *in vitro* reactions, and it seems somewhat redundant merely to give them more of the same from a doubtful source. A possible alternate function of transfer factor in cancer patients is to depress the level of blocking factors that interfere with effective immunity; this has been claimed in the treatment of breast cancer (Fujisawa *et al.*, 1978).

3.3. Tumor-Specific Antigens

Antigens are tumor-specific when they occur only in tumors, but the vexing question of true tumor specificity of antigens is difficult to examine effectively. With CMI, lymphocyte-mediated reactions may be set up to include controls with nonmalignant cells or tissue extracts. One attempts to use relevant normal cells or normal tissue, for example, normal hepatocytes or liver tissue, as a control for hepatocellular carcinoma (Halliday *et al.,* 1974a). The normal and malignant tissue should of course be from the same donor, to avoid spurious differences due to HLA and other nontumor antigens. For many cancers, the relevant control may be difficult to obtain, either because the appropriate cells form only a minority in a normal organ or because they are difficult to cultivate. A good normal control for melanoma is a problem.

The reexpression of normal fetal antigens in tumors is well known. Presumably, some of these could be immunogenic if tolerance had not been induced naturally (see Section 4.1).

To be quite precise, even the most carefully selected normal tissues, made into extracts of the same total protein concentration as the tumor extracts, are not adequate to prove tumor specificity of soluble tumor-associated antigens by methods such as LMI or LAI. Sensitized lymphocytes may fail to react positively with these control extracts, not because the relevant antigen is entirely absent, but because it is there at a concentration different from the optimum for detection.

4. Some Current Concepts Concerning Tumor Antigens

There is a current tendency to emphasize the complexity of the cancer problem; sometimes this is done with an air of despair that a solution can ever be found. A consequence of this attitude is that simple, straightforward concepts or findings are often dismissed as being naïve and unworthy of consideration. One may cite as examples two popular areas of research into tumor antigens: the characterization of antigens using xenogeneic rather than autochthonous immune responses and the question of antigenic variability during tumor growth and metastasis.

4.1. Immunoreactivity of the Autochthonous Host

Cancer patients respond immunologically to antigens of their tumors. This autochthonous response (detectable by various immune reactions between lymphocytes and allogeneic tumor material) may be against tumor-specific neoantigens or against normal tissue antigens. As noted above, the distinction between these choices may be difficult to make. The best-known examples of oncofetal "antigens" (carcinoembryonic antigen and α-fetoprotein) are not immunogenic in the autochthonous host; thus, though they are useful tumor markers, they tell us nothing about the immunobiology of cancer.

When injected into xenogeneic animals, human tumor cells induce responses against normal and tumor-associated antigens of many kinds. Much work has gone into preparing and characterizing the resulting antibodies from rabbits, monkeys, and mice. Serum antibodies can be rendered apparently tumor-specific by absorption with normal tissue. Murine monoclonal antibodies are exquisitely homogeneous and specific, and certain of these recognize molecules that seem to be part of the human tumor-cell membrane. Antibodies can be used to isolate these cell components as purified "tumor antigens." Many of these studies are described in other chapters.

If human tumor markers, detected and defined by xenogeneic phenomena, are not subsequently investigated for reactivity in the species of origin (man), their functional relevance to the host immune system remains obscure. To call these substances "tumor antigens" could be misleading. Furthermore, as the observed pattern of cell-surface antigens defined with reference to xenogeneic antibodies becomes increasingly complex, the tumor-type-specific antigens, common to all tumors of a given type and immunogenic in the autochthonous host, tend to be overlooked. These are the antigens that are important in immunodiagnosis now and that must be considered in relation to immunotherapy in the future.

4.2. Antigenic Constancy or Variability in Cancer

There is no doubt that tumor cells are highly variable in their antigenic constitution. Metastatic cells may differ from the primary tumor, and even cells from different areas of a tumor mass may be different from each other, as judged by several criteria (reviewed by Fidler and Kripke, 1980). These criteria include the ability to stimulate resistance of mice to tumor challenge with chemically induced sarcomas, a system much criticized for its artificiality. Heterogeneity of tumor antigens is an obviously important property to bear in mind if one is contemplating the manipulation of the host immune system as part of cancer therapy.

In contrast, certain tumor antigens appear to be qualitatively homogeneous and relatively invariable. These are the type-specific antigens that are readily solubilized from tumor tissue and are recognized not only by autochthonous but also by allogeneic lymphocytes *in vitro*. Most of the melanoma extracts used in our LAI studies (Halliday *et al.*, 1975, 1980; Noonan *et al.*, 1977) were made from metastatic tumor tissue. The reaction of these extracts with allogeneic lymphocytes of patients with melanoma was unrelated to stage of tumor development or presence of metastases. Thus, patients with only primary melanomas had responded *in vivo* to antigens common to primary tumors and to secondary metastatic tumors. From the diagnostic point of view, this constancy is a fortunate state of affairs. Immunodiagnosis would hardly be possible if all tumor antigens were as capricious as indicated by the studies referred to above.

5. Serum Blocking Factors

Specific blocking factors (BFs) were originally discovered in the serum of tumor-bearing subjects and had the property of inhibiting related reactions of CMI *in vitro*. Lymphocyte cytotoxicity with tumor target cells was the reaction employed (I. Hellström *et al.*, 1969). The general validity of this concept has been amply confirmed, and extended to other examples of CMI. Thus, BFs were shown to operate in the reaction of LAI (Halliday and Miller, 1972; Halliday *et al.*, 1974a–c) with tumor antigens. The existence of BFs related to melanoma is well documented (I. Hellström *et al.*, 1973; Halliday *et al.*, 1975, 1980).

5.1. Nature of Blocking Factors

The development of ideas regarding the molecular nature of BFs has been reviewed (K. E. Hellström *et al.*, 1977), and will therefore be described only briefly here. Some of the properties of BFs are consistent with those of antitumor antibodies or tumor antigens, produced during tumor growth and circulating in the blood. In several situations, BFs were suggested to be antigen–antibody complexes. Evidence from the Hellström laboratory relied on the dissociation and reassociation of the complex after treatment of BFs with acidic buffers (Sjögren *et al.*, 1971); studies of the Baldwin group involved the synthesis of BFs from partially purified tumor antigen and antibody (Baldwin *et al.*, 1972).

A novel type of BF was detected in 1976 in the serum of mice bearing chemically induced tumors. This was a tumor-specific molecule with a molecular weight of 56,000, with binding affinity for tumor cells and for antitumor antibody (Nepom *et al.*, 1976). Some properties of this material were similar to those of antigen-specific suppressor factors described in other systems.

5.2. Suppressor Factors

The best-characterized suppressor factors are those produced by mice rendered tolerant to defined antigens. Antigen-specific factors can be obtained by extracting or incubating thymus cells from these mice, and the factors are usually detected by their ability to inhibit the induction of the appropriate immune response *in vivo*. Production of these factors by suppressor T cells is partly coded by the *I-J* subregion within the major histocompatibility complex (MHC) of the mouse. An interesting outcome of this is the demonstration of the reduction of tumor growth by administration of anti-I-J antiserum, thought to act by antagonizing suppressor T cells (Greene *et al.*, 1977).

A bridge directly connecting BF and T-suppressor factors was made by observations in our laboratory. As a result of earlier work of Dr. Frances Noonan (Noonan and Halliday, 1980), it was shown that BFs of virus-induced tumor-bearing mice were strain-restricted in LAI; furthermore, they contained I-J determinants of the MHC and existed in a molecular-weight range of 40,000–50,000 (Koppi and Halliday, 1981). By definition, BFs are efferent inhibitors, acting on the expression of immunoreactivity *in vitro*. This appears to be a new role for the antigen-specific T-suppressor factors.

The results cited above were obtained with leukocytes of mice bearing virus-induced tumors, reacting with tumor extracts *in vitro*. The source of the extract was not strain-restricted, allogeneic tumor extracts being entirely suitable. Blocking was demonstrated by adding tumor-bearing serum. Being strain-restricted in their action, presumably because of their relationship to the MHC, tumor BFs of mice interact only with syngeneic lymphocytes in LAI. Thus, although CMI can be demonstrated readily with allogeneic tumor extracts (related to the same virus), blocking by serum is more selective and requires matching of the cell donor and serum donor.

Methylcholanthrene-induced tumors induced BFs with similar properties. It was not possible here to demonstrate strain-restriction of BFs, since the tumors themselves are strain-restricted (i.e, grow only within inbred mouse strains).

5.3. Possible Relationship to Human Leukocyte Antigen

Our earlier studies of LAI in human cancer suggested that both the tumor antigens and BFs were restricted only by tumor type. In many instances, the only requirement for the demonstration of BFs in melanoma, for example, was for the leukocytes, antigen, and serum to be derived from melanoma patients. Results were published showing LAI reactions with entirely allogeneic mixtures (Halliday et al., 1974b). Later attempts to use the detection of BFs in serum as a diagnostic procedure were disappointing. A more thorough investigation has shown that while the blocking of LAI by autochthonous tumor-bearer serum was regularly observed, blocking by allogeneic serum was unpredictable (Halliday et al., 1980).

One might speculate that the reason for these negative results is that, as in the mouse, human BFs need to be recognized by a compatible self-marker on reactive lymphocytes. In man, this might be one of the HLA-DR specificities, analogous to the mouse Ia system. If so, matching of the haplotype of leukocyte donor and serum donor should provide the necessary conditions for BFs to act. It is already clear that as in the experimental system of murine virus-induced tumors, there is no requirement for HLA matching with the tumor donor from whom the antigenic extracts are derived.

5.4. Specificity of Blocking Factors

Tumor specificity of BFs in LAI related to experimental murine tumors is easily demonstrated, since one can work within a single strain of inbred mice. In this way, the leukocyte donor and serum donor are perfectly matched, and any differences in BFs must be tumor-related. Tumor-specific BFs are found with individual chemically induced tumors (Halliday et al., 1974a), and these BFs are different from the ones produced with a virally induced tumor (Koppi and Halliday, 1981).

With human tumors such as melanoma, the tumor specificity is more difficult to discern, since it may be superimposed on another form of restriction based on HLA (see Section 5.3). At present, we can only say that fresh sera from melanoma patients never block the activity of leukocytes from colorectal-carcinoma patients and vice versa (Halliday et al., 1980). The observation that melanoma sera may or may not block allogeneic melanoma leukocytes could be a result of (1) an additional requirement for HLA compatibility or (2) a finer specificity in BFs due to their relationship to particular melanoma antigens.

A phenomenon recently observed with murine tumors (Yamauchi et al., 1979) may clarify the last statement. Growth of the related chemically induced sarcomas S1509a and SaI induced both cytotoxic T cells and suppressor T cells (with I-J determinants). Injection of solubilized tumor antigens from these sarcomas induced only suppressor cells. The cytotoxic cells were equally active against either sarcoma, but the suppressor cells inhibited the cytotoxic reaction against only the homologous tumor. The results suggested that there are two types of antigenic determinants on the two tumors; cross-reactive determinants are recognized by cytotoxic T cells and unique determinants by suppressor T cells. If one can imagine a similar situation with LAI and BFs in human melanoma, this would involve the generation in the host of cross-reactive lymphocytes that recognize the common melanoma antigen and of suppressor lymphocytes that recognize determinants of more restricted distribution. The latter cells could be the source of BFs able to block some allogeneic LAI reactions but not others.

Occasionally, it is possible to demonstrate tumor-type specificity of BFs in an intrinsically matched situation: the single patient with a double malignancy. Such a patient, with a past history of primary melanoma and breast carcinoma, had a tumor recurrence and was studied for CMI and BFs by the LAI reaction (Gardner et al., 1975). Leukocytes reactive with both types of tumor extract were detected, reflecting her past experience of both tumors. Only BFs related to melanoma were found in her serum, corresponding to the clinical diagnosis of her recurrent tumor. These BFs did not affect the LAI reaction with the other tumor extract, so were specific for tumor type.

6. Conclusion

In vitro reactions of CMI are particularly suitable for revealing some of the properties of melanoma antigens. As the tumor grows, certain of these antigens induce cellular and humoral changes in the host. The cellular immune response, as detected by rapid laboratory reactions such as LAI, regularly reveals the melanoma-associated antigens common to tumors of this type, both primary and metastatic. Whether or not these antigens are potentially important in tumor rejection is not known. The presence of tumor also leads to humoral BFs. By analogy with the better-characterized BFs of mouse tumors, some of the melanoma-associated BFs in man may be antigen-specific suppressor-cell products controlled by the histocompatibility complex.

An improvement in our knowledge of tumor antigens and the host immune response will lead to the immediate practical goal of immunodiagnosis and ultimately to a better understanding of cancer. Melanoma will continue to play an important role in this development.

ACKNOWLEDGMENTS. I thank Dr. Annette Maluish, Dr. Frances Noonan, and Mrs. Thelma Koppi and many clinical colleagues for their collaboration. The work in this laboratory was continually facilitated by the Queensland Melanoma Project (Dr. Neville Davis, coordinator), and by support from the Queensland Cancer Fund, the University Cancer Research Fund, and the National Health and Medical Research Council of Australia.

References

Avis, F., Avis, I., Newsome, J. F., and Haughton, G., 1976, Antigenic cross-reactivity between adenocarcinoma of the breast and fibrocystic disease of the breast, J. Natl. Cancer Inst. 56:17.
Baldwin, R. W., Price, M. R., and Robins, R. A., 1972, Blocking of lymphocyte-mediated cytotoxicity for rat hepatoma cells by tumour-specific antigen–antibody complexes, Nature (London) New Biol. 238:185.

Burger, D. R., Vandenbark, A. A., Finke, P., Malley, A., Frikke, M., Black, J., Acott, K., Begley, D., and Vetto, R. M., 1977, Assessment of reactivity to tumor extracts by leukocyte adherence inhibition and dermal testing, *J. Natl. Cancer Inst.* **59**:317.

Creemers, P., 1977, The role of leukocyte subpopulations in the indirect leukocyte adherence inhibition assay in the mammary tumor virus system, *Eur. J. Immunol.* **7**:48.

Dunn, I. S., and Halliday, W. J., 1980, Interactions between T and B lymphocytes and macrophages in the production of leukocyte adherence inhibition factor, *Cell. Immunol.* **52**:48.

Fidler, I. J., and Kripke, M. L., 1980, Tumor cell antigenicity, host immunity and cancer metastasis, *Cancer Immunol. Immunother.* **7**:201.

Fujisawa, T., Waldman, S. R., and Yonemoto, R. H., 1978, Transfer factor *in vitro* abrogation of blocking factors and amplification of immunoreactivity directed to soluble tumor-associated antigens in the leukocyte adherence inhibition assay, *Cancer Immunol. Immunother.* **4**:77.

Gardner, M. A. H., Maluish, A. E., Halliday, W. J., and Clunie, G. J. A., 1975, Immunodiagnosis of a metastasis in a patient with a history of double malignant disease, *Med. J. Aust.* **1**:446.

Goldrosen, M. H., and Howell, J. H., 1979, International workshop on leukocyte adherence inhibition, *Cancer Res.* **39**:551.

Goldrosen, M. H., Russo, A. J., Howell, J. H., Leveson, S. H., and Holyoke, E. D., 1979, Cellular and humoral factors involved in the mechanism of the micro-leukocyte adherence inhibition reaction, *Cancer Res.* **39**:587.

Greene, M. I., Dorf, M. E., Pierres, M., and Benacerraf, B., 1977, Reduction of syngeneic tumor growth by an anti-I-J alloantiserum, *Proc. Natl. Acad. Sci. U.S.A.* **74**:5118.

Grosser, N., and Thomson, D. M. P., 1975, Cell-mediated antitumor immunity in breast cancer patients evaluated by antigen-induced leukocyte adherence inhibition in test tubes, *Cancer Res.* **35**:2571.

Halliday, W. J., 1979, Historical background and aspects of the mechanism of leukocyte adherence inhibition, *Cancer Res.* **39**:558.

Halliday, W. J., and Miller, S., 1972, Leukocyte adherence inhibition: A simple test for cell-mediated tumour immunity and serum blocking factors, *Int. J. Cancer* **9**:477.

Halliday, W. J., Halliday, J. W., Campbell, C. B., Maluish, A. E., and Powell, L. W., 1974a, Specific immunodiagnosis of hepatocellular carcinoma by leucocyte adherence inhibition, *Br. Med. J.* **2**:349.

Halliday, W. J., Maluish, A. E., and Isbister, W. H., 1974b, Detection of anti-tumour cell mediated immunity and serum-blocking factors in cancer patients by the leucocyte adherence inhibition test, *Br. J. Cancer* **29**:31.

Halliday, W. J., Maluish, A. E., and Miller, S., 1974c, Blocking and unblocking of cell-mediated anti-tumor immunity in mice, as detected by the leukocyte adherence inhibition test, *Cell. Immunol.* **10**:467.

Halliday, W. J., Maluish, A. E., Little, J. H., and Davis, N. C., 1975, Leukocyte adherence inhibition and specific immunoreactivity in malignant melanoma, *Int. J. Cancer* **16**:645.

Halliday, W. J., Koppi, T. A., Kahn, J., and Davis, N. C., 1980, Leukocyte adherence inhibition: Tumor specificity of cellular and serum-blocking reactions in human melanoma, breast cancer and colorectal cancer, *J. Natl. Cancer Inst.* **65**:327.

Hellström, I., and Hellström, K. E., 1973, Some recent studies on cellular immunity to human melanomas, *Fed. Proc. Fed. Am. Soc. Exp. Biol.* **32**:156.

Hellström, I., Hellström, K. E., Pierce, G. E., and Yang, J. P. S., 1968, Cellular and humoral immunity to different types of human neoplasms, *Nature (London)* **220**:1352.

Hellström, I., Hellström, K. E., Evans, C. A., Heppner, G. H., Pierce, G. E., and Yang, J. P. S., 1969, Serum-mediated protection of neoplastic cells from inhibition by lymphocytes immune to their tumor-specific antigens, *Proc. Natl. Acad. Sci. U.S.A.* **62**:362.

Hellström, I., Hellström, K. E., Bill, A. H., Pierce, G. E., and Yang, J. P. S., 1970, Studies on cellular immunity to human neuroblastoma cells, *Int. J. Cancer* **6**:172.

Hellström, I., Warner, G. A., Hellström, K. E., and Sjögren, H. O., 1973, Sequential studies on cell-mediated tumor immunity and blocking serum activity in ten patients with malignant melanoma, *Int. J. Cancer* **11**:280.

Hellström, I., Hellström, K. E., Van Belle, G., and Warner, G. A., 1977, Leukocyte-mediated reactivity to human tumors as detected by the leukocyte adherence inhibition test. I. Demonstration of tumor type-specific reactions, *Am. J. Clin. Pathol.* **68**:706.

Hellström, K. E., Hellström, I., and Nepom, J. T., 1977, Specific blocking factors—are they important?, *Biochim. Biophys. Acta* **473**:121.

Herberman, R. B., and Holden, H. T., 1979, Natural killer cells as antitumor effector cells, *J. Natl. Cancer Inst.* **62**:441.

Holáň, V., Hašek, M., Bubeník, J., and Chutná, J., 1974, Antigen-mediated macrophage adherence inhibition, *Cell. Immunol.* **13**:107.

Holt, P. G., Roberts, L. M., Fimmel, P. J., and Keast, D., 1975, The LAI microtest: A rapid and sensitive procedure for the demonstration of cell-mediated immunity *in vitro*, *J. Immunol. Methods* **8**:277.

Koppi, T. A., and Halliday, W. J., 1981, Regulation of cell-mediated immunologic reactivity to Moloney murine sarcoma virus-induced tumors, *J. Nat. Cancer Inst.* **66**:1089.

Koppi, T. A., Maluish, A. E., and Halliday, W. J., 1979, The cellular mechanism of leukocyte adherence inhibition, *J. Immunol.* **123**:2255.

Leveson, S. H., Howell, J. H., Paolini, N. S., Tan, M. H., Holyoke, E. D., and Goldrosen, M. H., 1979, Correlations between the leukocyte adherence inhibition microassay and *in vivo* tests of transplantation resistance, *Cancer Res.* **39**:582.

Maluish, A. E., and Halliday, W. J., 1979, Hemocytometer leukocyte adherence inhibition technique, *Cancer Res.* **39**:625.

Marti, J. H., Grosser, N., and Thomson, D. M. P., 1976, Tube leukocyte adherence inhibition assay for the detection of anti-tumour immunity. II. Monocyte reacts with tumour antigens via cytophilic anti-tumour antibody, *Int. J. Cancer* **18**:48.

McCoy, J. L., Maluish, A. E., Halliday, W. J., and Herberman, R. B., 1980, Leukocyte migration inhibitory factor and leukocyte adherence inhibition assays, in: *Manual of Clinical Immunology*, 2nd ed. (N. R. Rose and H. Friedman, eds.), pp. 252–260, American Society for Microbiology, Washington.

Mortensen, R. F., 1979, Detection of cellular immunity to murine sarcoma virus-induced tumours by leukocyte adherence inhibition, *J. Natl. Cancer Inst.* **62**:157.

Mortensen, R. F., and Elson, L. M., 1980, Leukocyte adherence inhibition response to murine sarcoma virus-induced tumors. I. Cell requirements, specificity, lack of H-2 restriction, and role of antibody, *J. Immunol.* **124**:2316.

Nepom, J. T., Hellström, I., and Hellström, K. E., 1976, Purification and partial characterization of a tumor-specific blocking factor from sera of mice with growing chemically induced sarcomas, *J. Immunol.* **117**:1846.

Noonan, F. P., and Halliday, W. J., 1980, Genetic restriction of the serum factor mediating tolerance in trinitrochlorobenzene hypersensitivity, *Cell. Immunol.* **50**:41.

Noonan, F. P., Halliday, W. J., Wall, D. R., and Clunie, G. J. A., 1977, Cell-mediated immunity and serum blocking factors in cancer patients during chemotherapy and immunotherapy, *Cancer Res.* **37**:2473.

O'Connor, R., MacFarlane, J. K., Murray, D., and Thomson, D. M. P., 1978, A study of false positive and negative responses in the tube leucocyte adherence inhibition (tube LAI) assay, *Br. J. Cancer* **38**:674.

Powell, A. E., Sloss, A. M., Smith, R. N., Makley, J. T., and Hubay, C. A., 1975, Specific responsiveness of leukocytes to soluble extracts of human tumors, *Int. J. Cancer* **16**:905.

Powell, A. E., Sloss, A. M., and Smith, R. N., 1978, Leukocyte adherence inhibition: A specific assay of cell-mediated immunity dependent on lymphokine-mediated collaboration between T-lymphocytes, *J. Immunol.* **120**:1957.

Russo, A. J., Douglass, H. O., Leveson, S. H., Howell, J. H., Holyoke, E. D., Harvey, S. R., Chu, T. M., and Goldrosen, M. H., 1978, Evaluation of the microleukocyte adherence inhibition assay as an immunodiagnostic test for pancreatic cancer, *Cancer Res.* **38**:2023.

Sjögren, H. O., Hellström, I., Bansal, S. C., and Hellström, K. E., 1971, Suggestive evidence that the "blocking antibodies" of tumor-bearing individuals may be antigen–antibody complexes, *Proc. Natl. Acad. Sci. U.S.A.* **68**:1372.

Smith, T., 1979, The Queensland Melanoma Project—an exercise in health education, *Br. Med. J.* **1**:253.

Vandenbark, A. A., Greene, M. H., Burger, D. R., Vetto, R. M., and Reimer, R. R., 1979, Immune response to melanoma extracts in three melanoma-prone families, *J. Natl. Cancer Inst.* **63**:1147.

Winter, M., Nelson, D. S., and Milton, G. W., 1980, Leucocyte adherence inhibition test for the detection of cell-mediated immunity to malignant melanoma, *Aust. N. Z. J. Med.* **10**:405.

Yamauchi, K., Fujimoto, S., and Tada, T., 1979, Differential activation of cytotoxic and suppressor T cells against syngeneic tumors in the mouse, *J. Immunol.* **123**:1653.

10

Antigens in Human Melanomas Detected by Using Monoclonal Antibodies as Probes

Karl Erik Hellström and Ingegerd Hellström

1. Introduction

Some of the first evidence that human patients can react immunologically to their own tumors was obtained during the late 1960s when both humoral and cellular immune responses to putative tumor antigens were first reported (for reviews, see Herberman, 1974; K. E. Hellström and Brown, 1979). However, the nature of the antigens that were the targets in the reactions observed, and their degree of tumor specificity (if any), have been the subjects of much controversy.

Next to Burkitt lymphomas (G. Klein, 1973), melanomas are among the human neoplasms studied the most with immunological techniques. There are several reasons for this. Melanomas grow well *in vitro,* much better than, for example, carcinomas of the breast, lung, or colon, and are thus relatively easy to study. Furthermore, they occasionally undergo spontaneous regression, suggesting that at least some melanomas are immunogenic to the patients (I. Hellström and K. E. Hellström, 1972). Consequently, melanomas have been studied from the infancy of human tumor immunology, and the data that accumulated soon set them apart as interesting "models." Lymphocyte-mediated cytotoxicity, leukocyte-migration inhibition, and leukocyte-adherence inhibition (I. Hellström *et al.,* 1971; McCoy *et al.,* 1975; Halliday *et al.,* 1975) were demonstrated, primarily against antigens shared by most melanomas, but also against antigens characterizing subgroups of melanomas (I. Hellström and K. E. Hellström, 1973). Furthermore, antibodies were reported to be present in patient sera, both against antigens shared by melanomas (Morton *et al.,* 1968; Cor-

Karl Erik Hellström and Ingegerd Hellström • Division of Tumor Immunology, Fred Hutchinson Cancer Research Center, Seattle, Washington, 98104; Departments of Pathology (K. E. H.) and Microbiology/Immunology (I. H.), University of Washington, Seattle, Washington 98195.

nain *et al.,* 1975) and against antigens unique to the patients' own tumors (Lewis *et al.,* 1969). The shared, tissue-type-specific antigens of human tumors appeared, in the systems studied (particularly colon carcinomas), to be differentiation ("oncofetal") antigens, common to cells from tumors and embryos (I. Hellström *et al.,* 1970).

A problem in most of the early investigations was the question of antigen specificity. However, more recent serological studies by Shiku *et al.* (1976, 1977) have provided rather convincing evidence that tumor-specific antigens on human melanomas do indeed exist. In these studies, serum antibodies binding to the patients' own, autochthonous melanomas were measured, and the specificity of this binding was established on the basis of absorption studies with both autochthonous and allogeneic melanoma cells, as well as with cells from other tumors and with normal cells. Three different classes of antigens were defined. One (Class 1) is unique to the patients' own melanoma, another (Class 2) is shared by a number of different melanomas and a few other tumors, and a third (Class 3) is present on a variety of cultured cells, both normal and neoplastic.

Although the studies of Shiku *et al.* (1976, 1977) have gone a long way toward establishing antigen specificity, a problem has been the infrequent occurrence of antibodies in patient sera and their low titers. This hampers work aimed at detecting low levels of antigen expression in control tissues as well as investigations on the molecular nature of the target antigens. Furthermore, only those antigens that are immunogenic in man can be demonstrated by this approach, and there may be many antigens of potential interest for diagnosis and therapy that are not. There is a need, therefore, for techniques that would make it possible both to obtain high-titered antibodies to human melanoma antigens and to get antibodies even to those cell-surface molecules that are not immunogenic in the patients.

One approach to satisfy these needs is to use xenoimmunization procedures. Such procedures have been employed in tumor immunology for decades, with one of their most successful uses being for the identification of carcinoembryonic antigens (Gold and Freedman, 1965). Attempts to detect human melanoma-specific antigens in this way have provided suggestive evidence for antigens shared by many melanomas (Bystryn and Smalley, 1977). An inherent disadvantage of xenoimmunization, however, is that the sera obtained must be absorbed extensively to remove antibodies to normal tissue antigens. Furthermore, even after many absorptions, it is still difficult to make definitive conclusions about antigen specificity. Thus, many antigens first believed to be specific on the basis of data from xenoimmune sera later proved not to be so (K. E. Hellström and Brown, 1979).

The introduction by Köhler and Milstein (1975) of a technique by which monoclonal antibodies of defined specificity can be obtained has revolutionized tumor serology (K. E. Hellström *et al.,* 1980). It is now possible, at least in principle, to raise high-titered antibodies to antigens present on tumor cells but not on normal cells, including antigens that are not immunogenic in the tumor-bearing host. The hybridoma technique has recently been used to demonstrate antibodies to antigens associated with several different human neoplasms, including melanomas (Koprowski *et al.,* 1978; Yeh *et al.,* 1979; Woodbury *et al.,* 1980; Brown *et al.,* 1980, 1981; Carrel *et al.,* 1980; Dippold *et al.,* 1980), neuroblastomas (Kennett and Gilbert, 1979), and colon carcinomas (M. Herlyn *et al.,* 1979). In this chapter, we shall review the evidence for antigens of human melanomas, as detected by using this technique. A major question asked throughout this chapter concerns antigen specificity, a question that has still not been fully answered for many of the antigens described.

2. Methodology

Since the methods used often determine what one finds, we shall describe briefly the methods used in our laboratory. These methods have been reviewed in two recent publications (K. E. Hellström et al., 1980; I. Hellström et al., 1981a).

2.1. Establishment of Hybridomas

The methods used to establish hybridomas are based on the pioneering work from Milstein's laboratory (Köhler and Milstein, 1975, 1976; Köhler et al., 1976; Galfre et al., 1977), as further modified by various investigators (for a discussion, see K. E. Hellström et al., 1980). As a rule, mice are immunized, and the BALB/c mouse myeloma line P3-NS1/1-Ag4 (NS-1) or Sp2/0-Ag14 (Sp2/0) is generally used for fusion with the antibody-forming cells. NS-1 is a subline of MOPC21, a plasmacytoma, selected for loss of immunoglobulin heavy-chain synthesis and for resistance to azaguanine (Köhler et al., 1976). Sp2/0 is similarly resistant to azaguanine and differs from NS-1 in that it does not produce any immunoglobulin chains (Shulman et al., 1978). Polyethylene glycol (PEG) is normally employed as the fusing agent.

The immunization procedures used are most important for the type of response that is obtained (Stahli et al., 1980). As a rule, mice are immunized by an intraperitoneal injection of approximately 10^7 tumor cells and boosted 2 weeks later. At 3 days after boosting, their spleens are removed, and the spleen cells are suspended and mixed with NS-1 or Sp2/0 myeloma cells and spun down. To a pellet of spleen and myeloma cells, PEG is added. The cells are resuspended. The PEG is gradually diluted out, and the cells are centrifuged and resuspended in medium containing hypoxanthine, aminopterin, and thymidine (HAT medium). Normal thymocytes are added to this medium as feeder cells. Subsequently, aliquots of the cell suspension are dispensed into flat-bottomed microtest wells and incubated at 37°C.

Within 3 days, microscopic examination of the wells commonly reveals clusters of bright, refractile hybrid cells on a background of dead cells. At 7 days after the fusion, the hybrids are fed by replacing the medium with fresh HAT medium, and they are dense enough for testing about 4 days later.

2.2. Screening of Hybridomas

Since a minority of the hybrids (generally less than 1 in 500) will produce antibody of the desired specificity, it is necessary to be able to select these. The availability of rapid and sensitive techniques for detecting antibodies to tumor antigens is thus crucial for the success of the hybridoma technique. Screening of both fibroblasts and B cells from the same patient as the immunizing melanoma is desired, to quickly exclude many of those hybridomas that form antibodies to normal antigens, including human leukocyte antigen (HLA).

For adherent cells, binding assays employing radiolabeled reagents have proven very useful (Brown et al., 1979). Target cells are incubated first with samples of spent hybridoma culture medium, then with a rabbit anti-mouse immunoglobulin serum, and finally with ^{125}I-labeled protein A from *Staphylococcus aureus*. The incubation with the rabbit antiserum allows detection of antibodies that do not bind protein A directly, such as immunoglobulin M (IgM) and IgG$_1$. At the end of the assay, the plates are dried, and the ^{125}I-labeled protein A bound to the cells is detected by autoradiography (Parkhouse and Guarnotta, 1978). Enzyme-coupled reagents can also be employed (Engvall and Perlmann, 1971) and are preferred by some investigators. Cell membranes bound to plastic surfaces, rather than whole cells, may be used as well for screening.

An additional way of screening hybridomas has been introduced by Brown *et al.* (1980). It is based on the fact that radioimmunoprecipitation (RIP) techniques using protein A provide powerful tools for elucidating the nature of such protein antigens for which precipitating antibodies are available. As a first step, hybridoma supernatants are screened for the presence of IgG$_2$ antibodies, capable of binding to protein A. Second, those supernatants containing a certain level of IgG$_2$ antibodies (>4 μg/ml) are arranged in an 8 × 12 "matrix" pattern and then pooled in such a way that the horizontal rows are used to establish 8 pools and the vertical rows to establish another 12 pools. The 20 pools are then tested with the RIP technique. The localization on the matrix of a supernatant capable of precipitating a particular band can be determined, since the same supernatant is represented in both a horizontal and a vertical pool and is defined by the intersection between the two on the matrix. An advantage of this technique is that many of those hybridomas that produce antibodies to protein antigens can be detected and the apparent molecular weights of the respective antigens indicated. A disadvantage is that some biologically interesting antibodies may not be revealed, either because an antibody is not of a class that precipitates protein A, such as IgG$_1$, or because an interesting antigen is not a protein. The former problem may be rectified by adding an intermediary precipitating (e.g., rabbit) antibody as a sandwich. We feel that it is important not to use RIP assays exclusively for screening, but to use them in combination with binding assays.

Hybridomas selected for further studies on the basis of screening must be cloned, not only to ensure production of a single antibody specificity, but also to stabilize the antibody-producing phenotype. This is commonly done in microtest wells with a thymocyte feeder layer, single colonies being identified by microscopic examination (Nowinski *et al.*, 1979). It is important to freeze hybridomas at a very early state. By adding a large excess of normal thymocytes and using dimethylsulfoxide, as few as 100 hybridoma cells can be successfully preserved by freezing.

Although spent hybridoma culture medium can be used for serological tests, purified antibody is desirable for many applications. Spent medium from mass cultures of the hybridoma is one source of antibody. Alternatively, large amounts of antibody can be obtained by growing the hybridomas *in vivo* if contamination with small amounts of normal serum immunoglobulins can be tolerated. To do this, the hybridoma cells are inoculated intraperitoneally into syngeneic mice, where they grow as ascites tumors. Our methods for antibody purification have been published (Woodbury *et al.*, 1980).

The pattern of reactivity of a particular antibody on a panel of normal and neoplastic cells can be determined simply and directly by using purified, ^{125}I-labeled antibody in a binding assay. Knowing the specific radioactivity of the labeled antibody preparation, one can readily calculate the number of antibody molecules bound per cell. Labeled antibody can also be used to assess whether an antigen is expressed in normal tissues by testing intact cells or plasma-membrane preparations for binding of labeled antibody *in vitro*. Whether two monoclonal antibodies recognize the same antigenic determinant can be determined by incubating the target cells first with a saturating amount of one, unlabeled, antibody and then with another, labeled, antibody (Brown *et al.,* 1981).

2.3. Advantages in Using Monoclonal Antibodies for the Study of Tumor Antigens

Elucidation of the nature of tumor antigens is essential if we are to understand their origin and function. Antigens identified by monoclonal antibodies are particularly suited for structural studies, since they can be purified readily by immunoadsorption procedures. Protein antigens can be purified for molecular-weight determination, peptide mapping, and amino acid sequence analysis from as few as several million cells by the technique of RIP. The cells are surface-labeled, generally with ^{125}I, lysed with detergent, and the lysate incubated with the specific antibody. The antibody and bound antigen are isolated either by indirect immunoprecipitation or by adsorption to *S. aureus* (Kessler, 1975). Sodium dodecyl sulfate–polyacrylamide gel electrophoresis (SDS-PAGE) and subsequent autoradiography allow the molecular weight of the adsorbed antigen to be determined and give a substantial further purification. Monoclonal antibodies are also useful for the study of glycolipid antigens (Young *et al.,* 1979), although such antigens are often more difficult to investigate than are those of a protein nature.

In those cases where monoclonal antibodies can be raised to at least two determinants on the same antigen, an immunoradiometric assay often referred to as a "double-determinant immunoassay" (DDIA) can be used (Brown *et al.,* 1981a). In the DDIA, a cell-membrane lysate is first incubated with antibody to the first determinant in the presence of *S. aureus* organisms to which the antibody will quantitatively bind the antigen. Following incubation and pelleting of the bacteria by centrifugation, the bacteria are suspended in medium containing ^{125}I-labeled antigen-binding (Fab) fragments specific for the second determinant. The second antibody will measure the amounts of antigen bound to the bacteria. The specificity of any binding detected can be easily verified by competition experiments performed with unlabeled specific (or control) antibody. The DDIA has proven to be highly sensitive and accurate.

3. Various Antigens Identified by Monoclonal Antibodies to Human Melanomas

3.1. Antigens Restricted to a Subgroup of Melanomas

Yeh *et al.* (1979) immunized BALB/c mice with a short-term explant of a human melanoma, M1804, and fused spleen cells from the immunized mice with NS-1 cells. Three different hybridomas were selected for further studies (after they had been cloned). These hybridomas, referred to as 3.1, 3.2, and 3.3, form antibodies to an antigen that was found to be expressed much more on cultured cells from the immunizing melanoma than on any other cells used for screening, including cells from other melanomas, from tumors of different types, and normal fibroblasts. The antibodies have been extensively tested against peripheral-blood lymphocytes from many donors, and against B- and T-lymphoblast lines, to check, in particular, for reactivity to HLA including HLA-D [immune-associated (Ia)-like] antigens. All these tests were negative, as were tests of erythrocytes of blood groups A, B, and O, and of blood leukocytes from the M1804 patient.

Hybridoma 3.1 forms an IgG_1 antibody, while hybridomas 3.2 and 3.3 form IgG_{2a} and IgG_{2b} antibodies, respectively; a small amount of IgG_3 has also been detected among antibody purified from repeatedly cloned hybridoma 3.2. Cross-competition experiments with the three hybridomas have shown that the same antigenic determinant is being recognized by all three (Brown et al., unpublished findings). This determinant has been called 3.1 (Yeh et al., 1981). According to membrane immunofluorescence tests, it is present on more than 75% of cells from 2 of 30 immunizing melanomas tested (7%), with another 7% of melanomas expressing the antigen in 25–74% of the cells and 13% showing it in 1–24% of the cells. One of 24 melanomas tested for sensitivity to a complement-dependent cytotoxic effect of antibody 3.2 gave more than 75% target cell killing (M1804), while another 24% gave 15–74% killing (Hellström et al., unpublished findings).

Recent studies, in which ^{125}I-labeled 3.1 antibody was used in a direct binding assay, have shown that 6 of 39 cultured melanomas (15%) bound high levels of antibody, with another 18 melanomas (46%) giving intermediary levels and 15 melanomas (38%) being negative. Of 13 nonmelanoma tumor lines, 2 gave significant binding that could be competed out with unlabeled 3.1 antibody, but none was as high as that seen with the 6 highly reactive melanomas.

On the basis of the data that we have obtained, antigen determinant 3.1 cannot be described as a strict Class 1 antigen (Shiku et al., 1976), and it is, on face value, less specific than the individually unique antigens of chemically induced mouse sarcomas (Prehn and Main, 1957). One must take into account, however, that very sensitive binding assays were used to search for the expression of antigen 3.1 and that these assays were employed to test a large variety of cells, using a high-titered antibody. The individually unique antigens of chemically induced mouse sarcomas, on the other hand, have been detected with transplantation tests, which are relatively insensitive and allow for the examination of only a limited amount of tumor samples at the same time. Studies on low-titered antibodies in patient sera, on which the concept of "Class 1 antigens" was established, also suffer from the disadvantage that low degrees of antigenic cross-reactivity may be missed. Rather than calling the 3.1 antigen a "Class 1" or "Class 2" antigen, we prefer, therefore, to label it as a melanoma-subgroup-specific antigen that is strongly expressed by 10–15% of cultured human melanomas.

Monoclonal IgG_{2a} (3.2) antibody specific for 3.1 gives strong complement-dependent cytotoxicity (Yeh et al., 1979, 1981), and 3.2 antibody can act in consort with human lymphocytes (as a source of K cells) to give antibody-dependent cellular cytotoxicity (I. Hellström et al., 1981b).

Recently, Yeh et al. (1981) have established a series of clones of melanoma M1801. In this tumor, approximately 40% of the cells express antigen 3.1, according to assays with the membrane immunofluorescence technique. The clones were tested for the expression of antigen 3.1 and also for the expression of melanoma-associated antigen p97, defined by another set of monoclonal antibodies and described in Section 3.3. In addition to membrane immunofluorescence techniques, direct binding of ^{125}I-labeled antibody, complement-dependent cytotoxicity, and absorption methods were employed. Both 3.1-positive and 3.1-negative clones were identified. Progeny of the negative clones consistently were negative for antigen 3.1, while recloning experiments with an antigen-3.1-positive clone showed that it could give rise to negative daughter cells in addition to (a majority of) positive cells. Cells that had lost the expression of the 3.1 determinant still expressed antigen p97. Analogous data were then obtained with clones from melanoma M1804, in which originally about 98% of the cells express antigen 3.1. Yeh *et al.* (1981) concluded from this that the expression of antigen 3.1 is under genetic control and that it can be lost during tumor progression (Foulds, 1961), perhaps as a result of chromosomal rearrangement or loss.

The chemical nature of antigen 3.1 remains unknown. Methods used to detect protein antigens on melanoma cells, such as p97 (see Section 3.3), have given negative results. We believe, therefore, that antigen 3.1 is a glycolipid rather than a protein, but have not yet investigated whether this is really the case. The fact that 3.1, one of the most interesting antigens so far identified in human melanomas, was detected by using binding assays and would not have been detected had the screening been done only with the RIP assay illustrates the need to incorporate binding assays in the routine testing of newly derived hybridomas.

Recent studies, performed with binding assays on tumor biopsy material, have shown that antigen 3.1, unexpectedly, is expressed not only in melanomas but also in several normal human tissues (Brown *et al.*, 1981c). Since samples of the melanoma used for the immunization are not available, it is not possible to know whether this tumor, prior to culturing, expressed much higher levels than any normal tissues. The fact, however, that normal tissues can express fairly large amounts of an antigen *in vivo*, when this antigen is strongly expressed only on cells from a small subgroup of melanoma *in vitro* indicates the need to always study tissues prior to culturing. The reason for the discrepancy in antigen 3.1 expression *in vivo* as compared to *in vitro* remains unknown.

3.2. Antigens Expressed by Melanomas to the Exclusion of Other Tumors and Normal Tissues

Studies initiated in the late 1960s and discussed in Section 1 provided the first evidence that melanomas share tumor-type-specific antigens (I. Hellström and K. E. Hellström, 1972). Therefore, one may expect that monoclonal antibodies can be raised to antigens that are shared by melanoma and absent from both other tumors and normal tissues. One has to realize, however, that the exact specificity of these antibodies cannot be predicted, since the assays used in the past were far less precise than those that can be used with monoclonal antibodies. They would have detected neither low levels of cross-reactivity with other tumors nor the presence of high amounts of "melanoma antigens" on certain normal cell populations.

Koprowski *et al.* (1978) were the first to immunize mice with human melanoma and establish hybridomas forming antibodies to antigens detected on the immunizing cells. Hybridomas were isolated that form antibodies to antigens detected on most cultured human melanomas tested, but not on cultures from other tumors or normal cells. Although some of these hybridomas recognize an HLA-D (Ia-like) antigen also expressed on B cells (D. Herlyn *et. al.*, 1979), other hybridomas form antibodies that are melanoma-specific as far as tested, or shared by melanomas and some astrocytomas (Mitchell *et al.*, 1980; Kuprowski and Steplewski, 1981). Even if it has not been excluded that the specific monoclonal antibodies identify an antigen that is expressed in small amounts by certain other tumors or in high amounts by some normal stem cells, these antibodies are still of great interest in that they define antigens that are expressed much more by cells from melanomas and sometimes astrocytomas than by cells from any other of a multitude of normal and neoplastic tissues tested. Since some of these hybridomas define antigens that are detectable *in vivo*, they are of great potential interinterest for diagnosis and therapy.

Imai *et al.* (1981) have described monoclonal antibodies to a very large cell surface antigen (molecular weight above 250,000) which appears to be specific for cultured human melanomas. A similar (identical?) antigen has been demonstrated by Morgan *et al.* (1981). It has not yet been excluded whether normal cells contain small amounts of these antigens, and their expression *in vivo* needs to be investigated. Carrel *et al.* (1980) have described other monoclonal antibodies, which they report are specific for human melanomas with the exclusion of cells from other tumors and normal cells. However, the differences in antibody-binding activity among different cells so far published are relatively small, and the possibility remains that some amounts of the antigens are also present on nonmelanoma cells.

Loop *et al.* (1982) have recently identified a hybridoma, 6.1, that forms an IgM antibody that recognizes an antigen that is shared by approximately 50% of human melanomas tested with binding assays and RIP tests. The antigen has an apparent molecular weight of 155,000 on SDS-PAGE and is hence referred to as p155. Testing of human melanoma biopsies, prior to culturing, has revealed that p155 is present *in vivo*. Antigen p155 has not been detected, so far, in nonmelanoma tissues—including samples of a variety of carcinomas as well as cultivated skin fibroblasts and biopsy material from various normal human organs—with one exception: several samples of kidney carcinomas were found to demonstrate some binding when tested with indirect binding assays and one breast carcinoma gave a band of molecular weight 60,000 and one of 250,000–300,000 when tested with the anti-p155 antibody in an RIP assay. It needs to be established whether p155 is present on normal melanocytes. An antigen of the same approximate molecular weight has recently been described by Dippold *et al.* (1980).

Other antigens are shared by melanoma cells and normal melanocytes and are therefore cell-type-specific rather than tumor-specific. Dippold *et al.* (1980) have established a monoclonal antibody, R24, that defines such an antigen, present on all melanomas, on normal melanocytes, and on some astrocytomas,and another antibody, 4.2, with the same specificity has recently been described (Yeh *et al.*, 1982). As will be further discussed in Section 4, such antibodies may be useful for diagnosis and for certain forms of therapy, even though the antigen is not tumor-specific at all.

Before concluding this section, we would like to point out that an antigen may be believed, in the view of a certain amount of data, to be melanoma-specific, but later may prove not to be so, after it has been investigated with more sensitive techniques or when more control tumors and tissues have been examined. Therefore, the difference between (some of) the antigens described in this section and those described in the following section may be more apparent than real.

3.3. Antigens with a Relative (but Not Absolute) Specificity for Melanoma Cells

Some antigens are shared by many tumors and normal cells, but are expressed substantially more in melanomas than in other cells. One of these antigens, which has been denoted p97, has been studied extensively.

Antigen p97 was first identified in an experiment in which a BALB/c mouse had been immunized with cells from melanoma line SK-MEL 28, a line originally chosen for immunization because it expresses a Class 1 antigen (Shiku et al., 1976). Hybridomas were established from the spleen of an immunized mouse. One of these hybridomas, 4.1, was found to form an IgG_1 antibody that was detected by its ability to bind to SK-MEL 28 cells as compared to normal human skin fibroblasts (Woodbury et al., 1980). Further studies were performed in which the 4.1 antibody was directly labeled with ^{125}I and used in a binding assay with a variety of target cells. It appeared that many melanomas and some nonmelanoma tumors could bind significant amounts of the labeled antibody, while a variety of normal cells did not bind any antibody detectable over the background levels of the assays (Woodbury et al., 1980).

RIP assays were then performed with SDS-prepared membrane lysates that were run on PAGE. They showed that the antigen identified by hybridoma 4.1 has an apparent molecular weight of 97,000 (Woodbury et al., 1980). The molecular weight was estimated from comparison with a marker, rabbit phosphorylase B, which, according to sequencing data, has a molecular weight of 97,400 (Titani et al., 1977).

Subsequent work led to the identification of three more hybridomas forming antibody that recognizes p97. One of these hybridomas, 96.5, forms an IgG_2 antibody to the determinant recognized by hybridoma 4.1 that we have called p97[a] (Brown et al., 1981a). Another hybridoma, 118.1, forms an antibody to a different determinant on the p97 molecule, p97[b] (Brown et al., 1981a). The latter antibody does not compete with antibodies (4.1 or 96.5) to the first p97 determinant, but binds strongly to p97 isolated by using one of these two antibodies. A hybridoma, 8.2, was recently identified that forms an IgG_1 antibody to a third p97 determinant, p97[c] (Brown et al., 1981b).

Extensive searches have recently been made for the presence of p97 in various normal and neoplastic cells (Woodbury et al., 1981; Brown et al., 1981a,b,c). They have been performed in three different ways, and the results have been in good agreement, although the introduction (Brown et al., 1981a) of techniques more sensitive than the original binding and RIP assays (Woodbury et al., 1980) showed that p97 is more widely distributed than it was first believed to be. First, RIP techniques were used to test an extensive material of tumors and normal tissues (Woodbury et al., 1981). It appeared that cell-membrane preparations from most (90%) cultured melanomas, and from 50% of melanoma biopsies, contained detectable p97, and that membranes from cultures or biopsies of other tumors also contained p97, albeit in smaller amounts and less frequently. Using the same approach, p97 was not detected in a variety of tissues from normal adults. It was found, however, in some human fetal tissues obtained from abortions, particularly in fetal colon, which contained almost as much p97 as could be detected in the more p97-rich melanomas. Woodbury et al. (1981) concluded, therefore, that p97 is best labeled as an oncofetal (or differentiation) antigen.

Second, binding assays were performed (Brown *et al.*, 1981a,b) in which Fab fragments were used rather than whole antibody, as a way to increase the sensitivity; the Fab fragments were chosen because of their inability to bind nonspecifically to constant-fragment (Fc) receptors present on many cells. Fab fragments prepared from an anti-p97 antibody were labeled with ^{125}I and similar fragments from a control antibody were labeled with ^{131}I, so that the binding of specific vs. nonspecific fragments could be compared. To increase the precision of the assay, it was regularly ascertained that a binding denoted as specific could be competed out by unlabeled anti-p97 antibody. Using this assay, it became clear that p97 is also present on a variety of normal cells, including cultivated fibroblasts and peripheral-blood leukocytes. However, cells from most melanomas were shown to express much larger amounts of p97 than did cells from any of the various control tissues examined (Brown *et al.*, 1981a,b,c), 300,000–400,000 p97 molecules per cell being detected in some melanomas, as compared to less than 5,000 molecules per cell for a large variety of control cell populations.

Third, a DDIA was developed (as described in Section 2.3) and used to measure p97 in cell-membrane lysates prepared from a large variety of tissues; this assay could be employed because of the availability of monoclonal antibodies to different determinants of p97. It was shown (Brown *et al.*, 1981) that although p97 is expressed in virtually all cells, many melanomas, and some other tumors, have up to 100 times greater amounts of p97 than those detected among a large spectrum of normal adult tissues. Among the normal tissues, uterus and vagina were found to have a relatively high amount of p97, while liver, peripheral-blood leukocytes, kidneys, gut, lung, and brain have given very low binding. Certain fetal tissues, particularly fetal colon, were found to contain relatively high levels of p97, confirming the finding made by the RIP technique (Woodbury *et al.*, 1981).

The availability of monoclonal antibodies to more than one determinant of p97 has recently made it possible to study the combined effect of antibodies to two different determinants (p97[a] and p97[b]), in the presence of complement (I. Hellström *et al.*, 1981c). It was found that cells from many of those melanomas that express moderate to small amounts of p97 were not sensitive to a complement-dependent cytotoxic effect of either antibody 96.5 (to p97[a]) or 118.1 (to p97[b]). However, if the two antibodies were combined, a strong cytotoxic effect was commonly observed. This effect was synergistic, while the combination of either antibody 96.5 or 118.1 with an antibody to a different antigen had only an additive effect. These findings are similar to those reported by Howard *et al.* (1978), who studied the killing of rat cells by the combination of two alloantisera to the same antigen. Both sets of data have been attributed to a greater ability to bind complement when two IgG molecules are in close proximity by binding to different determinants of the same antigen molecule. It is interesting that nonmelanoma tumors, or normal cells, have not shown any synergistic cytotoxicity in the presence of the two antibodies. Therefore, had p97 been studied only with complement-dependent cytotoxicity techniques, rather than with highly sensitive binding assays, such as DDIA, it may have been erroneously characterized as an antigen confined to melanomas. One should also realize from these findings, however, that an antigen, such as p97, that is not truly tumor-specific may be made to operationally function as if it were—the amount of the same antigen expressed in normal cells may be too small for these cells to be damaged by antibody and complement. This might be utilized therapeutically.

Studies on the molecular nature of p97 have been initiated recently. They have shown that p97 is a glycoprotein which is synthesized by melanoma cells. (Brown *et al.*, 1981b). A fragment of molecular weight 40,000 can be cleaved off from this molecule by using papain (Brown *et al.*, 1981b). This fragment carries all three antigenic determinants so far detected on p97 (a, b, and c). A partial amino acid sequencing of the N-terminal end of p97 has been recently performed (Brown *et al.*, 1982). It shows a substantial homology between p97 and serum transferrin. Antibodies to denatured p97 bind significantly to serum transferrin and to lactotransferrin, while antibodies to native p97 do not. Like transferrin, p97 can bind iron (Brown et al., 1982). Thus p97 is one of the first cell membrane antigens of human neoplasms for which one has obtained information as to molecular structure and also some suggestive evidence as to possible function.

Antigens with a distribution similar to that of p97 have recently been described also from other laboratories, although these antigens have not been studied as extensively. Thus, a glycoprotein with a molecular weight of approximately 94,000, which is expressed in melanomas and certain other tumors, has recently been identified (Reisfeld *et al.*, 1980; Imai *et al.*, 1980; Dippold *et al.*, 1980). The relationship of some of these antigens to p97 is so far unclear. Competition experiments, as well as sequential RIP assays, have been performed on supernatants identifying the 94,000 antigen detected by Imai *et al.* (1980). They indicate that this antigen is not identical with p97 (Brown *et al.*, unpublished findings). On the other hand, there is recent evidence that p97 and the gp95 antigen of Dippold *et al.* (1980) are the same (Brown *et al.*, 1981b).

It has to be realized that only after testing with highly sensitive techniques could it be shown that p97 is present in small amounts on normal cells. If only relatively crude techniques had been employed, and if high-titered monoclonal antibodies had not been available for analysis, probably the only cells found to express p97 would have been those from about 30% of melanomas. If so, p97 would have been inadvertently labeled as a melanoma-specific antigen. It is possible that some of the "melanoma-specific" tumor antigens defined by monoclonal antibodies and studied by less sensitive assays than those employed for p97 may likewise be present on nonmelanoma cells. The same may hold true for antigens previously defined by antibodies in patient sera and for antigens studied with various tests for cell-mediated antitumor immunity.

A fourth antigen, p210, has been detected in melanomas and, also in relatively high amounts, in a variety of other tumors as well as in fetal and adult human brain (Loop *et al.*, 1982). Both binding assays with cultivated cells and RIP tests with cultivated cells and biopsy material have been employed in these studies. Antigen p210 appears to be substantially less specific than p97 due to the high amounts present in normal brain.

Table I summarizes data on the five antigens defined by our group by using the monoclonal-antibody technique.

4. Future Goals

The hybridoma technique has been used since around 1978 to analyze cell-surface antigens of human melanoma, and most of the work has been done in the few years since.

TABLE I

Summary of Antigens to Which Our Group Has Made Monoclonal Antibodies

Hybridomas defining antigen					
Designation	Name	Antibody class	Molecular nature	Specificity	First described by:
3.1	3.1	IgG₁	Unknown (glycolipid?)	Strongly only in cultured melanomas and strongest in 10% of melanomas. Normal tissues in vivo.	Yeh et al. (1979)
	3.2	IgG₂ₐ (IgG₃ contamin)			
	3.3	IgG₂ᵦ			
p97	4.1	IgG₁ (to p97ᵃ)	Glycoprotein, mol. wt. 97,000; 40,000 fragment can be cleaved off with papain.	All human cells, but strongest in tumor and fetal cells, with some melanomas having up to 100 times more p97 than cells from any adult normal tissue.	Woodbury et al. (1980), Brown et al. (1980)ᵃ
	96.5	IgG₂ₐ (to 97ᵃ)			
	118.1	IgG₂ₐ (to p97ᵇ)			
	8.2	IgG₁ (to 97ᶜ)			
p155	6.1	IgM	155,000-mol. wt. (glyco?)protein	Strongest in cells from 50% of melanomas.	Loop et al. (1981)
p210	5.1	IgG₁	210,000-mol. wt. (glyco?)protein	Melanomas, other tumors, normal adult brain.	Loop et al. (1981)
4.2	4.2	IgM	Glycolipid	Melanomas	Yeh et al. (1982)ᵇ

ᵃSame antigen subsequently described as gp 95 by Dippold et al. (1980).
ᵇAntigen 4.2 found to be the same as R₂₄, previously described by Dippold et al. (1980).

During this short period of experience, the technique has proved to be excellent for investigating those tumor-associated antigens that are immunogenic in mice, and the specificity and molecular nature of some of these antigens have been delineated. Some antigens, e.g., 3.1, have a relative specificity for a subgroup of melanomas, while others, e.g., p210, are not tumor-specific at all. Antigen p97, the antigen studied the most, was found not to be malanoma-specific, but still to have a sufficiently strong association with melanomas to stand out as a potentially interesting marker (see further below). Other antigens may possibly be specific for melanomas as a group, although we feel that final conclusions on this point should await further investigations. One antigen, defined by hybridoma R24 (Dippold et al., 1980), is not specific for tumor since normal melanocytes have it, but is still of great interest in that it is expressed by all melanomas and absent from the majority of other tumors; antigen 4.2 to which we have recently raised a monoclonal antibody (Yeh et al., 1982) appears to be the same as R24 (unpublished).

We shall now comment, under different headings, on some issues that we believe are important and on which much work will probably be done over the next few years.

4.1. Continued Studies on the Specificity and Nature of Antigens Defined by Available Monoclonal Antibodies and the Establishment of Hybridomas Forming Antibodies to Previously Unidentified Melanoma Antigens

First of all, exchange of reagents among various groups working with monoclonal antibodies to human melanomas is much needed. In addition to giving the field a much firmer basis than human tumor immunology has had in the past, it should be timesaving, since the same antigens may otherwise be investigated under different names, leading to unnecessary duplication of effort.

Once monoclonal antibodies are available to antigens that either are absent from all normal cells or are present there only in small concentrations, they can be used for a variety of purposes, as described below. The first priority continues to be, therefore, to characterize more rigorously the specificity of those antigens to which we already have monoclonal antibodies defining antigen expression in quantitative terms and to continue to raise hybridomas defining new melanoma antigens of even better specificity (if possible). The need to do both is obvious from the fact that the melanoma antigen studied the most, p97, is present, albeit in small amounts, in all human cells.

If an antigen is expressed on melanoma cells and on normal melanocytes, such as the one identified by hybridoma R24 (Dippold et al., 1980), it may still be a useful target for therapy. For example, antibody to such an antigen may be useful for removing melanoma cells from samples of bone marrow, as further discussed in Section 4.6.

If, on the other hand, large amounts of an antigen are present in some critical stem cells, the amount of antibody needed for tumor therapy may cause unacceptable side effects; it may even be lethal. Such an antigen may still be "useful" as a diagnostic marker and perhaps also for showing tumor localization in vivo, but it would not be a suitable target for therapy.

4.2. Attempts to Raise Monoclonal Antibodies to Antigens Recognized by Melanoma Patients

In view of the evidence, cited in Section 1, that human melanomas can induce in patients both cell-mediated and humoral immune responses to putative tumor antigens, it should be possible to establish hybridomas forming antibodies to those antigens. Such antibodies would be most useful for characterizing the respective antigens. So far, however, it has not been possible to show that melanoma patients form antibodies to any of the antigens identified by mouse hybridomas. Relatively little effort has gone into elucidating this important question, however, so definitive conclusions should not be made. The best possibility to study this may come from the hybridization of lymphocytes derived from human patients, rather than from immunized mice. Harvesting of lymphocytes subsequent to tumor removal, perhaps 2–3 days after a boost with irradiated tumor, might be optimal for this. Whether mouse or human myeloma cells are used as partners in the hybridization may be less important except for the fact that human–human hybridomas are known to be more stable than human–mouse hybridomas. The recent success in obtaining human–human hybridomas (Olsson and Kaplan, 1980; Croce et al., 1980) is very encouraging in this context.

One advantage of using patient lymphocytes for hybridization should be that the high frequency of hybridomas that recognize antigens of normal human cells should be decreased. Since the antigens likely to be recognized would be such that are normally immunogenic in man, they may be good targets for therapy. Another advantage with human antibodies is that they should be better than mouse antibodies for therapeutic purposes, since they could be given with less risk of complications, such as serum sickness.

A disadvantage of human hybridization is, on the other hand, that only those antigens that are immunogenic in the tumor patients will be detectable. It is possible that patients do not form antibodies to many tumor markers that could be of interest for diagnosis and therapy. This may be either because they lack lymphocyte clones capable of distinguishing the antigens as nonself or because a given antigen easily induces a suppressor-cell response. Therefore, even if it becomes possible to make human hybridomas that form antibodies to some antigens of human tumors, there will still be a need to search for human tumor markers by immunization of mice.

4.3. Further Use of Monoclonal Antibodies to Study the Molecular Nature of Tumor Antigens

The availability of monoclonal antibodies should greatly facilitate the purification of human tumor-associated antigens by immunoadsorption. Such purification should aid molecular studies on the respective antigens. The use of monoclonal antibodies to different determinants of the same antigen (Brown et al., 1981b) may be valuable in this context. One can, for example, investigate whether the same determinants are present on antigens derived from different normal and neoplastic tissues or whether the combination of the determinants differs. One may also be able to isolate and further study antigen fragments, which carry only one determinant, and this may facilitate many types of structural work.

For those tumor antigens that are proteins, it may be highly worthwhile to isolate antigens from various tissues (normal and neoplastic) and compare the isolates, e.g., by peptide mapping and by amino acid sequencing of the N-terminal end. Sequencing techniques should also elucidate the relationship of different tumor antigens to each other and to normal cell antigens. The information so obtained may guide us toward understanding what cellular functions, if any, a given antigen may have. Some strides in this direction have already been made for antigen p97 (Brown *et al.*, 1982) as discussed above.

One should realize that purified tumor antigens are of interest not only for molecular studies but also, perhaps, from a more practical point of view. Thus, a tumor antigen isolated by monoclonal antibody or — even better — synthesized *in vitro* after its molecular structure is known and the gene cloned, offer possibilities for therapy by being used for active immunization. It may be possible, for example, to establish human antibodies to an antigen first isolated by using a mouse monoclonal antibody by either immunizing human subjects (when that can be ethically justified) or by sensitizing with the antigen *in vitro* to induce the formation of human antibodies. As an alternative, primate antibodies could probably be obtained by immunization.

Tumor antigen or synthetic peptides may also be used for the induction of cell-mediated immune reactions. By coupling it to proper carriers, it may be possible to develop procedures by which cytotoxic and helper responses are induced to a greater extent than are such responses mediated by suppressor cells.

4.4. Monoclonal Antibodies for Diagnosis

One of the obvious uses of monoclonal antibody is for developing immunoassays of circulating antigen that might be applicable to the monitoring of patients with tumor. Such antigens that are easily released into the circulation are likely to be of the greatest value in this respect. Possibly, assays of sera can also be employed for the screening of seemingly healthy individuals for tumor. The latter will depend on the degree of antigen specificity, however. A high frequency of false positives would probably be seen with antigens that are expressed in normal cells, and this would then make a test of serum samples useless for diagnostic purposes.

Employment of monoclonal antibodies for histopathological diagnosis on tissue sections is also worthy of consideration. The antibodies most useful for this purpose would be such as can distinguish between different histological types of melanoma (e.g. between nodular and superficial spreading melanoma), and such as can distinguish between primary and metastatic melanoma. To what extent such antibodies can be raised remains to be investigated. The best way to screen for them is probably to test hybridoma supernatants (obtained after immunizing with primary or metastatic tumor) on histological sections, using peroxidase-anti-peroxidase techniques.

4.5. Tumor Localization *in Vivo*

One of the potentially most important clinical uses of monoclonal antibodies is for tumor localization. Radiolabeled antibodies have been employed for this for a long time (for a discussion, see Goldenberg *et al.*, 1980). The problem in the past has been to obtain an antibody of sufficient specificity to be of practical value. Once a specific antibody is available, on the other hand, procedures can probably be developed for using it to detect tumor masses with sufficient accuracy to be of clinical help. Monoclonal antibodies to antigens of very high specificity are obviously preferred; that is, the best antibodies are likely to be those that define antigens specific for subgroups of melanomas (e.g., antibodies to antigen 3.1) or specific for melanomas in general. However, even a widely distributed antigen, such as p97, may be specific enough for localization studies, since all that is needed is that the antigen be expressed substantially more on tumor cells than on normal tissues. By injecting a labeled control immunoglobulin to check for nonspecific uptake and using computerized procedures for subtraction of that uptake, localization of the specific antibody in tumor masses may be detected. Obviously, no antibodies should be injected into patients until the risk of complications has been thoroughly evaluated.

In a recent study (Larsen *et al.*, to be published), radiolabeled anti-p97, or control, antibody was injected intravenously into patients with metastatic melanoma, and antibody localization verified both by scanning techniques and by measuring uptake of specific versus control antibody in biopsies of tumor and normal tissue. Evidence of selective localization of anti-p97 antibody in tumor tissue was obtained.

4.6. Therapy by Infusion of Monoclonal Antibodies (Given Alone)

Some monoclonal antibodies may be useful for therapy. For those antibodies that, on the basis of specificity studies, are of interest, one can consider giving the antibody either alone or after it has been complexed with some antitumor agent. We shall first discuss antibody given alone. In this case, antibodies to be chosen are primarily those that are either cytotoxic in the presence of complement or that can serve as lymphocyte-dependent antibodies in consort with K cells (I. Hellström *et al.*, 1981b). Some already available IgG_2 mouse antibodies to the 3.1 antigen (antibody 3.2 and 3.3) or to p97 (antibody 96.5) are cytotoxic in the presence of complement (Yeh *et al.*, 1979; I. Hellström *et al.*, 1981c), and antibody 3.2 can give antibody-dependent cellular cytotoxicity (I. Hellström *et al.*, 1981b). The effectiveness of mouse monoclonal antibodies to utilize human complement for target-cell killing needs to be better studied, however, before predictions can be made as to their possible therapeutic usefulness *in vivo*. Human antibodies (whenever they can be developed) may be ultimately preferable, also because of a lesser risk of side effects.

As discussed in Section 3.3, there is recent evidence from studies on p97 that a strong synergistic effect can be obtained by using two or more antibodies to different determinants on the same antigen molecule, when either antibody alone has only borderline activity (I. Hellström *et al.*, 1981c). This should be an impetus to raise IgG_2 antibodies to more than one determinant also of other tumor antigens.

Other uses of monoclonal antibodies may be for removing free circulating tumor antigens or antigen–antibody complexes. This may be best achieved by *ex vivo* immunoadsorption procedures, binding the antibodies to a solid phase through which plasma is passed. Possibly, the antibodies may instead be injected in order to create immune complexes in antibody excess. The rationale for the latter two approaches is to remove antigens (or complexes) that are immunosuppressive, e.g., as a result of their activating a suppressor-cell response. Therefore, they deserve to be considered only for antibodies defining tumor antigens that are recognized as targets for an immune response in patients and where the presence of free antigen or complexes makes this response inefficient. So far, no antigens of this type have been identified with the monoclonal-antibody technique.

One of the earliest therapeutic uses of monoclonal antibody that may be considered will be for removing contaminating tumor cells from human bone-marrow samples, since attempts in this direction may already be feasible. The bone marrow is particularly sensitive to high-dose chemotherapy. Therefore, the possibility is being tried of removing a bone-marrow sample prior to such therapy and returning it later. The problem that the sample may contain living tumor cells might be solved by destroying such cells with specific antibody and complement (or by using cell-sorting procedures). Monoclonal antibodies that are substantially more cytotoxic to melanoma cells than to any crucial population of normal bone-marrow cells are potential candidates for use in such therapy. It is obvious that any antibody to be used for such a procedure must first be tested for lack of reactivity with any subpopulations of normal bone-marrow cells.

4.7. Monoclonal Antibodies as Carriers of Therapeutic Agents

In many cases, it may be advantageous to use monoclonal antibodies to transport toxic substances to a growing tumor rather than to give the antibodies alone. Such toxic substances include ricin A chains or diphtheria toxin, which, when attached to a cell membrane, will kill the cell to which they are attached, but which will not affect cells to which they are not (Gilliland *et al.*, 1980; Jansen *et al.*, Casellas *et al.*, 1981). One problem with this approach is the fact that cells expressing an antigen defined by a given monoclonal antibody may be quickly selected, since they would not be killed by an agent that affects only the cells to which it would bind. However, the extent to which antigens can be lost probably varies for different antigens. By using a combination of monoclonal antibodies to several different antigens at the same time, the problem can be minimized.

Other toxic substances worthy of consideration are those that have a more distant effect, including chemotherapeutic drugs. Some encouraging results have already been obtained by using conventional antibodies as carriers of drugs (Ghose and Blair, 1978; Sela *et al.*, 1979). There have, however, been two problems in doing this in the past. First, the antibodies used have had a low degree of tumor specificity. Second, the biological effects observed have not been much greater when antibodies were given bound to drug than when either agent was given alone. The problem with specificity may be solved by using a proper monoclonal antibody, while the problem of getting a conjugate with high selective toxicity is more difficult to tackle. The choice of the right agent to bind to the monoclonal antibody would be the important one.

One should also consider using antibodies to carry into tumors such agents as can improve the level of local antitumor reactivity. This includes agents that can induce delayed-hypersensitivity reactions and that can turn off suppressor-cell-mediated responses. It is noteworthy that considerable success has been obtained in treating human tumors localized to the skin by a combination of systemic sensitization with an agent such as dinitrochlorobenzol, followed by a topical application of the sensitizing agent over the tumor area (E. Klein, 1968). This success has probably been due to the fact that many tumor cells are more sensitive than normal cells to a cytotoxic effect of activated macrophages (and other inflammatory cells). Furthermore, natural killer (NK) cells may accumulate as an effect of macrophage activation and may be responsible for tumor-cell destruction as well. The obvious problem in employing this approach for tumors not situated in the skin has been to localize, to the tumor, the agent inducing the delayed-hypersensitivity reaction. By using monoclonal antibody as carrier for the sensitizer, this problem might be solved. It has to be realized, however, that the agent to be carried by the antibody may not, at all, be the sensitizer itself, but a "modified-self" molecule induced on the binding of the sensitizer to the proper host cell.

To make progress in this area, it is necessary to use animal models, in which monoclonal antibodies are available to tumor antigens. Preferably, these antigens should be similar to those encountered in human neoplasms. One model worthy of consideration comprises chemically induced mouse bladder carcinomas (Taranger *et al.*, 1972). These tumors have a shared antigen to which monoclonal antibodies have recently been raised (Hellström *et al.*, 1982).

4.8. Studies on the Loss of Tumor Antigens and Attempts to Take Such Losses into Account When Devising Therapy

Tumors normally undergo progression, during which there is a selection of spontaneously appearing cell variants that do not express a particular characteristic of the original neoplasm (Foulds, 1961). Losses of tumor antigens are examples of such progression and will complicate the use of immunotherapy aimed at destroying cells carrying a particular antigen (Yeh *et al.*, 1981). Because of such losses, it seems likely that even if methods could be developed for killing all cells expressing a particular tumor antigen, those cells would quickly be replaced by other cells lacking it.

One possible way out of this dilemma may be, as already pointed out above, to use antibodies to carry drugs that have a more generalized effect than, for example, ricin bound to a tumor-cell surface and that can also damage those tumor cells that lack the particular antigen. Chemotherapeutic drugs, agents that induce delayed-hypersensitivity reactions, and others fall into this category.

Another approach can be based on the fact that the same tumor cell often expresses more than one antigen to which monoclonal antibodies are available. For example, cells from some of the melanomas that we have ourselves studied express five antigens identified by monoclonal antibodies, 3.1, p97, p155, p210 and 4.2 (an probably express other antigens as well, to which monoclonal antibodies can be raised). It should be possible, therefore, to decrease the extent to which cell variants lacking antigens are selected by using a combination of antibodies to several antigens. This may have an added advantage: if a particular melanoma-associated antigen is shared by one subpopulation of normal cells, and a different melanoma antigen is shared by a different population of normal cells, a combination of antibodies to the two antigens may hurt the tumor cells more than the normal cell populations sharing only one of the two antigens with the tumor.

Antigen losses as a result of antigenic modulation (Old *et al.*, 1968) must be taken into account as well. An antigen that would easily modulate in the presence of the specific antibody would be a poor target for both tumor localization and therapy. The previously discussed antigens 3.1 and p97 do not appear to modulate in the presence of the respective antibodies (Hellström *et al.,* unpublished findings).

4.9. How Tumor-Specific Must an Antigen Be to Serve as a Target for Therapy?

The ideal tumor antigen is one that is entirely specific and the expression of which is intimately associated with the neoplastic behavior of the given tumor. To what extent such an antigen exists is uncertain, however, except for those cases where the antigen is coded for by a virus that also causes the neoplastic transformation (K. E. Hellström and Brown, 1979). No such virally related antigens have been demonstrated in human melanoma. Alternative candidates must therefore be considered.

Antigens of the "Class 1" type are, by definition, specific for an individual tumor. No such antigen has yet been defined by the monoclonal-antibody technique. The closest candidate is antigen 3.1, which is expressed most strongly by a small subgroup of melanomas (Yeh *et al.,* 1979). However, antigen 3.1 was unexpectedly detected in normal human tissue removed at surgery and tested prior to culturing (Brown *et al.,* 1981).

Antigens demonstrated by Koprowski *et al.* (1978), Mitchell *et al.* (1980), Carrel *et al.* (1980), and Imai *et al.* (1981), and reported to be melanoma-type-specific may be ideal candidates for tumor localization and therapy. However, it needs to be further substantiated whether any of these antigens is absolutely specific or whether the specificity is only relative. If the latter proves to be the case, the degree of cross-reactivity with normal (stem?) cells is likely to influence the practical usefulness of a given antigen.

Judging from our own data, we believe that the majority of human tumor antigens that will be detected by the monoclonal-antibody approach will prove to be differentiation ("oncofetal") antigens. The degree to which tumor cells and normal cells differ in the expression of a given antigen, and the type of normal cells that share it, will then decide whether the antigen is a suitable marker for tumor localization or a good target for therapy, or both. The p97 antigen seems to be a good candidate for both, since it is present in much greater amounts in some melanomas than in normal cells, and since bone marrow, liver, gut, kidneys, and blood express only low levels of p97, when studied at the whole-tissue level. An important caveat is, however, that we do not yet know whether any vitally important populations of stem cells, e.g., in the gut or bone marrow, express much p97; this is now being investigated.

Antigens shared by normal melanocytes and melanomas, e.g., the antigen defined by hybridoma R24 (Dippold *et al.,* 1980) or 4.2 (Yeh *et al.,* 1982), should also be considered, since a therapy-induced damage to normal melanocytes may be acceptable if, at the same time, melanoma cells can be destroyed. Of interest in this context is the finding of Bernstein *et al.* (1980) that anti-Thy-1 antibodies have an inhibitory effect *in vivo* on AKR lymphoma cells expressing the Thy-1 antigen. In this case, tumor destruction could be obtained without much side effect on the tumor-bearing host, even though its normal T cells and brain cells shared the Thy-1 antigen with the treated lymphoma.

5. Conclusions

Monoclonal mouse antibodies have been raised to various cell-surface antigens of human melanomas. Some of these antibodies define antigens that are relatively specific for subgroups of melanomas or possibly all melanomas while other antibodies are directed to antigens that are also present on cells from certain other tumors and on normal cells, such as some astrocytomas and normal melanocytes. The antigen studied the most, p97, is a glycoprotein of molecular weight 97,000 that is present on virtually all human cells but expressed up to 100 times stronger on cells from some melanomas than on any normal adult cells and that is related to serum transferrin. It is also expressed strongly on certain embryonic cells and is therefore best labeled as a differentiation (or oncofetal) antigen.

Even such antigens as are specific only from the quantitative point of view, e.g., p97, may prove to be useful as targets for tumor localization and therapy. However, this will be dependent on the extent to which the respective antigens are expressed in crucial normal stem-cell populations. Knowledge, in quantitative terms, of the specificity of the various cell-surface antigens that can be detected in human melanomas is urgently needed. Such knowledge is likely to have most important consequences for the diagnosis and therapy of human melanoma.

ACKNOWLEDGMENTS. The work of the authors cited herein was supported by Grants CA 14135, CA 19148, CA 19149, CA 25558, and CA 27841 from the National Institutes of Health and IM 241 and IM 43L from the American Cancer Society. The authors' experiments, as discussed in this chapter, were performed conjointly with Dr. Joseph P. Brown, Dr. Richard G. Woodbury, Dr. Kiyoshi Nishiyama, Dr. Ming-Yang Yeh, Charles E. Hart, and Stephen M. Loop, whose invaluable collaboration is gratefully acknowledged. This chapter was written when the authors were Humboldt Awardees working at the Deutches Krebsforschungszentrum (DKFZ) in Heidelberg, West Germany. Our sincere thanks are due to both the Humboldt Foundation and the DKFZ.

References

Bernstein, I. D., Tam, M. R., and Nowinski, R. C., 1980, Mouse leukemia therapy with monoclonal antibodies against a thymus differentiation antigen, *Science* **207**:68.

Brown, J. P., Tamerius, J. D., and Hellström, I. 1979, Indirect ^{125}I-labelled protein A binding assay for monoclonal antibodies to cell surface antigens, *J. Immunol. Methods* **31**:201.

Brown, J. P., Wright, P. W., Hart, C. E., Woodbury, R. G., Hellström, K. E., and Hellström, I., 1980, Protein antigens of normal and malignant human cells identified by immunoprecipitation with monoclonal antibodies, *J. Biol. Chem.* **255**:4980.

Brown, J. P., Woodbury, R. G., Hart, C. E., Hellström, I., and Hellström, K. E., 1981a, Quantitative analysis of melanoma-associated antigen p97 in normal and neoplastic tissues, *Proc. Natl. Acad. Sci. U.S.A.* **78**: 539.

Brown, J. P., Nishiyama, K., Hellström, I., and Hellström, K. E., 1981b, Structural characterization of human melanoma-associated antigen p97 using monoclonal antibodies, *J. Immunol.* **127**:157.

Brown, J. P., Hellström, K. E., and Hellström, I., 1981c, Use of monoclonal antibodies for quantitative analysis of antigens in normal and neoplastic tissues, *Clin. Chem.* **27**:1592.

Brown, J. P. Hewick, R. M., Hellström, I., and Hellström, K. E., Doolittle, R. F., and Dreyer, W. J., 1982, Human melanoma-associated antigen p97 is structurally and functionally related to transferrin, *Nature* (in press).

Bystryn, J.-C., and Smalley, J. R., 1977, Identification and solubilization of iodinated cell surface human melanoma associated antigens, *Int. J. Cancer* **20**:165.

Carrel, S., Accolla, R. S., Carmagnola, A. L., and Mach, J.-P., 1980, Common human melanoma-associated antigen(s) detected by monoclonal antibodies, *Cancer Res.* **40**:2523.

Casellas, P., H. E. Blythman, J. P. Brown, O. Gros, P. Gros, K. E. Hellström, I. Hellström F. K. Jansen, P. Poncelet and H. Vidal, 1981, *Protides of the Biological Fluids*, (ed. H. Peeters) (in press).

Cornain, S., de Vries, J. E., Collard, J., Vennegoor, C., Wingerden, I. V., and Rümke, P., 1975, Antibodies and antigen expression in human melanoma detected by the immune adherence test, *Int. J. Cancer* **19**:981.

Croce, C. M., Linnenbach, A., Hall, W., Steplewski, Z., and Koprowski, H., 1980, Production of human hybridomas secreting antibodies to measles virus, *Nature (London)* **288**:488.

Dippold, W. G., Lloyd, K. O., Li, L. T. C., Ikeda, H., Oettgen, H. F., and Old, L. J., 1980, Cell surface antigens of human malignant melanoma: Definition of six antigenic systems with mouse monoclonal antibodies, *Proc. Natl. Acad. Sci. U.S.A.* **77**:6114.

Engvall, E., and Perlmann, P., 1971, Enzyme linked immunosorbent assay (ELISA): Quantitative assay of immunoglobulin G, *Immunochemistry* **8**:871.

Foulds, L., 1961, Progression and carcinogenesis, *Acta Unio Int. Contra Cancrum* **17**:148.

Galfre, G., Howe, S. C., Milstein, C., Butcher, G. W., and Howard, J. C., 1977, Antibodies to major histocompatability antigens produced by hybrid cell lines, *Nature (London)* **266**:550.

Garrigues, H. J., Tilgen, W., Hellström, I., Franke, W., and Hellström, K. E., 1982. Detection of a human melanoma-associated antigen, p97, in histological sections of primary human melanomas, submitted for publication.

Ghose, T., and Blair, A. H., 1978, Antibody-limited cytotoxic agents in the treatment of cancer, *J. Natl. Cancer Inst.* **61**:657.

Gilliland, D. G., Steplewski, Z., Collier, R. J., Mitchell, K. F., Chang, T. H., and Koprowski, H., 1980, Antibody-directed cytotoxic agensts: Use of monoclonal antibody to direct the action of toxin A chains to colorectal carcinoma cells, *Proc. Natl. Acad. Sci. U.S.A.* **77**:4539.

Gold, P., and Freedman, S. O., 1965, Demonstration of tumor-specific antigens in human colonic carcinoma by immunological tolerance and absorption techniques, *J. Exp. Med.* **121**:439.

Goldenberg, D. M., Kim, E. E., DeLand, F. H., Bennett, S., and Primus, F. J., 1980, Radioimmunodetection of cancer with radioactive antibodies to carcinoembryonic antigen, *Cancer Res.* **40**:2984.

Halliday, W. J., Maluish, A. E., Little, J. H., and Davis, N. C., 1975, Leukocyte adherence inhibition and specific immunoreactivity in malignant melanoma, *Int. J. Cancer* **16**:645.

Hellström, I., and Hellström, K. E., 1972, Immunity to neuroblastomas and melaomas, *Annu. Rev. Med.* **23**:19.

Hellström, I., and Hellström, K. E., 1973, Some recent studies on cellular immunity to human melanomas, *Fed. Proc. Fed. Am. Soc. Exp. Biol.* **32**:156.

Hellström, I., Hellström, K. E., and Shepard, T. H., 1970, Cell-mediated immunity against antigens common to human colonic caricnomas and fetal gut epithelium, *Int. J. Cancer* **6**:346.

Hellström, I., Hellström, K. E., Sjögren, H. O., and Warner, G. A., 1971, Demonstration of cell-mediated immunity to human neoplasms of various histological types, *Int. J. Cancer* **7**:1.

Hellström, I., Hellström, K. E., Brown, J. P., and Woodbury, R. G., 1981a, Antigens of human tumors, particularly melanomas, as studied with the monoclonal antibody technique, in: *Monoclonal Antibodies and T cell hybridomas*, Vol. 3 (G. J. Hämmerling, *et al.*, eds. Elsevier/North-Holland, Amsterdam.

Hellström, I., Hellström, K. E., and Yeh, M.-Y., 1981b, Lymphocyte-dependent antibodies to antigen 3.1, a cell surface antigen expressed by a subgroup of human melanomas (submitted).

Hellström, I., Brown, J. P., and Hellström, K. E., 1981c, Monoclonal antibodies to two determinants of melanoma-antigen p97 act synergistically in complement-dependent cytotoxicity, *J. Immunol.* **127**:157.

Hellström, I., Rollins, N., Settle, S., Chapman, P., Chapman, W. H., and Hellström, K. E., 1982, Monoclonal antibodies to two mouse bladder carcinoma antigen, *Int. J. Caqncer* (in press).

Hellström, K. E., and Brown, J. P., 1979, Tumor antigens, in: *The Antigens* (M. Sela, ed.), pp. 1–82, Academic Press, New York.

Hellström, K. E., Brown, J. P., and Hellström, I., 1980, Monoclonal antibodies to tumor antigens, in: *Contemporary Topics in Immunobiology*, Vol. 11, (N. L. Warner, ed.), pp. 117–137, Plenum Press, New York.

Herberman, R. B., 1974, Cell-mediated immunity to tumor cells, *Adv. Cancer Res.* **19**:207.

Herlyn, D., Herlyn, M., Steplewski, Z., and Koprowski, H., 1979, Monoclonal antibodies in cell-mediated cytotoxicity against human melanoma and colorectal carcinoma, *Eur. J. Immunol.* **9**:657.

Herlyn, M., Steplewski, Z., Herlyn, D., and Koprowski, H., 1979, Colorectal carcinoma-specific antigen: Detection by means of monoclonal antibodies, *Proc. Natl. Acad. Sci. U.S.A.* **76**:1438.

Howard, J. C., Butcher, G. W., Galfre, G., and Milstein, C., 1978, Monoclonal anti-rat MHC (H-1) alloantibodies, *Curr. Top. Microbiol. Immunol.* **81**:54.

Imai, K., Glassey, M. C., Molinaro, G. A., and Ferrone, S., 1980, Monoclonal antibodies to human melanoma associated antigens, *Fed. Proc. Fed. Am. Soc. Exp. Biol.* **39**:351 (abstract).

Imai, K., Wilson, B. S., Kay, N. E., and Ferrone, S. 1981. Monoclonal antibodies to human melanoma cells: comparison of erological results of several laboratories and molecular profile of melanoma-associated antigens, in: *Monoclonal Antibodies and T Cell Hybridomas*, Vol. 3 (G. Hämmerling *et al.*, eds), Elsevier/North Holland, Amsterdam.

Jansen, F. K., Blythman, H. E., Carriere, D., Cassellas, P., Gros, O., Gros, P., Paolucci, E., Pau, B., Poncelet, P., Richer, G., Vidal, H., and Voisin, G. A., 1981, Assembly and activity of conjugates between monoclonal antibodies and the toxic subunit of ricin (immunotoxins), in: *Monoclonal Antibodies and T Cell Hybridomas*, Vol. 3 (G. J. Hämmerling, *et al.*, eds.), Elsevier/North-Holland, Amsterdam.

Kennett, R. H., and Gilbert, F., 1979, Hybrid myelomas producing antibodies against a human neuroblastoma antigen present on fetal brain, *Science* **203**:1120.

Kessler, S. W., 1975, Rapid isolation of antigens from cells with a *Staphylococcal* protein A-antibody adsorbent: Parameters of the interaction of antibody–antigen complexes with protein A, *J. Immunol.* **115**:1617.

Klein, E., 1968, Immunotherapy of cutaneus and mucosal neoplasms, *N. Y. State J. Med.* **68**:900.

Klein, G., 1973, The Epstein–Barr virus, in: *The Herpes Viruses* (A. Kaplan, ed.), p. 521, Academic Press, New York.

Köhler, G., and Milstein, C., 1975, Continuous culture of fused cells secreting antibodies of predefined specificity, *Nature (London)* **256**:495.

Köhler, G., and Milstein, C., 1976, Derivation of specific antibody-producing tissue culture and tumor lines by cell fusion, *Eur. J. Immunol.* **6**:511.

Köhler, G., Howe, S. C., and Milstein, C., 1976, Fusion between immunoglobulin-secreting and nonsecreting myeloma lines, *Eur. J. Immunol.* **6**:292.

Koprowski, H. Steplewski, Z., Herlyn, D., and Herlyn, M., 1978, Study of antibodies against human melanoma produced by somatic cell hybrids, *Proc. Natl. Acad. Sci. U.S.A.* **75**:3405.

Koprowski, H., and Steplewski, Z. 1981, Human solid tumor antigens defined by monoclonal antibodies, in: *Monodonal Antibodies and T Cell Hybridomas* Vol. 3 (G. J. Hämmerling *et al.*, eds), Elsevier/North Holland, Amsterdam.

Lewis, M. G., Ikonopisov, R. L., Nairn, R. C., Phillips, T. M., Hamilton-Fairley, G., Bodenham, D. C., and Alexander, P., 1969, Tumor-specific antibodies in human malignant melanoma and their relationship to extent of disease, *Br. Med. J.* **3**:547.

Loop, S. M., Nishiyama, K., Hellström, I., Woodbury, R. G., Brown, J. P., and Hellström, K. E., 1981, Two human tumor-associated antigens, p155 and p210, detected by monoclonal antibodies *Int. J. Cancer* **227**:775.

McCoy, J. L., Jerome, L. F., Dean, J. H., Perlin, E., Oldham, R. K., Char, D. H., Cohen, M. H., Felix, E. L., and Herberman, R. B., 1975, Inhibition of leukocyte migration by tumor-associated antigens in soluble extracts of human malignant melanoma, *J. Natl. Cancer Inst.* **55**:19.

Morgan, A. C., Galloway, D. R., and Reisfeld, R. A., 1981, *Hybridoma* **1**:27.

Mitchell, K., Fuhrer, P., Steplewski, Z., and Koprowski, H. 1980, Biochemical characterization of human melanoma cell surfaces: dissection with monoclonal antibodies. *Proc. Natl. Acad. Sci. U. S. A.* **77**:7267.

Morton, D. L., Malmgren, R. A., Holmes, E. C., and Ketcham, A. S., 1968, Demonstration of antibodies against human malignant melanoma by immunofluorescence, *Surgery* **64**:233.

Nowinski, R. C., Lostrom, M. D., Tam, M. R., Stone, M. R., and Burnette, W. N., 1979, The isolation of hybrid cell lines producing monoclonal antibodies against the p15(E) protein of ecotropic murine leukemia viruses, *Virology* **93**:111.

Old, L. J., Boyse, E. A., Geering, G., and Oettgen, H. F., 1968, Serologic approaches to the study of cancer in animals and man, *Cancer Res.* **28**:1288.

Olsson, L., and Kaplan, H. S., 1980, Human–human hybridomas producing monoclonal antibodies to predefined antigen specificity, *Proc. Natl. Acad. Sci. U.S.A.* **77**:5429.

Parkhouse, R. M. E., and Guarnotta, G., 1978, Rapid binding test for detection of alloantibodies to lymphocyte surface antigens, *Curr. Top. Microbiol. Immunol.* **81**:142.

Prehn, R., and Main, D., 1957, Immunity to methylcholanthrene induced sarcomas, *J. Natl. Cancer Inst.* **18**:768.

Reisfeld, R. A., Galloway, D., Imai, K., Ferrone, S., and Morgan, A. C., 1980, Molecular profiles of human melanoma associated antigens, *Fed. Proc. Fed. Am. Soc. Exp. Biol.* **39**:351 (abstract).

Sela, M., Hurmitz, E., and Maron, R., 1979, Use of antibodies for delivery of chemtherapeutic drugs, in: *The Role of Non-specific Immunity in the Prevention and Treatment of Cancer* (M. Sela, ed.), p. 481, Elsevier/North-Holland, New York.

Shiku, H., Takahashi, T., Oettgen, H. F., and Old, L. J., 1976, Cell surface antigens of human malignant melanoma. II. Serological typing with immune adherence assays and definition of two new surface antigens, *J. Exp. Med.* **144**:873.

Shiku, H. J., Takahashi, T., Resnick, L. A., Oettgen, H. F., and Old, L. J., 1977, Cell surface antigens of human malignant melanoma. III. Recognition of autoantibodies with unusual characteristics, *J. Exp. Med.* **145**:784.

Shulman, M., Wilde, C. D., and Köhler, G., 1978, A better cell line for making hybridoma secreting specific antibodies, *Nature (London)* **276**:269.

Stahli, C., Stachelin, T., Miggiano, V., Schmidt, J., and Häring, P., 1980, High frequencies of antigen-specific hybridomas: Dependence of immunization parameters and prediction by spleen cell analysis, *J. Immunol. Methods* **32**:297.

Taranger, L. A., Chapman, W. H., Hellström, I., and Hellström, K. E., 1972, Immunological studies on urinary bladder tumors of rats and mice, *Science* **176**:1337.

Titani, K., Koide, A., Hermann, J., Ericsson, L. H., Kumar, S., Wade., R. D., Walsh, K. A., Neurath, H., and Fisher, E. H., 1977, Complete amino acid sequence of rabbit muscle glycogen phosphorylase, *Proc. Natl. Acad. Sci. U.S.A.* **74**:4762.

Woodbury, R. G., Brown, J. P., Yeh, M.-Y., Hellström, I., and Hellström, K. E., 1980, Identification of a cell surface protein, p97, in human melanomas and certain other neoplasms, *Proc. Natl. Acad. Sci. U.S.A.* **77**:2183.

Woodbury, R. G., Brown, J. P., Loop, S. M., Hellström, K. E., and Hellström, I., 1981, Analysis of normal and neoplastic human tissues for the tumor-associated protein p97, *Int. J. Cancer* **27**:145.

Yeh, M.-Y., Hellström, I., Brown, J. P., Warner, G. A., Hansen, J. A., and Hellström, K. E., 1979, Cell surface antigens of human melanoma identified by monoclonal antibody, *Proc. Natl. Acad. Sci. U.S.A.* **76**:2927.

Yeh, M.-Y., Hellström, I., and Hellström, K. E., 1981, Clonal variation in expression of a human melanoma antigen defined by a monoclonal antibody, *J. Immunol.* (**126** :1312.

Yeh, M. -Y., Hellström, I., Abe, K., Hakomori, S., and Hellström, K. E., 1982, A cell surface antigen which is present in the gaglioside fraction and shared by human melanomas, *Int. J. Cancer* (in press).

Young, W. W., MacDonald, E. M. S., Nowinski, R. C., and Hakomori, S.-I., 1979, Production of monoclonal antibodies specific for two distinct steric portions of the glycolipid ganglio-*N*-triosylceramide (asialo GM$_2$), *J. Exp. Med.* **150**:1008.

11

The Nature and Significance of Melanoma Antigens Recognized by Human Subjects

PETER HERSEY AND WILLIAM H. MCCARTHY

1. Introduction

Since the reports of Lewis *et al.* (1969) and Morton *et al.* (1968), a number of studies have confirmed the presence of antibodies against melanoma cells in the sera of patients with melanoma. These studies have raised considerable controversy that centered initially on the cross-reactivity of antigens detected by human antisera between different melanoma cells and then on both the biological and biochemical nature of these antigens. With the application of more stringent criteria of tumor specificity and different assay techniques, there has been renewed debate on the specificity of many of these antigens for melanoma and whether they are the focus of tumor-related immune responses by patients with melanoma.

The extent to which these issues are unresolved is a reflection of the inherent difficulties involved in studies on human material, such as the availability of autologous tissues, the complexity and variety of antibodies in human sera, and the transient nature of some immune responses against tumor antigens. These difficulties are such that there has been understandable relief with the advent of monoclonal-antibody technology and its potential for solving many of the problems in this field.

Despite the difficulties involved, continued study of antigens which give rise to immune responses in human subjects appears essential to identify the structures on melanoma cells that may be important in control of tumor growth by the immune system. Precedents in the study of human leukocyte antigen (HLA) complex antigens also indicate that many of

PETER HERSEY • Medical Research Department, Kanematsu Memorial Institute, Sydney Hospital, Sydney, N. S. W. 2000, Australia.   WILLIAM H. MCCARTHY • Melanoma Unit, Department of Surgery, University of Sydney, Sydney Hospital, Sydney, N. S. W. 2000, Australia.

the private specificities recognized by homologous lymphoid cells are poorly recognized by xenogeneic lymphoid cells currently used for production of monoclonal antibodies (Zola, 1980). Similar difficulties in recognition of fine-structural alterations associated with malignancy may apply in studies on melanoma antigens. Recognition of such differences may be important for development of immunodiagnostic tests in melanoma and as a focus for immune responses in control of tumor growth.

In the following sections, some of the developments over the past decade in studies on melanoma antigens detected by human antisera are retraced. Particular emphasis is given to our studies using leukocyte-dependent antibody (LDA) assays and some of the applications that we see evolving from them. In addition, attention is given to an area of study of melanoma antigens that has been largely overlooked in discussion of their specificity and cross-reactivity. This relates to their functional importance, not only as a focus for immune responses against the tumor cell, but also as membrane components with important biological functions that may determine various aspects of tumor-cell behavior in the host. We consider that information on these aspects over the next decade may have a major impact on our ability to influence the clinical behavior of tumor growth in melanoma patients.

2. Heterogeneity of Tumor-Associated Antigens Recognized by Human Subjects on Melanoma Cells

2.1. Individual-Specific vs. Cross-Reactive Antigens

One of the first areas of dissent in studies on antibodies to melanoma cells related to whether they detected antigens common to all melanoma cells, as suggested by Morton *et al.* (1968, 1971a) and supported by Liao *et al.* (1978), or specific to individual cells (Lewis *et al.*, 1969; Lewis and Phillips, 1972; Bodurtha *et al.*, 1975; The *et al.*, 1975).

This debate was a natural sequel to previous studies on animal tumors in which it was shown that tumors of viral origin had common cross-reacting antigens whereas chemical-carcinogen-induced tumors commonly had tumor antigens unique to individual tumors (Old and Boyse, 1964; Old *et al.*, 1962).

It soon became apparent that the question of cross-reactivity of melanoma antigens was not to be resolved as simply as these studies suggested. Several groups found that antisera from human patients cross-reacted with only a proportion of allogeneic melanoma cells (Macher *et al.*, 1975; Hersey *et al.*, 1976a; Shiku *et al.*, 1976; Seibert *et al.*, 1977). Different antisera also reacted with different groups of melanoma cells in an overlapping pattern. These findings were consistent with the presence of antigenic determinants on several different membrane structures associated with melanoma and/or the presence of polymorphic determinants on one membrane component common to all the cells.

An alternative explanation was that the restricted cross-reactivity may have been due to the presence of multiple antibodies with specificity for individual (monomorphic) determinants on each melanoma cell.

2.2. Absorption Studies: Type I and II Melanoma Antigens

A common approach used by several groups to examine these alternatives was to retest the melanoma antisera after absorption on different melanoma cells. Removal of activity against only the absorbing cell and not other melanoma cells indicated that the antibodies were specific for private determinants on the absorbing cell (Type I antigens). If absorption on the one cell removed activity against other melanoma cells, this was evidence for antigenic determinants common to these cells (Type II antigens). Whether an antigen is truly individual-specific may depend on the number of allogeneic target cells against which the sera are tested. What appears as an individual-restricted antigen on the basis of tests against a limited number of melanoma cells may become a partially cross-reactive determinant if tests are conducted against a larger number of melanoma cells.

A possible example of this is the absorption studies on serum from a patient (J.T.) referred to elsewhere (Hersey *et al.*, 1976a). Absorption of this antiserum on an allogeneic melanoma cell line (MM200) resulted in loss of LDA activity against the absorbing cell but not other allogeneic melanoma cells. This antigen presumably cross-reacted with the autologous tumor cell from J.T. and hence was really a Type II antigen rather than a Type I antigen. The complexity of the antibodies in some human antisera was shown by further studies on this sera in that absorption on other melanoma cells resulted in loss of activity against a number of other melanoma cell lines but not the MM200 cell line. These results were found with several antisera from human patients and were consistent with the presence of antibodies against both "individual"-specific and partially cross-reactive antibodies.

The results of this study also suggested that some melanoma cell lines may express only Type II antigens in that no autologous reactivity was detected against them but partially cross-reactive antigens were detected with allogeneic sera. Results similar to those in these studies were reported by several groups using immune-adherence and mixed-hemadsorption assays (Macher *et al.*, 1975; Shiku *et al.*, 1976, 1977; Seibert *et al.*, 1977). Those of Shiku *et al.* (1976) were particularly important in that only sera with autologous reactivity were selected, which largely avoided the possibility that some of the reactions were due to antibodies against antigens of the major histocompatibility complex. In addition to detection of individual-specific determinants and partially cross-reacting determinants, these authors also defined an antibody that cross-reacted with a number of different cell types including xenogeneic cells (Shiku *et al.*, 1977).

3. Nature of Melanoma Antigens Detected by Human Subjects

3.1. Relationship to Viral Antigens

Results from the studies cited above provided little support for the presence of common cross-reactive determinants as described on virally induced tumors in animals. Whether the antigens are of viral origin has not, however, been adequately examined. Shiku *et al.* (1976) noted no loss of activity from human melanoma antisera (Type I or II) after they were absorbed on simian sarcoma virus (SSV), murine leukemia virus (MuLV), and endogenous cat viruses (RD114).

Antisera against a variety of C-type viruses and viral components were tested in LDA assays against melanoma cells in our laboratory. [Antisera were from Dr. Gallo, National Cancer Institute, and are referred to in Pullen and Hersey (1981).] Two antisera against disrupted SSV were positive against the MM200 cell line, but no reactivity was detected with antisera against baboon endogenous virus, SSV internal protein p27, gibbon ape leukemia virus, Moloney, Rauscher, and Gross MuLV, and the feline leukemia virus. The significance of the reactions with the SSV antisera is still under study. Preincubation of melanoma cells with the SSV antiserum (10-5B) did not inhibit binding of human red blood cells coated with human melanoma antisera to the melanoma target cells, which suggested that they were recognizing different determinants on the target cell. These experiments do not exclude the possibility that the human antisera were recognizing viral determinants different from those recognized by the rabbit antisera or that they were directed to viral-associated antigens such as the feline-oncornavirus-associated cell-membrane antigen (FOCMA) (Stephenson et al., 1977). Evidence for C-type viruses in melanoma is circumstantial (Parsons et al., 1974; Birkmayer et al., 1975), and whether oncogenic DNA viruses are involved appears to have received little attention.

3.2. Oncofetal Antigens

Studies by several groups suggest that some antigens on melanoma cells may be related to antigens expressed during fetal development. In our studies, this applied particularly to the antigens referred to as Type II, i.e., those expressed on groups of melanoma cells. Absorption of some human antisera on spleen and thymus cells from a 12-week- and a 16-week-old fetus removed reactivity completely against some melanoma cells but not against others; e.g., the serum J.T. still reacted with cells from the MM200 and MM170 lines, but lost reactivity against cells from three of the other cell lines (Hersey et al., 1976a). This pattern of reactivity was the same as that observed after absorption of this antiserum on one of the cell lines (MM127) and suggested that the antigens on the three cell lines cross-reacted with the fetal antigens. Similar results were obtained by absorption of several other antisera in this study (G, D, and Q). (Absorption of sera from normal pregnant women that reacted to melanoma cells was found to remove activity against all melanoma cells, suggesting that this activity was directed entirely against fetal antigens on the melanoma.)

On the basis of these results, it was possible that all partially cross-reactive antigens on melanoma cells may have been oncofetal antigens (OFAs) similar to previous descriptions of cross-reactivity of OFAs on tumors of similar histological type in animal models (Thompson and Alexander, 1973; Baldwin and Embleton, 1974).

Some of the OFAs detected by human antisera on melanoma cells cross-reacted with similar antigens on other histological types of carcinomas such as colon carcinoma. One such antigen that cross-reacted strongly with fetal brain tissue was described by Irie et al. (1976, 1979a). Immune responses to this antigen could be demonstrated in melanoma patients (Irie et al., 1979b) and appeared to relate to prognosis in the patient (Irie et al., 1979a; Jones et al., 1981). Antigens cross-reacting with those on fetal liver cells may also be detected on melanoma and other carcinoma cells and are immunogenic in man (Salinas et al., 1978).

Not all cross-reactive antibodies to melanoma cells appear to be removed by absorption on fetal tissues, as illustrated by studies on serum B.N. referred to (Hersey *et al.*, 1976a). Shiku *et al.* (1976) also found that absorption of Type I or II antisera on fetal lung did not remove their activity. It is possible to argue that in both instances, absorption on a wider range of fetal tissues and at different fetal ages may have identified fetal antigens to which these antisera reacted. It appears more likely, however, that some cross-reacting agents are unrelated to those expressed on fetal tissues.

3.3. Melanocyte Differentiation Antigens

A close similarity between antigens on gliomas and melanomas was shown by cross-reactivity of antibodies from patients with gliomas with both glioma and melanoma cells (Pfreundschuh *et al.*, 1978; Coakham *et al.*, 1980; Levy, 1978). Similarly, cross-reactive antigens between these tumor types were detected by several groups using monoclonal antibodies Herlyn *et al.*, 1980; Carrel *et al.*, 1980). The common determinants shared by melanoma and these tissues presumably reflect their common neuroectodermal origin and suggest that the structures identified in these reactions may be involved in differentiation of neuroectodermal tissue.

There is no firm evidence that melanoma patients develop immune responses to these antigens or to melanocyte-restricted differentiation antigens. This has been technically difficult to answer by *in vitro* studies due to the absence of a source of normal melanocytes at different stages of development. Absorption of two melanoma antisera on uveal-tract cells from an adult person and from a 16-week-old fetus did not remove activity against melanoma cell lines (Hersey *et al.*, 1979b). In direct tests in LDA assays against fetal eye melanocytes in culture, low titer activity was found, but absorption of the antisera on these cells did not remove activity against the MM200 melanoma cell line (unpublished data). Immunofluorescent or immunoperoxidase studies on histological sections have so far been unsatisfactory for detection of membrane antigens by these antisera.

Several clinical phenomena such as vitiligo and halo nevi appearing in melanoma patients may be evidence of immune responses against common differentiation antigens on melanocytes and tumor cells. Expression on tumor cells of differentiation antigens that cross-react with those on immature melanocytes may explain the patchy occurrence of vitiligo; e.g., an immune response induced by the tumor may affect only melanocytes in areas of the skin where division of these cells is most pronounced. This could occur in response to sunlight and so explain the appearance of patchy vitiligo in sun-exposed areas. Melanocyte division and differentiation may also occur in response to injury to the skin, and this may explain why many patients develop vitiligo at sites of split skin grafts and their donor sites. Whether other antigens on tumor cells are differentiation antigens is unknown, although it has been suggested that DRw antigens may have this role on melanoma cells (Winchester *et al.*, 1978; Herlyn *et al.*, 1980).

3.4. Relationship to Histocompatibility Antigens

A constant problem in studies on human antisera against allogeneic melanoma cells has been to know whether the reactions were due to contaminating alloantibodies resulting either from pregnancies or from transfusions of blood products. Many workers point to the higher incidence of detectable antibodies to melanoma cells in women and believe this to be due to the immunization against HLA antigens during pregnancy. In several large studies, repeated absorption on pooled platelets was found to remove activity against melanoma cells in a large proportion of the sera tested (Seibert *et al.*, 1977; Carrel and Mach, personal communication).

Different workers have adopted different approaches to exclude reactivity against histocompatibility antigens in studies on melanoma antigens. Shiku *et al.* (1976, 1977) selected sera that reacted only with autologous cells. In practice, however, this approach restricts the number of sera that can be studied, because autologous tumor is frequently unavailable either because of prior removal before referral or because of histopathological requirements. An approach adopted by many groups (Irie *et al.*, 1976), and one that we favor, is to absorb sera whenever possible against either phytohemagglutinin (PHA)- or Epstein–Barr virus (EBV)-transformed lymphocytes from the same allogeneic donor as the tumor cells to which the human antisera react. Absorption on pooled platelets is an alternative approach when EBV- or PHA-transformed cells from the tumor-cell donor are not available. This approach is theoretically less satisfactory because it assumes that reactions against melanoma cells are not due to expression of "alien" HLA antigens. The latter phenomena have been described in several experimental tumors (Invernizzi *et al.*, 1977; Garrido *et al.*, 1976), and these antigens may be the target for control of tumor growth by the immune system. The mechanism underlying appearance of these foreign HLA antigens is unknown, but may be due to alteration of the histocompatibility antigens by viral products (Schmidt *et al.*, 1980).

We have examined the possibility that partially cross-reactive Type II melanoma antigens are "alien" HLA antigens by testing human melanoma antisera from nontransfused patients against a panel of 15 PHA-transformed lymphocytes bearing a range of the most common HLA antigens. The antisera were absorbed prior to testing on two EBV-transformed cell lines that were autologous to melanoma cells to which the antisera reacted. No reactions were detected against this panel, which argued against aberrant or foreign HLA antigens as a frequent tumor-associated determinant on melanoma cells. These results were consistent with those of Curry *et al.* (1979), who showed that somatic hybrids deficient in human chromosome 6 (which coded for HLA antigens) still expressed a melanoma-tumor-associated antigen detected by rabbit antisera. McCabe *et al.* (1978) also showed that melanoma antigens detected by a rabbit antibody and by delayed-hypersensitivity skin testing of melanoma patients were separable from HLA antigen by an ultracentrifugation technique.

4. Tumor-Related Immune Responses to Melanoma Antigens

4.1. Changes in Leukocyte-Dependent Antibody Levels in Relation to Tumor Growth

Although the results cited above indicate that the nature of antigens recognized by human patients is poorly understood, their detection by a number of different laboratories

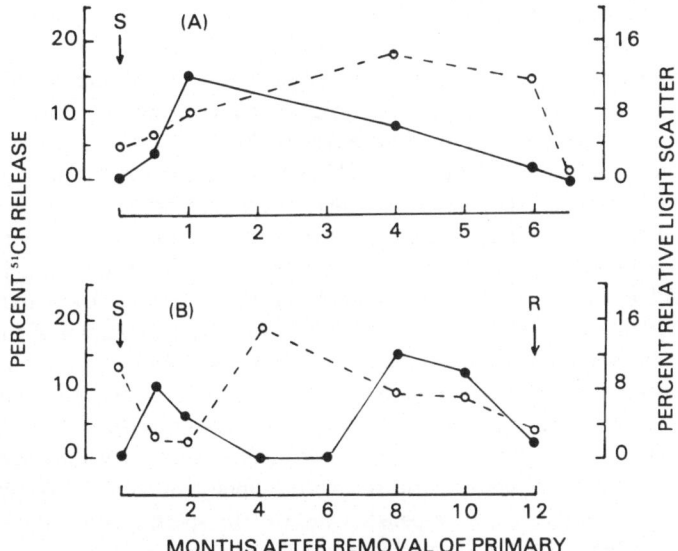

FIGURE 1. Patterns of LDA activity. (A) Appearance of LDA activity (●——●) in sera from a 55-year-old male after removal of a primary melanoma on the back followed by gradual disappearance of this activity. (O---O) Immune-complex levels detected in the nephelometer by monoclonal rheumatoid factor to IgG. $\left(\begin{smallmatrix} S \\ \downarrow \end{smallmatrix}\right)$ Surgical removal of melanoma. (B) Appearance of LDA activity after removal of primary melanoma on the scalp of a 35-year-old male. At 8 months after removal of the primary, LDA activity was again noticed in serum, and recurrent melanoma in cervical lymph nodes was detected 12 months later. Target cells were from allogeneic melanoma cell line MM200 (3×10^3). Effector/target-cell ratio 100 : 1. Serum dilutions shown: 1 : 10. Immune-complex levels were elevated prior to recurrence from melanoma and were undetectable at time of detection of recurrence $\left(\begin{smallmatrix} R \\ \downarrow \end{smallmatrix}\right)$.

using various assay systems appears to reaffirm their existence. Further evidence for tumor-related immune responses in melanoma patients was obtained in sequential studies of LDA and natural killer (NK)-cell activity in relation to surgical removal of localized melanoma. In initial studies on 33 patients with clinical Stage I or II melanoma, it was found that approximately one third of the patients had low or undetectable levels of LDA in their sera against the allogeneic melanoma cell line (MM200), which increased to maximal levels 1–4 weeks after surgical removal of the melanoma. These levels gradually receded over the next few months to undetectable levels (Hersey *et al.*, 1978b). This was referred to as a Pattern A response and is illustrated in Fig. 1A.

A proportion of these patients subsequently showed a rise in LDA activity prior to development of recurrences from melanoma, which disappeared by the time the recurrence was detected clinically. Figure 1B illustrates this sequence of changes in a 35-year-old male who developed metastases to regional lymph nodes 12 months after removal of a primary melanoma of the scalp. Immune-complex levels detected by a monoclonal rheumatoid factor in nephelometric assays (Whitsed *et al.*, 1979) were also noted to rise and then fall prior to detection of metastases, possibly due to the inability of this and the $[^{125}I]$-C1q precipitation assay to detect immune complexes in antigen excess. This transient LDA response (Pattern A) contrasted with patients who had either no detectable LDA or marked inhibitory activity against the NK activity of the effector cells in the assays (Pattern B) and with patients who had high constant titers of LDA activity that did not change in relation to tumor growth (Pattern C). The latter, with one exception, were multiparous women.

These patterns of antibody response have now been confirmed in studies on over 300 patients. Approximately 35% of the patients with Stage I or II melanoma had a Pattern A response, 10% had Pattern C, and the remainder had no detectable LDA in their unfractionated sera (Pattern B). Gel-filtration or membrane chromatography of the unreactive sera under acidic conditions (to dissociate immune complexes) revealed that immunoglobulin G (IgG)-containing fractions of the sera had detectable LDA activity in approximately 45% of the unreactive sera (approximately 20% of the sera overall).

The Pattern A responses were of particular interest, since they were seen equally in both men and women and were clearly related to tumor growth. Several questions were raised concerning this pattern of response. One was the specificity of the antibody. The relationship to tumor growth and occurrence in nontransfused males was evidence that the antibody was not directed to histocompatibility antigens on the MM200 target cells. This was further confirmed by absorption of EBV-transformed cells from donors of tumor cells to which the antisera reacted. Approximately 30% of these sera reacted with nonmelanoma carcinoma lines. Absorption of the latter sera on fetal brain or a mixture of fetal thymus and spleen cells resulted in loss of activity against both melanoma and nonmelanoma cells from two thirds of the sera. The remaining sera reacted against melanoma cells only. Approximately half the sera not cross-reacting with nonmelanoma carcinoma lost activity against melanoma cells after absorption of fetal brain, suggesting that in at least 50% the antibodies were directed to oncofetal antigens. The specificity of the sera the activity of which was not removed by absorption on fetal brain is unknown. Reactivity was not detected against four glioma lines or cultured fetal uveal-tract cells. Tests on several of these antibodies against an extended panel of nine melanoma cells showed a partially cross-reactive pattern observed with many of the high-titer melanoma sera. Cross-absorption studies with different melanoma cells on these antisera have not yet been carried out.

A number of other authors have described tumor-related antibody responses in melanoma patients. Lewis *et al.* (1969) and Lewis (1972) found that antibody was detected only in patients with localized diseases and disappeared on dissemination of the tumor. Similar results were reported by several other authors (Morton *et al.*, 1971a,b; Bodurtha *et al.*, 1975). Irie *et al.* (1979a) described three patterns of antibody response to the OFA-1 antigen in melanoma patients. A high constant pattern was associated with a good prognosis, whereas a rise in titer or low antibody levels were associated with a higher incidence of recurrence.

Tumor-associated immune responses in melanoma patients were not confined to changes in LDA activity. In a study of 154 patients with localized melanoma and 105 control subjects, it was found that NK activity in patients with Stage I melanoma frequently showed a transient increase after removal of the tumor. The increase in activity was relatively specific for melanoma cells in some patients, whereas in others it was detected against a variety of target cells. Patients with Stage II melanoma rarely showed an increase in NK activity after removal of tumor, and instead their NK activity appeared to decrease to low levels. Further details of the study are described in Hersey *et al.* (1980a).

4.2. Variation in Melanoma Leukocyte-Dependent Antibody Levels Due to Neutralization by Factors in Sera

A second question raised by the appearance of Pattern A Type II antibody responses in melanoma patients was why antibody was often undetectable or at low levels prior to surgical removal of melanoma. To answer this question, IgG was separated from sera (taken prior to surgical removal of melanoma) by gel-filtration or membrane chromatography under acidic conditions to dissociate immune complexes. The IgG fractions were found in all instances to have LDA activity to melanoma cells, which suggested that antibody was neutralized by factors in sera (Hersey *et al.*, 1978b; Murray *et al.*, 1977). These were subsequently shown to be low-molecular-weight glycoproteins that bound to concanavalin A (Con A) and were present in gel-filtration fractions of molecular weight less than 60,000 (60K). Inhibition was specific for melanoma LDA and was not detected against LDA to other cell-surface antigens (Murray *et al.*, 1978). The low molecular weight of the factors distinguished them from antiglobulins and antiidiotypes to melanoma antibodies described by Lewis *et al.* (1971, 1976) and the antiidiotype to melanoma antibody described in normal sera by Morgan *et al.* (1979). Low-molecular weight glycoproteins similar to those detected in sera were also identified in urea–acetate extracts of melanoma-cell membranes, which suggested that the serum factors were melanoma antigens shed from the cell surface (Hersey *et al.*, 1979b).

Surgical removal of melanoma was not the only procedure that resulted in "unblocking" of melanoma LDA *in vivo* in that it was shown that removal of these factors *in vivo* by plasmapheresis also resulted in the appearance of LDA in these patients (Hersey *et al.*, 1976b, 1978c; Hersey and Isbister, 1979).

4.3. Application of Melanoma Leukocyte-Dependent-Antibody-Inhibition Assays to Monitor Tumor Growth

Preliminary studies revealed that the levels of these melanoma LDA-inhibitory factors in the sera of melanoma patients appeared to correlate with tumor growth. Surgical removal of melanoma resulted in disappearance of the LDA-inhibitory activity from sera, whereas clinically detected recurrences from melanoma were preceded by the appearance of these factors in sera (Hersey *et al.*, 1978c).

These results were sufficiently encouraging to conduct a prospective study on the value of melanoma LDA-inhibition assays as markers of tumor growth in melanoma patients (Hersey *et al.*, 1980b). A total of 112 patients with melanoma and 41 patients with non-melanomatous carcinoma were included in the study. Low-molecular-weight fractions were obtained by gel-filtration of membrane chromatography of acidified sera and tested for their ability to inhibit LDA in ^{51}Cr-release cytotoxic assays. A panel of LDA was used consisting of three melanoma-"specific" antisera from melanoma patients and three nonmelanomatous antisera against carcinoembryonic antigen (CEA), β_2-microglobulin, and fetal antigens. Several melanoma antisera were used in the panel, since we have previously shown that the serum fractions from different patients often inhibited different antisera (Hersey et al., 1979a; Hersey and Isbister, 1979). The results showed that in patients with melanoma, approximately 70% had melanoma LDA-inhibitory activity detected in the low-molecular-weight fractions of their sera when these were tested against the panel of melanoma LDA. The specificity of the inhibitory activity for melanoma LDA was shown by failure of the serum fractions to inhibit nonmelanomatous LDA and by absence of inhibitory activity in equivalent serum fractions from nonmelanomatous carcinoma patients for melanoma LDA.

The levels of melanoma LDA-inhibitory activity in the serum fractions correlated with tumor growth as shown by clearance of the inhibitory activity after surgical removal of melanoma and reappearance in the serum of patients who subsequently developed recurrent melanoma. One example of these changes in LDA-inhibitory activity in the one patient is shown in Fig. 2. Inhibitory activity against melanoma LDA was not detected in 30% of patients known to have melanoma, which indicated that the assays could not be used to reliably exclude melanoma. However, the close correlation with tumor growth and the low number of false-positive results suggested that in the 70% of patients who released these factors, the assays would be of value to monitor the effectiveness of therapy and to detect recurrence of melanoma. Future studies in this area are directed to development of more portable assays and standardized sources of antisera for detection of these antigens in sera.

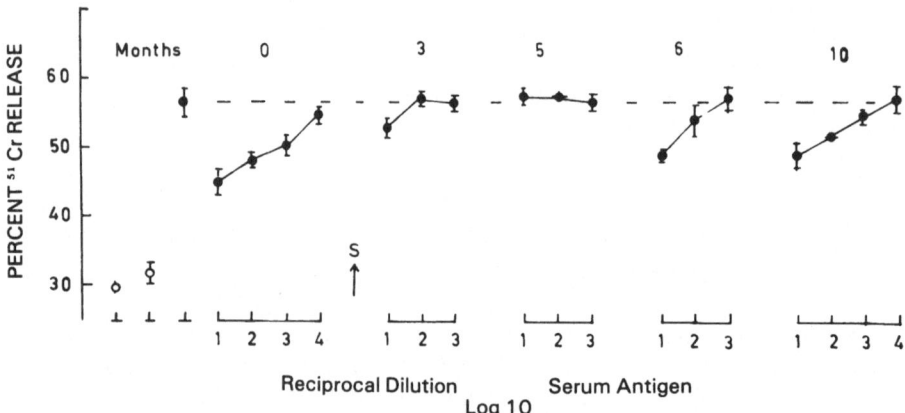

FIGURE 2. Reappearance of melanoma LDA-inhibitory activity in low-molecular-weight fractions of sera from a 43-year-old woman 6 months after removal of melanoma involving inguinal lymph nodes. Before surgery, the LDA-inhibition titer was 10^{-3}. This was cleared completely by 3–5 months after surgery $\left(\begin{smallmatrix} S \\ \uparrow \end{smallmatrix} \right)$. Cerebral metastasis was detected at 12 months. Reproduced from Hersey et al. (1980b) with the kind permission of the editors of Cancer Immunology and Immunotherapy.

5. Biochemical Nature of Melanoma Antigens

5.1. Antigens Defined in Melanoma-Cell-Membrane Extracts by Leukocyte-Dependent-Antibody-Inhibition Assays

Analysis of the biochemical structure of melanoma antigens is a prerequisite for answers to a number of questions raised by the studies referred to above on the specificity and cross-reactivity of melanoma antigens; e.g., isolation of these structures can help define whether individual antigenic determinants and the cross-reactive determinants are on the same molecules or different molecules in the membranes. Studies of antigens on breast-carcinoma cells provide an example of how these questions can be resolved by such studies. A common (20K) determinant on mammary carcinoma cells referred to as mammary-tumor-specific glycoprotein (MTGP) (Leung and Edgington, 1980) and individual specific determinants recognized by human antisera were both shown to be present on a 53K molecule isolated by monoclonal antibodies (Edgington and Leung, 1980).

Comparable information about the biochemical nature of melanoma antigens is as yet incomplete. Using inhibition of melanoma LDA assays, antigens from lactoperoxidase ^{125}I-labeled urea–acetate extracts of melanoma-cell membranes were found to bind Con A affinity columns and were isolated in small (15K) fractions on Biogel P100 columns. Examination of the 15K fractions by sodium dodecyl sulfate–polyacrylamide gel electrophoresis (SDS-PAGE) revealed fractions at 12K, 15K, 28K, and 60K (Hersey et al., 1979b). Passage of the 15K fraction from gel filtration over the IgG fraction of a melanoma antiserum (bound to Sepharose 4B) resulted in partial removal of the 15K and to a lesser extent the 28K fractions when rerun on SDS-PAGE. These results were similar to previous studies that suggested that the antigens detected by human LDA in the serum of melanoma patients were 15K glycoproteins that bound to Con A (Murray et al., 1978). Since the 15K molecule appeared too small to be a complete membrane component, it is possible that this was the terminal portion of a larger integral membrane component as described above for MTGP.

5.2. Comparative Studies on Melanoma Antigens

Estimates of the molecular weight of melanoma antigens by other workers have generally been much higher than 15K. Lewis and colleagues identified two melanoma-associated antigens in water-soluble extracts of plasma membranes by affinity chromatography on autologous antibody bound to Sepharose 4B. One fraction of 125K appeared to bind to the individual specific antibody, whereas an 80K fraction appeared to cross-react with those on other melanoma cells (Preddie et al., 1978a,b). Du Bois and Rossen (1980) used antisera from melanoma patients to identify antigens of 125K and 140 K in 3 M KCl extracts of a melanoma cell line, using double-antibody precipitation techniques. Antigens shed into the culture supernatants of melanoma-cell cultures were also found to be in the size range 80–150K by gel-filtration studies. An antiserum from a patient immunized with autologous melanoma cells that cross-reacted with a number of melanoma cells was used to define the antigens (Leong *et al.*, 1978).

Relatively large membrane components were identified in melanoma-cell membranes by other workers using quite different techniques. Lloyd *et al.* (1979) found that two major glycoproteins of 110K and 90K could be identified using methods that labeled the carbohydrate component of the glycoproteins. Mitchell *et al.* (1981) isolated an antigen recognized by a mouse monoclonal antibody of approximately 250K, but this consisted of subunits of 116K, 95K, 29K, and 26K. The 95K molecule was linked to the 116K molecule by noncovalent bonds. There was no information from the latter two studies as to whether these molecules were immunogenic in man.

Several studies have used cell-mediated reactions to define melanoma-tumor-associated antigens. Jehn *et al.* (1970) isolated a protein with β-electrophoretic mobility and a molecular weight probably less than 40K that stimulated cell division of autologous and allogeneic lymphocytes from melanoma patients. Hollinshead (1975) defined relatively large glycolipoproteins in ultrasonic extracts of melanoma cells that appeared specific for melanoma in delayed-hypersensitivity skin testing of human patients. Rather similar results were obtained by Roth *et al.* (1976) in delayed-hypersensitivity skin tests of 3 M KCl extracts of melanoma cells.

5.3. Association of β_2-Microglobulin with Melanoma Antigens

Several groups have shown that antigens detected in leukocyte-adherence inhibition (LAI) assays appeared to be associated with β_2-microglobulin in the cell membrane, but not with tumor antigen spontaneously shed from the tumor cell surface. Thomson *et al.* (1978) used anti-β_2-microglobulin affinity columns to purify antigen detected in papain extracts of melanoma cells by LAI tests. The antigen was detected in 70–190K fractions by gel filtration, and these were resolved by SDS-PAGE into subunits of approximately 50K, 40K, 25K, and 12K. Subsequent studies by Malley *et al.* (1979) indicated that the β_2-microglobulin was not associated with HLA antigens in the fractions containing melanoma antigens.

6. Biological Significance of Melanoma Antigens

6.1. Induction of Immune Responses against Tumor Growth

Apart from the use of melanoma antigens as markers of tumor growth, the main significance attributed to them has been their effectiveness as immunogens in inducing immune responses controlling tumor growth. This is a poorly understood area and probably involves a number of factors such as the number of "foreign" determinants available for recognition by lymphoid cells, the stability of the structures in the membrane, and their relationship to other structures in the membrane such as the DRw or HLA antigens (Hersey, 1977). The possible importance of the fluidity of antigens in the cell membrane and their rate of shedding from the tumor-cell surface was suggested by studies on murine lymphomata that showed that tumor cells with high metastatic potential released histocompatibility antigens into the supernatant at a faster rate than the nonmetastatic tumor cells (Davey *et al.*, 1976).

Evidence for the effectiveness of immune responses against particular types of antigens in control of tumor growth is limited. Immune responses against fetal antigens on some experimental chemical-carcinogen-induced tumors appeared ineffective in control of tumor growth, whereas those against individual-specific antigens on the tumors produced effective resistance to tumor growth (Baldwin *et al.*, 1974). In other models, immunization against fetal antigens produced resistance against tumor growth (Coggin and Anderson, 1974). Several studies suggest that immunization against fetal antigens in melanoma cells may have some role in control of melanoma growth. Irie *et al.* (1979a) and Jones *et al.* (1981) reported that melanoma patients with antibodies to OFA-1 (either naturally occurring or induced by immunization) had longer 5-year survivals than patients without such antibodies.

Studies to assess whether antibodies to various melanoma antigens in patients may have an influence on tumor growth are being evaluated in long-term prospective studies on over 300 patients. Preliminary analysis suggests that patients with high-titer melanoma LDA may have a significantly longer survival than patients with no LDA or a transient LDA response. Approximately one third of these sera have antibodies to OFA-1. The nature of the antigens detected by the antibodies in the other high-titer sera is as yet poorly defined, but presumably, like OF-1, may influence tumor growth by induction of immune responses in the tumor-bearing host.

In previous studies, an attempt was made to study the significance of immunization against fetal antigens during pregnancy in control of melanoma growth by epidemiological studies on survival from melanoma in previously pregnant women compared to women with no recorded pregnancies (Hersey *et al.*, 1977). A survey on a sample of 443 women suggested that survivals in the former group were longer than those in the latter, which supported the view that immunization against fetal antigens during pregnancy may protect against tumor growth. Subsequent analysis of a larger group of women indicated that the significance of the difference between the two groups was marginal (Shaw *et al.*, 1978). Similar surveys at another center failed to show significant differences in the two groups of women (Elwood and Coldman, 1978). These results suggest that the first sample of patients may not have been representative of the population at large or that changes in the treatment of patients may have obscured the effect of prior pregnancy on women with melanoma.

Evidence that certain other antigens on melanoma cells identified by a human antiserum (CHI) may have importance as "immunogens" in control of tumor growth is discussed in Section 6.3.

6.2. Antigens Recognized by Natural Killer Cells

Studies in animal tumor models (Keissling and Haller, 1978) and in melanoma patients (Hersey *et al.*, 1978a) suggest that NK activity may be an important mechanism in the control of tumor growth. The nature of the cell-membrane structures recognized by NK cells is poorly understood and may include oncofetal-related antigens on the cell surface (Hersey, 1979). Inhibition of binding of NK cells to their target cells was used to study the structures on tumor cells recognized by NK cells. These were shown to be glycoproteins of 140K, 160K, 190K, and 240K. The 140K molecules appeared to be common to a number of different target cells, whereas the 240K molecules had a more restricted expression (Roder et al., 1979). In other studies, NK-sensitive melanoma cells were found to release factors into the supernatants of cultured cells that selectively inhibited NK activity in ^{51}Cr-release cytotoxic assays. These factors appeared to be glycoproteins of 120–140K that bound to Con A or wheat germ lectin affinity columns (Zaunders et al., 1981). A logical extension of these studies will be the development of serological reagents against these structures that may then be used to evaluate the prognostic significance of their expression on tumor cells in relation to the clinical course of tumor growth.

6.3. Functional Importance of Melanoma Antigens; Assessment of Antigenic Phenotype of Melanoma Cells; Relationship to Clinical Behavior of Tumor Growth

The attention given to melanoma antigens over the past decade has focused largely on such factors as their specificity and cross-reactivity and the nature of the immune response induced against them. This emphasis has tended to overlook the fact that many of the structures recognized as antigens are most probably functional components of the cell membrane that may have important functions in the biology of the tumor cell. In the case of tumor antigens, these structures may be important determinants of such characteristics as invasiveness, metastatic potential, and spread to particular sites in the body. The function of certain of these structures could conceivably have more importance in determining the behavior of the tumor cell than the immune response directed against them. [An example of the function of certain tumor-associated antigens may be the report suggesting that human thymus leukemia-associated antigen (HThy-L) is an isoenzyme of adenosine deaminase (Chechik et al., 1980).]

To obtain information about the possible functional importance of melanoma antigens (as well as their immunogenicity), a program was initiated to "type" the antigens on melanoma cells from tumors removed at surgery. The presence or absence of certain antigens or combinations of antigens was then correlated with various clinical aspects of tumor growth. These included (1) duration to first recurrence, (2) duration to dissemination of tumor, (3) site of metastases, (4) duration to death, and (5) immune responses to the antigens in the patient.

The panel of antisera used to assess the antigen profile on melanoma cells (melanoma-cell-typing panel) in the intial studies included three antisera from melanoma patients that detected different cross-reacting antigens on allogeneic melanoma cells and antisera to β_2-microglobulin and CEA. [The latter antigen was shown to be present on a high proportion of melanoma cells (Morgan et al., 1977), although recent studies by Dent et al. (1980) suggest that the CEA on melanoma cells may not be "true" CEA; absorption of CEA

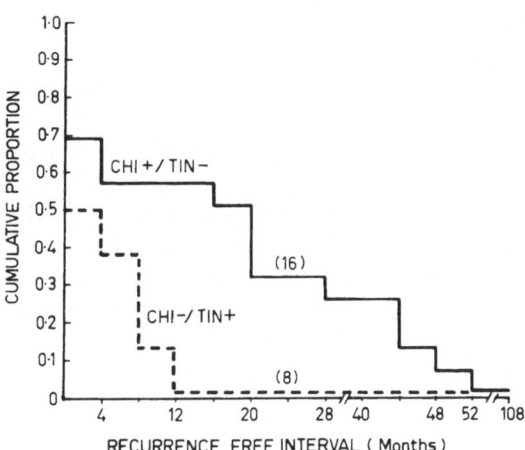

Figure 3. Relationship between the recurrence-free period after removal of primary melanoma and the expression of antigens detected by antisera CHI and TIN. Patients with tumors expressing antigens detected by CHI but not TIN had a significantly longer recurrence-free period than patients with tumors expressing antigens detected by TIN but not CHI. By log rank analysis, $\chi^2 = 4.11$ $(0.05 > p > 0.025)$. Reproduced from Werkmeister *et al.* (1980) with the kind permission of the editors of *Cancer Immunology and Immunotherapy*.

antisera on melanoma cells did not remove activity against colon carcinoma cells.] Antisera to DRw antigens were not included in the initial melanoma-cell-typing panel.

An interim analysis of the results of this program on tumors from 33 patients was of interest in that one of the human antisera (CHI) appeared to identify an antigen associated with a good prognosis in the patient (Werkmeister *et al.*, 1980). Patients with tumors expressing this particular antigen (CHI+ cells) had a longer recurrence-free interval after removal of the primary tumor than patients with tumors not expressing this antigen (CHI⁻ cells). There was a tendency for two antigens (CHI and TIN) to be reciprocally expressed on the tumor cells and for the expression of antigen TIN to be associated with a shorter recurrence-free period. The expression of CEA and β_2-microglobulin was not significantly associated with the recurrence-free period, but may become so (particularly for expression of β_2-microglobulin) in studies on a larger group of patients. Figure 3 illustrates the difference in the recurrence-free interval in patients with CHI+, TIN⁻ tumors compared to that in patients with CHI⁻, TIN+ tumors.

The basis for the association between expression of the antigen CHI on melanoma cells and the longer recurrence-free interval in the patients is unknown. We have examined the sera of these patients for LDA activity and their lymphoid cells for NK-cell activity against allogeneic melanoma target cells at several intervals in relation to surgical removal of the tumor. No significant difference in these assays was detected between patients having CHI+ and CHI⁻ tumors (such differences may be detected in studies on a larger number of patients). Similar comments also applied to analysis of the relationship between expression of these antigens and other tumor-related prognostic factors such as tumor thickness (Breslow, 1975). Another possibility is that the antigen detected by CHI antisera was a differentiation antigen expressed only on more "mature" melanocytes. The growth rate and invasiveness of melanoma cells arising at that stage of differentiation may consequently have been less than that of melanomas arising from cells at a less differentiated stage and that perhaps expressed the antigen TIN.

These studies are being continued with an expanded panel of antisera to obtain a more complete antigenic phenotype of melanoma cells. Particular interest has been given to the relationship between expression of DRw antigens on melanoma cells (Winchester *et al.*, 1978; Wilson *et al.*, 1979) and their clinical behavior. Previous studies have shown that both DRw and HLA antigens are important determinants of the function of lymphoid cells (Munro and Bright, 1976; Bergholtz and Thorsby, 1978), and it is conceivable that they may play a role in recognition of tumor antigens on melanoma cells by lymphoid cells. Because of the analogy with the expression of DRw antigens on precursor but not mature cells of the erythroid and myeloid series, Winchester *et al.* (1978) suggested that they may be involved in differentiation of melanocytes. Certain of the OFAs such as OFA-1, may also be involved in differentiation of melanocytes and hence be important determinants of certain characterisitcs of melanoma behavior such as the frequent occurrence of cerebral or subcutaneous metastases.

7. Summary Table

A synopsis os the present information about melanoma antigens recognized by antibody responses of patients with melanoma is given in Table I. Although Type I and II antigens are now recognized, the table illustrates that there is considerable uncertainty in most of the other areas. The biochemical studies indicate that there may be more uniformity of results than generally expected. Antigens defined by cell-mediated reactions are not included.

8. Conclusions

One of our aims in the preceding sections was to draw attention to the many areas of agreement in studies on melanoma antigens. This appeared necessary in that a surprising degree of skepticism is expressed in some quarters as to whether patients recognize tumor-associated antigens on melanoma cells and related aspects. Such views appear hard to sustain in view of the published work referred to over the past decade. Perhaps most important in this context are those studies showing that immune responses in many melanoma patients were related to growth of the tumor. This was evidenced by the appearance of (antibody) responses in patients with recurrent disease and disappearance of the response after removal of the tumor. These changes were observed in at least one third of cases in sequential studies on large numbers of patients with localized melanoma.

With respect to the nature of the antigens detected in these responses and their specificity for melanoma, there is perhaps more justifiable room for doubt. Even on these points, however, there is more consensus than many would expect; e.g., by various assay methods, several groups confirmed that some melanoma antigens appeared restricted in their expression to individual specific tumors as suggested initially by Lewis and his colleagues. Similiarly, there seems little doubt that some melanoma antigens show wider cross-reactivity among different melanoma cells. Totally cross-reactive antigens, however, do not appear to be recognized by human antisera.

TABLE I

Classification and Summary of Melanoma Antigens Recognized by Human Antisera

Serological type	Biological nature	Biochemistry (mol.wt.)	Biological significance	
			Protective tumor immune responses	Determinant of tumor-cell behavior
Type I (individual-specific)	Unknown	125K[a]	Unknown	Unknown

Type II (partially cross-reactive)	1. Oncofetal
	    OFA-1
	    Liver-associated
	    Other
		80K[a]
		125K[b], 140K[b],
		80–150K[d]
				Favorable prognosis of CHI[+] tumors[c] (otherwise unknown)

	2. Differentiation
	    Neuroectodermal
	    Epithelial
	3. Other
	    Alien HLA?
	    Viral?
		110K[e], 90K[e]
		250K[f]
		15[g]		

[a]–[h]References: [a]Preddie et al. (1978a,b); [b]Du Bois and Rossen (1980); [c]Werkmeister et al. (1980); [d]Leong et al. (1978); [e]Lloyd et al. (1979); [f]Mitchell et al. (1980); [g]Hersey et al. (1979b); [h]Jones et al., 1981.

It is also agreed that certain of the partially cross-reactive antigens are similar to antigens expressed on various fetal tissues. Some of the latter are expressed on a variety of carcinomas, whereas others may be restricted to melanoma, fetal eye tissue, and fetal brain. Whether these antigens are oncofetal or differentiation antigens may be difficult to decide. Not all the partially cross-reactive antigens appear related to fetal antigens in that the reactivity of a number of sera against partially cross-reactive antigens was not removed by absorption on fetal tissue.

The absence of controversy concerning the nature of the latter antigens is more a reflection of inadequate study of their nature than concordance of results. A frequently expressed opinion is that they are related to differentiation antigens of melanocytes and that their heterogeneity is a reflection of melanoma development at different stages of differentiation. This hypothesis is attractive in explaining the frequent occurrence of vitiligo in melanoma patients at sites where melanocyte proliferation may occur. More substantial support has come from the frequent reactions of monoclonal antibodies produced against melanoma antigens with other tumors of neuroectodermal origin. Similar comments apply to two other candidates for a role as tumor-associated melanoma antigens, namely, HLA antigens and oncogenic viral antigens. Several studies appear to exclude a role for "alien" HLA antigens as tumor antigens in melanoma, whereas studies on viral antigens on melanoma cells are insufficient to draw conclusions.

Given the variety of techniques that have been used in biochemical studies on melanoma antigens, it is surprising that there is any concordance of results in this area. In several studies where human antisera were used to define the antigens, they were frequently shown to be glycoprotein molecules in the 110–125K range and in the 80–90K range. Similar results were reported using carbohydrate labeling methods and monoclonal-antibody techniques. The latter techniques show promise of helping to resolve many questions in these areas. such as whether the low-molecular-weight antigens defined in our studies are cleavage products of the larger molecules described by others.

We conclude from the findings discussed above that worthwhile progress has been made in studies on melanoma antigens detected by human subjects and that these form a substantial basis for further progress in these areas. The application of these findings in practical management of patients such as monitoring of tumor growth or in immunotherapy has received limited attention. Initial studies, however, show promise that worthwhile benefits may be expected in both areas. The results of prospective studies on over 100 melanoma patients using LDA-inhibition assays to detect melanoma antigens in sera suggest that detection of these antigens may be useful to assess effectiveness of therapy and to detect recurrence from melanoma. Similarly, the reports of Irie and colleagues suggest that immunization with certain antigens expressed on melanoma cells (OFA-1) may provide effective resistance against tumor growth in melanoma patients.

The studies cited above could be considered as belonging to conventional tumor immunology. A new area of study that could become increasingly important over the next decade is that relating certain antigens to functional aspects of the tumor. Our report of an association between the expression of an antigen on melanoma cells and the recurrence-free interval in the patient may be one example of detection of a functionally important antigen on melanoma cells. Precedents for the association of certain antigens with biological behavior of tumor cells have been established in several animal tumor models. One such model was described by Shearman and Longenecker (1980a,b), who selected variants of a Marek's disease lymphoma that metastasized selectively to the liver. Cell-surface structures were identified by monoclonal antibodies that were specific for the latter variants. These antibodies were shown to inhibit metastasis of the tumor cells to the liver. Schirrmacher and Bosslet (1980a,b) described several variants of a chemically induced DBA/2 mouse lymphoma that had different metastasizing potential that was associated with different tumor-associated antigens on their surface. Variants with no detectable tumor antigens metastasized to the spleen.

The mechanisms underlying these phenomena are unknown. Possibilities would include matching of recognition structures on the tumor cell and the normal host tissues at the site of metastasis; e.g., similar structures (differentiation antigens?) on tumor cells and neural cells may facilitate cerebral metastases. Alternatively, the tumor cell may recognize structures on endothelial cells of blood vessels in certain sites similar to that postulated to occur between T lymphocytes and vessels of the "T-dependent" lymph-node areas (Ritter and Morris, 1980).

Melanoma appears to be an ideal human tumor model to identify similar structures in the cell membrane that influence the clinical behavior of the tumor; e.g., melanoma in human subjects shows wide variability in metastatic potential. Metastases also occur frequently in certain regions such as the brain and subcutaneous tissue that are infrequent sites of metastasis for other common tumors. The selective spread of ocular melanoma to the liver is a further example of clinical phenomena peculiar to this tumor. We suggest that in the present decade, a major challenge will be the identification of cell-membrane components that confer metastatic potential on melanoma cells and that determine the sites to which they spread. Continued study of melanoma antigens recognized by the immune responses of human patients may facilitate these studies as well as identify the major antigens that are associated with protective immune responses by the host against tumor growth. This information may assist pathologists to assess the prognosis of melanoma in individual patients more accurately and allow clinicians to carry out immunotherapy programs with specific objectives in each patient.

ACKNOWLEDGMENTS. The authors' investigations referred to herein were supported by grants from the National Health and Medical Research Council, the New South Wales State Cancer Council, and the Clive and Vera Ramaciotti Foundation, and by NCI Contract NOI-CB-74120. We wish to thank Mrs. Murray, Mrs. Edwards, Miss Ruell, and Dr. Werkmeister for their contribution to these studies. We wish to thank Professor Milton for permission to study the patients under his care.

References

Baldwin, R. W., and Embleton, M. J., 1974, Neoantigens on spontaneous and carcinogen induced rat tumours defined *in vitro* lymphocytotoxicity assays, *Int. J. Cancer* **13**:433.

Baldwin, R. W., Glaves, D., and Vose, B. M., 1974, Immunogenecity of embryonic antigens associated with chemically induced rat tumours, *Int. J. Cancer* **13**:135.

Bergholtz, B. O., and Thorsby, E., 1978, HLA-D restriction of the macrophage-dependent response of immune human T lymphocytes to PPD *in vitro:* Inhibition by anti HLA-DR antisera, *Scand. J. Immunol.* **8**:63.

Birkmayer, G. D., Hammer, C., Eberhard, H. D., and Brendel, W., 1975, A tumour specific antigen associated witb reverse transcriptase in human melanoma, *Behring Inst. Mitt.* **56**:107.

Bodurtha, A. J., Chee, D. O., Lauciuse, J. F., Mastrageco, M. J., and Prehn, R. T., 1975, Clinical and immunological significance of human melanoma cytotoxic antibody, *Cancer Res.* **35**:189.

Breslow, A., 1975, Tumor thickness, level of invasion and node dissection in stage I cutaneous melanoma, *Ann. Surg.* **182**:572.

Carrel, S., Accolla, R. S., Carmagnola, A. L., and Mach, J. P., 1980, Common human melanoma-associated antigen(s) detected by monoclonal antibodies, *Cancer Res.* **40**:2523.

Chechik, B. E., Schrader, W. P. and Daddona, P. E., 1980, Identification of human thymus-leukaemia-associated antigen as a low-molecular weight form of adenosine deaminase, *J. Natl. Cancer Inst.* **64**:1061.

Coakham, H. B., Kornblith, P. C., Quindlen, E. A., Pollack, L. A., Wood, W. C., and Hartnett, C. C., 1980, Autologous humoral response to human gliomas and analysis of certain cell surface antigens: *In vitro* study with use of microcytotoxicity and immune adherence assays, *J. Natl. Cancer Inst.* **64**:223.

Coggin, J. H., Jr., and Anderson, N. G., 1974, Cancer differentiation and embryonic antigens: Some central problems, *Adv. Cancer Res.* **19**:106.

Curry, R. A., Quaranta, V., Pellegrino, M. A., and Ferrone, S., 1979, Serologically detectable human melanoma-associated antigens are not genetically linked to HLA-A & B antigens, *J. Immunol.* **122**:2630.

Davey, G. C., Currie, G. A., and Alexander, P., 1976, Spontaneous shedding and antibody induced modulation of histocompatibility antigens on murine lymphomata: Correlation with metastatic capacity, *Br. J. Cancer* **33**:9.

Dent, P. B., Carrel, S., and Mach, J. P., 1980, Detection of new cross-reacting carcinoembryonic antigen(s) on cultured tumor cells by mixed hemadsorption assay, *J. Natl. Cancer Inst.* **64**:309.

Du Bois, D. B., and Rossen, R. D., 1980, A melanoma specific antigen identified by immunoprecipitation with human sera. Proceedings of the 4th International Conference of Immunology, Abstract 10.1.16.

Edgington, T. S., and Leung, J., 1980, A candidate human breast tumor-specific membrane glycoprotein antigen, Proceedings of the 4th International Congress of Immunology, Abstract 10.1.17.

Elwood, J. M., and Coldman, A. J., 1978, Previous pregnancy and melanoma prognosis, *Lancet* **2**:1000.

Fidler, I. J., 1973, Selection of successive tumor lines for metastasis, *Nature (London) New Biol.* **242**:148.

Garrido, F., Festenstein, H., and Schirrmacher, V., 1976, Further evidence for derepression of H-2 and Ia-like specificities of foreign haplotypes in mouse tumour lines, *Nature (London)* **261**:705.

Herlyn, M., Clark, W. H., Mastrangelo, M. J., Dupont, G., Elder, D. E., Larossa, D., Hamilton, R., Bondi, E., Tuthill, R., Steplewski, Z., and Koprowski, H., 1980, Specific immunoreactivity of monoclonal anti-melanoma antibodies, *Cancer Res.* **40**:3602.

Hersey, P., 1977, Recent views on tumour antigens and their relation to host defence mechanisms, *Aust. N. Z. J. Med.* **7**:526.

Hersey, P., 1979, Natural killer cells: A new cytotoxic mechanism against tumours? *Aust. N. Z. J. Med.* **9**:464.

Hersey, P., and Isbister, J., 1979, Developments in immune complex therapy and its application to cancer, in: *Human Cancer Immunology* (B. Serrou and C. Rosenfeld, eds.), pp. 135–166, Elsevier/North-Holland, Amsterdam.

Hersey, P., Honeyman, M., Edwards, A., Adams, E., and McCarthy, W. H., 1976a, Antigens on melanoma cells detected by leucocyte-dependent antibody assays of human melanoma antisera, *Int. J. Cancer* **18**:564.

Hersey, P., Isbister, J., Edwards, A., Murray, E., Adams, E., Biggs, J., and Milton, G. W., 1976b, Antibody dependent cell mediated cytotoxicity against melanoma cells induced by plasmapheresis, *Lancet* **1**:825.

Hersey, P., Morgan, G., Stone, D., McCarthy, W. H., and Milton, G. W., 1977, Prior pregnancy as a protective factor against death from melanoma, *Lancet* **1**:451.

Hersey, P., Edwards, A., Milton, G. W., and McCarthy, W. H., 1978a, Relationship of cell-mediated cytotoxicity against melanoma cells to prognosis in melanoma patients, *Br. J. Cancer* **37**:505.

Hersey, P., Edwards, A., Murray, E., McCarthy, W. H., and Milton, G. W., 1978b, Sequential studies of melanoma leukocyte dependent antibody activity in melanoma patients, *Eur. J. Cancer* **14**:629.

Hersey, P., Murray, E., Ruygrok, S., Edwards, A., and Milton, G. W., 1978c, Blocking factors against melanoma leukocyte-dependent antibody: Relationship to disease activity in melanoma patients, *Aust. N. Z. J. Surg.* **48**:26.

Hersey, P., Murray, E., and Edwards, A., 1979a, Leukocyte dependent antibody assays in melanoma patients, in: *Immunodiagnosis of Human Cancer* (R. B. Herberman, ed.), pp. 599–604, Elsevier/North-Holland, New York.

Hersey, P., Murray, E., Werkmeister, J., and McCarthy, W. H., 1979b, Detection of a low molecular weight antigen on melanoma cells by a human antiserum in leukocyte dependent antibody assays, *Br. J. Cancer* **40**:615.

Hersey, P., Edwards, A., and McCarthy, W. H., 1980a, Tumour related changes in natural killer cell activity in melanoma patients: Influence of stage of disease, tumour thickness and age of patient, *Int. J. Cancer* **25**:187.

Hersey, P., Murray, E., and McCarthy, W. H., 1980b, Evaluation of antibody inhibition assays of melanoma antigens in sera to monitor tumor growth in melanoma patients, *Cancer Immunol. Immunother.* (in press).

Hollinshead, A. C., 1975, Analysis of soluble melanoma cell membrane antigens in metastatic cells of various organs and further studies of antigens present in primary melanoma, *Cancer* **36**:1282.

Invernizzi, G., Carbone, G., Mesachini, A., and Parmiani, G., 1977, Multiple foreign non-H-2 determinants on the surface of a chemically induced murine sarcoma, *J. Immunogenet.* **4**:97.

Irie, R. F., Irie, K., and Morton, D. C., 1976, A membrane antigen common to human cancer and fetal brain tissues, *Cancer Res.* **36**:3510.

Irie, R. F., Giuliano, A., Golub, S., and Morton, D. C., 1979a, Humoral antibodies to oncofetal antigen, in: *Immunodiagnosis of Human Cancer* (R. B. Herberman, ed.), pp. 587–596, Elsevier/North-Holland,

Irie, R. F., Giuliano, A. E., Golub, S. H., and Morton, D. L., 1979b, Oncofoetal antigen: A tumour associated fetal antigen immunogenic in man, *J. Natl. Cancer Inst.* **63**:367.

Jehn, U. W., Nathanson, L., Schwartz, R. S., and Skinner, M., 1970, *In vitro* lymphocyte stimulation by a soluble antigen from malignant melanoma, *N. Engl. J. Med.* **283**:329.

Jones, P. C., Sze, L. L., Liu, P. Y., Morton, D. L., and Irie, R. F. 1981, Prolonged survival for melanoma patients with elevated IgM antibody to oncofetal antigens, *J. Natl. Cancer Inst.* **66**:249.

Keissling, R., and Haller, O., 1978, Natural killer cells in the mouse: an alternative immune surveillance mechanism?, in: *Contemporary Topics in Immunobiology*, Vol. 8 (N. L. Warner, ed.), pp. 171–179, Plenum Press, New York.

Leong, S. P., Cooperband, S. R., Sutherland, C. M., Krementz, E. T., and Deckers, P. J., 1978, Detection of melanoma antigens in cell free supernatants, *J. Surg. Res.* **24**:245.

Leung, J. P., and Edginton, T. S., 1980, Radioimmunoassay for tissue distribution of a human mammary tumor-specific glycoprotein, *Cancer Res.* **40**:662.

Levy, W. L., 1978, Specificity of lymphocyte-mediated cytotoxicity in patients with primary intracranial tumours, *J. Immunol.* **121**:903.

Lewis, M. G., 1972, Immunology of human malignant melanoma, *Ser. Haematol.* **5**:44.

Lewis, M. G., and Phillips, T. M., 1972, The specificity of surface membrane immunofluorescence in human malignant melanoma, *Int. J. Cancer* **10**:105.

Lewis, M. G., Ikonopisov, R. L., Nairn, R. C., Phillips, T. M., Hamilton Fairley, G., Bodenham, D. C., and Alexander, P., 1969, Tumour specific antibodies in human malignant melanoma and their relationship to the extent of the disease, *Br. Med. J.* **3**:547.

Lewis, M. G., Phillips, T. M., Cook, K. B., and Blake, J., 1971, Possible explanation of loss of detectable antibody in patients with disseminated malignant melanoma, *Nature (London)* **232**:52.

Lewis, M. G., Hartman, D., and Jerry, L. M., 1976, Antibodies and antibodies in human malignancy: An expression of deranged immune regulation, *Ann. N. Y. Acad. Sci.* **276**:316.

Liao, S. K., Leong, S. P. L., Sutherland, C. M., Dent, P. B., Kwong, P. C., and Krementz, E. T., 1978, Common human melanoma membrane antigens detected by mixed hemadsorption microassay with serum from a patient undergoing immunotherapy with autologous tumour cells, *Cancer Res.* **38**:4395.

Lloyd, K. O., Travassos, L. R., Takahashi, T., and Old, L. J., 1979, Cell surface glycoproteins of human tumor cell lines: Unusual characteristics of malignant melanoma, *J. Natl. Cancer Inst.* **63**:623.

Macher, E., Muller, C. H. R., Sorg, G., Gassen, A., and Sorg, C., 1975, Evidence for cross-reacting membrane associated specific melanoma antigens as detected by immunofluorescence and immune adherence, *Behring Inst. Mitteil.* **56**:86–90.

Malley, A., Burger, D. R., Vandenbark, A. A., Frikke, M., Finke, P., Begley, D., Acott, K., Black, J., and Vetto, M. R., 1979, Association of melanoma tumor antigen activity with β_2 microglobulin, *Cancer Res.* **39**:619.

McCabe, R. P., Ferrone, S., Pellegrino, M. A., Kern, D. H., Holmes, E. C., and Reisfelo, R. A., 1978, Purification and immunologic evaluation of human melanoma associated antigens, *J. Natl. Cancer Inst.* **60**:773.

Mitchell, K. F., Fuhrer, J. P., Steplewski, Z., and Koprowski, H., 1981, Structural characterization of the "melanoma-specific" antigen detected by monoclonal antibody 69115 Nu-4-B, *Mol. Immunol.* **18**:207.

Morgan, G., McCarthy, W. H., and Hersey, P., 1977, Detection of carcinoembryonic-like antigen on melanoma cells by leukocyte-dependent antibody assays, *Br. J. Cancer* **36**:446.

Morgan, A. C., Rossen, R. D., and Twomey, J. J., 1979, Naturally occuring circulating immune complexes: Normal human serum contains idiotype–antiidiotype complexes dissociable by certain IgG antiglobulins, *J. Immunol.* **122**:1672.

Morton, D. L., Malmgren, R. A., Holmes, E. C. and Ketcham, A. S., 1968, Demonstration of antibodies against human malignant melanoma by immunofluorescence, *Surgery* **65**:233.

Morton, D. L., Holmes, E. C., Eilber, F. R., and Wood, W. C., 1971a, Immunological aspects of neoplasia: A rational basis for immunotherapy, *Ann. Intern. Med.* **74**:587.

Morton, D. L., Eilber, R. F., and Malmgren, R. A., 1971b, Immune factors in human cancer: Malignant melanoma skeletal and soft tissue sarcomas, *Prog. Exp. Tumor Res.* **14**:25.

Munro, A., and Bright, S., 1976, Products of the major histocompatibility complex and their relationship to the immune response, *Nature (London)* **264**:145.

Murray, E., McCarthy, W. H., and Hersey, P., 1977, Blocking factors against leucocyte-dependent melanoma antibody in the sera of melanoma patients, *Br. J. Cancer* **36**:7.

Murray, E., Ruygrok, S., McCarthy, W. H., Milton, G. W., and Hersey, P., 1978, Analysis of serum blocking factors against leukocyte dependent antibody in melanoma patients, *Int. J. Cancer* **21**:578.

Old, L. J., and Boyse, E. A., 1964, Immunology of experimental tumours, *Annu. Rev. Med.* **16**:167.

Old, L. J., Boyse, E. A., Clark, D. A., and Carswell, E. A., 1962, Antigenic properties of chemically induced tumours, *Ann. N. Y. Acad. Sci.* **101**:80.

Parsons, P. G., Goss, P., and Pope, J. H., 1974, Detection in human melanoma cell lines of particles with some properties in common with RNA tumour viruses, *Int. J. Cancer* **13**:606.

Pfreundschuh, M., Shiku, H., Takahashi, T., Ueda, R., Ransohoff, J., Oettgen, H. F., and Old, L. J., 1978, Serological analysis of cell surface antigens of malignant brain tumors, *Proc. Natl. Acad. Sci. U.S.A.* **75**:5122.

Preddie, E., Hartmann, D., and Lewis, M. G., 1978a, Human tumor specific antigens. 1. An allogeneic antigen from patient "PY" melanoma tumor cell plasma membranes, *Cancer Biochem. Biophys.* **2**:161.

Preddie, E., Hartmann, D., Persad, S., Khosraui, M., and Lewis, M., 1978b, Isolation of an autologous tumor-specific antigen from tumor cell plasma membranes of a human melanoma patient, *Cancer Biochem. Biophys.* **2**:199.

Pullen, S., and Hersey, P., 1981, Reactivity of antisera to antigens of C type viruses with leukocytes from patients with acute leukaemia, *Pathology* **13**:289.

Ritter, M. A., and Morris, R. J., 1980, Thy-1 antigen: Selective association in lymphoid organs with the vascular basement membrane involved in lymphocyte recirculation, *Immunology* **39**:85.

Roder, J. C., Ahrlund-Richter, L., and Jondal, M., 1979, Target–effector interaction in the human and murine natural killer system: Specificity and xenogeneic reactivity of the solubilized natural killer–target structure complex and its loss in a somatic cell hybrid, *J. Exp. Med.* **150**:471.

Roth, J. A., Slocum, H. K., Pellegrino, M. A., Holmes, E. C., and Reisfeld, R. A., 1976, Purification of soluble human melanoma-associated antigens, *Cancer Res.* **36**:2360.

Salinas, F. A., Shiekh, K. M., and Chandor, S. B., 1978, Serological reactivity in cancer patients to human and mouse fetal liver cells, *Cancer Res.* **38**:401.

Schirrmacher, V., and Bosslet, K., 1980a, Tumor metastases and cell-mediated immunity in a model system in DBA/2 mice. X. Immunoselection of tumor variants differing in tumor antigen expression and metastatic capacity, *Int. J. Cancer* **25**:781.

Schirrmacher, V., and Bosslet, K., 1980b, Changes in expression of tumor-associated transplantation antigens within cloned tumor cell lines, Proceedings of the 4th International Conference of Immunology, Abstract 10.3.38.

Schmidt, W., Festenstein, H., and Atfield, G., 1980, Serologic and immunochemical studies on the cell membrane alloantigens of K36 on AKR spontaneous leukaemia, *Transplant. Porc.* **12**:29.

Seibert, E., Sorg, C., Happle, R., and Macher, E., 1977, Membrane associated antigens of human malignant melanoma. III. Specificity of human sera reacting with cultured melanoma cells, *Int. J. Cancer* **19**:172.

Shaw, H. M., Milton, G. W., Farago, G., and McCarthy, W. H., 1978, Endocrine influences on survival from malignant melanoma, *Cancer* **42**:669.

Shearman, P. J., and Longenecker, B. M., 1980a, Selection for virulence and organ-specific metastasis of her-pesvirus-tranferred lymphoma cells, *Int. J. Cancer* **25**:363.

Shearman, P. J., and Longenecker, B. M., 1980b, An organ specific metastasis-associated antigen detected by monoclonal antibodies, Proceedings of the 4th International Congress of Immunology, Abstract, 10.1.51.

Shiku, H., Takahashi, T., Oettgen, H. F., and Old, L. J., 1976, Cell surface antigens of human malignant melanoma. II. Serological typing with immune adherence assays and definition of two new surface anti-gens, *J. Exp. Med.* **144**:873.

Shiku, H., Takahashi, T., Resnick, L. A., Oettgen, H. F., and Old, L. J., 1977, Cell surface antigens of human malignant melanoma. III. Recognition of autoantibodies with unusual characteristics, *J. Exp. Med.* **145**:784.

Stephenson, J. R., Essex, M., Hino, S., Aaronson, S. A., and Hardy, W. D., Jr., 1977, Feline oncornavirus-associated cell-membrane antigen (FOCMA): Distinction between FOCMA and the major virion glyco-protein, *Proc. Natl. Acad. Sci. U.S.A.* **74**:1219.

The, T. H., Huighes, H. A., Schrafforot Koops, H., Lamberts, H. B., and Nieweg, H. O., 1975, Surface antigens on cultured malignant melanoma cells as detected by membrane immunofluorescence method with human sera: Lack of tumor-specific reactions on melanoma lines, *Ann. N. Y. Acad. Sci.* **254**:528.

Thomson, D. M. P., and Alexander, P., 1973, A cross-reacting embryonic antigen in the membrane of rat sarcoma cells which is immunogenic in the syngeneic host, *Br. J. Cancer* **27**:35.

Thomson, D. M. P., Ralich, J. E., Weatherhead, J. C., Friedlander, P., O'Connor, R., Grosser, N., Shuster, J., and Gold, P., 1978, Isolation of human tumour-specific antigens associated with β_2 microglobulin, *Br. J. Cancer* **37**:753.

Werkmeister, J., Edwards, A., McCarthy, W. H., and Hersey, P., 1980, Prognostic significance of expression of antigens on melanoma cells, *Cancer Immunol. Immunother.* **9**:233.

Whitsed, H., McCarthy, W. H., and Hersey, P., 1979, Nephelometric detection of circulating immune com-plexes using monoclonal rheumatoid factor, *J. Immunol. Methods* **29**:311.

Wilson, B. S., Indiveri, F., Pellegrino, M. A., and Ferrone, S., 1979, DR (Ia-like) antigens on human melanoma cells: Serological detection and immunochemical characterization, *J. Exp. Med.* **149**:658.

Winchester, R. J., Wang, C. Y., Gibofsky, A., Kunkel, H. G., Lloyd, K. O., and Old, L. J., 1978, Expression of Ia-like antigens on cultured human malignant melanoma cell lines, *Proc. Natl. Acad. Sci. U.S.A.* **75**:6235.

Zaunders, J., Werkmeister, J., McCarthy, W. H., and Hersey, P., 1981, Characterization of antigens recog-nized by natural killer cells in cell culture supernatants, *Br. J. Cancer* **43**:5.

Zola, H., 1980, Monoclonal antibodies against cell membrane antigens—current state of the art and potential for use in the diagnostic laboratory, *Pathology* **12**:539.

12

Cellular and Humoral Studies of Malignant Melanoma

ARIEL HOLLINSHEAD, KEITH TANNER, AND
W. DANIEL KUNDIN

1. Work by Others

Recent studies have provided additional information with regard to antigenic properties of melanoma cells. Some of these studies have been performed using material shed into culture media during the growth of melanoma cells. Reisfeld *et al.* (1980) describe melanoma-associated antigens (MAAs) shed in the culture media of radiolabeled melanoma cells, which react with polyclonal antimelanoma xenoantisera. MGP-1, a subunit of a larger structure, was described an antigen with a molecular weight of 240,000 that was exclusive to melanoma cells, and MGP-2, a single-chain antigen with a molecular weight of 94,000, was found to be present on melanoma cells, carcinoma cells, and fetal melanocytes. It was found that radiochemically pure antigens had different charge properties. In a recent review, these authors described the many variables to be considered in the evaluation of MAAs (Ferrone and Pellegrino, 1979). Gupta *et al.* (1979a) studied the antigenic activity of spent serum-free, chemically defined media by monitoring complement fixation and immune adherence. This group described two distinct antigens, namely, oncofetal antigen and tumor-associated antigen, (TAA). In a further study (Gupta and Morton, 1980), this group described the same TAA, derived from the M14 melanoma cell line after radiolabeling with ^{125}I in radioimmunoassays (RIAs) with patient sera. Positive antibodies (positive antibody was defined as $\geq$ 1 : 100 serum dilution) were in 65% of melanoma sera, 36% of carcinoma sera, and 15% of normal sera. Spent media of melanoma cell lines, or tumor extracts (63% of both), gave 50% inhibition, but little or no inhibition was seen using the spent media of sarcoma (0%), colon or breast cell lines (17%), or extracts of fetal and

ARIEL HOLLINSHEAD, KEITH TANNER, AND W. DANIEL KUNDIN • Division of Hematology and Oncology, Department of Medicine, The George Washington University Medical Center, Washington, D.C. 20037.

normal tissues (0%). The authors suggest that TAA is expressed by a majority of melanomas and that melanoma patients have the highest antibody to TAA. They found that immunologically similar antigens are expressed by breast cancer, testicular cancer, and ovarian cancer. Morgan et al. (1980) performed studies with inhibitors of glycosylation that indicated that the carbohydrate moieties of the MGP-1 and MGP-2 described by Reisfeld and co-workers (see above) are required for shedding, but not for intercalation and expression on the cell surface. Whether the carbohydrate moieties are required for antigenic expressions of various types by the separated MAAs needs to be studied. It would be of interest to know more about the chemical nature of the antigens described by Gupta.

Using hybridoma monoclonal antibodies to antigens present on the same M14 melanoma cell lines, Saxton et al. (1980) have been defining the types of hybridoma antibodies that bind preferentially to melanoma cell lines. Similarly, Yeh et al. (1979) have studied hybrid cells of mouse NS-1 myeloma and spleen cells from M1804-melanoma-cell-immunized BALB/c mice and have found three hybrids that produced antibody to melanoma cells. Antibodies from two of the clones were cytotoxic to M1804 cells and to 2 of 11 allogeneic melanomas, but were not cytotoxic to control cells, suggesting identification of an MAA for some, but not all, melanomas. This is consistent with some of our own studies that suggest that not all metastatic tissues from melanoma patients contain the same TAA. Many problems compound the identification of antigens; for example, Liao et al. (1979) found that cultured cells adsorb serum components from culture media and, to further compound the problem, normal human adult serum and fetal cat serum antigens are cross-reactive. In addition, we have often found that antisera directed against whole cells do not react with separated, purified TAA. This observation was also made by Otterstrom (1979) in studies of murine UV-induced skin tumors. He identified a 76,000-molecular-weight tumor-rejection antigen for this system and thought to use antiserum directed against whole cells for isolating the antigen by antibody-affinity chromatography. Unfortunately, the antiserum did not react with this tumor-rejection antigen. This is not unusual, since most TAAs exist in very small amounts on the cell surface and are usually blocked or masked by non-specific materials. In our studies, we have found that most of the material in spent media of those particular melanoma cell lines that are well defined for containing TAA consist mainly of nonspecific normal antigens and immune complexes, thus making spent media, in our experience, a difficult source for isolation of TAA. Nonspecific complexes present on the cell surface have other effects. Winkelhake et al. (1979) purified radiolabeled mouse antibodies to melanoma cells by affinity chromatography and detected approximately 9 $\times$ 10^6 melanoma antigenic sites per cell; the antibody blocked the binding of melanocyte-stimulating hormone, and it was suggested that this and other activities by antibody may play a role in tumor progression.

Other workers have also defined MAAs. Carey et al. (1979) described a unique autologous cell-surface melanoma-related glycoprotein, unrelated to β_2-microglobulin of the human leukocyte antigen (HLA) complex. Ishii and Mavligit (1979) used a double-antibody RIA and detected MAAs in all but one melanoma extract, while normal tissue and nonmelanoma tumor extracts were negative. MAA was also found in 8 of 13 melanoma-patient sera. This particular MAA is defined as a glycoprotein with an estimated molecular weight of 40,000 that does not cross-react with either β_2-microglobulin or bacillus Calmette Guérin (BCG) preparations. Stuhlmiller and Seigler (1979) used complement-dependent microcytotoxicity assays and found melanoma-cell-membrane TAAs on all membranes tested thus far. They claim that this antigen is not detectable on normal peripheral-blood leukocytes, erythrocytes, adult skin fibroblasts, epithelial cells, fetal fibroblasts, T- or B-lymphoblastoid cell lines, or tumors of nonmelanoma origin.

Many investigators have been examining the humoral changes and nonspecific immunological changes related to melanoma. Van Der Giessen et al. (1978) as well as other groups have found that leukocytes from patients with invasive or late-state melanoma have higher levels of immunoglobulin G (IgG) and complement inclusions and have shown that these complexes are loosely bound; Raji-cell reactive material is in the first fraction of gel filtration with a molecular weight of greater than 350,000. Our studies and those of other groups agree with these findings; our Raji-cell reactive material was in the heavy, nonsolubilized cell-membrane material and in the half of the first Sephadex G200 peak, as well as at the very top of the cathodic end of separations performed by discontinuous-gradient polyacrylamide gel electrophoresis (PAGE). On the other hand, Van Wingerden et al. (1978) measured the circulating immune complexes (CICs) in melanoma patients by means of a granulocyte phagocytosis test; leukocyte suspensions were incubated with appropriate sera for 90 min at $37°C$, washed, fixed, and assayed by indirect immunofluorescence (IF) for either human IgG or complement, and the numbers of positive cells (with 5 or more fluorescent granules) per 1000 cells studied were 48 for tumor-bearing patients, 26 for tumor-free patients, and 10 for controls. These authors found no correlation between the stages of tumor-bearing patients and their CIC levels, and they also observed that individual CIC levels did not fall after surgery. Lewis et al. (1979) have described differences in the types of antibody during tumor progression, and in elution studies found that antimembrane antibody decreased and anticytoplasmic antibody increased during the period of tumor progression. Ninger et al. (1979) evaluated three erythrocyte (E)-rosette assays in melanoma patients, before surgery and at the 3- to 6-month postsurgical period, and found that the active erythrocyte-rosette-forming cells (E RFC) and the 29 E-rosette assays were not superior to total E RFC in demonstrating differences in immune status. State I patients did not differ from controls (69% for both), but the mean percentages of cells counted in the total E RFC were lower for Stage II (64.9%) and Stage III (59.6%) patients. Thatcher et al. (1979) found that surface Ig staining cells and serum IgA, IgM, and IgG levels of 16 patients with advanced melanoma were not significantly different from control values. In patients on BCG or Corynebacterium parvum immunotherapy, both the null-cell counts and phytohemagglutinin blastogenesis median stimulation indexes were significantly lower than controls. Treatment with C. parvum caused significant increases in relative E RFC counts and decreases in erythrocyte–antibody (EA) RFC values. Jassem et al. (1979) also studied serum components. Except for a slight IgA decline and IgM rise observed in females with malignant melanoma, and a decrease in IgG, IgA, and IgM in patients with advanced malignancy, none of the differences was significant. This group also studied autoimmune antibodies, and no antinucleus antibodies were found in serum (diluted 1 : 20); serum of patients with early-stage melanoma had more anti-smooth muscle antibodies than the control sera studied. West (1979) has presented evidence that primary aberrations in E RFC from cancer patients might be, in part, the result of an increase in constant-fragment (Fc)-receptor-bearing T cells with fragile interactions with sheep red blood cells.

These and other studies are important in understanding how to predict the harmful effects of chemotherapy or immunotherapy. Helander et al. (1979) have reported that prolonged BCG therapy may result in an enhanced risk of dissemination of malignant melanoma. Natali *et al.* (1980) have studied HLA-d-related (HLA-DR) antigens, which mediate immune recognition processes. They studied HLA-DR monoclonal antibodies by immunofluorescence vs. 14 explanted melanoma tumors and found levels that varied from 15 to 90%, whereas 13 nevi studied were all negative. Hersey *et al.* (1980) studied the effect of tumor growth on natural killer (NK)-cell activity in ^{51}Cr- release assays before and at intervals after surgical debulking of localized melanoma. NK activity directed against melanoma cells was maximal at 2–4 weeks after the removal of the tumor in Stage I patients with melanoma, and then NK decreased to normal levels. The NK at the 2- to 4-week level was directly related to the thickness of the tumor. NK activity in Stage II melanoma patients did not increase, but fell to low levels after removal of the tumor, and was not related to the thickness of the primary melanoma. It was not clear why, but these authors found that NK activity showed a significant increase with age. Vandenbark *et al.* (1979) studied 40 members of three melanoma-prone families and found that members with close exposure to melanoma patients for 10 years or more had significantly higher leukocyte-adherence inhibition (LAI) test responses. Further, they found that the elevated LAI responses were not genetically determined and suggested the presence of transmissible melanoma-associated material capable of immunizing individuals with prolonged close exposure to melanoma patients.

These and other earlier studies of the cellular and immunological aspects of melanoma provide important information, and it is to be hoped that as time progresses, we will be able to assemble the bits and pieces for an improved understanding of this malignancy.

2. Work by Our Group

For several years, our group has been involved in identifying separated cell-membrane components that produce cell-mediated immune (CMI) reactivity, after study of the entire spectrum of separated, soluble membrane components from malignant tissues and counterpart fetal and benign and normal adult tissues. The way in which our studies differ from those of others rests on the facts that (1) we started with carefully washed membrane preparations from washed, counted viable cells, for all our initial work; and (2) our goals were directed toward finding antigens appropriate for immunotherapy, rather than immunodiagnosis, and therefore we were interested in identifying only those separated components that induce CMI responses, initially *in vivo*, and when the techniques became available, *in vitro* as well. We review here basic aspects of a large study, reported elsewhere (Hollinshead *et al.*, 1982).

The new developments in technology have permitted us to perform experiments in the laboratory with a view to helping those who are interested in developing diagnostic or monitoring tests for melanoma. The initial skin tests in carefully chosen postoperative or untreated advanced-stage, nonanergic patients with highly purified antigens free from nucleic acids and nonidentical to major HLA antigens, single- and double-diffusion studies, lymphocyte-migration inhibition (LMI) tests, IF studies, initial attempts at RIA, separations by preparative electrophoresis for larger-scale purification of melanoma TAAs, and other studies are described elsewhere (Char *et al.*, 1974, 1977; Gorodilova and Hollinshead, 1975; Gorodilova *et al.*, 1976; Hollinshead, 1975a,b, 1978, 1979a,b; Hollinshead *et al.*, 1974, 1980). The improved techniques of affinity chromatography have been of great assistance in better characterization of the antigens we have identified. Therefore, trusting that our observations will be helpful to others, in Section 2.1 we have summarized the characteristics of melanoma-cell-membrane antigens that induce melanoma-related CMI responses, and we have summarized the characteristics of xenogeneic hyperimmune antisera to one of these antigens that appears to be tumor-associated. In Section 2.2, we summarize our experiences during pilot specific-active immunotherapy studies (Hollinshead *et al.*, 1980) on the use of a nonspecific test to follow humoral and cell-related immunological changes, in individual and serial testing of melanoma patients. This nonspecific test parameter is called the Cancer Serum Index (CSI) and has been described elsewhere (Hollinshead *et al.*, 1977; Hollinshead and Chuang, 1978). Briefly, 100 μg protein each of coded serum samples was separated by discontinuous-gradient PAGE, and the gels were removed from the tubing and stained with Coomassie brilliant blue. Densitometry tracings were made of test sample standards and controls using a Gelman ACD-13 densitometer. The areas of α_1-acid glycoprotein (AGP) and thyroxin-binding prealbumin (PA) peaks were measured, and the index was determined by dividing AGP area by PA area.

2.1. Specific Cellular and Humoral Immunity

Antigens identified by our methods and the electrophoretic mobility, chemical composition, stability, and a comparison with standard proteins are shown in Table I. Only one of these antigens appeared to be tumor-associated, and it elicited positive delayed cutaneous hypersensitivity reactions (DCHRs) mainly in melanoma patients with early-stage systemic and ocular melanoma (where the tumor is confined to one site), with approximately 88% of nonanergic patients responding. Only 37% of patients with advanced stages of melanoma were skin-test-positive, with approximately 3% positivity seen in patients with other types of cancer. As shown in Table I, some nonspecific antigens that induce CMI responses were also identified, but positive reactions were elicited in only 48% of patients with early-stage melanoma, with a more marked response seen in 72% of patients with advanced stages of melanoma; however, these particular antigens produced positive skin-test responses in patients with breast cancer, and as delineated in footnote[j] to Table I, also reacted in double immunodiffusion with the antigen separated from fetal black skin cell membranes as well as from separated ductal breast-cancer cell membranes (Hollinshead, 1973, 1975a; Hollinshead *et al.*, 1974, 1977). As shown, the chemical composition of melanoma TAA is as a fairly high-molecular-weight glycolipoprotein. This antigen is fairly stable, but sometimes after preparative isotachophoresis or preparative gel electrophoresis, the carbohydrate splits off, and, as shown in Table I, the antigen migrates toward the anode. It is difficult to ascribe a particular molecular weight to this antigen without equilibrium ultragradient centrifugation studies with a large amount of highly purified antigen, and we have ascribed higher priority to the use of this antigen in other studies at present. However, as shown, the relative migration of haptoglobin type 2.2 and hemopexin suggests the possible molecular-weight range of the lipoprotein portion.

The partial specificity of melanoma TAA was described in earlier studies (Hollinshead, 1978). Double immunodiffusion–immunoelectrophoresis (ID-IE) techniques were used to better define the TAA. As shown in Table II, our results before affinity chromatography of xenographic hyperimmune antisera prepared to partially purified melanoma TAA were fairly good. In the double-ID studies, 52 melanoma preparations were positive,

TABLE I

Characteristics of Melanoma-Cell-Membrane Antigens That Induce Melanoma-Related Cell-Mediated Immune Responses

Purified antigens	Electrophoretic mobility (cm distance from tracking dye on gradient PAGE)[a]	Chemical composition[b]	Stability in pure form[c]			Migration in relation to proteins of known molecular size[d]
			Room temp. for 2 hr	4°C for 1 week	−70°C for 6 months	
Melanoma TAA[e]	9.3 (without carbohydrate, migrages to 8.0)	glycolipoprotein	+	±	+	β-Lipoprotein products: migrates 9.6–9.95; unknown Haptoglobin type 2.2: migrates 8.9; mol. wt. 400,000
Nonspecific antigens[f] b2	5.6,5.8	Protein	+	+	+	Hemopexin: migrates 6.2; mol. wt. 57,000
Nonspecific antigens[f] b4	4.4, 4.6	Lipoprotein	+	+	+	Gc globulin: migrates 5.1–5.45; mol. wt. 51,000 AGP: migrates 4.0; mol. wt. 40,000
b6	3.2	Protein	+	+	+	Thyroxin-binding PA: migrates 3.4; mol. wt. 61,000

[a] The tracking dye (TD) was bromphenol blue (molecular weight 670); PAGE stacked gels: 3.5, 4.75, 7, and 10%; calculations adjusted for relationship of TD to marker albumin in control PAGE.

[b] Individual gels were stained with Coomassie brilliant blue, oil red 0, and periodic acid–Schiff.

[c] As tested by reseparation on sodium dodecyl sulfate–PAGE for intact band and by DCHR and LMI test for CMI activity.

[d] Estimation of precise migration of serum components on control gels; identification of specific components by reactions with monospecific antisera in gel double diffusion.

[e] Elicits a positive DCHR mainly in patients with early-stage systemic and ocular melanoma.

[f] These antigens are more broadly reactive, giving positive reactions in some patients with early-stage systemic melanoma, but mainly in patients with advanced stages of melanoma; they also produce some positive responses in patients with other malignancies, but mainly in patients with breast cancer. Antigens b2 and b6 cross-react in double ID with separated fetal black skin antigen; b4 shares ID-IE reactivities with material from the same PAGE region as separated ductal-breast-cancer cell membranes, but the antigens are not comparable for electrophoretic mobility.

TABLE II

Characteristics of Xenogeneic Hyperimmune Antisera to Melanoma Tumor-Associated Antigen[a]

Double immunodiffusion tests: positive with partially purified melanoma TAA from 3 amelanotic melanoma, 41 primary melanoma, and 8 of 9 melanoma liver metastases

Before affinity chromatography of antisera:

Also positive to:	extracts from cell membranes of 2 of 18 breast cancers, white blood cells, 1 of 15 lung cancers, 2 of 8 colon cancers.
Negative to:	extracts from cell membranes of fetal black skin, fetal white skin, fetal intestine, normal lung tissue from a melanoma patient, MCF breast-cancer cell line, whole and fractionated AB pooled sera, 16 of 18 breast-cancer extracts, 14 of 15 lung-cancer extracts, 6 of 8 colon-cancer extracts, AA-1 bladder cell line, J-82 bladder-cell line, angioma herpes-simplex-virus-acute-infected WI-38 cells, WI-38 cell, 42 nevi extracts, ovarian-cancer TAA, normal ovarian tissue, white skin, black skin, adenocarcinoma lung TAA, colon-cancer TAA, fibrosarcoma of breast, meningioma cell line, acute lymphocytic leukemia, gastric cancer, hemopexin, AGP, transferrin

After affinity chromatography of antisera: [b]

Negative to:	the aforenamed extracts of 18 breast cancers, 1 lung and 2 colon cancers, white blood cells, and AB pooled sera.
Positive to:	melanoma TAA from each of 29 tumors, with classic precipitin lines of identity

[a] The antisera were prepared in albino New Zealand rabbits inoculated monthly $\times$ 5 with 15 μg TAA glyco-lipoprotein plus a faint second band; the 4th-month bleeding of one of the rabbits was partially absorbed and used before and after affinity chromatography procedures, in the tests described in the table.

[b] Antisera also show melanoma-cell-associated positive reactions as determined by indirect immunofluorescence to controlled tests in triplicate with wet tumor tissue imprints from 19 melanoma, 7 breast-tumor, and 8 lung-tumor fresh specimens, as well as to one melanoma TAA-containing cell line (Gi), using antisera to squamous-cell TAA and ABO pooled normal sera as controls. Of 20 melanoma preparations, 17 were positive.

and numerous and repeated tests with a number of control extracts (Table II) were negative; however, six preparations were positive, and the precipitin bands suggested that all these extracts shared a cross-contaminant. After affinity chromatography to free the antisera from the cross-contaminant present on white blood cells, we repeated a battery of tests including positive and negative extracts used in the previous study, and these results are shown in the lower portion of Table II. Although we would by no means designate our antigen as specific, at this point, with the methods used, the antigen initially identified by *in vivo* testing appeared to be, at least in part, tumor-associated. Although our initial work with indirect IF testing was not extensive, the antisera appeared to produce immunofluorescing properties and some of the cells appeared to have the type of fluorescence described as positive (Lewis and Phillips, 1972). Recent studies using antisera after affinity chromatography indicate a fairly precise association with melanoma cells (see footnote *b* to Table II). Recent studies with postaffinity human hyperimmune melanoma TAA antisera are described elsewhere (Hollinshead *et al.*, 1982).

In some of our earlier studies, we also looked for TAA on various melanoma cell lines in tissue culture, after growth in chemically defined, serum-free media, and identified certain melanoma cell lines that, at that passage level and under the conditions of culture, contained melanoma TAA. Of greater interest was the question of whether or not TAA from primary melanoma cells also existed on metastatic melanoma cells, and in earlier studies (Hollinshead, 1975b) we reported that primary TAA appeared to be present in some but not all adrenal, lung, and liver metastases. Positive responses to metastatic TAA in different stages were distributed differently from that of primary melanoma TAA,

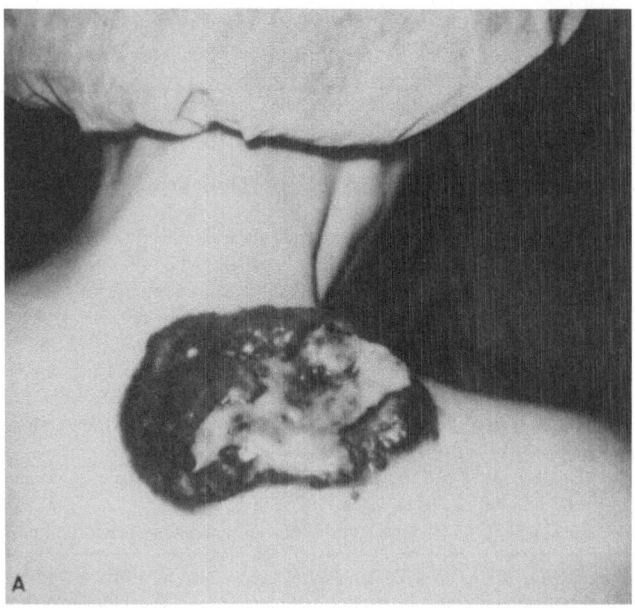

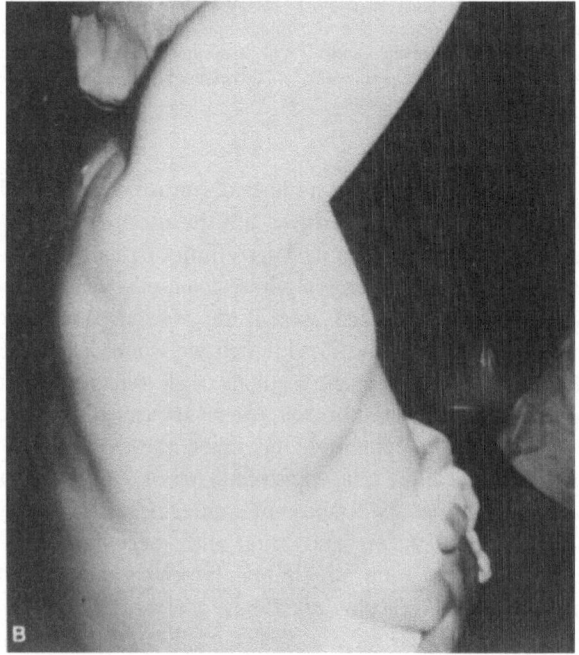

Figure 1. Patient with a large primary melanoma tumor (A) who subsequently developed large metastatic tumors under the arm (B). These tumors were the sources for cell membranes used for separation of TAA for comparative studies. Photographs courtesy of *Cancer* [see Hollinshead *et al.* (1982)].

namely, approximately 47% of patients with Stages I and II and 33% of patients with Stage III or IIIa. This suggested to us that either primary TAA was missing from metastatic tissues, although the PAGE profiles indicated the presence of some form of the antigen, or the configuration or structural composition of the antigen might have altered somewhat in some of the metastatic tissues or was present in complex form attached to antibody. In our studies of these and other forms of cancer, as a general rule, we see larger quantities of antigen–antibody complexes present in the larger primary tissues and also in metastatic tissues. To study this question further, we obtained a large amount of primary tumor and a large amount of metastatic tumor from the same individual; as shown in Fig. 1, this individual had a large primary tumor and developed large metastatic tumors under the arm. Cells, membranes, and affinity separated soluble TAA were processed from these tumors for simultaneous testing in 23 patients with various stages of melanoma. Of 12 patients with early-stage disease, 10 (83%) were positive to primary TAA, whereas only 5 (42%) of these 12 melanoma patients (2 of whom were not positive to primary TAA) gave responses to the metastatic melanoma TAA. Of 11 patients with metastatic melanoma, 4 (36%) gave positive responses to primary TAA and 5 patients (45%) (1 of these also responding to primary TAA) were positive for metastatic melanoma TAA. These studies suggested that there might be differences, but the results of sequential immunizations (booster studies) conducted at that time suggested that conversion to a positive response to primary TAA might be possible (Hollinshead et al., 1980, 1982).

As reported in Section 1, Reisfeld et al. (1980) have suggested that the carbohydrate portion of the melanoma TAA is loosely bound. Our experience suggests that the intact glycolipoprotein produces the greatest response in vivo. However, work by others on a different antigen suggests that it is the protein rather than the carbohydrate that is the important part of the antigenic determinant (Morris et al., 1975). In these studies (Morris et al., 1975), IgG and the divalent $F(ab')_2$ and univalent $F(ab')$ antigen-binding fragments of anti-carcino-embryonic antigen (CEA) all produced equivalent inhibition curves, and thus increased avidity to bivalent binding to a single antigen molelcule would not explain the sensitivity observed in the CEA assay; the authors conclude that the high sensitivity implicated the protein rather than the carbohydrate as an important antigenic determinant of CEA. The presence of specific antimelanoma IgG as well as native common melanoma antigen has been reported by others (Kristensen et al., 1976), and the possibility of further analysis of antigenic sites for melanoma TAA should be studied. Subsequent work has suggested the presence of immunoreactive IgG in all and IgM in some melanoma sera (Gupta et al., 1979b). Others are also studying the possibility of antibodies against melanoma by the somatic-cell hybrid method (Koprowski et al., 1978). Klingler et al. (1977) have reported a spectrum of atypical melanosomal proteins in human malignant melanoma. One of these antigens was tumor-associated and shown to produce activity in LMI studies. The antigen was associated with membranous organelles and not with soluble cytoplasmic material (Kerney et al., 1977). Carrel et al. (1980) have described monoclonal antibodies that appear to be directed against common melanoma antigens present in membrane-enriched fractions from melanoma cell line Me43. Other organelles contain antigenic materials; for example, microsomal antigens were shown to produce responses in vivo (Klingler et al., 1977). The development and production of antigens during the course of transformation and during different phases of individual cell growth must be studied in detail. Studies of NK cells and studies with highly purified radiolabeled antigens or mon-

TABLE III

Cancer Serum Indexes of Stage IV Melanoma Patients Treated by Cytoreductive Surgery and Immunochemotherapy[a]

Patient No.	Dates and Cancer Serum Indices							
31	12/4/78 1.1	2/05/79 1.8	4/22/80 1.7					
32	11/8/77 1.8	2/14/78 1.7	2/27/78 1.7	5/10/78 1.9	7/24/78 1.9	11/20/78 1.6	4/17/79 3.0	8/28/79 5.3
33	1/16/80 4.5	1/18/80 4.3	4/09/80 2.9					
34	11/28/78 1.6	3/05/79 4.7	4/03/79 5.7	4/05/79 5.5				
35	9/12/78 0.7	9/25/78 1.5	10/23/78 1.8	11/27/78 1.6	2/21/79 1.5			
36	4/14/76 1.9	2/10/77 1.5	5/23/77 1.8	11/10/77 1.4	11/18/77 1.6	11/20/78 1.5	2/14/79 1.7	3/22/79 1.8
37	2/20/80 6.3	2/27/80 6.0						
38	1/19/79 4.5	2/16/79 1.9						
40	9/28/78 1.5	11/08/78 1.4	1/08/79 1.8	2/27/79 2.4	3/13/79 5.8	3/20/79 4.5		
41	6/28/78 1.7	8/02/78 2.4	9/20/78 2.5	1/23/79 2.3	1/30/79 2.1	2/07/79 2.6	2/18/79 3.1	
42	6/22/77 1.5							
43	4/27/77 2.1	10/20/78 10.8	1/16/79 5.8	1/22/79 6.6				
44	12/20/76 1.8							

Patient								
45	8/31/77 2.1	9/21/77 3.4	1/11/77 4.4	1/30/78 6.3	2/12/78 4.8	2/27/78 4.0	9/18/78 5.1	10/19/78 7.5
	10/23/78 7.9	1/25/79 12.3	1/30/79 21.0					
46	7/14/76 4.2	9/01/76 3.4	9/14/76 3.5	4/11/77 4.5	5/26/77 5.4			
47	10/16/78 9.8	10/19/78 12.2						
48	11/26/76 2.4	11/29/76 2.4	1/26/77 3.0	2/07/77 2.0	2/15/77 4.4	4/11/77 2.1	4/18/77 2.9	8/31/77 2.6
	10/04/77 3.0	11/21/77 4.0	2/08/78 5.2					
49	10/13/78 2.4							
50	4/02/76 2.8	5/17/76 4.4	5/20/76 6.0	6/08/76 10.6	6/16/76 7.7	6/23/76 3.4	6/30/76 3.8	8/04/76 9.2
	9/15/76 5.4	10/21/76 18.5	11/29/76 2.7					
51	8/28/79 2.2	11/19/79 4.6		1/14/77 5.7	2/18/77 48.5			
52	2/08/76 2.7	2/27/76 3.8	3/26/76 1.9	5/12/76 2.1	6/09/76 1.4	6/16/76 2.1	6/23/76 2.5	8/02/76 3.0
	9/02/76 3.1	9/14/76 4.0	10/21/76 3.5					
53	3/17/76 2.7	4/17/76 1.8	9/01/76 2.2					
54	7/17/78 11.9	9/12/78 9.5						
55	5/10/79 1.3							

a Data are for Patients 31–38 and 40–55 (see Hollinshead et al., 1982). Significance of CSI: normal, 1.14 (S.D. 0.37); elevated, > 2.0; highly significant, > 2.5.

ospecific antibodies or both, in double competitive assays, may permit a better understanding of the biology and clinical responsiveness in melanoma patients. Our clinical observations (Arlen et al., 1977; Hollinshead et al., 1980, 1982; Hollinshead and Stewart, 1979) and those of Stein et al. (1979) have contributed additional information of value.

2.2. Nonspecific Humoral Immunity

The humoral changes as well as the cellular changes are important, and the studies of certain serum proteins are more useful in understanding prognosis. Thus, the artificial separation of CMI and humoral immune parameters should be replaced by humoral–systemic immunity (HSI) evaluations. In Table III, we list the results of retrospective studies performed on sera collected from Stage III melanoma patients. Previous studies (Hollinshead and Chuang, 1978; Hollinshead et al., 1977) indicated that a Cancer Serum Index (CSI) might be useful in following tumor load and in assessing the effects of therapy. As shown in Table III, a number of retrospective observations were possible. Patient 31 was free of tumor after surgical debulking plus immunochemotherapy and remains free of disease. Patient 32 had no evidence of disease for 2 years and then, by clinical examination and by X-ray, was seen to develop a retroperitoneal mass. However, the CSI shows a rise 7 months before the recurrence was detectable clinically. Following second surgery and further immunochemotherapy, the CSI decreased to 2.9, and as of September 1980, there is no evidence of disease for 6 months. Patient 33 responded to therapy, but shows a significant CSI 1 month before clinical detection of progression. Patient 34 did not respond to chemotherapy (0.7 to 1.8) but the addition of immunotherapy had a slight effect. Patient 35 has CSIs within normal limits and has had no evidence of disease. A positive CSI was evident for Patient 36 4 months before clinical evidence of reappearance of disease. We have only one serum for Patient 37, 2 weeks after surgical debulking. Similarly, for Patient 38, we have only one serum specimen taken 4 months prior to expiration. In Patient 40, the CSIs, reflect low levels at the time of 80% regression of tumor, but are elevated 1 month prior to detection of liver metastases and are highly significant at the time of liver metastasis. Patient 41 had complete clinical regression for a period of 1 year; however, the CSIs, were slightly elevated after the 2nd month and were significantly high 4 months before detection of gastrointestinal metastases. The one serum sample for Patient 42 indicates successful excision of a scar recurrence. The CSI for Patient 43 indicated a highly elevated CSI prior to detection of brain metastases, followed by lower but highly significant CSIs, indicating a lack of response to treatment. Again, we have only one serum for Patient 44, 2 weeks postsurgery. A total of 11 serum samples from Patient 45 show partial, unsatisfactory reactions to treatment and a progressive, steadily rising CSI, reflective of metastatic spread, prior to expiration. Serum samples were available for Patient 46 during the early period of treatment with no clinical evidence of disease; however, the CSI did not return to normal, and suggests a failure of complete response to combination treatment. Patient 47 expired within 2 months as a result of liver metastases, and the highly significant CSIs reflect the tumor load. Patient 48 had elevated CSIs for a period of 1 year, but the CSI levels became highly significant during the 2nd year, and this patient expired at the end of 2 years with visceral metastases. We have only one serum for Patient 49, who showed a 60% reduction in mass postsurgery, and this is reflected in the significant but not elevated CSI for the serum taken at that time.

The serial sera for Patient 50 are of great interest. The clinical notes indicate a 90% reduction in tumor load by 8 months and at that time a weight gain of 40 pounds. Responses to the first, second, and third courses of immunochemotherapy are reflected in shifts to lower, but still elevated, CSIs, followed by escape from therapy and massive tumor load at the time of expiration. Patient 51 was a 28-year-old man with visceral metastases who had an elevated CSI, with a highly significant CSI at least 1 month prior to expiration. Patient 52 had an elevated CSI, but responded to therapy, as shown in the progressive CSIs, then developed significantly positive indexes prior to expiration. This patient showed an 80% regression in lymph nodes 4 months after the initiation of immunochemotherapy, and this is reflected in a CSI of 1.4 at that period. Clinically, Patient 53 showed no response, but there appeared to be a slight improvement, after which the CSI once again elevated. Patient 54 showed no response to therapy and expired within 3 months, with rapid progression, as indicated by the elevated CSI. There is only one serum sample for Patient 55, taken at the time when the patient was free of disease.

There are no serum samples available for Patients 39 and 56.

We consider the foregoing observations of the parallel between the CSIs and tumor load as well as response to therapy to be highly useful and practical, and we plan to continue the use of this monitor in our next study.

Thus, tumor-associated and more broadly reactive melanoma-cell-membrane antigens have been separated, identified, and characterized using *in vivo* (DCHR) and *in vitro* (ID-IE, LMI) methods. Highly purified melanoma TAA and hyperimmune antibody purified by affinity chromatography were useful in further characterization using ID-IE, IF, and DCHR. Melanoma TAAs from primary and some metastatic sources may share sequences that produce common antigenic reactions, but there are indications of some differences in reactivity, indicating the possible usefulness of polyvalent, allogeneic melanoma TAA for use in specific-active immunotherapy. Whether antibody to melanoma TAA will be useful in carrying drugs to tumor sites awaits sophisticated coupling experiments. In the future, the interference by large amounts of nucleoprotein cell-membrane inhibitory material may be dealt with by use of (1) preliminary antiinhibitor passive immunotherapy, especially in patients with advanced disease, or (2) drugs such as cis-platinum that strip off these inhibitors. In current clinical studies, we find the use of plasmapheresis following immunochemotherapy to be useful in therapy of melanoma patients with advanced disease.

Further, the manner in which ordinary serum proteins predict anergy (fall in PA), inflammation (rise in AGP), or tumor load (ratio of AGP to PA) should be understood in relation to the presence or absence of the nucleoprotein inhibitors as well as to TAA levels and to the more broadly reactive antigens. The interplay between cellular and humoral changes is gradually being understood as a result of the work by many groups. We await the results of cooperative cross-comparisons of our antigens with those identified by other groups.

References

Arlen, M., Hollinshead, A. C., and Scherrer, J., 1977, Tumor-specific immunity in patients with malignant melanoma, *Surg. Forum* **27**:168–169.

Carey, T. E., Lloyd, K. O., Takahashi, T., Travassos, L. R., and Old, L. J., 1979, AU cell-surface antigen in human malignant melanoma: Solubilization and partial characterization, *Proc. Natl. Acad. Sci. U.S.A.* **76**(6):2898–2902.

Carrel, S., Accolla, R. S., Carmagnola, A. L., and Mach, J.-P., 1980, Common human melanoma-associated antigen(s) detected by monoclonal antibodies, *Cancer Res.* **40**:2523–2528.

Char, D. V., Hollinshead, A. C., Cogan, D. G., Ballantine, R. J., Hogan, M. J., and Herberman, R. B., 1974, Cutaneous delayed hypersensitivity reactions to soluble melanoma antigen in patients with ocular malignant melanoma, *N. Engl. J. Med.* **291**:274–277.

Char, D. V., Hollinshead, A. C., and Herberman, R. B., 1977, Skin tests with soluble melanoma antigens in patients with choroidal tumors, *Cancer* **40**:1650–1654.

Ferrone, S., and Pellegrino, M. A., 1979, Serological detection of human melanoma-associated antigens, in: *Immunodiagnosis of Cancer,* Vol. 9, Part I (R. B. Herberman and R. W. McIntire, eds.), pp. 588–632, Marcel Dekker, New York.

Gorodilova, V. A., and Hollinshead, A. C., 1975, Melanoma antigens that produce cell-mediated immune responses in melanoma patients: Joint US–USSR study, *Science* **190**:391–392.

Gorodilova, V. V., Hollinshead, A. C., and Babakova, S. V., 1976, Cell immunity reaction in patients with melanoma, *Vopr. Oncol.* **12**:1–5.

Gupta, R. K., and Morton, D. L., 1980, Specificity by radioimmunoassay of tumor-associated antigen isolated from spent culture medium of a human melanoma cell line, *Fed. Proc. Fed. Am. Soc. Exp. Biol.* **39**:1144 (abstract).

Gupta, R. K., Irie, R. F., Chee, D. O., Kern, D. H., and Morton, D. L., 1979a, Demonstration of two distinct antigens in spent tissue culture medium of a human malignant melanoma cell line, *J. Natl. Cancer Inst.* **63**(2):347–356.

Gupta, R. K., Silver, H. K., Reisfeld, R. A., and Morton, D. L., 1979b, Isolation and immunochemical characterization of antibodies from the sera of cancer patients which are reactive against human melanoma cell membranes by affinity chromatography, *Cancer Res.* **39**:1683–1695.

Helander, I., Nordman, E., Hakkinen, I. P., and Toivanen, A., 1979, Prolonged BCG treatment of melanoma: Does it suppress the immune capacity?, *Br. J. Dermatol.* **101**(4):421–427.

Hersey, P., Edwards, A., and McCarthy, W. H., 1980, Tumor-related changes in natural killer cell activity in melanoma patients: Influences of stage of disease, tumor thickness and age of patients, *Int. J. Cancer* **25**(2):187–194.

Hollinshead, A. C., 1975a, Delayed hypersensitivity reactions to soluble membrane antigens of human malignant melanoma cells in patients with systemic and ocular melanomas, *Fed. Proc. Fed. Am. Soc. Exp. Biol.* **34**:1042.

Hollinshead, A. C., 1975b, Analysis of soluble melanoma cell membrane antigens in metastatic cells of various organs and further studies of antigens present in primary melanoma, *Cancer* **36**:1282–1288.

Hollinshead, A. C., 1978, Active-specific immunotherapy, in: *Immunotherapy of Human Cancer,* pp. 213–233, Raven Press, New York.

Hollinshead, A. C., 1979a, Skin tests to identify TAA of melanoma for use in immunotherapy and to produce antisera to purified TAA for the development of radioimmunoassay, in: *Compendium of Assays for Immunodiagnosis of Human Cancer* (R. B. Herberman, ed.), pp. 605–610, Elsevier/North-Holland, New York.

Hollinshead, A. C., 1979b, Melanoma tumor rejection antigen and its interrelationship with inhibitory or suppressor substances *in vivo* and *in vitro,* Symp. Abst. No. 6, Proc. VII Mtg. Intl. Oncodevelopmental Bio. and Med: Tumour Markers, Guilford, U. K.

Hollinshead, A. C., and Chuang, C. Y., 1978, Evaluation of the relationships of prealbumin components in sera of patients with cancer, (Natl. Cancer Inst. Monogr. **49**:187–192.

Hollinshead, A. C., and Stewart, T. H. M., 1979, Specific-active immunotherapy and specific-active immunoprophylaxis in lung cancer, in: *Advances in Medical Oncology Research and Education,* Vol. 6, *Basis for Cancer Therapy 2* (Moore, ed.), pp. 85–94, Pergamon Press, New York.

Hollinshead, A. C., Jaffurs, W., Alpert, L., and Herberman, R., 1973, Specific soluble membrane antigen of malignant and normal breast cells: Delayed hyper-sensitive skin reactions in cancer patients, Proc. II Intl. Sym. of Cancer Detection and Prevention, Bologna, Italy, pp. 647–654.

Hollinshead, A. C., Herberman, R., Jaffurs, W., Alpert, L., Minton, J. P., and Harris, J. E., 1974, Soluble membrane antigens of human malignant melanoma cells, *Cancer* **34**:1235–1243.

Hollinshead, A. C., Chuang, C. Y., Cooper, E. H., and Catalona, W. J., 1977, Interrelationship of prealbumin and alpha$_1$-acid glycoprotein in cancer patient sera, *Cancer* **40**(6):2993–2998.

Hollinshead, A. C., Stewart, T. H. M., Yonemoto, R., Arlen, M., and Takita, H., 1980, Immunotherapy of advanced disease, in: *Tumor Progression* (R. G. Crispin, ed.), pp. 289–300, Elsevier/North-Holland, New York.

Hollinshead,, A. C., Arlen, M., Yonemoto, R., Cohen, M., Tanner, K., Kundin, W. D., and Scherrer, J., 1982, Pilot studies using melanoma tumor-associated antigen (TAA) in specific-active immunochemotherapy of malignant melanoma *Cancer* **49:** in press.

Hughes, L. E., Kearney, R., and Tully, M., 1970, A study in clinical cancer immunotherapy, *Cancer* **26:**269–278.

Ishii, Y., and Mavligit, G., 1979, Soluble melanoma antigen: Its characterization and diagnostic detection by radioimmunoassay, in: *Compendium of Assays for Immunodiagnosis of Human Cancer,* Vol. 1 (R. B. Herberman, ed.), pp. 591–596, Elsevier/North-Holland, New York.

Jassem, J., Moszkowska, G., Mlodkowska, A., and Jaskiewicz, J., 1979, IgG, IgA and IgM levels and the presence of autoimmune antibodies against nuclei and smooth muscle in patients with malignant melanoma, *Pol. Tyg. Lek.* **34**(21):813–816.

Kerney, S. E., Montague, P. M., Chretien, P. B., Nicholson, J. M., Ekel, T. M., and Hearing, V. J., 1977, Intracellular localization of tumor-associated antigens in murine and human malignant melanoma, *Cancer Res.* **37:**1519–1524.

Klingler, W. G., Montague, P. M., Chretien, P. B., and Hearing, V. J., 1977, Atypical melanosomal proteins in human malignant melanoma, *Arch. Dermatol.* **113:**19–23.

Koprowski, H., Steplewski, Z., Herlyn, D., and Herlyn, M., 1978, Study of antibodies against human melanoma produced by somatic cell hybrids, *Proc. Natl. Acad. Sci. U.S.A.* **75**(7):3405–3409.

Kristensen, E., Langvad, E., and Reimann, R., 1976, Humoral immunity in malignant skin melanoma: Isolation of melanoma specific IgG from melanoma metastases, *Eur. J. Cancer* **12:**945–950.

Lewis, M. G., and Phillips, T. M., 1972, The specificity of surface membrane immunofluorescence in human malignant melanoma, *Int. J. Cancer* **10:**105–111.

Lewis, M. G., Phillips, T. M., Noble, P. B., and Hartmann, D. P., 1979, Immune derangement in patients with malignant melanoma, *J. Cutan. Pathol.* **6**(3):201–207.

Liao, S. K., Rahman, A. F., Kwong, P. C., and Dent, P. B., 1979, A simple microassay for detection of antibodies to fetal calf serum and related antigens and its application to the serological definition of human tumor antigens, *J. Immunol. Methods* **27**(2):111–125.

Morgan, A. C., Halloway, D. M., Imai, K., Ferrone, S., and Reisfeld, R. A., 1980, The effects of inhibitors of glycosylation on the shedding and cell surface expression of human melanoma-associated antigens, *Fed. Proc. Fed. Am. Soc. Exp. Biol.* **39:**351 (abstract).

Morris, J. E., Egan, M. L., and Todd, C. W., 1975, The binding of carcinoembryonic antigen by antibody and its fragments, *Cancer Res.* **35:**1804–1808.

Natali, P. G., Cordiali, P., Cavalieri, R., Di Filippo, F., Quaranta, V., Pellegrino, M. A., and Ferrone, S., 1980, Reactivity of HLA-DR monoclonal antibodies with freshly explanted melanoma cells, but not with nevi cells, *Fed. Proc. Fed. Am. Soc. Exp. Biol.* **39:**684 (abstract).

Ninger, E., Zemanova, D., Kovarik, J., and Lauerova, L., 1979, Evaluation of three E-rosette assays in melanoma patients, *Cancer Immunol. Immunother.* **6**(2):121–124.

Otterstrom, J. R., 1979, Research on the nature of tumor rejection antigens of an ultraviolet light induced murine skin tumor, *Diss. Abstr. Int. B* **40**(4):1695B.

Reisfeld, R. A., Galloway, D., Imai, K., Ferrone, S., and Morgan, A. C., 1980, Molecular profiles of human melanoma associated antigens, *Fed. Proc. Fed. Am. Soc. Exp. Biol.* **39:**351 (abstract).

Saxton, R. E., Burk, M., Meier, S., and Morton, D. L., 1980, Hybridoma monoclonal antibody: Use in defining unique antigens on human melanoma cells, *Fed. Proc. Fed. Am. Soc. Exp. Biol.* **39:**1144 (abstract).

Stein, J. A., Adler, A., Czernobilsky, B., Goldfarb, A. J., Rozin, R. R., Teva, Z., and Stavorovsky, M., 1979, Cutaneous response to autochthonous tumor cells in breast cancer and melanoma patients by active immunization, *Proceedings of the Serono Symposia,* Vol. 16, *Tumor-Associated Antigens and Their Specific Immune Response* , pp. 343–353.

Stuhlmiller, G., and Seigler, H. F., 1979, Melanoma cell membrane tumor-associated antigens in: *Compendium of Assays for Immunodiagnosis of Human Cancer,* Vol. 1 (R. B. Herberman, ed.), pp. 591–596, Elsevier/North-Holland, New York.

Thatcher, N., Swindell, R., and Crowther, D., 1979, Effects of repeated *Corynebacterium parvum* and BCG therapy on immune parameters: A weekly study of melanoma patients. II. Changes in serum immunoglobulins and lymphoid cell subpopulations, *Clin. Exp. Immunol.* **36**(3):456–464.

Vandenbark, A. A., Greene, M. H., Burger, D. R., Vetto, R. M., and Relmer, R. R., 1979, Immune response to melanoma extracts in three melanoma-prone families, *J. Natl. Cancer Inst.* **63**(5):1147–1151.

Van Der Giessen, M., The, T. H., Schraffordt Kiips, H., Van Wingerden, I., and Rumke, P. H., 1978, Detection, isolation and characterization of immune complexes in malignant melanoma, *Protides Biol. Fluids Proc. Colloq.* **26**:341–344.

Van Wingerden, I., The, T. H., Van Der Giessen, M. and Rumke, P. H., 1978, Demonstration of circulating immune complexes in melanoma patients by means of a granulocyte phagocytosis test, *Protides Biol. Fluids Proc. Colloq.* **26**:345–348.

West, W. H., 1979, E-rosette formation in immunodiagosis, in: *Immunodiagnosis of Cancer*, Vol. 9, Part 2 (R. B. Herberman and R. W. McIntire, eds.), pp. 704–721, Marcel Dekker, New York.

Winkelhake, J. L., Elcombe, B. M., and Hodach, A., 1979, Immunological block to synthetic alpha-melanocyte-stimulating hormone–melanocyte interaction by antibodies isolated from cell column immunoadsorbents, *Cancer Res.* **39**(8):3058–3064.

Yeh, M. Y., Hellström, I., Brown, J. P., Warner, H. A., Hansen, J. A., and Hellström, K. E., 1979, Cell surface antigens of human melanoma identified by monoclonal antibody, *Proc. Natl. Acad. Sci. U.S.A.* **76**(6):2927–2931.

13

Immunodiagnosis of Human Melanoma: Detection of Circulating Melanoma-Associated Antigens by Radioimmunoassay

Yoshifumi Ishii and Giora M. Mavligit

1. Introduction

Immunodiagnosis of cancer may provide a powerful ancillary tool for more accurate staging and judicious clinical management of patients with neoplastic disease. This is particularly true in disease categories where a high incidence of complete clinical remission can be achieved by the current therapeutic modalities. Under these circumstances, with subclinical disease in all likelihood still present, an accurate secondary tumor staging is crucial for evaluation, planning, and monitoring of further treatment. The use of a sensitive immunodiagnostic procedure under these circumstances may detect evidence for the presence of minute amounts of actively growing residual tumor, as reflected by spontaneous release of tumor antigens into the circulation (Alexander, 1974).

Heterologous antiserum raised against human melanoma has been shown to distinguish melanoma-associated antigens (MAAs) from other nonspecific cellular components (Metzgar *et al.*, 1973; Stuhlmiller and Seigler, 1975; Fritze *et al.*, 1976; Jehn *et al.*, 1970). More recently, monoclonal antibody against human melanoma cells has been developed and used to define MAAs on the cell surfaces (Steplewski *et al.*, 1979; Yeh *et al.*, 1979). As in the case of carcinoembryonic antigen (CEA) and α-fetoprotein (AFP) determination,

Yoshifumi Ishii and Giora M. Mavligit • Department of Developmental Therapeutics, M. D. Anderson Hospital and Tumor Institute, Houston, Texas 77030.

the use of such xenoantiserum carries the potential for immunodiagnosis, once the purification of the relevant antigens is achieved (Herberman, 1976). Several groups including ours have reported that MAAs can be extracted in an antigenic form either by using hypertonic KCl or by low-frequency sonication or limited papain digestion (Mavligit *et al.*, 1973; Hollinshead *et al.*, 1974; Thomson *et al.*, 1976). These extracts may therefore provide a suitable source of antigenic material to raise specific antibodies in heterologous animals. We wish to report on our preliminary experience with the development of radioimmunoassy (RIA) using KCl-extracted MAAs and antimelanoma xenoantiserum and its use for immunodiagnosis of human melanoma.

2. Materials and Methods

2.1. Antigen Preparation

Fresh tumor and normal tissues were finely minced and washed thoroughly with phosphate-buffered saline (PBS), and 1 volume of tissue fragments was suspended in 9 volumes of 3 M KCl (Reisfeld *et al.*, 1971). Suspensions of leukocytes and leukemia cells were also washed and resuspended in 3 M KCl. The mixture was gently stirred for 20 hr at $4°C$ and spun at $100,000g$ for 1 hr. The supernatant was collected, dialyzed against PBS, and recentrifuged at $100,000g$ for 1 hr. The supernatant was again collected, concentrated, and stored at $-80°C$ until use.

2.2. Antisera

Anti-human leukocyte serum (ALS) was prepared by repeated immunization of rabbits with 1×10^8 pooled human leukocytes mixed with Freund incomplete adjuvant. The γ-globulin fraction of ALS was coupled with a Sepharose 4B column (Porath *et al.*, 1973). A 10-mg aliquot of the crude melanoma extract obtained from a single melanoma patient was loaded onto the column, and the effluent was collected. This procedure was repeated until the effluent no longer showed any reactivity with ALS in Ouchterlony double diffusion. The final effluent was dialyzed against PBS and filtered through a Millipore membrane. Rabbits were immunized weekly with 2 mg of the ALS-absorbed melanoma antigen emulsified with Freund incomplete adjuvant for 4 weeks. The animals were bled 10 days after the last injection. Next, 1 volume of the antiserum was absorbed with 2 volumes of normal human serum (HNS) and with 3 volumes of mixed normal tissue extracts (10 mg/ml). The resulting immunoprecipitates were removed by centrifugation at $100,000$ g for 1 hr. This serum showed no reactivity with NHS and normal tissue extracts in double diffusion and immunoelectrophoresis and was used as a specific anti-human melanoma serum (AHMS). The preimmune normal rabbit serum (NRS) was similarly absorbed and served as a control. Rabbit antisera to mouse B16 melanoma cells were prepared by immunizing rabbits weekly with 2×10^7 cultured B16 cells for 4 weeks. The serum was absorbed with mouse red cells, spleen cells, and liver homogenate and was used as anti-mouse melanoma serum (AMMS).

2.3. Radioiodinated Melanoma-Associated Antigens

Antigenic materials were separated from crude human melanoma extracts by using a Sepharose 4B column coupled with unabsorbed AHMS. Bound material was eluted from the column with 3 M KCNS, dialyzed against PBS, and concentrated to 1 mg/ml. The sample was redialyzed against 0.5 M phosphate buffer (pH 7.5), and 20 μg of the protein was labeled with ^{125}I by the chloramine T method. Since the reagent was still reactive with rabbit anti-NHS serum in radiobinding assay, the labeled reagent was passed through a Sepharose 4B column coupled with anti-NHS antibodies. The unbound fraction was collected and further applied to a Sepharose 4B column coupled with concanavalin A (Con A). Since, as will be described later, the Con-A-bound fraction that was eluted by adding to the column 0.5 M D-methylmannoside had a strong MAA activity, it was used as labeled MAAs for RIA. Radiolabeled MAAs were similarly purified from mouse B16 melanoma extract by using AMMS and Con-A-coupled Sepharose 4B affinity columns.

2.4. Radioimmunoassy

MAAs were detected by measuring the ability of a test sample to inhibit the direct binding reaction of labeled MAAs with antimelanoma antisera. Dilution of teh antimelanoma serum (AMS) required to bind 50% of the labeled MAAs was defined from a titration curve. A 100-μl aliquot of appropriately diluted AMS was mixed with 100 μl tissue extracts or melanoma sera and incubated at 37°C for 1 hr and at 4°C for 20 hr. Labeled MAAs (30,000 cpm) were then added to each test tube, and the mixture was incubated at 37°C for 2 hrs. Antigen–anitbody complexes were precipitated by adding an excess of goat anti-rabbit immunoglobulin (IgG). A 10-μl aliquot of undiluted NRS was added to all tubes to provide carrier immunoglobulin. After incubation at 37°C for 1 hr and at 4°C for 20 hr, immunoprecipitates were washed twice with PBS, and their radioactivity was counted in a Packard gamma counter. The results were expressed in terms of precentage inhibition of the binding reaction.

2.5. Sodium Dedecyl Sulfate–Polyacrylamide Gel Electrophoresis

For sodium dodecyl sulfate–polyacrylamide gel electrophoresis (SDA-PAGE), 50 μl of a 1 : 5 dilution of the antiserum was incubated with labeled antigens, and the radioactivity bound to the antiserum was precipitated by adding 300 μl 10% *Staphylococcus aureus* Cowan I (SACI) to the mixture (Cullen and Schwartz, 1976). After 30 min at 37°C, the bacteria were washed three times with PBS, suspended in 200 μl 50 mM Tris-CHl (pH 7.0) containing 2% SDS with or without 5% mercaptoethanol, heated in a boiling water bath for 4 min, and centrifuged at 4000 g for 20 min. The supernatant was collected and loaded onto a 10% SDS–polyacrylamide tube gel (Laemmli, 1970). The gel was electrophoresed at 3 mA/tube. After electrophoresis, the get was cut into 2-mm slices, and the radioactivity of the slices was measured. Protein standards and their molecular weights were phosphorylase B (94,000), bovine serum albumin (67,000), ovalbumin (43,000), carbonic anhydrase (30,000), trypsin inhibitor (20,100), and α-lactalbumin (14,4000).

3. Results

3.1. Melanoma-Associated Antigens in B16 Mouse Melanoma and in Sera of B16-Melanoma-Bearing Mice

Table I shows that labeled MAAs can be partially purified by sequential chromatographic separation using AMMS and Con-A-coupled Sepharose 4B affinity columns. Labeled MAAs that could be bound to both AMMS and Con A were used for radioimmunoprecipitation (RIP) in this study, and it was found that 47.5% of the labeled MAA preparations were specifically bound to the antiserum.

Similar experiments were conducted to partially purify MAAs from unlabeled B16 melanoma extract. MAA activity in each fraction was monitored by RIA using labeled MAA preparations and AMMS. As can be seen in Table II, MAAs were copurified with tyrosinase by using a Con A affinity column. However, MAAs were separated from tyrosinase by the following purification step using an AMMS-coupled Sepharose 4B column, since the latter activity was found exclusively in the unbound fraction of the column effluent.

MAA activity in fractions obtained from each purification step was estimated more quantitatively by RIA using different concentrations of the sample (Fig. 1). MAA activity in Con-A-bound material was found to be 4 times higher than that in the crude KCl extract

TABLE I

Purification of Iodinated Melanoma-Associated Antigens from B16 Melanoma Extract

Column[a]	Added cpm	AMS	NRS	Specific binding
AMMS	111,263	42,046	23,162	18,884 (16.97%)
Con A				
Unbound	45,099	3,904	1,750	2,154 (4.78%)
Bound	23,530	12,061	877	11,184 (47.53%)

[a]Bound protein to an AMS-coupled Sepharose 4B column was iodinated by the chloramine T method and separated into unbound and bound fractions by Con A affinity-column chromatography.

TABLE II

Purification of Melanoma-Associated Antigens from B16 Melanoma

Column[a]	Fraction	Protein (mg/ml)	MAAs (% inhibition)	Dopa oxidation ($A475 \times 10^3$)
Crude	—	2.0	74.06	26
Con A	Unbound	2.0	21.91	10
	Bound	2.0	93.06	42
Con A	Unbound	0.4	30.99	33
+ AMMS	Bound	0.08	69.38	0

[a]Affinity column coupled with either Con A or AMMS.

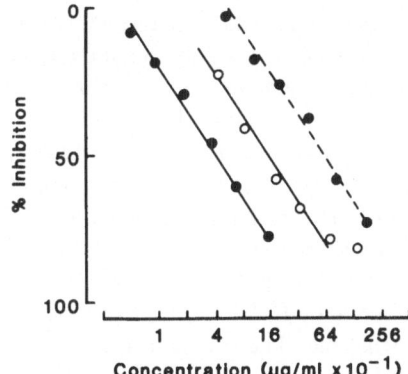

FIGURE 1. Standard inhibition curve. (●——●) Crude B16 melanoma extract; (O——O) Con-A-bound fraction; (●——●) Con-A- and AMMS-bound fraction.

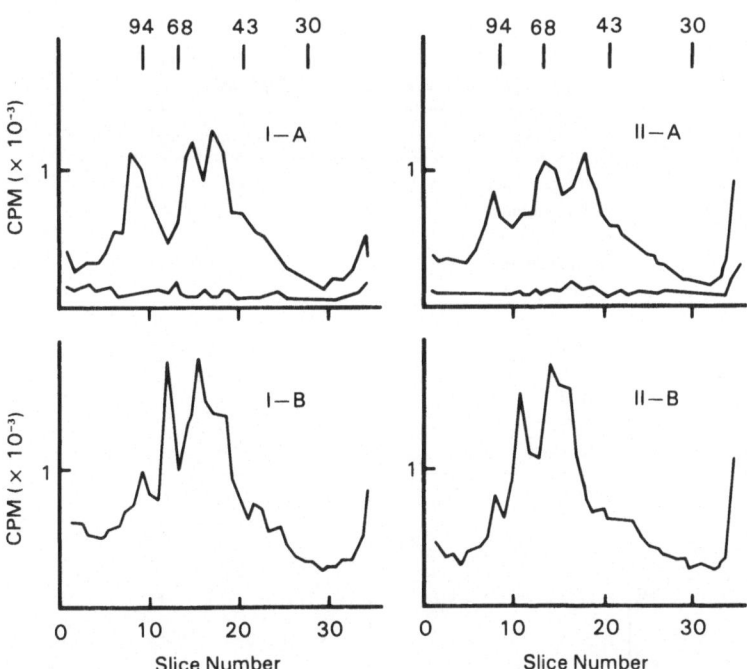

FIGURE 2. SDS-PAGE profiles of labeled MAAs precipitated with AMMS (A). Original [^{125}I]-MAA was run in the parallel gels (B). Electrophoregrams were compared for reduced (I) and nonreduced samples (III).

of B16 melanoma. Wehn the Con-A-bound fraction was further pruified by an AMMS-coupled Sepharose 4B column, 16-fold purification of MAAs was achieved when compared to the crude melanoma extract.

Molecular-weight profiles of labeled MAAs were analyzed by RIP and SDS-PAGE (Fig. 2). AMMS precipitated two major components with molecular weights of 68,000 and 54,000 from the labeled MAA preparation. A relatively small peak around the 94,000 gel region was also noticed. These three antigenic components were thought to be glycoproteins because of their ability to adhere to Con A, and furthermore, they appeared not to have disulfide bonds in their structure because their electrophoretic mobilities in SDS-PAGE were not influenced by the reducing condition.

Tissue distribution of MAAs as measured by RIA is shown in Table III. MAAs exist largely in B16 melanoma tissue and to much lesser extent in Harding–Passey (HP) allogeneic melanoma. Syngeneic C57BL fetal tissue and normal tissues including skin and brain showed less than 7% of MAA activity compared to that in B16 melanoma tissue.

Finally, MAAs possibly present in sera of B16-melanoma-bearing C57BL mice were detected by RIA. Sera were collected from mice carrying different weights of growing B16 melanoma. The results in Fig. 3 show a parallel relationship between the tumor burden and the amount of circulating MAAs. This may provide a rational basis for clinical immunodiagnosis among melanoma patients by using a similar assay system.

TABLE III

Distribution of Melanoma-Associated Antigens
among Various Tissues in C57BL Mice

Tissue types	MAAs (units/mg)[a]
B16 melanoma	120
HP melanoma	12
Fetus	5
Normal tissues	
Kidney	3
Liver	5
Skin	7
Lung	3
Brain	1
Spleen	4
Red cell	0

[a]MAAs in 1 μg purified antigen preparation ($= 2$ units).

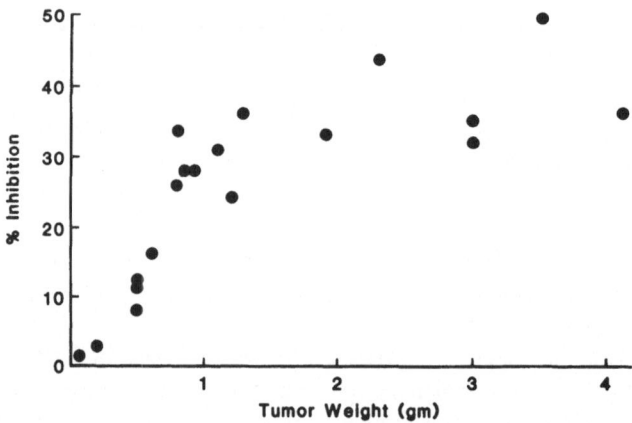

FIGURE 3. Circulating B16 melanoma antigen in tumor-bearing C57BL mice.

3.2. Melanoma-Associated Antigens in Human Melanoma and Immunodiagnosis in Melanoma Patients

Antigenic material that reacted with AHMS was separated by an AHMS-coupled Sepharose 4B affinity column, radioiodinated by the chloramine T method, and further purified by a Con-A-coupled Sepharose 4B column, Contaminating serum proteins, mostly serum albumin, were removed by passing the labeled sample through a Sepharose 4B column coupled with anti-NHS. After partial purification, 42–45% of a labeled MAA sample could be bound to either unabsorbed or absorbed AHMS (Table IV).

RIP and SDS-PAGE analysis of immunoprecipitates formed between labeled MAAs and AHMS disclosed that AHMS precipitated two major components with molecular weights of 37,000 and 31,000, respectively (Fig. 4). An additional small peak was also found around the 80,000 region. These components seemed to be glycoproteins and to have no disulfide bonds because of the same reasons described above.

To assess a possible relationship between MAAs detected by AHMS and human leukocyte antigen *(HLA)* complex antigens or antigens cross-reacting with bacillus Calmette Guérin (BCG) (Minden *et al.,* 1976), labeled MAA, were reacted with rabbit antisera to either β_2-microglobulin (β_2m) or BCG (Table V). We found negligible binding between labeled MAAs and these antisera, suggesting that AHMS detects neither HLA(A,B,C) nor BCG-related cross-antigens.

Tissue distribution of MAAs in different human tumor and normal tissues was studied by RIA using KC1 extracts of these tissues. First, KC1 extracts of melanoma, muscle, erythrocytes, and leukocytes were obtained from a single melanoma patient and were tested for MAA activity (Fig. 5). While the melanoma extract showed a strong reactivity with AHMS, autologous normal-cell extracts contained less than 7% MAA activity compared to that in the melanoma extract. Several melamona extracts (2 mg/ml) obtained from different melanoma patients were similarly tested, and all but one showed strong inhibition of the binding of labeled MAAs to AHMS. Nonmelanoma tumors and normal tissues showed less than 10% MAA content (Fig. 6).

Sera from 45 melanoma patients with various stages of the disease were tested by RIA for the detection of putative circulating MAAs. Sera from normal donars and colon-cancer patients (Dukes' D) with high serum CEA levels served as controls. As shown in Fig. 7, there is a correlation between disease staging and amounts of circulating MAAs. While control sera always showed 15% or less inhibition, melanoma sera frequently showed more than 15% inhibition, especially in patients with Stage IV disease (Table VI).

TABLE IV

Purification of Radioiodinated Melanoma-Associated Antigens by Affinity Chromatography

Affinity column coupler	Fraction	Antimelanoma serum[a]	
		Unabsorbed	Absorbed
AHMS	Bound	61.45	15.20
Anti-NHS	Unbound	21.23	20.11
Con A	Unbound	4.00	4.07
	Bound	44.84	42.31

[a] Values are expressed as percentages of bound relative to total radioactivity.

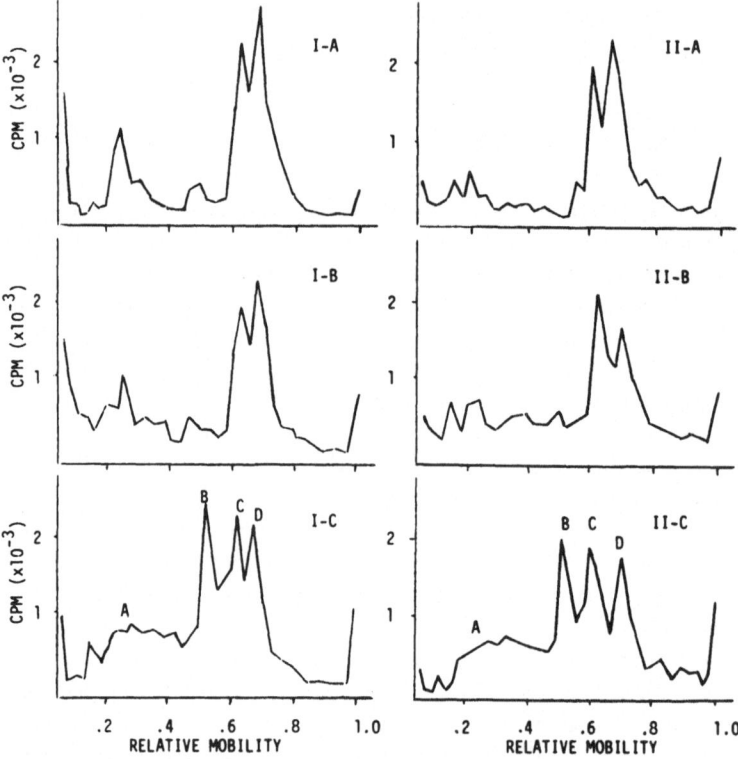

FIGURE 4. SDS-PAGE profiles of [125I]-labeled MAAs precipitated with either unabsorbed (A) or absorbed AHMS (B). Original [125I]-MAA was run in the parallel SDS gels (C). Electrophoregrams were compared for nonreduced (I) and reduced samples (II). Molecular-weight peaks: (A) 80,000; (B) 50,000; (C) 37,000; (D) 31,000.

TABLE V
*Reactivity of Melanoma-Associated Antigens
with Different Antisera[a]*

Antiserum to:	[125I] Antigen	Specific binding (%)
Melanoma	MAA	43.39
Leukocytes	MAA	2.83
NHS	MAA	0.28
β_2m	MAA	0.31
	β_2m	61.10
BCG		
Serum 1	MAA	0.87
Serum 2	MAA	1.07
gp70	MAA	0.22
	gp70	72.63

[a] A 100-μl aliquot of antiserum (1 : 10 dilution) was incubated with labeled antigens (20,000 cpm). Immune complexes were precipitated with either anti-IgG antibodies or SACI.

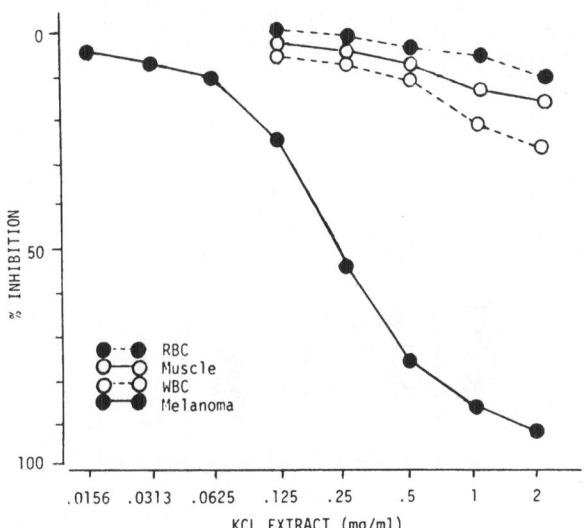

FIGURE 5. MAAs in different tissues and cells from a single melanoma patient.

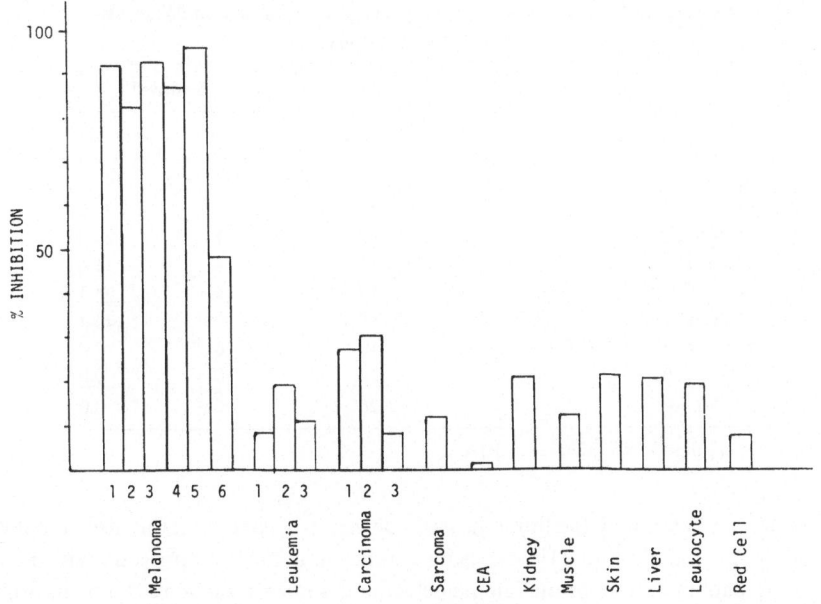

FIGURE 6. Tissue distribution of MAAs.

4. Discussion

A variety of tumor-associated antigens have been found in the blood circulation of patients with malignant neoplastic disease (Herberman, 1976). Sensitive RIA techniques are now available for detecting minute amounts of circulating CEA or AFP (Shuster *et al.*,

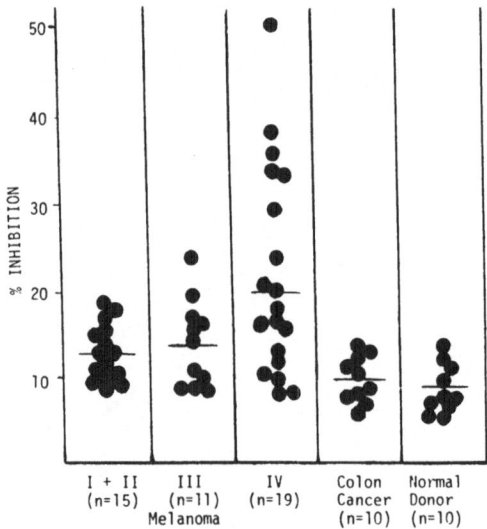

FIGURE 7. Detection of MAAs in melanoma sera.

TABLE VI

Detection of Melanoma-Associated Antigens in Melanoma Sera by Radioimmunoassay

		Positive[a]	
Sera	Number	Number	%
Melanoma			
Stage I	10	2	20.0
Stage II	5	1	20.0
Stage III	11	4	36.4
Stage IV	19	13	68.4
TOTALS:	45	20	44.4
Colon cancer (Dukes' D)	10	0	0.0
Normal donors	10	0	0.0
TOTALS:	20	0	0.0

[a]More than 15% inhibition in RIA.

1978), which can potentially facilitate the early detection of cancer. In the case of malignant melanoma, Viza and Phillips (1975), using counterimmunoelectrophoresis with xenantibodies to the papain extract of melanoma cells, have shown positive reactions in approximately 20% of melanoma patients' sera. Carrel and Theilkaes (1973) detected MAAs in melanoma patients' urine. Furthermore, Grosser and Thomson (1976) showed by using leukoycte-adherence inhibition (LAI) tests that sera of patients with advanced melanoma contained an excess of MAAs that could block LAI reactivity of patients' leukocytes. On the basis of these reports and since cultured melanoma cells release antigenic components *in vitro* either spontaneously (Grimm *et al.*, 1976) or when they are incubated with specific antibodies (Nordquist *et al.*, 1977), one can safely assume that shedding of human MAAs from growing melanoma cells into the blood circulation of tumor-bearing hosts also occurs *in vivo* as is the case in an animal tumor model (Alexander, 1974).

The results of our preliminary innunodiagnostic testing demonstrate that MAAs circulate in the blood of some but not all patients with malignant melanoma. The amounts of circulating MAAs appear to correlate with the tumor burden, and sera of patients with disseminated melanoma contain much more MAAs than sera from patients with localized tumor. This is further confirmed by animal experiments in which the content of MAAs in sera of B16-melanoma-bearing mice was directly related to the weight of growing tumor. However, we could detect considerable levels of circulating MAAs only in 20–68% of sera from melanoma patients who had localized or disseminated tumors, indicating the limited usefulness of this assay system for initial diagnosis and staging of this maligancy. The reason we could not detect serum MAAs in all patients could be related to the relative insensitivity of RIA developed in this study. It could also be related to MAA heterogeneity; i.e., there may be more than one MAA released by growing melanoma (Ferrone and Pellegrino, 1978), and the AHMS used in this study may be directed against some MAA but not against the other. Alternatively, some MAAs may not be shed in sufficient amounts by the growing melanoma cells, resulting in a relatively low concentration of circulating MAAs. Furthermore, nonmeasurable MAAs could be theoretically related to the presence of antibodies in patients' own sera that can interfere with the serological detection of circulating MAAs. In fact, it has been shown that a considerable amount of immune complexes exists in melanoma sera, particularly after treatment with BCG and attenuated tumor cells (Theofilipoulos et al., 1977). To rule out this possibility, we may have to measure circulating MAAs after presplitting of such putative immune complexes by appropriate procedures.

SDS-PAGE analysis of immunoprecipitates formed between AHMS and baleled MAAs demonstrated that AHMS reacted with two major glycoproteins with molecular weights of 37,000 and 31,000, respectively. The lack of reactivity between MAAs and anti-β_2m serum suggests that the MAAs are unrelated to HLA (A,B,C) antigens. On the other hand, these two components (38,000 and 37,000) resemble HLA-D-related (HLA-DR) antigens in terms of their molecular weights and their ability to bind to *Lens culinaris* hemagglutinin (lentil lectin). Some cultured melanoma cell lines have recently been demonstrated to express immune-associated (Ia)-like (DR) antigens on their cell membrane; (Wilson et al., 1979). Nevertheless, we have not yet tested the reactivity of our MAA preparations with anti-Ia serum. This has to be done and compared with the reactivity of anti-Ia serum against 3 M KC1 extracts of autologous B lymphocytes, which have been reported to express Ia-like antigens on their cell surfaces (Koyama et al., 1977). We also need to determine whether the MAAs are tumor-specific or organ-specific.This would be best achieved by testing the reactivity of AHMS against normal human melanocytes. It is hoped that this work, now under way, will probide important information on the biological and immunochemical nature of MAAs.

References

Alexander, P., 1974, Escape from immune destruction by the host through shedding of surface antigens: Is this a characteristic shared by malignant and embryonic cells), *Cancer Res.* **34**:2077.

Carrel, S., and Theilkaes, L., 1973, Evidence for a tumour-associated antigen in human malignant melanoma, *Nature (London)* **242**:609.

Cullen, S. E., and Schwartz, B. D., 1976, An improved method for isolation of H-2 and Ia alloantigens with immunoprecipitation induced by protein A-bearing staphylocci, *J. Immunol.* **117**:136.

Ferrone, S., and Pellegrino, M. A., 1978, Antigens and antibodies in malignant melanoma, in: *The Handbook of Cancer Immunology* (H. Waters, ed.), pp. 291–327, Garland STPM Press, New York.

Fritze, D., Kern, D. H., Drogemuller, C. R., and Pilch, Y. H., 1976, Production of antisera with specificity for malignant melanoma and human fetal skin, *Cencer Res.* **36**:458.

Grimm, E. A., Silver, K. B., Roth, J. A., Chee, D. O. Gupta, R. K., and Morton, D. L., 1976, Detection of tumor-associated antigen in human melanoma cell line supernatants, *Int. J. Cancer* **17**:559.

Grosser, N., and Thomson, D. M. P., 1976, Tube leukocyte (monocyte) adherence inhibition assay for the detection of anti-tumor immunity. Ill. "Blockade" of monocyte reactivity by excess free antigen and immune complexes in advanced cancer patients, *Int. J. Cancer* **18**:58.

Herberman, R. B., 1976, Immunologic approaches to the diagnosis of cancer, *Cancer* **37**:549.

Hollinshead, A. C., Herberman, R. B., Jaffurs, W. J., Alpert, L. K., Minton, J. P., and Harris, J. E., 1974, Soluble membrane antigens of human malignant melanoma cells, *Cancer* **34**:1235.

Jehn, U. W., Nathanson, L., Schwartz, R. S., and Skinner, M., 1970, *In vitro* lymphocyte stimulation by a soluble antigen from malignant melanoms, *N. Engl. J. Med.* **283**:329.

Koyama, K., Nakamuro, K., Tanigaki, N., and Pressman, D., 1977, Alloantigens of human lymphoid cell lines; "human IA-like antigent" alloantigenic activity and cell line, organ and tissue distribution as determined by radioimmunoassay, *Immunology* **33**:217.

Laemmli, U. K., 1970, Cleavage of structural proteins during the assembly of the head of bacteriophage T4, *Nature (London)* **227**:680.

Mavligit, G. M., Ambus, U., Gutterman, J. U., and Hersh, E. M., 1973, Antigen solubilized from human solid tumours: Lymphocyte stimulation and cutaneous delayed hypersensitivity, *Nature (London) New Biol.* **243**:188.

Metzgar, R. S. Bergoc, P. M., Moreno, M. A., and Seigler, H. F., 1973, Brief communication: Melanoma-specific antibodies produced in monkeys by immunization with human melanoma cell lines, *J. Natl. Cancer Inst.* **50**:1065.

Minden, P., Sharpton, T. R., and McClatchy, J. K., 1976, Shared antigens between human malignant melanoma cells and Mycobacterium bovis (BCG), *J. Immunol.* **116**:1407.

Nordquist, R. E., Anglin, J. H., and Lerner, M. P., 1977, Antibody-induced antigen redistribution and shedding from human breast cancer cells, *Science* **197**:366.

Porath, J., Aspberg, K., Drevin, H., and Axeń, R., 1973, Preparation of cyanogen bromide-activated agarose gels, *J. Chromatogr.* **86**:53.

Reisfeld, R. A., Pellegrino, M. S., and Kahan, B. D., 1971, Salt extraction of soluble HL-A antigens, *Science* **172**:1184.

Shuster, J., Thompson, D. M. P., and Gold, P., 1978, Immunodiagnosis, in: *Immunological Aspects of Cancer* (J. E. Castro, ed.), pp. 283–312, MTP Press, Lancaster.

Steplewski, Z., Herlyn, M., Herlyn, D., Clark, W. H., and Koprowski H., 1979, Reactivity of monoclonal anti-melanoma antibodies with melanoma cells freshly isolated from primary and metastatic melanoma, *Eur. J. Immunol.* **9**:94.

Stuhlmiller, B. M., and Seigler, H. F., 1975, Characterization of a chimpanzee anti-human melanoma antiserum, *Cancer Res.* **35**:2132.

Theofilopoulos, A. N., Andrews, B. S., Marshall, M. U., Morton, D. L., and Dixon, F. J., 1977, The nature of immune complexes in human cancer sera, *J. Immunol.* **119**:657.

Thomson, D. M. P., Gold, P., Freedman, S. O., and Shuster, J., 1976, The isolation and characterization of tumor-specific antigens of rodent and human tumors, *Cancer Res.* **36**:3518.

Viza, D., and Phillips, J., 1975, Identification of an antigen associated with malignant melanoms, *Int. J. Cancer* **16**:312.

Wilson, B. S., Indiveri, F., Pellegrino, M. A., and Ferrone, S., 1979, DR (Ia-like) antigens on human melanoma cells, *J. Exp. Med.* **149**:658.

Yeh, M. Y., Hellström, T., Brown, J. P., Warner, G. A., Hanson, J. A. and Hellström, K. E., 1979, Cell surface antigens of human melanoma indentified by monoclonal antibody, *Proc. Natl. Acad. Sci. U.S.A.* **79**:2927.

14

The Association between Antigens of Human Malignant-Melanoma Cells and *Mycobacterium bovis* (BCG)

PERCY MINDEN, PETER J. KELLEHER, AND LINDA K. WOODS

1. Introduction

Antigenic components shared between *Mycobacterium bovis* (BCG) and certain experimental and human tumors have been demonstrated by a variety of methods (Borsos and Rapp, 1973; Minden *et al.*, 1974; Bucana and Hanna, 1974; Minden *et al.*, 1976a; McCoy *et al.*, 1978; Lewis *et al.*, 1976; Holan *et al.*, 1979). There are also data suggesting that other microorganisms have determinants in common with some tumors (Minden *et al.*, 1976b; Minden, 1976; James *et al.*, 1976; Kwapinski *et al.*, 1978). With respect to human tumors, there is evidence that antigens from human malignant melanoma (Bucana and Hanna, 1974; Minden *et al.*, 1976a) and acute myeloid leukemia (Minden *et al.*, 1976b) are shared with or are similar to antigens in BCG.

The occurrence of common antigens among bacteria and tumors resembles in some ways the known cross-reactivity between mammalian tissue antigens and microorganisms. For example, components of streptococci cross-react with heart and kidney tissues (Kaplan and Suchy, 1964; Kaplan and Svec, 1964) and anitgens in human erythrocytes are shared by components of gram-negative organisms (Springer, 1967). Some gram-negative bacteria are related to blood-group-active substances and so-called isoantibodies have their origin in

PERCY MINDEN AND PETER J. KELLEHER • Department of Medicine, National Jewish Hospital and Research Center, Denver, Colorado 80206. LINDA K. WOODS • Surgical Oncology Laboratory, Denver General Hospital, Denver, Colorado 80204.

the immunological response to cross-reactive bacterial antigens (Geobel et al., 1943; Muschel and Osawa, 1959). Similar relationships exist between bacteria and histocompatibility antigens; e.g., streptococcal and staphylococcal organisms share antigenic specificities with some transplantation antigens (Rapaport, 1972; Rapaport and Chase, 1964; Chase and Rapaport, 1965).

The antigenic relationship between tumor cells and bacteria is of particular interest because bacteria and bacterial components can be used for the therapy of some animal and human tumors (Bast et al., 1976; Ribi et al., 1976; Hersh et al., 1978; Mathe et al., 1979). The mechanism or mechanisms underlying bacterial immunotherapy are not completely understood but have been attributed to a "nonspecific" potentiation of immune mechanisms (Old et al., 1961; Weiss, 1972; Baldwin and Pimm, 1978). A more satisfactory understanding of the relationship between bacteria and tumors is needed because of the possibility that successful bacterial therapy may be the result of "specific" stimulation due to shared or cross-reacting antigenic stimuli. In addition, this kind of antigenic relationship may be responsible for the observations that normal animals and humans frequently display immune responses to many kinds of tumor-associated antigens (TAAs) (Bias et al., 1972; Herberman and Aoki, 1972; Minden et al., 1976c; Brunda and Minden, 1977; Herberman and Holden, 1979).

2. Shared Antigens between *Mycobacterium bovis* (BCG) and the Guinea Pig Line-10 Hepatocarcinoma

Antigens shared by BCG and tumor cells were first reported between BCG and the line-10 hepatocarcinoma of strain-2 guinea pigs (Borsos and Rapp, 1973; Minden et al., 1974; Bucana and Hanna, 1974). This line of investigation was instigated by the fact that the line-10 tumor responded to therapy with BCG (Rapp, 1973) and because this experimental tumor has been used as a model for the development of immunotherapy protocols for human tumors (Rapp, 1976; Zbar et al., 1976). In experiments carried out in this laboratory, soluble antigenic components were prepared from BCG and from line-10 cells (Minden et al., 1974). They are referred to as BCG-S and SA-10. Antibodies in sera from rabbits immunized with disrupted BCG (anti-BCG) and line-10 cells emulsified in incomplete Freund's adjuvant (anti-line-10) were found to bind both radiolabeled BCG-S [^{125}I]-BCG) and SA-10 ([^{125}I]-SA-10). In these and subsequent studies described below, radiolabeled antigen–antibody complexes were precipitated with heterologous antiimmunoglobulins. Binding of [^{125}I]-BCG by anti-BCG could be inhibited both by preincubation of antisera with unlabeled BCG-S and by absorption of anti-BCG with line-10 cells. The reaction between [^{125}I]-SA-10 and anti-line-10 was similarly diminished by unlabeled BCG-S. Neither of these reactions was affected by absorption of antisera with normal guinea pig tissues. In addition, antigens in *Listeria monocytogenes* were found to share antigens with line-10, but not with line 1 cells, which is a syngeneic tumor with distinct tumor-specific antigens (Minden et al., 1976c). There was a strong suggestion that line-10 cells also had antigens in common with *Brucella abortus* and *Salmonella typhimurium.* Bucana and Hanna (1974), using immunoelectronmicroscopy, demonstrated antigens on line-10 cell surfaces that bound to anti-BCG. Absorption of anti-BCG with lyophilized BCG reduced reactivity to tumor cells. Experiments providing similar conculsions have been reported by others (Borsos and Rapp, 1973; McCoy *et al.,* 1978). There is now evidence from many laboratories using different techniques that BCG shares antigens with line-10 cells. Of possible significance, both BCG and *L. monocytogenes* have therapeutic effects against this tumor (Bast *et al.,* 1976; Brunda *et al.,* 1980).

The evidence in favor of shared antigens between BCG and line-10 cells was substantial but not entirely conclusive. The data derived from all these experiments, although statistically significant, sometimes showed only small differences between experimental and control groups. The line-10 and BCG antigens are known to consist of many components, only a few of which may be critical for the kind of binding and inhibition studies that were attempted. Such antigenic complexities undoubtedly account for the limited percentage of labeled antigens bound by antibodies in sera from immunized animals and the sometimes small reduction in binding noted in some of the inhibition and absorption experiments. Isolation of specific antigens and antibodies for the reactions described above was therefore needed to evaluate further the significance of the antigenic relationships between BCG and line-10 cells.

The question as to whether line-10 components shared with BCG constituted determinants directly concerned with the biological activity of this tumor was important because these components could possible influence the antitumor effects of BCG. For example, "nonspecific" bacterial immunotherapy might be the outcome of specific shared or cross-reacting immunological stimuli. In the broader view, if sharing of antigens between tumor cells and microorganisms is widespread, the possibility exists that microorganisms could be selected in a specific way for immunotherapy or prophylaxis of some tumors. It is tempting to speculate that such shared antigens may account for the many scattered reports of apparently beneficial effects on neoplasms of concurrent infections (Nauts *et al.,* 1946; Ruckdeschel *et al.,* 1972).

To approach these questions, we carried out affinity-chromatography studies to try and isolate these components and to determine whether antigens shared by line-10 cells and BCG exerted antitumor effects *in vivo.* Ascites fluid (AF) from line-10 tumor-bearing animals, which is known to contain soluble line-10 TAAs (Detrick-Hooks *et al.,* 1976), was passed through an immunoadsorbent to which a purified preparation of antibodies to BCG had been coupled (Ferguson *et al.,* 1978). Less than 0.1% of the protein in AF bound to these antibodies. These "shared antigens" were eluted and were designated Sh-ag-10. When these antigens were mixed with viable line-10 cells and injected intradermally into strain-2 guinea pigs, tumor growth was completely suppressed in 75% of the animals tested. There was specific immunity to subsequent challenges with line-10 cells. Furthermore, radiolabeled Sh-ag-10 bound to antibodies in antisera raised to line-10 cells and to BCG (Minden *et al.,* 1980). It was not clear whether Sh-ag-10 consisted exclusively of structures related to BCG and line-10 cells. Isolation and *in vivo* testing of components of Sh-ag-10 by various separation procedures are under way to define with certainty the characteristics of the common antigens. These experiments, however, provided the first convincing evidence in support of the biological importance of antigens shared by bacteria and tumors.

3. Shared Antigens between BCG and Human Malignant-Melanoma Cells

Results of experiments using line-10 cells prompted studies to investigate the antigenic relationships between BCG and human malignant-melanoma cells. This tumor has also been reported to be responsive to BCG clinically (Hersh *et al.*, 1978). Similar to the experiments described for the line-10 guinea pig system, groups of rabbits were immunized with BCG and with melanoma cells that were derived from five patients (antimelanoma). Some of the melanoma cells had been grown in tissue culture (Quinn *et al.*, 1977). When sera were reacted with [^{125}I]-BCG as described above, there were, as expected, considerable increases in binding by antisera from rabbits immunized to BCG, and there were substantial increases in binding by some of the antimelanoma sera as well. Control sera made by immunizing rabbits with acute and chronic lymphatic leukemia cells, normal human spleen cells, sheep red blood cells, and ovalbumin showed no or only minor increases. When anti-BCG and antimelanoma sera were preincubated with unlabeled soluble BCG (BCG-S), there was a significant decrease in binding to [^{125}I]-BCG (Minden *et al.*, 1976a).

When anti-BCG was similarly reacted with radiolabeled KCl extracts of melanoma cells ([^{125}I]-mel), many anti-BCG sera showed considerable increases in binding. It is known that soluble KCl extracts of melanoma cells consist of several solubilized cellular components including some that appear to be tumor-specific (McCoy *et al.*, 1975). When anti-BCG was absorbed with normal human spleen cells, there was no change in binding to [^{125}I]-BCG or [^{125}I]-mel.

When anti-BCG and antimelanoma were preincubated with unlabeled BCG-S, there was a considerable reduction in their capacity to bind to [^{125}I]-mel. Binding of [^{125}I]-mel was evaluated further after absorption of these antisera with human melanoma cells, with a tissue-culture line of autologous lymphocytes, by normal allogeneic human lymphocytes, and by preincubation of antisera with BCG-S. The decreases in binding in these reactions are indicated in Fig. 1. The only appreciable reduction in binding was by melanoma cells

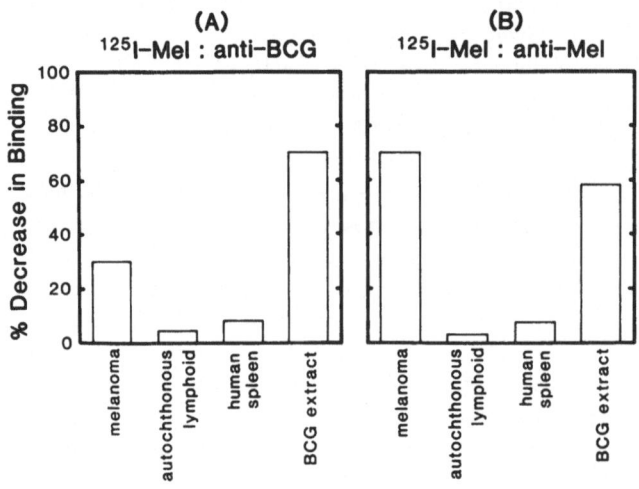

FIGURE 1. Binding of [^{125}I]-mel by anti-BCG (A) and antimelanoma (B) after absorption or preincubation with melanoma, normal cells, and BCG-S. Autochthonous lymphoid cells were derived from the same patient whose melanoma cells were used to prepare [^{125}I]-mel and antimelanoma. BCG-S was incubated with antisera before addition of [^{125}I]-mel.

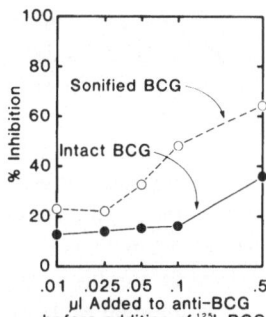

FIGURE 2. Inhibition of binding of anti-BCG to [^{125}I]-BCG by unlabeled intact and sonified BCG. From Minden and Mathews (1980), courtesy of *Cancer Research*.

and BCG. It was of considerable interest that there was no change in binding to [^{125}I]-BCG or [^{125}I]-mel when the antimelanoma sera were absorbed with autologous lymphocytes. The latter were tissue-cultured autologous lymphocytes that originated from one of the patients whose melanoma cells were studied this way. This finding, in additon to the fact that binding to BCG was not found by sera from rabbits immunized with normal human spleen cells or lymphatic leukemia cells, but only by sera from rabbits immunized with melanoma cells, made most unlikely the influence of antibodies to histocompatibility antigens that may have been present in the KC1 extracts of the melanoma cells. In other studies, BCG-specific antibody has been demonstrated to bind to surfaces of cultured human melanoma cells by immunoelectronmicroscopy (Bucana and Hanna, 1974). Absorption of anti-BCG with BCG reduced the reactions.

In summary, reactions between the two kinds of radiolabeled antigens derived from BCG and melanoma cells, and the two kinds of antisera (anti-BCG and antimelanoma), were inhibited after the sera were preincubated with unlabeled BCG-S and after they were absorbed with intact melanoma cells. Altogether, antigens in melanoma cells that were derived from each of the five patients studied were shown to share antigenic components with BCG-S.

In contrast to the results of studies in this laboratory are several reports where antibodies to melanoma-associated antigens were not removed after absorption of antisera with BCG (Liao *et al.*, 1979; Brüggen *et al.*, 1978; Shiku *et al.*, 1976). In our studies, absorptions were carried out with disrupted BCG because it is known that intact mycobacteria are enclosed with a tough lipid-containing coat (Raffel, 1961). We have observed that even the reactions between [^{125}I]-BCG and anti-BCG are inhibited poorly by intact BCG as compared to an equivalent amount of BCG that was desrupted by sonication, thereby exposing antigenic determinants unavailable on surfaces of intact BCG (Minden and Mathews, 1980) (see Fig. 2). This would probably account for the discrepancies noted by other investigators.

It has been reported that when human malignant-melanoma cells are grown in tissue culture, soluble antigens with specificity for melanoma tumors are released into the spent tissue-culture medium (Gupta *et al.*, 1979). Experiments were therefore carried out similar to the ones in which AF from tumor-bearing guinea pigs was employed. In this case, spent tissue-culture medium was passed through an immunoadsorbent made of a purified anti-BCG preparation. The components of culture fluid that bound to anti-BCG were eluted, concentrated, and radiolabeled. This material is referred to as Sh-ag-mel.

When radiolabeled and subjected to electrophoresis in sodium dodecyl sulfate (SDS)–polyacrylamide gels, it consisted of four major and three minor bands (see Fig. 3). When reacted with various antisera, it was found to bind to sera from rabbits that had been immunized with melanoma cells or with BCG to a significantly greater extent than by samples of normal rabbit serum (NRS) (see Fig. 4). It has not been possible to carry out *in vivo* type experiments with Sh-ag-mel comparable to those described above with Sh-ag-10, but the implications that Sh-ag-mel is also of biological importance are most intriguing. More information about the biological and physicochemical characteristics of Sh-ag-mel is needed before this impression is confirmed.

Additional evidence that favors the biological importance of antigens shared by melanoma cells and bacteria is presented below.

4. *In Vitro* Immunization against Human Malignant-Melanoma Cells with Bacterial Extracts

It has been shown that lymphocytes from normal persons can become immunized to a variety of tumor cells by exposure to tumor cells *in vitro* (Sharma and Terasaki, 1974). Since close antigenic relationships between BCG and melanoma cells have been demonstrated, studies were carried out to see whether BCG and other bacterial antigens could

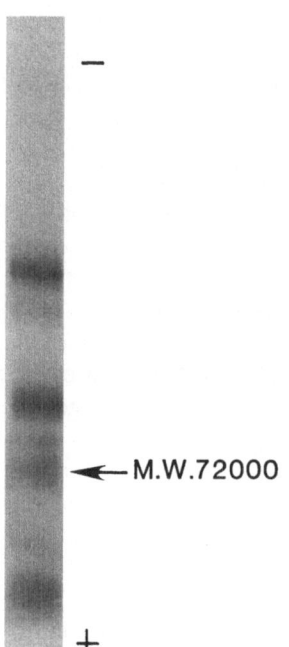

— M.W.72000

FIGURE 3. Electrophoresis of [^{125}I]-Sh-ag-mel in 10% SDS–polyacryl-amide gel. (←) indicates molecular-weight marker.

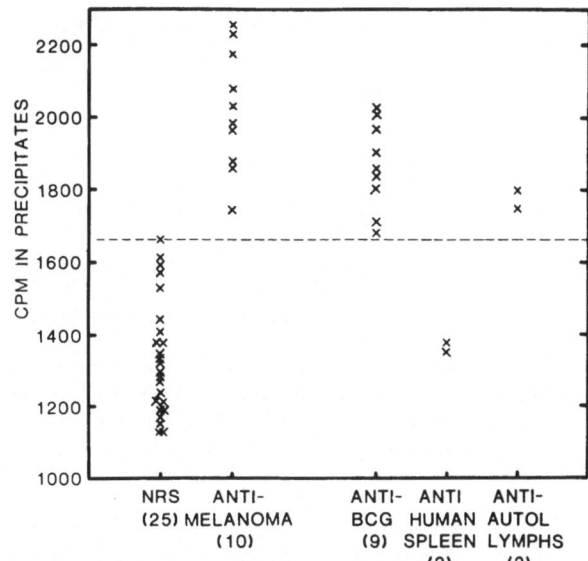

FIGURE 4. Binding by 1 : 5 dilutions of a variety of antisera to [^{125}I]-Sh-ag-mel. The numbers of rabbit sera tested are indicated in parentheses. (----) Greatest antigen binding by NRS.

similarly immunize lymphocytes from normal persons *in vitro* against melanoma cells. It was found that not only was this possible, but also the cytotoxicity of bacterial-immunized lymphocytes was sometimes greater than when lymphocytes were sensitized by melanoma cells alone. Peripheral-blood lymphocytes were obtained from 12 normal tumor-free persons and purified over Ficoll-Hypaque. These were then sensitized with melanoma cells grown in tissue culture that had been treated with mitomycin C or with various concentrations of extracts of BCG, *Listeria monocytogenes* (LM), *Escherichia coli* (EC), and *Staphylococcus aureus* (SA). The cytotoxicity of *in-vitro*-sensitized cells was then measured by a ^{51}Cr-release assay using radiolabeled melanoma cells (Sharma *et al.*, 1977, 1979). Results were compared with the capacity of the same cells to kill normal lymphoblastic target cells.

It was found that BCG-sensitized lymphocytes from 11 of the 12 normal donors caused a greater release of ^{51}Cr from labeled melanoma cells than from labeled control lymphoblasts. LM-sensitized cells from all the 7 donors tested were also cytotoxic to melanoma cells. In contrast, lymphocytes from only a few donors treated with SA and no lymphocytes from donors treated with EC were rendered cytotoxic to melanoma cells. Data from several experiments are summarized in Fig. 5.

A control study was carried out to evaluate the possible mitogenic effects of the bacterial extracts. Lymphocytes from some of the donors were pretreated with the mitogens phytohemaglutinin (PHA), pokeweed mitogen (PWM), and concanavalin A (Con A). PHA-treated leukocytes from 4 of 10 persons, PWM-treated cells from 3 of 5 donors, and lymphocytes from 1 of 6 donors treated wtih Con A became cytotoxic to melanoma cells. The degree of cytotoxicity, however, was lower and more variable than that produced by the bacterial extracts. This would minimize the possibility that the cytotoxicity initiated by the bacterial extracts was entirely due to mitogenic effects.

We also considered that the cytotoxic reactions observed between effector and target

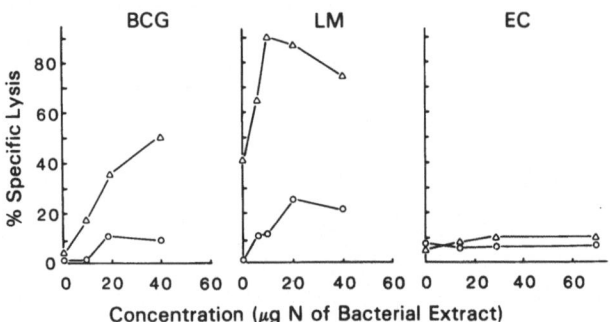

FIGURE 5. *In vitro* immunization of lymphocytes from normal donors against human malignant-melanoma cells with extracts of BCG, *Listeria monocytogenes* (LM), and *Escherichia coli* (EC). Sensitized lymphocytes were tested against melanoma target cells (△) and against normal lymphoblasts (○). The percentage specific lysis of ^{51}Cr-labeled melanoma cells was then measured. Modified from Sharma *et al.* (1977), courtesy of *Nature*.

cells might have been due to histocompatibility differences. When allogeneic lymphocytes were tested as target cells, however, there was considerably less cytotoxicity and sometimes no specific ^{51}Cr release, suggesting that the cytotoxicity observed against melanoma cells was not directed toward the histocompatibility antigens of the tumor target cells.

In other experiments, soluble extracts prepared from other microorganisms, e.g., *Salmonella typhimurium, Pseudomonas Spp., Bordetella pertussis,* and *Candida albicans,* were also found to generate cytotoxicity directed to tissue-cultured human malignant-melanoma cells. It is too early to evaluate the underlying mechanism(s) and the full potential for *in vitro* sensitization of lymphocytes. However, cross-reactivity between bacterial and melanoma-associated antigens may be involved. A full understanding of this cross-reactivity may provide insights into the mechanisms by which cytotoxic lymphocytes may be generated in patients during bacterial immunotherapy and perhaps in normal persons as a result of exposure to environmental microorganisms.

5. Antibodies to Melanoma-Cell and BCG Antigens in Sera from Tumor-Free Individuals and from Melanoma Patients

Antibodies to mycobacteria and other bacterial antigens are found universally in sera from normal humans (Minden and Farr, 1975). Since there is a broad range of shared or cross-reactive antigens among mycobacteria and unrelated microorganisms (Minden *et al.*, 1972), it is conceivable that an immune response by normal humans and animals to mycobacteria was induced by exposure to taxonomically unrelated microorganisms ubiquitous in the environment. Antibodies in sera from patients with various neoplasms have often been observed that react with antigens derived from their own tumors or from tumors of the same histological types (Hellström *et al.*, 1968). Humoral responses to tumor-associated antigens have similarly been noted in sera from normal humans and animals (Bias *et al.*, 1972; Herberman and Aoki, 1972; Brunda and Minden, 1977). These are often referred to as "natural" or nonspecific. Cytotoxic reactions by lymphoid cells from normal animals and humans to many kinds of tumor cells have also been reported (Herberman *et al.*, 1975). In one study, sera from normal, tumor-free humans were investigated to see whether they contained antibodies that could react with a KCl extract of melanoma cells as well as with BCG antigens (Minden *et al.*, 1976d). If this were the case, perhaps immunological reactions by normal humans to melanoma antigens might reflect previous sensitization by microorganisms.

Melanoma cells that had been grown in tissue culture were treated with 3 M KCl. These KCl extracts had been used in other experiments including some to investigate antigenic relationships between human malignant-melanoma cells and BCG (Minden *et al.*, 1976a). The primary interactions between labeled test antigens and antibodies in human sera were analyzed by precipitation of ^{125}I-labeled antigen–antibody complexes with anti-human immunoglobulin.

Sera from 63 patients with malignant melanoma were obtained shortly after surgery and before the patients were started on a chemoimmunotherapy program. Of these 63 patients, 13 had Stage I disease, 4 had Stage II, 29 had Stage III, and 17 had Stage IV. Ages ranged from 21 to 72 years. There were 41 male and 22 female patients. Control sera were from 50 healthy subjects, most of whom were personnel at the National Jewish Hospital and Research Center. Sera were not obtained from subjects who had been in contact wtih human tumors in the laboratory.·

When sera from all the patients and normal subjects were tested for their capacity to bind [^{125}I]-BCG and [^{125}I]-mel, there was a wide range in their capacity to bind both radiolabeled antigens (Fig. 6). As a group, sera from patients with melanoma bound [^{125}I]-BCG

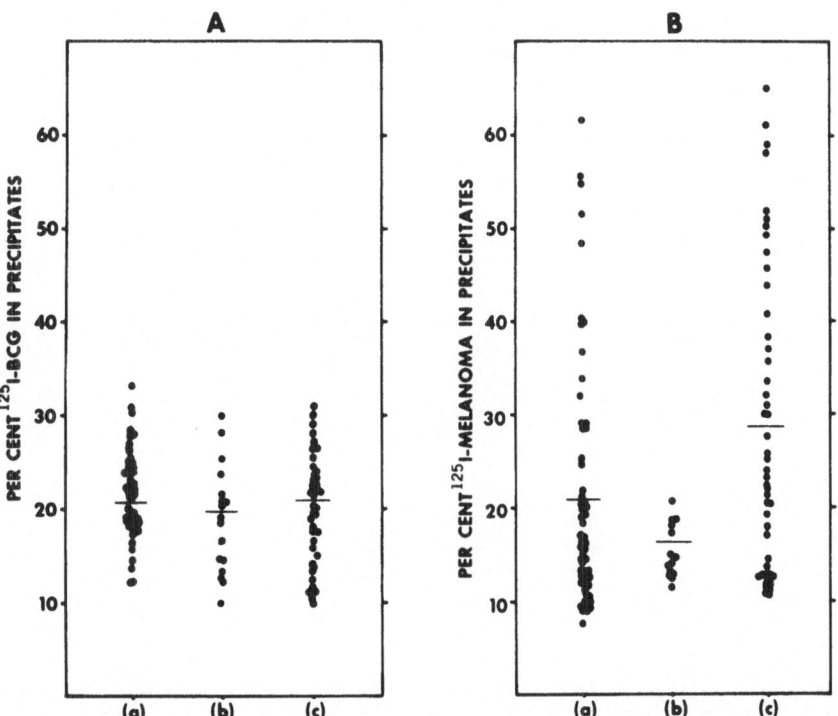

FIGURE 6. Results of binding tests using [^{125}I]-BCG (A) and [^{125}I]-mel (B) expressed as percentages of labeled antigens bound by 0.1 ml of a 1 : 5 dilution of whole serum. (a) All melanoma (63); (b) Stage IV melanoma (17); (c) no disease (50). From Minden *et al.* (1976d), courtesy·of *Nature (London)*.

to about the same extent as did sera from normal subjects. The capacity of sera from 17 patients with Stage IV disease to bind [^{125}I]-BCG was less than that of normal sera. When the same sera were reacted wtih [^{125}I]-mel, antibodies in normal sera bound more antigen than did sera from the melanoma patients ($p < 0.025$). This large difference makes it unlikely that immunity to HLA or blood-group antigens that might have been present in the KCl extract employed could account for the binding observed, although this possibility has not been ruled out. When sera from patients with Stage IV disease were compared with normals, they had significantly lower ($p < 0.005$) binding values. Lowered antidody levels to other antigens have been shown when circulating antigen, soluble antigen–antibody complexes, or antiidiotype antibodies are present, and this may have been the case in some patients with far-advanced melanoma (Rowley et al., 1973).

Of further interest were experiments undertaken to evaluate the specificity of the binding data. Sera from 11 melanoma patients and from 7 normal persons were preincubated wtih 300 μg nitrogen (N) unlabeled BCG-S. Control samples were incubated with buffer. At 24 hr later, [^{125}I]-BCG and [^{125}I]-mel were added, and binding capacities of the antisera were determined. The percentage decrease of binding is shown in Table I. As expected, unlabeled BCG-S considerably inhibited the binding to [^{125}I]-BCG. To a lesser extent, it also reduced the binding by most of the antisera to [^{125}I]-mel. This was compatible with

TABLE I

Percentage Decrease of Binding of [^{125}I]-BCG and [^{125}I]-Mel by Sera from Normal Subjects and Patients with Malignant Melanoma after Preincubation of Sera with 300 μg N Unlabeled Soluble BCG[a]

Antiserum donors no.	[^{125}I]-BCG antigen	[^{125}I]-Mel antigen
Normal human		
1	54.5	2.4
2	31.5	7.0
3	70.6	22.8
4	58.2	3.2
5	29.3	0.4
6	55.5	42.7
7	36.6	19.9
Melanoma patient		
1	29.2	2.9
2	57.2	10.6
3	47.7	0,4
4	40.6	1.2
5	62.7	28.0
6	57.1	23.2
7	48.7	20.4
8	49.1	6.3
9	50.1	32.5
10	50.7	5.9
11	30.7	1.6

[a]From Minden et al., (1976-d), courtesy of Nature (London). Percentage decrease = [(cpm in precipitates after preincubation with BCG-S/(cpm in precipitates after preincubation with buffer) −1] × 100.

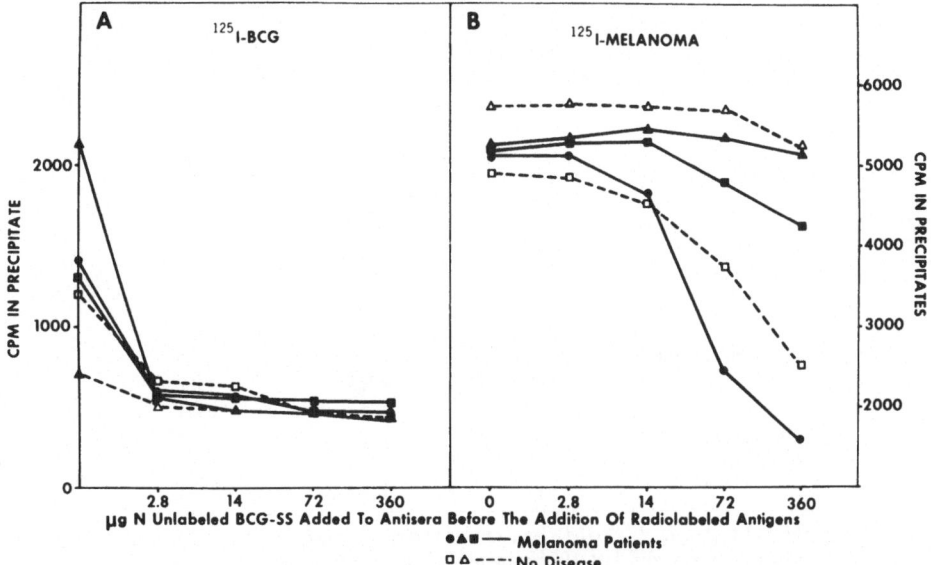

FIGURE 7. Inhibition of binding of [^{125}I]-BCG (A) and [^{125}I]-mel (B) by sera from normal (□, △) and melanoma patients (■, ▲, ●) after preincubation of sera with dilutions of BCG-S. From Minden *et al.* (1976d), courtesy of *Nature (London)*.

previous observations that antigenic components are shared between BCG and melanoma cells (Bucana and Hanna, 1974; Minden *et al.*, 1976a).

Inhibition studies were carried out in greater detail using sera from three melanoma patients and two normal individuals. Serial dilutions of unlabeled BCG were tested for their capacity to inhibit binding of [^{125}I]-BCG and [^{125}I]-mel to dilutions of antisera. Controls consisted of buffer added to the diluted antisera. After overnight incubation, labeled BCG and melanoma antigens were added, and binding to these antigens was determined. As little as 2.8 μg N unlabeled BCG-S inhibited the binding by normal and melanoma antisera to [^{125}I]-BCG, and with increasing amounts there was slightly more inhibition (see Fig. 7). When [^{125}I]-mel was the antigen, there was similar inhibition of binding by four of the five sera tested, but more BCG-S was required. As shown in Fig. 7, 72 μg N caused slight inhibition and 300 μg was considerably more effective.

Sera from two melanoma patients, two normal subjects, and two patients with active tuberculosis were then absorbed with 3×10^7 intact melanoma cells, or with 2×10^8 normal human spleen cells, and then reacted with [^{125}I]-mel (Table II). Sera from patients with tuberculosis were included because they generally have greater capacities to bind [^{125}I]-BCG than do sera from normal subjects (Bardana *et al.*, 1973). After absorption with melanoma cells, there was a marked reduction in binding to [^{125}I]-mel by all the sera. Absorption of the same sera with normal human spleen cells showed only slight decreases, except for normal serum No. 1, where there was a more moderate decrease in binding. There was no reduction in binding to [^{125}I]-BCG after absorption with 3×10^7 melanoma cells (not shown in Table II). It would appear, however, that because of antigenic simi-

TABLE II

Binding of [¹²⁵I]-Mel by Sera from Normal Persons and from Patients with Malignant Melanoma and Tuberculosis after Absorption with Melanoma and Spleen Cells[a]

	Cpm in precipitates absorbed with:		
Antiserum donors no.	Unabsorbed	Melanoma cells[b]	Normal spleen cells[c]
Normal human			
1	7546	1827	5681
2	7983	1847	7742
Melanoma patient			
1	7408	1963	7352
2	7034	1762	6831
Tuberculosis patient			
1	5373	1695	5269
2	1834	1520	1798

[a]From Minden *et al.* (1976d), courtesy of *Nature (London)*.
[b]Absorption was with 3×10^7 melanoma cells for 1.0 ml serum.
[c]Absorption was with 2×10^8 normal human spleen cells for 1.0 ml serum.

larities between BCG and melanoma cells, antibodies to melanoma-associated antigens could have been induced in normal persons by exposure to mycobacteria or other microorganisms in the environment. Antibodies to TAAs in sera from normal persons would not therefore be "natural," but they would be an expected response to stimulation by cross-reactive antigens in bacteria.

6. Concluding Remarks

Antigens shared by human malignant cells and BCG have been isolated. Several investigations have been reviewed in which the biological importance of these antigens is strongly implicated. As a result of the *in vivo* antitumor effects demonstrated by antigens similarly shared by BCG and the line-10 guinea pig hepatocarcinoma, an understanding of the full relationship between bacterial and melanoma antigens deserves serious and continued attention.

Antigens shared by other tumor cells and bacteria may be widespread, and immune responses, whether cellular or humoral, might then exist in normal humans to many tumors. It is possible that normal humans may respond immunologically to tumor antigens just as they respond to bacterial antigens. Whether the finding of natural killer (NK) cells in humans (Herberman and Holden, 1979) has anything to do with stimulation by bacterial antigens is an intriguing question that has not been investigated. NK cells may possibly be the cellular counterpart of "natural" antibodies. In mouse experiments, pathogen-free animals have been reported to have little or no NK activity, whereas when they were moved to conventional quarters, they quickly developed considerable NK activity (Clark *et al.*, 1979). Immune responses by normal humans or animals to tumor antigens conceivably are not "natural" or "nonspecific," but could be specific responses to direct stimulation by microbial antigens.

Accordingly, immune responses by patients to tumor antigens may sometimes represent an elevation of an "isoimmune" state, rather than a new actively acquired immune response. Such a response may be of relevance in influencing the course of neoplastic disease. Of even greater significance, immune reactions to TAAs by normal individuals may be important in influencing the incidence or course of spontaneously arising neoplasms.

ACKNOWLEDGMENTS: This work was supported by Grant CA-15446 awarded by the National Cancer Institute, Department of Health, Education and Welfare (P.M.), and by Grant AI-00048, National Institutes of Health, Department of Health, Education and Welfare (P.J.K.) The authors are grateful to Drs. R. S. Farr and G. E. Moore for their advice and encouragement.

References

Baldwin, R. W., and Pimm, M. V., 1978, BCG in tumor immunotherapy *Adv. Cancer Res.* **28**:91.

Bardana, E. J., McClatchy, J. K., Farr, R. S., and Minden, P., 1973, Universal occurrence of antibodies to tubercle bacilli in sera from non-tuberculous and tuberculous individuals, *Clin. Exp. Immunol.* **13**:65.

Bast, R. C., Bast, B. S., and Rapp, H. J., 1976, Critical review of previously reported animal studies of tumor immunotherapy with nonspecific immunostimulants, *Ann. N. Y., Acad. Sci.* **277**:60.

Bias, W. B., Santos, G. W., Burke, P. J., Mullins, G. M., and Humphrey, R. L., 1972, Cytotoxic antibody in normal human serums reactive with tumor cells from acute lymphocytic leukemia, *Science* **178**:304.

Borsos, T., And Rapp, H. J., 1973, Antigenic relationship between *Mycobacterium bovis* (BCG) and a guinea pig hepatoma, *J. Natl. Cancer Inst.* **51**:1085.

Brüggen, J., Sorg, C., and Macher, E., 1978, Membrane associated antigens of human malignant melanoma. V. Serological typing of cell lines using antisera from nonhuman primates, *Cancer Immunol. Immunother.* **5**:53.

Brunda, M. J., and Minden, P., 1977, Antibodies to bacterial and tumor derived antigens in sera from normal guinea pigs, *J. Immunol.* **119**:1374.

Brunda, M. J., Mathews, H. L., Ferguson, H. R., McClatchy, J. K., and Minden, P., 1980, Immunotherapy of the guinea pig line-10 hepatocarcinoma with a variety of non-viable bacteria, *Cancer Res.* **40**:3211.

Bucana, C., and Hanna, M. G., Jr., 1974, Immunoelectronmicroscopic analysis of surface antigens common to *Mycobacterium bovis* (BCG) and tumor cells, *J. Natl. Cancer Inst.* **53**:1313.

Chase, R. M., Jr., and Rapaport, F. T., 1965, The bacterial induction of homograft sensitivity. I. Effects of sensitization with group A streptococci, *J. Exp. Med.* **122**:721.

Clark, E. A., Russell, P. H., Egghart, M., and Horton, M. A., 1979, Characteristics and genetic control of NK-cell-mediated cytotoxicity activated by naturally acquired infection in the mouse, *Int. J. Cancer.* **24**:688.

Detrick-Hooks, B., Smith, H. G., Bast, R. C., Jr., Dunkel, V. C., and Borsos, T., 1976, Naturally soluble tumor antigens from guinea pig hepatomas: Isolation and partial characterization, *J. Immunol.* **116**:1324.

Ferguson, H. R., McClatchy, J. K., Sharpton, T. R., and Minden, P., 1978, Immunological method to differentiate between antigens of tubercle bacilli, other mycobacterial species, and non-acid fast bacteria, *Infect. Immunity* **22**:101.

Goebel, W. F., Shedlovsky, T., Lavin, G. I., and Adams, M. H., 1943, Heterophile antigen of pneumococcus, *J. Biol. Chem.* **148**:1.

Gupta, R. K., Irie, R. F., Chee, D. O., Kern, D. H., and Morton, D. L., 1979, Demonstration of two distinct antigens in spent tissue culture medium of a human malignant melanoma cell line, *J. Natl. Cancer Inst.* **63**:347.

Hellström, I., Hellström, K. E., Pierce, G. E., and Yang, J. P. S., 1968, Cellular and humoral immunity to different types of human neoplasms, *Nature (London)* **220**:1352.

Herberman, R. B., and Aoki, T., 1972, Immune and natural antibodies to syngeneic murine plasma cell tumors, *J. Exp. Med.* **131**:94.

Herberman, R. B., and Holden, H. T., 1979, Natural killer cells as antitumor effector cells, *J. Natl. Cancer Inst.* **62**:441.

Herberman, R. B., Nunn, M. E., and Lavrin, D. H., 1975, Natural cytotoxic reactivity of mouse lymphoid cells against syngeneic and allogeneic tumors. I. Distribution of reactivity and specificity, *Int. J. Cancer* **16**:216.

Hersh, E. M., Gutterman, J. U., Mavligit, G. M., Granatek, C. H., Rossen, R. D., Rios, A., Goldstein, A. L., Patt, Y. Z., Rivera, E., Richman, S. P., Bottino, J. C., Farquhar, D., Morris, D., and Ezaki, K., 1978, Clinical rationale for immunotherapy and its role in cancer treatment, in *Immunotherapy of Human Cancer*, p. 83, Raven Press, New York.

Holan, V., Chutna, J., and Harsek, M., 1979, Cross-reactivity between bacillus Calmette–Guérin and Rous virus-induced sarcoma detected in rats by tube leukocyte adherence inhibition assay, *Cancer Res.* **39**:593.

James, K., Willmott, N., Milne, I., and McBride, W. H., 1976, Antitumor antibodies and immunoglobulin class and subclass levels in *Corynebacterium parvum*-treated mice, *J. Natl. Cancer Inst.* **56**:1035.

Kaplan, M. H., and Suchy, M. L., 1964, Immunologic relation of streptococcal and tissue antigens. II. Cross-reactions of antisera to mammalian heart tissue with a cell wall constituent of certain strains of group A streptococci, *J. Exp. Med.* **119**:643.

Kaplan, M. H., and Svec, K. H., 1964, Immunologic relation of streptococcal and tissue antigens. III. Presence in human sera of streptococcal antibody cross-reactive with heart tissue: Association with streptococcal infection, rheumatic fever and glomerulonephritis, *J. Exp. Med.* **119**:651.

Kwapinski, G., Oliver, H., Kwapinski, E., and Stein, M., 1978, Microbial-like antigens in human leukemia, *Onocology* **35**:263.

Lewis, M. G., Jerry, L. M., Rowden, G., Phillips, T. A., Shibatan, H., and Capele, A., 1976, Some effects of oral administration of BCG on immune responses in cancer patients, in *BCG in Cancer Immunotherapy* (G. Lamoureux, V. Portelance, and R. Turcotte, eds.), pp. 339–358, Grune and Stratton, New York.

Liao, S. K., Kwong, P. C., Thompson, J. C., and Dent, P. B., 1979, Spectrum of melanoma antigens on cultured human malignant melanoma cells as detected by monkey antibodies, *Cancer Res.* **39**:183.

Mathe, G., Florentin, I., Bruly-Rossel, M., Kiger, N., and Olsson, L., 1979, Systemic immunotherapy of cancer minimal residual disease: Clinical status and new experimental data approaches, in *Adjuvant Therapy of Cancer II* (S. E. Jones and S. E. Salmon, eds.), p. 87, Grune and Stratton, New York.

McCoy, J. L., Jerome, L. F., Dean, J. H., Perlin, E., Oldham, R. K., Char, D. H., Cohen, M. H., Felix, E. L., and Herberman, R. B., 1975, Inhibition of leukocyte migration by tumor-associated antigens in soluble extracts of human malignant melanoma, *J. Natl. Cancer Inst.* **55**:19.

McCoy, J. L., Bradhorst, J., and Hanna, M. C., Jr., 1978, Leukocyte migration inhibition of tumor antigen and purified protein derivative reactivity in guinea pigs sensitized to line-10 hepatocarcinoma and BCG, *J. Natl. Cancer Inst.* **60**:693.

Minden, P., 1976, Shared antigens between animal and human tumors and microorganisms, in: *BCG in Cancer Immunotherapy* (G. Lamoureux, V. Portelance, and R. Turcotte, eds.), pp. 73–81, Grune and Stratton, New York.

Minden, P., and Farr, R. S., 1975, The universal presence of antibodies to microorganisms in sera from normal persons (editorial), *Chest* **68**:749.

Minden, P., and Mathews, H. L., 1980, Suppression and immunotherapy of the guinea pig line-10 hepatocarcinoma mediated by heat-killed disrupted *Mycobacterium bovis* (BCG). *Cancer Res.* **40**:3214.

Minden, P., McClatchy, J. K., Cooper, R., Bardana, E. J., Jr., and Farr, R. S., 1972, Shared antigens between *Mycobacterium bovis* (BCG) and other bacterial species, *Science* **176**:57.

Minden, P., McClatchy, J. K., Wainberg, M., and Weiss, D. W., 1974, Shared antigens between *Mycobacterium bovis* (BCG) and neoplastic cells, *J. Natl. Cancer Inst.* **53**:1325.

Minden, P., Sharpton, T. R., and McClatchy, J. K., 1976a, Shared antigens between human malignant melanoma cells and *Mycobacterium bovis* (BCG), *J. Immunol.* **116**:1407.

Minden, P., Gutterman, J. U., Sharpton, T. R., and McClatchy, J. K., 1976b, Antigenic relationships between human acute myeloid leukemia cells and *Mycobacterium bovis* (BCG), in Proceedings of the XIIth Joint Meeting: U.S.–Japan Cooperative Medical Science Program, Tokyo, p. 429.

Minden, P., Sharpton, T. R., and McClatchy, J. K., 1976c, Shared antigens between bacteria and guinea pig line-10 hepatocarcinoma cells, *Cancer Res.* **36**:1680.

Minden, P., Gutterman, J. U., Hersh, E. M., Jarrett, C., and McClatchy, J. K., 1976d, Antibodies to melanoma cell and BCG antigens in sera from tumour-free individuals and from melanoma patients, *Nature (London)* **263**:774.

Minden, P., Mathews, H. L., and Kelleher, P. J., 1980, Suppression of the line-10 guinea pig hepatocarcinoma by antigens related to both *Mycobacterium bovis* (BCG) and the tumor, *J. Immunol.* **125**:2685

Muschel, L. H., and Osawa, E., 1959, Human blood group substance B and *Escherichia coli* 086, *Proc. Soc. Exp. Biol. Med.* **101**:614.

Nauts, H. C., Swift, W. E., and Coley, B. L., 1946, Treatment of malignant tumors by bacterial toxins as developed by the late William Coley, M.D., reviewed in the light of modern research, *Cancer Res.* **6**:205.

Old, L. J., Benacerraf, B., Clarke, D. A., Carswell, E. A., and Stockert, E., 1961, The role of the reticuloendothelial system in the host reaction to neoplasia, *Cancer Res.* **21**:1281.

Quinn, L. A., Woods, L. K., Merrick, S. B., Arabasz, N. M., and Moore, G. E., 1977, Cytogenetic analysis of twelve human malignant melanoma cell lines, *J. Natl. Cancer Inst.* **59**:301.

Raffel, S., 1961, Tuberculosis in *Immunity*, 2nd ed., p. 412, Appleton-Century-Crofts, New York.

Rapaport, F. T., 1972, The biological significance of cross-reactions between histocompatibility antigens and antigens of bacterial and/or heterologous mammalian origin in: *Transplantation Antigens* (B. E. Kahan and R. A. Reisfeld, eds.), pp. 182–209, Academic Press, New York.

Rapaport, F. T., and Chase, R. M., Jr., 1964, Homograft sensitivity induction by group A streptococci, *Science* **145**:407.

Rapp, H. J., 1973, A guinea pig model for tumor immunology, *Isr. J. Med. Sci.* **9**:366.

Rapp, H. J., 1976, Immunotherapy of experimental cancer as a guide to the treatment of human cancer, *Ann. N. Y. Acad. Sci.* **276**:550.

Ribi, E., Milner, K. C., Granger, D. L., Kelly, M. T., Yamamoto, K., Brehmer, W., Parker, R., Smith, R. F., and Strain, S. M., 1976, Immunotherapy with nonviable microbial components, *Ann. N. Y. Acad. Sci.* **277**:228.

Rowley, D. A., Fitch, F. W., Stuart, F. P., Köhler, H., and Cosenza, H., 1973, Specific suppression of immune responses, *Science* **181**:1133.

Ruckdeschel, J. C., Codish, S. D., Stranahan, A., and McKneally, M. F., 1972, Post operative empyema improves survival in lung cancer. Documentation and analysis of a natural experiment, *N. Engl. J. Med.* **287**:1013.

Sharma, B., and Terasaki, P. I., 1974, *In vitro* immunization to cultured human tumor cells, *Cancer Res.* **34**:115.

Sharma, B., Tubergen, D. G., Minden, P., and Brunda, M. J., 1977, *In vitro* immunisation against human tumour cells with bacterial extracts, *Nature (London)* **267**:845.

Sharma, B., Brunda, M. J., and Minden, P., 1979, Generation of cytotoxic lymphocytes against human tumor cells *in vitro* by various soluble microbial extracts, *J. Natl. Cancer Inst.* **63**:341.

Shiku, H., Takahashi, T., Oettgen, H. F., and Old, L. J., 1976, Cell surface antigens of human malignant melanoma. II. Serological typing with immune adherence assays and definition of two new surface antigens, *J. Exp. Med.* **144**:873.

Springer, G. F., 1967, The relation of microbes to blood group-active substances, in *Cross-Reacting Antigens and Neo-Antigens* (J. Trenton, ed.), pp. 29–47, Williams and Wilkins, Baltimore.

Weiss, D. W., 1972, Nonspecific stimulation and modulation of the immune response and of states of resistance by the methanol-extraction residue fraction of tubercle bacilli, *Natl. Cancer Inst. Monogr.* **35**:157.

Zbar, B., Ribi, E., Kelly, M., Granger, D., Evans, C., and Rapp, H. J., 1976, Immunologic approaches to the treatment of human cancer based on a guinea pig model, *Cancer Immunol. Immunother.* **1**:127

15

Monoclonal Antibodies to Human Melanoma-Associated Antigens: Elicitation and Evaluation with Immunochemically Defined Antigen Preparations

ALTON C. MORGAN, JR.

1. Introduction

Rapid advancements have been made in the production of monoclonal antibodies with the advent of hybridoma technology, originally described by Köhler and Milstein (1975). Among these advances has been the production of monoclonal reagents to viral antigens (Wiktor and Koprowski, 1978), histocompatibility antigens (Galfre *et al.*, 1977), haptens (Köhler and Milstein, 1976; Bottcher *et al.*, 1980), and other cell-surface antigens (Milstein *et al.*, 1979). The latter category includes antibodies to human tumor-associated antigens (TAAs); the production of such antibodies is a prominent goal of many investigators. The use of intact tumor cells for both elicitation and evaluation of hybridoma products has been a hallmark of most of these research efforts.

To improve the efficiency of production of monoclonal antibodies to TAAs, we have used immunologically and biochemically defined antigen preparations for both elicitation and screening of hybridomas. This work was the result of both serological and biochemical studies of TAA components isolated from spent culture medium of human melanoma cells utilizing polyclonal xenoantisera. These results, obtained in our laboratory, are reviewed

ALTON C. MORGAN, JR. • Department of Molecular Immunology, Scripps Clinic and Research Foundation, La Jolla, California 92037.

in Chapter 17. To summarize briefly: We identified two glycoprotein components in the spent culture medium of human melanoma cells. The first of these has a molecular weight of 240,000 and is shed only by melanoma cells. The second component has a molecular weight of 94,000 and is elaborated by both melanoma and carcinoma cell lines as well as cultured human fetal melanocytes, but not by lymphoid or fibroblastoid cultures. Distinct biochemical differences exist between these two antigens and other nontumor specific components, allowing their separation and purification. This chapter details the utilization of immunochemically defined antigen preparations for elicitation and evaluation of hybridomas to TAAs and describes some of the hybridomas produced by these approaches.

2. Elicitation of Tumor-Associated-Antigen-Specific Hybridomas with Immunochemically Defined Antigens

Our results and those of other investigators indicated that though intact tumor cells are immunogenic in xenoimmunizations, the vast majority of hybridomas produced recognize determinants *not* unique to either the immunizing tumor cell or other tumor cells of the same histological origin. The relatively rare occurrence of hybridomas secreting antibody to tumor-specific molecules in fusions from whole-cell immunizations may suggest that most of the repertoire of antigen-reactive B cells in the immunized animal is directed to a relatively few immunodominant molecules on tumor cells. It would thus appear advantageous to (1) use immunogens devoid of these immunogenic, non-tumor-specific components, but yet enriched in the less immunogenic, tumor-specific molecules; and (2) ensure that these tumor-specific components are presented in the most immunogenic form. The first criterion was met by using soluble antigen preparations from melanoma cells grown in chemically defined medium (CDM), i.e., either spent culture medium or isotonic urea extracts. These antigen preparations are naturally devoid of human leukocyte antigen (HLA)-A, B, C, and HLA-D-related (DR) antigens and can be depleted of another highly immunogenic component, fibronectin, by passage over gelatin–Sepharose 4B. To fulfill the second criterion of presentation of these antigens in their most immunogenic form, they were bound to either *Lens culinaris* hemagglutinin (LeH)–Sepharose 4B or polyclonal rabbit anti-melanoma cell antibody (anti-MAA) previously adsorbed to protein A–Sepharose 4B (PAS). Both adsorbents were shown to be effective in the production of rabbit antisera to human histocompatibility and tumor antigens (Wilson *et al.*, 1978; Galloway *et al.*, 1981).

Hybridomas elicited by one such immunochemically defined immunogen were assayed for binding to melanoma or lymphoid cell targets by an [^{125}I] *Staphylococcus aureus* protein A ([^{125}I]-SpA) radioimmunometric antibody-binding assay (McCabe *et al.*, 1979) and compared to hybridomas from a fusion elicited with intact melanoma cells from which the insolubilized immunogen was derived. Figure 1 shows the binding of hybridomas produced by immunization of mice with intact cells. It is evident that although many hybridomas react preferentially with melanoma cells, none binds epitopes that are not expressed to some degree on lymphoid cells. The complete lack, in this fusion, of antibodies that bind tumor-associated components may be only fortuitous, since other investigators have been able to raise tumor-specific monoclonal antibodies using intact cells as immunogens. However,

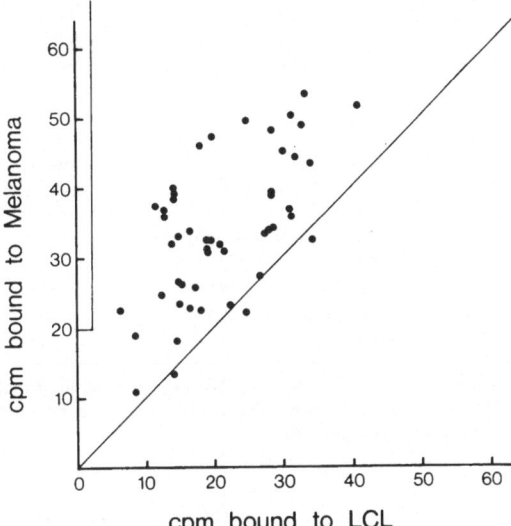

FIGURE 1. Specificity of hybridomas elicited by whole cells. Each hybridoma supernate was assayed vs. 2 × 10⁵ M21 melanoma or FO LCL lymphoid cells. Binding was detected by consecutive incubations with a 1:250 dilution of rabbit anti-mouse immunoglobulin (Ig) and [¹²⁵I]-SpA.

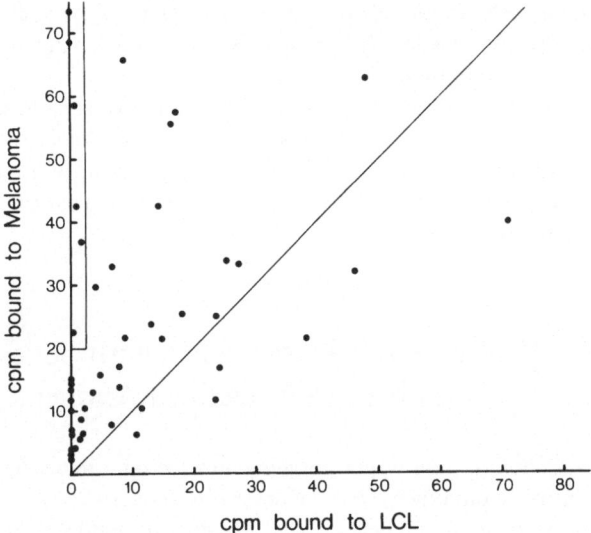

FIGURE 2. Specificity of hybridomas elicited by an immunochemically defined immunogen. Hybridomas, produced with CDM bound to rabbit anti-MAA adsorbed to PAS, were screened by the protocol described in the Fig. 1 caption.

these data at least demonstrate that the occurrence of such antibodies is relatively rare. In contrast, Fig. 2 shows results obrained by screening hybridomas induced by spent-culture-medium components bound to anti-MAA antibody adsorbed onto PAS. Of 50 hybridomas that were prescreened on CDM, 6 bound specifically to melanoma cells. A summary of our experience to date with these types of immunogens is presented in Table I. Other immunogens like urea extract, depleted of fibronectin and adsorbed onto LeH–Sepharose 4B, proved even more effectve eliciting tumor-specific hybridomas (Fusion No. 1). In addition, immunization of a mouse with urea extract bound to anti-MAA–PAS resulted in almost 50% of the positive hybridomas secreting antibody to tumor-associated molecules (Fusion

TABLE I

Evaluation of Hybridomas with Solid-Phase Immunochemically Defined Antigens

Fusion No.	Immunogen	Wells with hybrids	Percentage of hybrids[a] positive vs.:			
			CDM	Cells	Both targets	Specific[b]
1	Urea extract/Lch–Sepharose 4B	1590	13.1	5.2	5.0	3.7
2	CDM/anti-MAA–PAS	132	18.1	14.4	14.3	4.5
4	Urea extract/anti-MAA–PAS	400	14.5	12.3	12.0	5.8
5	Whole cells	336	27.0	25.6	24.1	0

[a] Hybridoma supernates binding 2.5-fold background or more as measured with P3 × 63 Ag8.
[b] Hybridoma supernates binding 10,000 cpm or more to melanoma but 500 cpm or less to lymphoid cells after subtraction of background.

No. 4). Immunization with CDM adsorbed onto the same carrier yielded fewer hybrids secreting antibody to TAAs (Fusion No. 2). By comparison, immunization of mice with intact cells produced the highest percentage of hybrids that secreted antibody binding to melanoma cells or solid-phase CDM. However, none of these antibodies recognized tumor-specific molecules.

These results indicate that it is not necessary to use highly purified tumor-specific immunogens to elicit a high percentage of hybridomas secreting antibodies to tumor-specific antigens; it is sufficient for this purpose to remove immunodominant, non–tumor-specific contaminants and to present these antigen preparations in insolubilized form adsorbed onto immunogenic carriers.

3. Evaluation of Hybridomas with Solid-Phase, Immunochemically Defined Antigens

Solid-phase target antigens have become increasingly popular for the evaluation of antibody binding because of several characteristics: (1) they can be defined by either serological or immunochemical methods, e.g., indirect immunoprecipitation techniques; (2) their reproducibility is superior to that of intact cells; and (3) they require fewer manipulations. We have found that a variety of soluble antigen preparations are quite suitable for screening hybridomas once they are adsorbed to polyvinyl microtiter wells. The first and most widely applicable target antigen proved to be spent culture medium from a melanoma cell line (M14), grown in chemically defined medium. Our earlier results with polyclonal xenoantisera to melanoma cells indicated that this antigen source was enriched in tumor-specific components and devoid of histocompatibility antigens (Morgan *et al.*, 1980). This fact made it possible to assay for tumor-specific antibody in these polyclonal xenoantisera without previous absorption with pooled lymphoid cells or erythrocytes. This characteristic proved advantageous in screening hybridomas, since only primary screening against CDM was required for selection, as opposed to the usual method of screening against both melanoma and lymphoid cells. As shown in Table I, most of the hybrids that were preselected with CDM also bound to determinants on melanoma cells. In addition, most of the hybrids positive vs. CDM, when tested against melanoma and lymphoid targets, bound to antigens that were at least preferentially expressed on melanoma cells (Figs. 1 and 2).

One of our major concerns in using CDM for selection of hybridomas was whether the hybridomas selected would secrete antibodies that recognized only molecules found in spent culture medium but not on the cell surfaces of melanoma cells. Previous data obtained with polyclonal xenoantisera made to melanoma cells had indicated that at least 70–80% of the components of CDM were derived from the cell surface (Morgan *et al.*, 1980). This question was reexamined by screening hybrids from Fusion No. 1 against both intact cells and CDM (Fig. 3). It was apparent that many of the hybrids from this fusion recognized determinants preferentially expressed on one or the other target. However, this was not generally the case, since immunization with other chemically defined immunogens produced about 80% of hybrids that reacted with both intact cells and CDM (see Table I). Thus, this concern proved not warranted, but demonstrated that certain immunogens may evoke the production of antibodies that recognize only shed or secreted molecules. Indeed, such antibodies may be invaluable as diagnostic or prognostic probes of patients' sera, where recognition is required of molecules that may have an altered conformation or constitute a degraded form of cell-surface structure.

Other types of solid-phase antigen preparations have been found useful for screening hybrids. The serological definition of these targets is summarized in Table II. The melanoma-specific glycoprotein of molecular weight 240,000 (240K), recognized by antibody 9.2.27 (see Section 4), is readily detected on intact cells, on membranes, in cell-surface extracts, or in CDM. In contrast, the common tumor antigen of molecular weight 94,000 (94K) is shed at high levels into CDM, but is present at low levels on intact cells, membranes, or cell-surface glycoproteins of melanoma cells. In contrast to these tumor antigens, the expression of human histocompatibility antigens (HLA-DR and HLA-A,B,C) is restricted to cells or to cell-surface-derived preparations and is not found in CDM. Interestingly, β_2-microglobulin (β_2m), the light chain of the HLA-A,B,C antigen complex, though detected on cells and cell-surface-derived targets, is found in relatively large amounts in CDM in free form, not complexed to the heavy chain of the histocompatibility

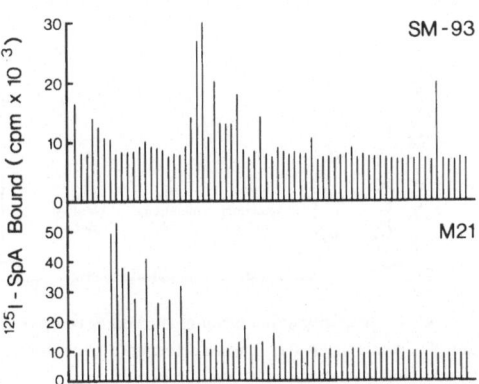

FIGURE 3. Reactivity of hybridomas elicited by an immunochemically defined immunogen with either CDM or whole cells. Hybridomas, produced by immunizing mice with a 4 M urea extract of M14 melanoma cells adsorbed onto LcH–Sepharose 4B, were assayed vs. CDM (SM-93) and M21 melanoma cells.

TABLE II

Evaluational Solid-Phase Antigens for Screening of Monoclonal and Polyclonal Xenoantisera

	Monoclonal antibody[a]					Polyclonal antisera[a]		Background (cpm)	Optimal antigen density (µg/well)
Antigen source	α240K	α94K	αHLA-DR	αHLA-A,B,C	α β₂m	αMAA	αFN[b]		
CDM	17.6	34.0	1.3	1.8	24.0	23.0	1.4	1200	3
Cells	12.0	5.3	7.0	8.4	8.9	13.6	7.5	4272	—
Urea extract	10.5	10.8	1.6	4.5	5.4	19.0	15.3	2459	10
Membranes	7.4	4.6	3.1	1.8	2.5	7.8	5.4	4336	1

[a]Percentage of antibody positive vs. the various target antigens.   [b](FN) Fibronectin.

complex or to other components. Fibronectin, which is normally detected in both CDM and other antigen preparations, is readily removed by affinity chromatography as evidenced by the lack of binding to CDM. It is obvious by inspection of the data presented in Table II that hybridoma antibody binding to the 240K and 94K glycoproteins, characterized in our laboratory, is most easily discriminated on solid-phase CDM. On the other hand, CDM may not be an appropriate screening tool for some tumor antigens that are integral membrane components. However, our results certainly indicate that a suitable source of antigen can be produced that will have the characteristic of being relatively enriched either in shed or secreted molecules or, alternatively, in peripheral or integral membrane components. Soluble antigen preparations are also valuable as solid-phase targets because they can readily be depleted of those molecules that may be immunogenic in xenoimmunizations, thus eliminating the selection of hybrids secreting non-tumor-specific antibodies.

4. Characteristics of Monoclonal Antibodies Elicited and Selected with Immunochemically Defined Antigens

As detailed above, a number of antibodies from Fusion No. 1 failed to react with intact cells. Three of these antibodies, Nos. 2, 33, and 41, were selected for further characterization. Figure 4 illustrates that these antibodies indeed did not bind either to lymphoid cells

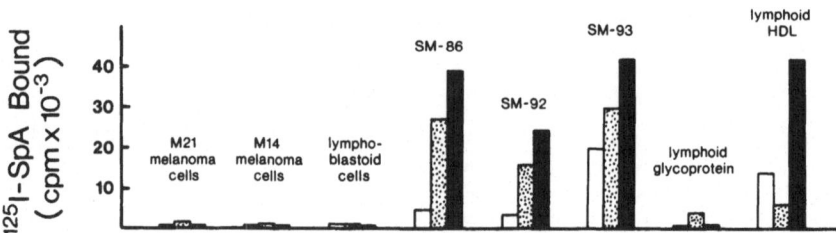

FIGURE 4. Specificity of monoclonal antibodies reactive with shed or secreted antigens. Hybridomas Nos. 2, 33, and 41 from Fusion No. 1 were screened against intact melanoma and lymphoid cells as well as solid-phase targets from melanoma cells and lymphoid cells.

or th M21 and M14 melanoma cells from which the CDM is derived. In contrast, Antibody Nos. 33 and 41 bound well to the original screening target, CDM-92, as well as to other batches of CDM. Antibody No. 2 bound only to CDM-93. The molecules recognized by these antibodies appeared to be tumor-associated, since the antibodies did not bind to gly-coproteins derived from lymphoid cells. However, to make certain that non-cell-surface lymphoid components were included, we also utilized high-density lipoproteins derived from lymphoid cells and isolated by KBr flotation (Allison *et al.,* 1977). Reactivity of Antibody Nos. 2 and 41 was found with this antigen preparation, while Antibody No. 33 did not bind. Antibody No. 33 thus requires further characterization to determine whether it is tumor-specific.

In marked contrast to Antibody No. 33, Antibody 9.2.27, derived from the same cell fusion, was highly reactive with intact cells, and thus its specificity could be more easily assessed by binding to a variety of cultured cell lines (Morgan *et al.,* 1981). As shown in Fig. 5, this antibody was reactive with all melanoma cell lines tested, but unreactive with cultured carcinoma or lymphoid or fibroblastoid cultures. Indirect immunoprecipitation of labeled glycoprotein derived from M21 melanoma cells with Antibody 9.2.27 and SDS-PAGE analysis revealed a two-chain structure with the lower band having a molecular weight of 240K (Fig. 6). ^{35}S-labeling studies and other biochemical characteristics suggest that the higher-molecular-weight component is proteoglycan that associates with the 240K

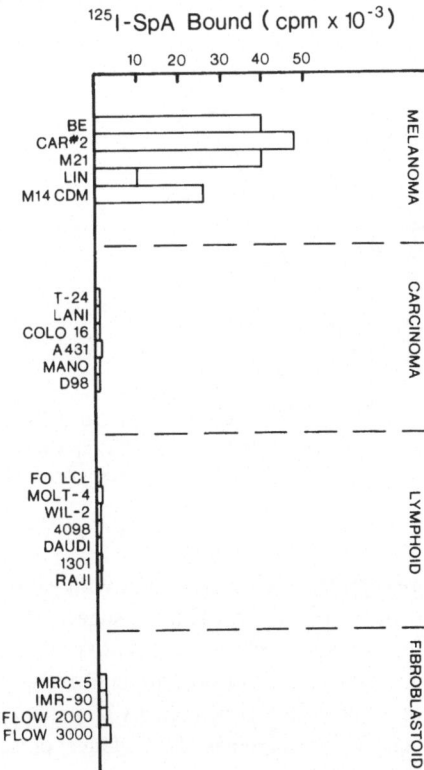

FIGURE 5. Specificity of monoclonal Antibody 9.2.27. Monoclonal Antibody 9.2.27, derived from Fusion No. 1, was assayed against the indicated target cells.

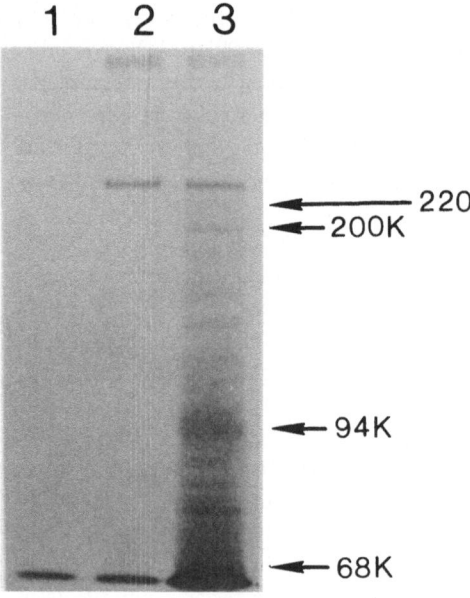

FIGURE 6. Molecular nature of glycoproteins reactive with monoclonal Antibody 9.2.27. Cell-surface glycoprotein, prepared from M21 melanoma cells, (3×10^5 cpm) was reacted with Antibody 9.2.27–PAS. After washing, antigen was eluted and electrophoresed on a 5% acrylamide–0.135% bis-acrylamide sodium dodecyl sulfate slab gel at 30 mA/gel. (1) P3 $\times$ 63 Ag8 control; (2) Antibody 9.2.27; (3) polyclonal rabbit anti-MAA (No. 6522). Molecular-weight standards: human plasma fibronectin, myosin, phosphorylase B, bovine serum albumin.

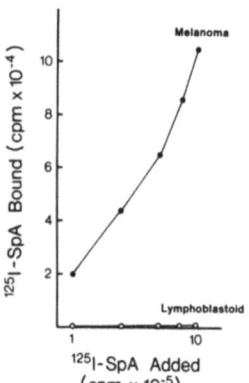

FIGURE 7. Expression of 240K glycoprotein on melanoma and lymphoid cells. [^{125}I]-SpA was added in increasing amounts to cells previously exposed to saturating levels of Antibody 9.2.27 and rabbit anti-mouse Ig.

glycoprotein. Binding studies with saturating levels of monoclonal antibody, second antibody, and [^{125}I]-SpA (Fig. 7) suggest that the apparent specificity of the 240K glycoprotein for melanoma cells is not quantitative, since the antigen is expressed at least 100-fold more on melanoma than on lymphoid cells. Preliminary results with indirect immunofluorescence on histological sections of patient tumors indicate that Antibody 9.2.27 is reactive only with melanomas (D. O. Chee, personal communication).

5. Conclusions

The antibodies that were elicited and selected by using the immunochemically defined antigen preparations detailed above represent the extremes of a spectrum of antibodies. Each of these may find uses in diagnosis, prognosis, or radioimaging of human melanomas. Regardless, we have demonstrated that immunochemically and serologically defined antigen preparations, adsorbed onto the proper carrier vehicles, can be more effective than whole cells in inducing antibody responses to tumor-specific molecules. This approach represents an attractive alternative not only because it requires less investment of time and materials to produce desired antibodies, but also because antibodies of unique specificity can be produced that may not have been induced or selected with intact cells. Our results demonstrate this fact, since many antibodies are elicited to tumor-specific components once immunodominant non-tumor-specific components are removed from the immunogens. Those molecules that were lacking or removed by affinity chromatography from our immunogens did not represent all the non-tumor-specific components. Indeed, it may not be necessary or, for that matter, even desirable to remove all the non-tumor-specific components from immunogens, since they may have some useful adjuvant effect. In summary, the use of immunochemically defined antigens as immunogens and targets in screening assays offers a powerful and versatile tool for tailoring the process of antibody elicitation and selection to obtain the desired monoclonal antibodies.

ACKNOWLEDGMENTS. The author's research cited herein was supported by USPH Service Grant CA 28420 and Grant IM-218 of the American Cancer Society. The author thanks J. Brock and C. Hockman for their excellent technical assistance. This chapter is Publication No. 2409 from the Department of Molecular Immunology, Scripps Clinic and Research Foundation.

References

Allison, J. P., Pellegrino, M. A., Ferrone, S., Callahan, G. N., and Reisfeld, R. A., 1977, Biologic and chemical characterization of HLA antigens in human serum, *J. Immunol.* **118**:1004.

Bottcher, I., Ulrich, M., Hirayama, N., and Ovary, Z., 1980, Production of monoclonal mouse IgE antibodies with DNP-specificity by hybrid cell lines, *Int. Arch. Allergy Appl. Immunol.* **61**:248.

Galfre, G., Howe, S. C., Milstein C., Butcher, G. W., and Howard, J. C., 1977, Antibodies to major histocompatibility antigens produced by hybrid cell lines, *Nature (London)* **266**:550.

Galloway, D. R., McCabe, R. P., Pellegrino, M. A., Ferrone, S., and Reisfeld, R. A., 1981, Tumor-associated antigens in spent medium of human melanoma cells: Immunochemical characterization with xenoantisera, *J. Immunol.* **126**:62.

Köhler, G., and Milstein, C., 1975, Continuous cultures of fused cells secreting antibody of predetermined specificity, *Nature (London)* **256**:495.

Köhler, G., and Milstein, C., 1976, Derivation of specific antibody producing tissue culture and tumor lines by cell fusion, *Eur. J. Immunol.* **6**:511.

McCabe, R. P., Quaranta, V., Frugis, L., Ferrone, S., and Reisfeld, R. A., 1979, A radioimmunometric antibody binding assay for evaluation of xenoantisera to melanoma associated antigens. *J. Natl. Cancer Inst.* **62**:455.

Milstein, C., Galfre, G., Secher, D. S., and Springer, T., 1979, Monoclonal antibodies and cell surface antigens, *Cell Biol. Int. Rep.* **3**:1.

Morgan, A. C., Jr., Galloway, D. R., Wilson, B. S., and Reisfeld, R. A., 1980, Human melanoma associated antigens: A solid-phase assay for detection of specific antibody, *J. Immunol. Methods* **39**:233.

Morgan, A. C., Jr., Galloway, D. R., and Reisfeld, R. A., 1981, Production and characterization of monoclonal antibody to a melanoma-specific glycoprotein, *Hybridoma* **1**:17.

Wiktor, T. J., and Koprowski, H., 1978, Monoclonal antibodies against rabies virus produced by somatic cell hybridization: Detection of antigenic variants, *Proc. Natl. Acad. Sci. U.S.A.* **75**:3938.

Wilson, B. S., Pellegrino, M. A., Reisfeld, R. A., and Ferrone, S., 1978, A simple method for production of specific xenoantisera to human histocompatibility (HLA-A,B,C) antigens, *Transplant. Proc.* **10**:741.

16

The Significance of Circulating Immune Complexes in Patients with Malignant Melanoma

T. M. PHILLIPS, W. D. QUEEN, AND M. G. LEWIS

1. Introduction

There is increasing evidence that malignancy in both humans and experimental animal models can elicit the formation of host-mediated immune reactions directed against the growing neoplasm (Aoki *et al.,* 1976; Klein, 1975; Mastrangelo *et al.,* 1974; Old *et al.,* 1968). It is thought that the basis for the promotion of these reactions is configurational changes in glycosylated proteins and lipids of the tumor-cell plasma membrane that distinguish them as being different and therefore antigenic. However, if such immune reactions can be promoted, then the question still remains: why cannot the host control the growth of the tumor and the course of the disease? Several mechanisms have been suggested to explain this situation, such as the possibility that the tumor antigens are weak and do not elicit a strong host reaction, that tumor antigen-shedding may "soak up" the antibody in the form of circulating immune complexes, and that there are present circulating "blocking factors" that interact with the various components of the host's immune system and block their reactivity. Such blocking factors have also been cited as being circulating immune complexes that are able to react with and neutralize primed lymphocytes (Baldwin *et al.,* 1972; Baldwin and Robbins, 1976; Hellström *et al.,* 1969; Hellström and Hellström, 1970; Pyrhonen *et al.,* 1976; Sjögren *et al.,* 1971).

The study of the mechanisms involved in metastasis of tumor cells has also shed light on the role of the circulating antibody and its effect on tumor cells in the bloodstream.

T. M. PHILLIPS AND W. D. QUEEN ● Department of Medicine, George Washington Medical Center, Washington, D. C. 20037   M. G. LEWIS ● Department of Pathology, Stritch School of Medicine, Loyola University, Maywood, Chicago, Illinois 60153.

Studies in animals have revealed that cytotoxic antibodies may interact with and prevent tumor cells from settling in the endothelial beds of the capillaries (MacFadden, 1976; O'Neil, 1976). These experiments were performed in primed animals and have had some confirmation in the human situation (Hellström and Hellström, 1970). However, many other reports cite that antibody formation, especially of the noncytotoxic type, may help tumor cells by protecting them from lymphocyte attack. Such antibodies may either attach directly to the tumor antigens or interact and neutralize the primed lymphocytes via constant-fragment (Fc) receptors. In a similar vein, the role of circulating immune complexes has been suggested as being responsible for neutralization of the lymphocyte action and in one report has been shown to be the "blocking factor" reported in many other studies (Baldwin *et al.*, 1972). Studies on humoral immunity in humans have revealed the presence of several different types of antibodies, directed against many different antigens. Studies have shown the presence of cytotoxic membrane-directed antibodies as well as those directed against cytoplasmic components, fetal antigens, and other nonspecific or non-tumor-related material (Bodurtha *et al.*, 1975; Canevari *et al.*, 1975; deVries *et al.*, 1975; Lewis *et al.*, 1973, 1978b; Morton *et al.*, 1968; Old *et al.*, 1968; Whitehouse, 1973). In addition, the presence of antiimmunoglobulins has been demonstrated in long-standing tumor-bearing hosts and in situations where the host's antibody-mediated response has been in existence for a considerable period of time (Bartfield, 1969; Pyrhonen *et al.*, 1976; Lewis *et al.*, 1971b, 1976, 1978c).

It is becoming clear that the old arguments about antibodies being either "good" or "bad" are invalid and that the role of the circulating antibody has to be reviewed in the light of the clinical situation and the extent of the disease. The production of tumor-directed antibodies will depend on many factors such as the nutritional status of the patient, the degree of expression of the tumor antigens, and whether necrosis has released other internal components that become recognized as antigenic. Due to the abundance of these components, they often become the main target for the host immune attack. In such cases, the leaking of this type of material into the bloodstream via the lymphatics and the intracellular spaces would provide an antigenic stimulus from which the host would form a wide array of both beneficial and detrimental antibodies (Lewis *et al.*, 1978a). These antibodies would in turn produce a variety of circulating immune complexes that would both potentiate the immune response through macrophage processing and macrophage–T cell (Yoshida and Andersson, 1972) interaction or cause lymphocyte blocking effects (Sinclair, 1978). This latter process could occur either through interaction of the antibody with activated Fc receptors or through the antigen, in excess, reacting with the antigen receptors on the surface of the primed lymphocyte (Nussenzweig, 1974; Uhr and Phillips, 1966). In addition, the production of such antibodies and their resulting complexes would elicit the formation of antiimmunoglobulins such as rheumatoid factors (anti-Fc) (Waaler, 1940) and serum agglutinators [anti-F(ab')^2] (Waller *et al.*, 1968; Hartmann, 1976) in an attempt to remove the circulating immune debris. It is now known that the rheumatoid factors may bind complement into their aggregates, which could be a problem if these deposits were to settle in the beds of the fine capillary networks (Baum *et al.*, 1964). The action of such large antiimmunoglobulins coupled to an existing immune complex would quickly block kidney filtration (Gilboa *et al.*, 1979) and lead to the immunopathological state of glomerulonephritis associated either with the antiimmunoglobulin or with immune-complex deposition (Poskitt *et al.*, 1974; Lewis *et al.*, 1971a; Olsen *et al.*, 1979; Sutherland *et al.*, 1974).

The formation of the immune complexes and their composition, along with their ability to bind complement, are important in their role in tissue damage and cell blockage. The components of circulating immune complexes may be used to study the events taking place during the progression of a growing neoplasm, as defined by the host's immune system. The isolated complex components may be used to localize the site of antibody attack and the antigens used to study their effectiveness in producing either lymphocyte priming or as hypersensitivity reagents. In either case, the reagents recovered would be indicative of the host's own recognition of the *in vivo* situation.

In this chapter, we wish to outline a system for the detection and recovery of circulating immune complexes in human malignant melanoma and attempt to define the roles of the different responses leading to the production of such complexes. From these studies, it has been possible to show that other immunological processes are in action at the same time as the tumor growth, and the multiassay system for immune-complex detection and analysis has the advantage that it is able to distinguish between tumor-directed responses and those of another nature.

2. Physicochemical Properties of Immune Complexes

2.1. Formation of Immune Complexes

Although the *in vivo* formation of immune complexes has not been fully demonstrated, there are considerable data on their formation *in vitro*. Laboratory studies have shown that complexes are formed according to the classic precipitin curve described by Heidelberger (1956), wherein the formation of different types of complexes is determined by the availibility of the two reacting agents (Fig. 1). This reaction is dependent on the ionic conditions of the surrounding media, the pH, and the strength (avidity) and specificity (affinity) of the two reactants for each other. At equilibrium, the reactants form large aggregates that precipitate out of solution. At either end of the curve, there exist soluble complexes in either antigen or antibody excess. These complexes are reversible and in the *in vivo* state are probably unstable, breaking up and re-forming as they interact with either more antigen or more antibody. Thus, the *in vivo* situation probably reflects a situation wherein the complexes oscillate in size between medium and small, each eliciting a different effect on the host's immune system. These effects could be potentiation of the immune response through macrophage processing via attachment of the complexes to the cell's Fc receptors or blocking of the primed lymphocytes through the same mode of attachment. This latter situation may also arise through antigen attachment to antigen receptors on the primed lymphocytes.

2.1.1. Bonding Forces Involved in Immune-Complex Formation

The interaction between antigen and antibody is dependent on the closeness of fit (affinity) that the antibody receptors have for the structural configuration that constitutes the antigen determinant on the antigen molecule. There are four main types of forces

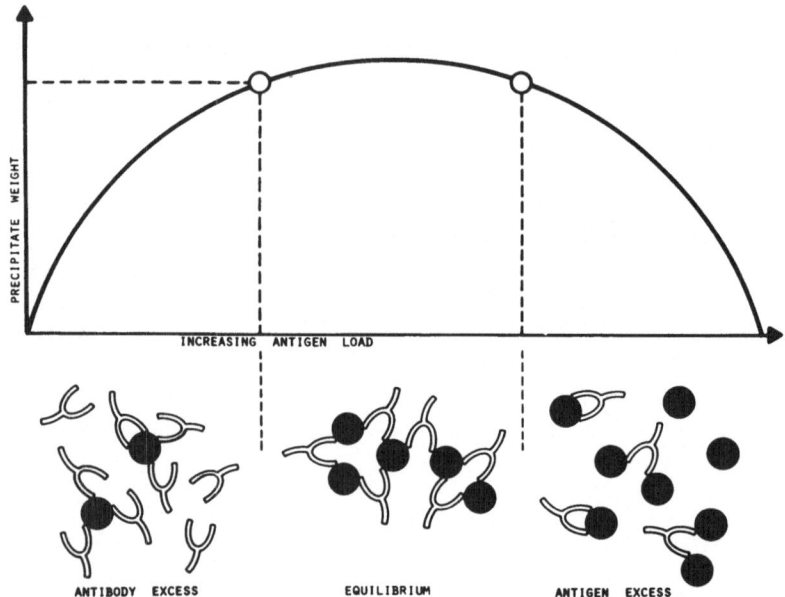

FIGURE 1. Microprecipitin curve. Relationship between the classic precipitin curve as described by Heidelberger (1956) and the formation of immune complexes.

involved in the bonding of antigen–antibody complexes, and the forces will be described in detail in order of diminishing importance (Fig. 2).

2.1.1a. Van der Waal Forces. These are the most important forces involved in the formation of complexes. They are formed when the "electron clouds" of the two reactive sites interact and form dipoles through a temporary disturbance of the electron clouds in both molecules. These dipoles are responsible for forming attractive forces between the two molecules that result in their drawing into close proximity with each other. When the dipoles swing back through equilibrium, they set up oscillatory forces that in turn make the attractive force inversely proportional to the 7th power of the distance, thus creating a force that increases as the distance between the molecules lessens.

2.1.1b. Coulombic Forces. These forces arise as a result of the attraction between two ionic groups of opposite charge, strategically placed on the two interacting molecules. A common example of such attraction is that between an amino group on one molecule for a carboxyl group on another. If both groups are ionized, the attractive force is inversely proportional to the square of the distance between the groups on the interacting molecules. Again, the closer the two groups, the stronger the bonding forces.

2.1.1c. Ion Attractive Forces. This is essentially a force associated with an antibody and a protein antigen and is formed between two hydrophobic amino acid side groups in aqueous solution. The water molecules in contact with these groups are not H-bonded and are at a higher energy state than the two hydrophobic groups. If the hydrophobic groups can come close enough to exclude all the water, then the two lower-energy groups will prefer to stay in close proximity rather than disperse into the surrounding high-energy solution.

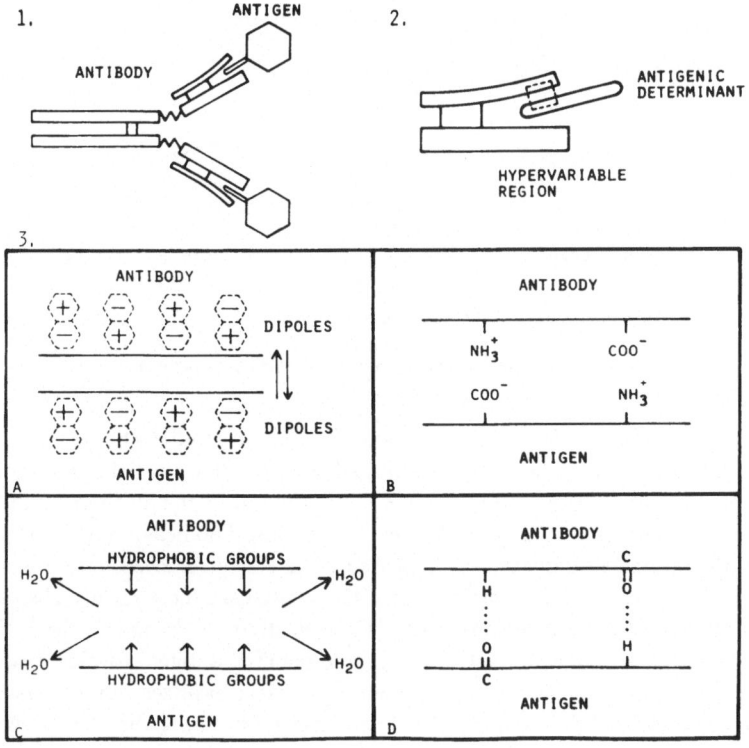

FIGURE 2. Types of bonding involved in antigen–antibody reactions. (1) Diagrammatic representation of a hypothetical antigen–antibody complex. (2) Enlarged view of the hypervariable region of the antibody and the antigenic determinant. The small square is magnified in (3). (3) (A) Van der Waal forces. Oscillating dipoles (+/−) form attractive forces between the antibody and the antigen. (B) Coulombic forces. Attractive forces between ionized amino and carboxyl groups of exposed amino acid side chains. (C) Ion attractive forces. Bonding formed between two hydrophobic amino acid side groups during close contact of the antibody with the antigen. (D) Hydrogen-bond forces. Attractive forces formed between hydrophillic groups of the two reacting molecules.

2.1.1d. Hydrogen-Bond Forces. These weak bonds are formed between hydrophilic groups on the two interacting molecules and are reversible. Bonding is by electron interaction and therefore, close proximity of the two molecular reactive sites is required for maximum binding capacity to be reached.

2.1.2. Fate of Circulating Immune Complexes According to Size

The fate of all immune complexes will be determined by their size (Fig. 3), which in turn is dependent on their composition; antibody-excess complexes will bind to cell Fc receptors more readily than those at equilibrium or in antigen excess and are removed by Fc-bearing cells. The binding of complement (see Section 2.2) will also determine the size, charge, and fate of each individual complex. In our experience, the complexes isolated from our melanoma patients could be divided into three main types: light (3–7 S), medium

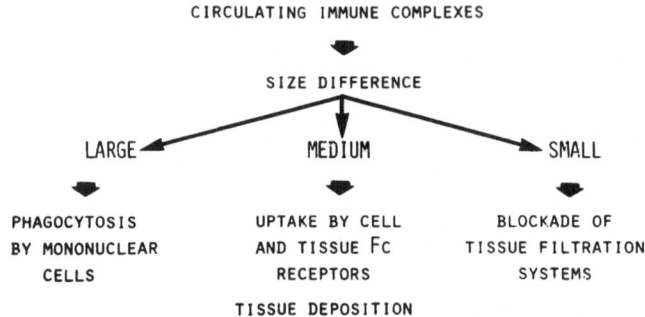

FIGURE 3. Effect of size of immune complexes on their fate.

(15–30 S), an heavy (32–50 S). It was found by elution studies (Feltkamp and Boode, 1971) performed on skin, kidney, and lymph-node biopsies that the light and medium complexes were often found deposited in the fine capillaries, while the medium complexes comprised the most abudant material in kidney depositions. The heavy complexes sometimes were found deposited in kidneys, but appeared to be easily removed by the mononuclear cells and were rarely seen as vessel deposits. The complexes most readily observed in the glomeruli of the tumor-bearing host were of the medium type, and of these, 30% were shown to contain antitumor antibody and its corresponding antigen. Elution studies on cell suspensions of lymph nodes from patients with primary, localized, and metastatic melanoma also demonstrated (Lewis *et al.,* 1980) the changes in tumor-directed antibodies with the progression of the disease (Table I). These changes correlated with the composition of the circulating immune complexes at the three different stages studied.

2.2. Interaction of Circulating Immune Complexes with Complement

At present, we have been able to determine several areas where circulating immune complexes may interact with and activate complement (C) (Fig. 4). In the classic pathway, there is interaction at the $C'1q$, $C'3$, and $C'5$ levels of the cascade. However, immune complexes may also act as activated particles that react with the $C'3$ convertase system to cause activation of the alternate pathway.

TABLE I

Incidence of Antitumor-Antibody Production in Lymph Nodes Draining Malignant Melanomas

Tumor stage	Type of antibody produced	
	Membrane-directed	Cytoplasm-directed
Primary	19/20 (100%)	0/20 (0%)
Localized	21/35 (60%)	13/35 (37%)
Widespread	3/28 (11%)	25/28 (89%)

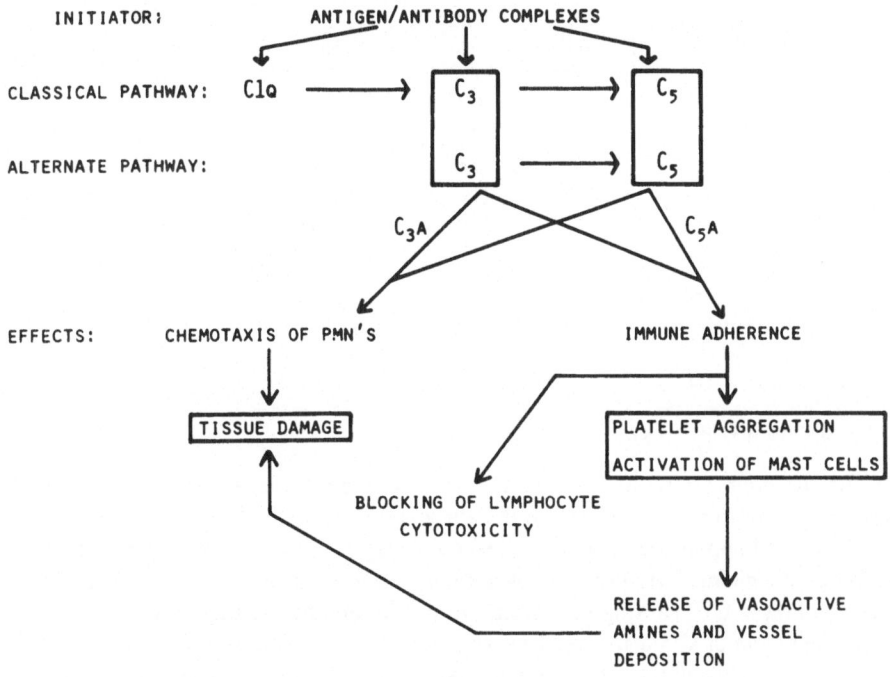

FIGURE 4. Interaction of immune complexes with the complement cascade.

2.2.1. Classic Pathway Activation

Once an antigen–antibody reaction has taken place and the molecular changes associated with the antibody hinge-region swing have further acted on the Fc region of the antibody and rendered it active for complement binding, $C'1q$ becomes attached to the complex by ionic attraction. During this process, $C'1q$ is thought to become structurally altered, which effects $C'1r$, causing it to undergo cleavage. This action activates $C'1s$ to complete the formation of the activated C1 complex. The activated C1 complex reacts with $C'4$, causing its cleavage and the binding of $C'2$; the resulting $C'4b,2a$ complex then attaches to the immune complex. The $C'4b,2a$ complex is actually $C'3$ convertase, a precurser to $C'3$ activation.

Once $C'3$ has been activated and cleaved, the resulting complex, $C'4b,2a,3b$, becomes known as $C'5$ activator and acts on $C'5$ to produce $C'5a$ and b, the b portion being incorporated into the $C'4b,2a,3b$ complex. The rest of the components of the complement cascade are bound in a numerical manner. The immunopathological properties of complement binding to immune complexes arise from the chemotactic and immune adherent properties of both the bound components and the cleaved by-products. The chemotactic by-products $C'3a$ and $C'5a$ are the cause of many immune-complex-mediated immunopathological conditions due to their ability to attract polymorphonuclear cells, especially neutrophils and eosinophils, to the site of immune-complex deposition.

TABLE II
Molecular Weight and Properties of Complement Components

Component	Molecular weight	Effect
C'4b,2a	300,000	Activation of C'3
C'4b,2a,3b	471,000	Activation of C'5
C3a	8,900	Anaphylatoxin + chemotaxis
C'3b	172,500	Immune adherence
C'5a	15,000	Anaphylatoxin + chemotaxis
C'5b,6,7	365,000	Chemotaxis

2.2.2. Alternate-Pathway Activation

The circulating immune complex may act as an activated aggregate or particle that can trigger the properdin activation of the alternate pathway. This is especially true when the antigen is a lipopolysaccharide complexed in antigen excess. There is also evidence that human immunoglobulin A (IgA) complexes may initiate activation of the complement system by binding to C'3, causing its convertion to C'3b and thus acting as a priming system for the production of C'5 activator. In such a case, the complex would act as an activated particle, able to activate the alternate pathway without properdin. The size and effects of complex bound components of the complement cascade are summarized in Table II.

2.3. Interaction of Immune Complexes with Cells and Tissues

Circulating immune complexes may interact with cells and tissues of the host in several different ways. The main interaction is via binding to Fc receptors or Fc-receptor-like structures on the plasma membranes of different types of cells in the bloodstream and with tissues also bearing similar structures. The macrophage appears to be the main cell type with which interaction takes place, again via the Fc receptors but also through activated C'3 receptors (Mantovani *et al.*, 1972); in either case, the macrophage appears to endocytose the complexes and remove them from the circulation. There is evidence that such complexes may be processed by the engulfing macrophage and, in cases of antigen excess, process the antigen, thus producing a stimulatory effect (Vansnick *et al.*, 1978). Binding by Fc receptor has also been indicated in the case of eosinophils (King *et al.*, 1979) and neutrophils (Movat, 1979; Ann, 1980), which are usually attracted to complement-binding complexes that have become deposited in the vessel walls.

We have studied the binding of immune complexes to the surfaces of autologous platelets in our patients with malignant melanoma and have found that 21% with metastatic disease have circulating immune complexes that are able to bind to the surface of autologous platelets and cause platelet aggregation (Sacher *et al.*, 1980). Immunofluorescent-labeled complexes of known composition were used to study platelet uptake of immune complexes. In our studies, we found that autologous platelets will actively take up certain types of immune complexes, but that there are certain requirements before such a phenomenon can take place. Aggregating complexes are usually composed of IgG and glycoprotein antigens that have bound complement to the C′3b level. We also noted that activated C′3 was required before the platelets could be aggregated. Further immunofluorescent studies revealed that isolated IgG Fc could bind to the surface of platelets, but only after it had been aggregated and had bound complement. In such an event, minute amounts of the isolated, washed complex could induce large numbers of washed, autologous platelets to aggregate, thus forming small discrete thrombi. Another event that accompanied the platelet aggregation was the release of vasoactive amines, which in turn alters the vascular permeability and aids the endothelial deposition of the complexes.

Similar studies on kidney glomeruli and the choroid plexus of cancer patients with immune complexes detectable at death revealed that complement-activated Fc labeled with fluorescein could be demonstrated in the endothelium of vessels of both organs (Foidart *et al.*, 1979; Globus and Wilson, 1979). The specificity of this localization was confirmed by the abolition of the staining by prior treatment of the sections with unlabeled Fc.

To date, our tissue studies have suggested that several organs may become the target for immune-complex deposition, and work is progressing to prove the incidence and mechanisms whereby the complex deposition takes place in these areas. Our investigations have now widened to include the kidney glomeruli, the skin capillary bed, the ciliary body of the eye (Rao, personal communication), the choroid plexus of the brain, and the alveolar bed of the lung. The suggestion has arisen that in cases on oncology patients in a state of stress, the coronary vessels may also be a prime target for complex deposition following interaction with platelets and the formation of microthrombi.

3. Detection and Isolation of Immune Complexes

There are several different techniques available for the detection of circulating immune complexes, but individually they give information about only one aspect of the complex and do not give a full picture of all the available complexes and their individual properties. In our laboratory, we utilize a multifacet assay system (Fig. 5) to glean from the available complexes as much data as possible. Circulating immune complexes may be detected by three main types of assays: (1) methods that utilize the binding of complement components; (2) physicochemical separation techniques; and (3) immunological techniques. The collective data from all these techniques may then be used to piece together a reasonable picture of the spectrum of different complex types present and their ability to bind complement and potentially cause immunopathological conditions (Fig. 6).

3.1. Techniques That Utilize the Binding of Complement Components

This series of assays includes the C′1q–binding assay (Zubler *et al.*, 1976), the Raji-cell assay (Theofilopoulos *et al.*, 1976), and polyethylene glycol (PEG) precipitation (Creighton *et al.*, 1975; Pesce *et al.*, 1980; Haskova *et al.*, 1978; Phillips and Lewis, 1980).

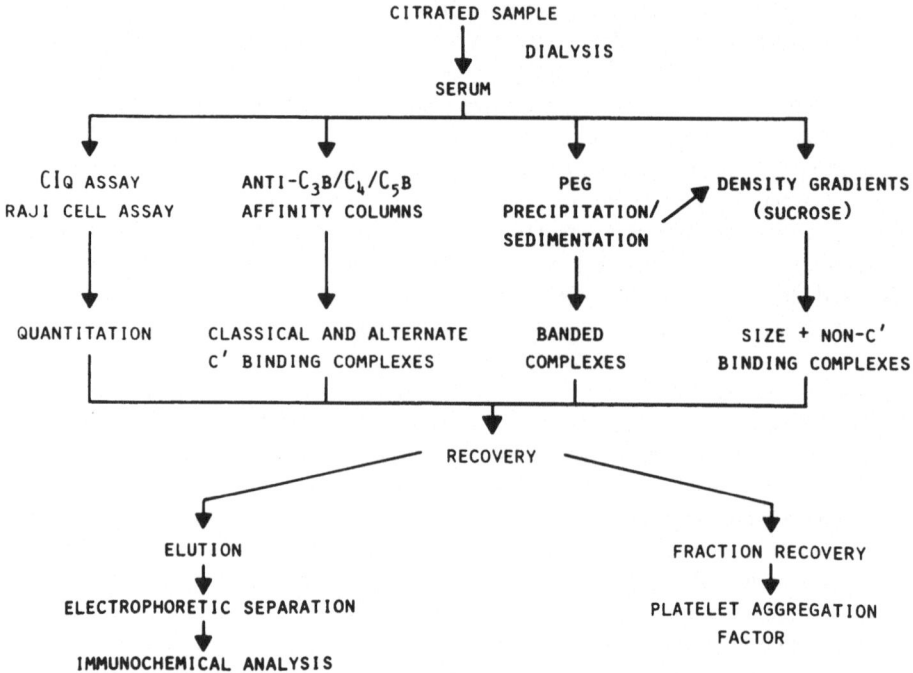

FIGURE 5. Georgetown University multiassay system for the detection of immune complexes. The system is a multifacet analytical one for the total detection of different types of circulating immune complexes.

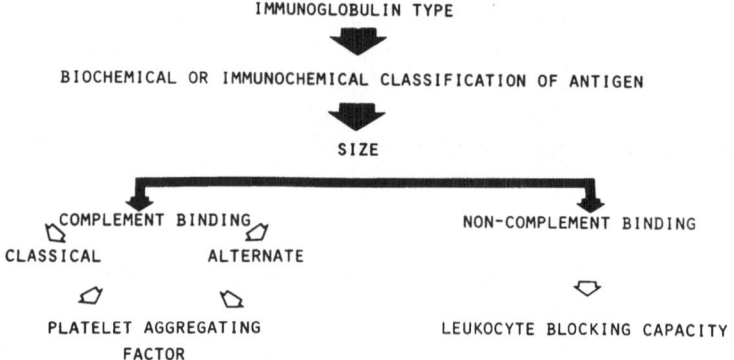

FIGURE 6. Classification of circulating immune complexes. The scheme outlines the data produced for each individual complex by the Georgetown University system.

3.1.1. C'1q-Binding Assay

Human C'1q is isolated by the method of Heusser *et al.* (1973) and the isolated material stored in vapor-phase liquid nitrogen at $-136°C$ until ready to be iodinated by the lactoperoxidase method. The working life of this reagent is considered to be 1 week. The assay (Fig. 7) is performed by adding 100 μl of sample to 100 μl ethylenediamine tetraacetic acid (EDTA) buffer (0.4 M, pH 7.5) and incubating for 30 min at 37°C followed by cooling to 0°C prior to the addition of 5 μl of a 200 μg/ml solution of the labeled C'1q. This mixture is incubated for 1 hr at 4°C, and the resulting complexes are precipitated by the addition of 1 ml PEG of molecular weight 6000. The precipitate is separated by centrifugation at 10,000 g for 10 min at 4°C, washed twice in cold normal saline, and the precipitate–supernatant counted in a gamma counter.

3.1.2. Raji-Cell Assay

This assay involves the incubation of immune-complex-containing samples with a lymphoblastoid cell line that is rich in receptors for C'3b (Fig. 8). A 100-μl sample is mixed with 1×10^6 Raji cells and incubated for 30 min at 37°C. After the incubation, the cells are washed five times in Hank's medium and incubated with 100 μl 5 mg/ml ^{125}I-labeled heat-aggregated human IgG prepared from Sigma Cohn fraction II, to saturate the binding sites. In all cases, ultracentrifuge-purified normal sera were used as controls. A quantitative curve is made up by incubating the labeled IgG with known amounts of heat-aggregated, unlabeled IgG and the results expressed in μg/ml aggregated globulin/ml sample. Inhibition of the labeled globulin binding is considered evidence of complex binding.

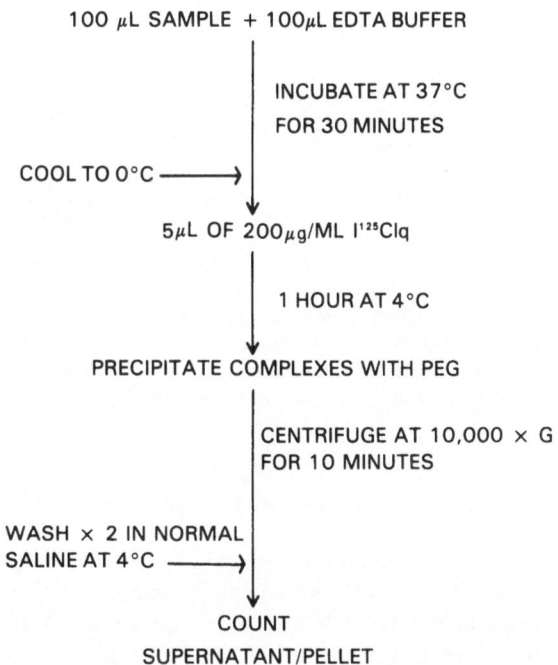

FIGURE 7. C1q-assay flowchart.

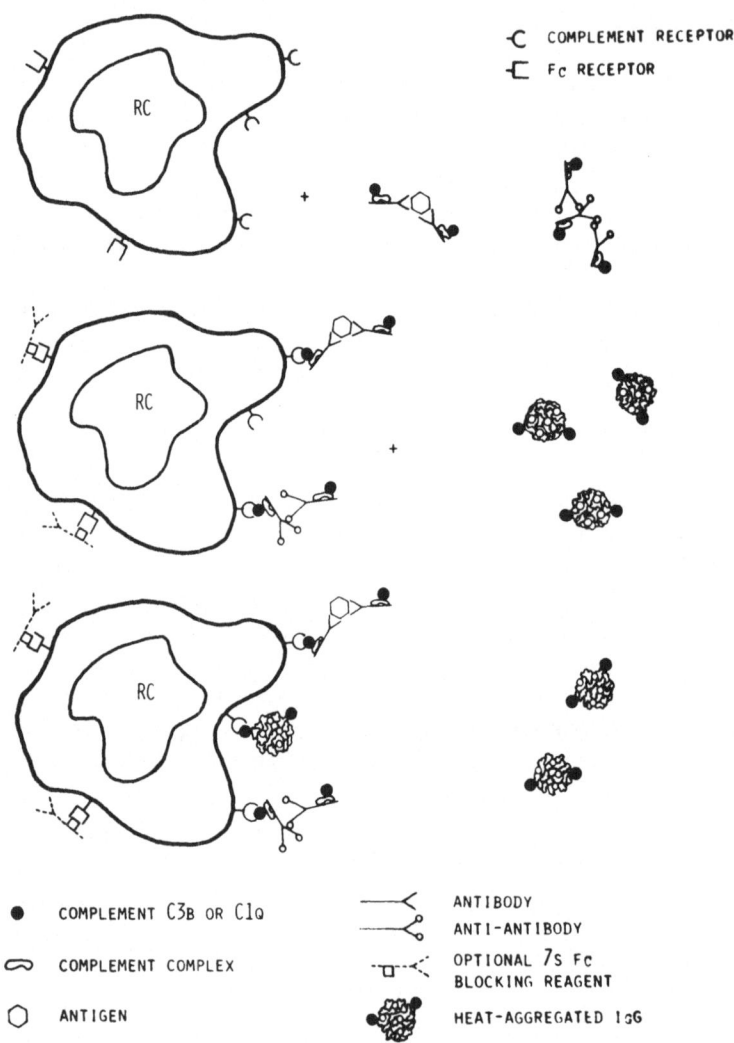

FIGURE 8. Raji-cell assay. The Raji cell (RC) is a lymphoblastoid cell carrying complement and Fc surface receptors. Circulating immune complexes of either antigen–antibody or antibody–antiimmunoglobulin are bound to cell via fixed complement. Quantitation of complex uptake is performed by adding complement-binding, heat-aggregated IgG. The degree of inhibition of the radiolabeled IgG uptake is quantitatively measured in a gamma counter. Modification of this assay includes preincubation of the Raji cell with a 7 S Fc-blocking reagent to inhibit Fc binding of the radiolabeled IgG.

3.1.3. Polyethylene Glycol Precipitation

Immune complexes binding C′1q may be precipitated with a low percentage of PEG. In our assay, 100 μl of test sample is incubated with a final volume of 3% PEG and allowed to remain at 4°C for 30 min, to precipitate the complexes. The precipitate is washed three times by centrifugation at 10,000 g for 10 min in cold saline and the final precipitate measured by turbidometry in a spectrophotometer. The results are expressed in $\mu g/ml$ and calculated by comparison with a curve formed from measurements made on known amounts of aggregated human IgG.

3.2. Techniques That Use Physicochemical Properties

This section includes PEG precipitation–sedimentation (Phillips and Lewis, 1980) and sucrose-density-gradient studies (Steensgard and Jacobsen, 1979).

3.2.1. Polyethylene Glycol Precipitation–Sedimentation

PEG-precipitated complexes are usually a mixture of different immune-complex types as well as contaminating nonimmune, noncomplexed materials that may hinder the analysis. In order that such interfering materials may be identified and removed, we have developed a PEG gradient system that separates the different precipitated materials by weight. A 100-μl sample is mixed with an equal volume of 6% PEG (molecular weight 6000) to give a final percentage of 3% PEG. The sample is mixed and the precipitation allowed to proceed for 30 min at 22°C. The precipitate is removed by centrifugation at 15,000g for 5 min, washed three times in cold saline, and layered onto a 4-ml 10–40% PEG gradient (molecular weight 20,000). This gradient is then spun at 30,000g for 30 min, and the resulting bands (Fig. 9) are recovered in a Beckman fraction-recovery system. Three main zones are usually seen: a light zone containing free C'1q and immunoglobulin fragments, a medium zone that contains the majority of the medium- and low-molecular-weight complexes, and a heavy zone that consists of aggregated immunoglobulin and complexes composed of immunoglobulin and antiimmunoglobulin such as rheumatoid factor. Once recovered, the zones may be sized by sucrose-density-gradient studies or dissociated by acid or chaotropic elution and analyzed by biochemical and immunochemical means.

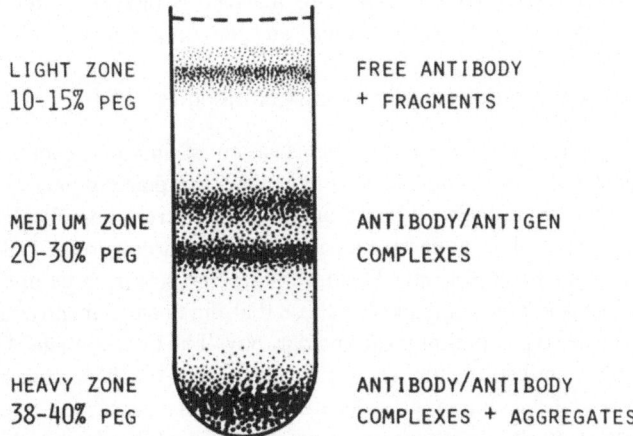

FIGURE 9. PEG sedimentation tube. The diagram shows the typical postcentrifugation localization of PEG-precipitated materials on a 10–40% PEG gradient (molecular weight 20,000) centrifuged at 30,000g for 30 min at 22°C.

3.2.2. Sucrose-Gradient Studies

This technique is useful in determining the size of complexes and for the detection of non-complement-binding complexes. A 100-μl sample is layered onto the top of a 10–40% sucrose gradient and spun at 48,000g for 18 hr. The formed bands are again isolated on a fraction-recovery system and retained for dissociation and biochemical and immunochemical analysis. To determine the molecular weight of these complexes, a reference tube is set up onto which purified immunoglobulins are placed as reference markers for determination of the sedimentation rate of the test complexes.

3.3. Immunological Techniques

This section covers affinity chromatography for the collection of all types of complement-binding complexes with solid-phase antibodies specific for the complement components.

3.3.1. Affinity Chromatography for the Isolation of Complexes by Complement Binding

To assess the complement binding in all immunoglobulins types of immune complexes, affinity chromatography using solid-phase antibodies directed against human C′3b, C′4, and C′5b may be used to capture the complexes via these bound complement components (Fig. 10). The sample is cascaded over either Sephadex or polyacrylamide beads to which one of the aforementioned antibody systems has previously been covalently bound (Inman and Dintzis, 1969). During the passage of the sample through the column, the complexes containing the bound complement components become attached to the immobilized antibodies in the column matrix. While the unreacted material passes through. The bound material is recovered by passing an acid buffer at pH 2.5 through the column and collecting the material that is eluted. This material is then ready for separation into its respective components prior to biochemical and immunochemical analysis.

3.3.2. Affinity Chromatography against Antibodies

The aforedescribed system for the isolation of immune complexes by antibodies directed against the different bound complement components may also be extended to include solid-phase antibodies directed against the different immunoglobulin classes. The principle is the same, but the complexes are isolated according to the antibody class and not their ability to bind complement. This technique has proven to be useful when detecting non-complement-binding complexes or those that bind complement weakly and dissociate during the former type of affinity chromatography. The disadvantage of this system is that the immobilized antibodies often exert a strong affinity for the complexed antibodies they are extracting and the elution often denatures the tertiary structure of the eluted complex antibody. Alternatively, the affinity binding of the immobilized antibody to the circulating immune complex is so strong that the complex formed between the circulating immune complex and the solid-phase antibody cannot be broken, rendering the antibody unrecoverable.

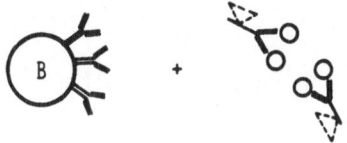 SAMPLE CONTAINING IMMUNE COMPLEX
ADDED TO IMMOBILIZED ANTISERA

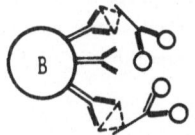 IMMUNE COMPLEXES BOUND TO
IMMOBILIZED ANTISERA

ACID OR CHAOTROPIC ELUTION

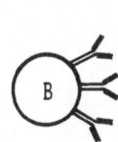 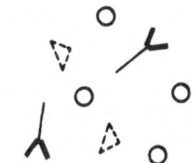 BOUND COMPONENTS FREED BY THE
ACTION OF THE ELUTING AGENT AND
RECOVERED FOR IMMUNOCHEMICAL
ANALYSIS

 IMMOBILIZED ANTISERUM

 ANTIBODY FROM IMMUNE COMPLEX

 COMPLEMENT COMPONENT

 ANTIGEN FROM IMMUNE COMPLEX

FIGURE 10. Affinity chromatography for the isolation of complement-binding immune complexes.

4. Dissociation and Separation of Immune-Complex Components

4.1. Dissociation of Immune Complexes

In our experience, the isolated complexes from either the PEG or sucrose gradients may be dissociated with recovery of viable antibody and antigen by either of two methods: (1) acid or (2) chaotropic-ion dissociation. The chaotropic-ion dissociation appears to give better results, but, as with all dissociation techniques, some damage to the tertiary structure of both the antibody and the antigen is sustained.

4.1.1. Acid Dissociation

Immunoprecipitates may be solubilized at both extremes of the pH scale (Kleinschmidt and Boyer, 1972), but many proteins appear to be denatured at the high pH range. Acid dissociation is the most popular form of treatment, and in this study we used a series of different acid combinations in an attempt to find the gentlest techniques for the recovery of the components in an active form. Isolated complexes were treated with dilute hydrochloric acid, glycine, and hydrochloric acid–glycine mixtures (Kabat amd Mayer, 1971; Ruoslahti, 1976), and it was found that citric acid at pH 2.5–3.0 gave the best results (Phillips and Draper, 1975). A combination of citric-acid-buffered saline at pH 2.5 was eventually adopted for dissociation of high-affinity complexes, while the less avid complexes responded well to chaotropic elution.

4.1.2. Chaotropic Dissociation

Chaotropic ions interact with and dissociate immune precipitates by ionic substitution. The chaotropes react in the order $SCN^- > I^- > Br^- > Cl^-$ and must be used in high molar concentrations (Dandliker *et al.*, 1967). Avrameas and Ternynck (1976) have shown that laboratory-constructed complexes of IgG and anti-IgG may be dissociated by iodine, bromide, and chloride salts, but the best results were obtained by using 2 M iodide. This treatment also appeared to result in the least denaturing effects on both the antibody and the antigen.

We have found that the gentlest dissociation method is to incubate the isolated complex in a 4 M solution of polyvinylpyrrolidone (PVP)–iodine for 30 min at 22°C. During this incubation, the free ions compete with the electrons binding the complex components and neutralize their attractiveness. As the complex dissociates, the presence of the PVP helps to maintain the structure of the complex components.

4.2. Separation of the Dissociated Complex Components

Separation and recovery of the individual complex components may be achieved by either agarose-block electrophoresis or thin-layer chromatography (TLC).

4.2.1. Agarose-Block Electrophoresis

The dissociated complex is placed into a slot cut in a 1% agarose block (1 inch × 3 inches × 1 inch deep) made up in barbital–acetate buffer, pH 8.6. The agarose is Sigma type III, high endosmotic flow, and the buffer is used at a strength of 0.05 M barbital. A current of 1 mA/cm is passed through the plate, and the components are allowed to migrate along the horizontal axis. During the electrophoresis, the antigens usually migrate toward the anode, while the highly charged antibodies either migrate a short way toward the cathode or are actively carried along with the ionic backflow caused by endosmosis in the gel. The separated components are recovered by scanning the gel with a UV lamp and recovering the opaque spots. The spots are cut from the gel plate and the isolated components removed from the gel by gentle diffusion into saline at 4°C for 16 hr.

4.2.2. Thin-Layer Chromatography

This technique is used in conjunction with the complexes that had been dissociated by chaotropic-ion treatment. Separation is achieved by placing the complex–chaotropic solution into a TLC plate composed of Sephadex G200 superfine beads and running the plate in a PVP–iodine buffer at an angle of 30° until the yellow buffer runs over the edge of the plate. The electrophoresis running conditions for this phase are a potential of 1 mA/cm in barbitol–acetate buffer 0.5 M, pH 8.6. This process also helps to neutralize the affects of the elution buffer and prepare the components for typing by immunochemical means.

4.3. Techniques Used to Characterize the Isolated Complex Components

These techniques include indirect immunofluorescence to localize the isolated antibodies against both intact autologous and allogeneic tumor cells, immunodiffusion–counter current electrophoresis to check the specificity of the isolated antigens against the types of antibodies, and double countercurrent immunoelectrophoresis to type the isolated, dissociated complexes without subjecting the components to physicochemical isolation.

4.3.1. Indirect Immunofluorescence

This technique is performed in the same manner as described by Phillips and Lewis (1970), using the isolated antibodies from the complexes. Briefly, the antibodies are incubated for 30 min at room temperature with either living tumor cells or snap-frozen tumor cells. The former are used to detect membrane-associated antigens, while the latter are used to detect cytoplasmic antigens. Following the antibody incubation, the cells or smears of frozen cells are washed three times in phosphate-buffered saline (pH 7.2, 0.01 M PO_4) and the bound antibodies detected by applying a goat anti-human IgG conjugated to fluorescein isothiocyanate (isomer I). This reagent is applied for a further 30 min and finally extensively washed prior to microscopic examination. In both cases, the material under investigation is mounted in phosphate-buffered glycerol, pH 8.6.

Examination is performed with a Leitz orthoplan microscope equipped with an HBO 100 mercury lamp, a 490 interference excitation filter, and a 525 nm secondary filter. The basic patterns of membrane and cytoplasmic staining (Fig. 11) were recorded in both the autologous and the allogeneic situations.

4.3.2. Immunodiffusion and Counterelectrophoresis

Immunodiffusion is performed by matching the isolated complex antigens and preparations from the membranes and the cytoplasm of the tumor cells against the isolated, complexed antibodies. Crude tumor-cell-membrane fractions are prepared by hypotonic lysis and ultracentrifugation. The supernatant following a 3-hr 30,000g spin is labeled as membrane-rich and the pellet as cytoplasm-rich. Agarose plates are prepared at 1% in 0.1 M tricine buffer and a series of six peripheral wells cut around a larger central well (standard Ouchterlony immunodiffusion). The antibody is placed into the central well, and the antigens, at varying concentrations, are placed into the peripheral wells. The plates are

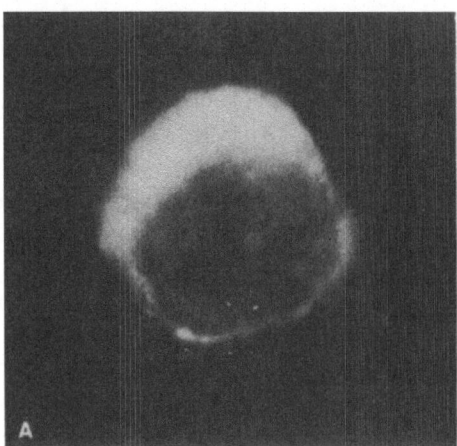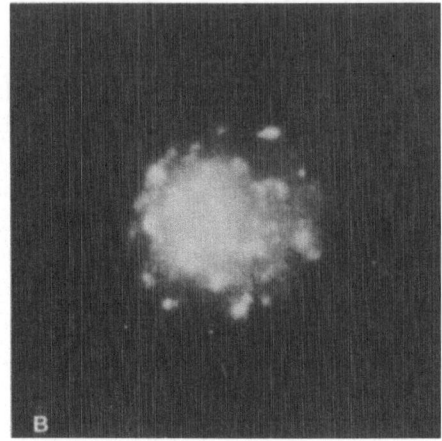

FIGURE 11. Immunofluorescence patterns on melanoma cells. (A) Cytoplasmic localization of isolated, complexed antibody on autologous or allogeneic snap-frozen melanoma cells; (B) plasma-membrane localization of isolated, complexed antibody against autologous melanoma tumor cells.

allowed to react for 72 hr in a moist atmosphere at 4°C, following which they are examined under opaque light and the reaction lines recorded.

In those reaction sets where no precipitin lines are observed at 72 hr, the reagents are tested by countercurrent electrophoresis. This technique has an additional advantage over immunodiffusion in that reactions are of an all-or-nothing type. The electrical current forces approximately 90% of the two reactants together, giving a greater concentration gradient in which precipitation can occur. During this process, the antibodies are swept back toward the cathode by the endosmotic flow through the gel, while the negatively charged antigens are carried by the electrical flow toward the anode (Fig. 12). If the wells are filled with the antibody on the anodal side and the antigen on the cathodal side, then during the electrophoresis the two reactants are forced together, thus increasing their chances of interaction. The final result is a line of precipitin formed between the two reactants. This technique, however, has more inherent technical problems than the immunodiffusion technique and still holds a secondary role to the latter.

4.3.3. Double Countercurrent Immunoelectrophoresis for the Analysis of Immune-Complex Components

This technique (Fig. 13) is performed by the modification described by Phillips and Lewis (1980) of the original technique described by Phillips and Draper (1975). Immune complexes from the PEG or sucrose gradients are treated with either 0.33 M citrate or 4 M PVP–iodine and placed in the center well in a 1% agarose plate. The plate is made up of high-endosmotic agarose in a 0.5 M barbital–acetate buffer at pH 8.6. The plate is electrophoresed at 10 mA/cm for 1 hr, and two peripheral wells are cut on the anodal and cathodal sides of the central well, along the electrophoresis tract. Antibodies from the iso-

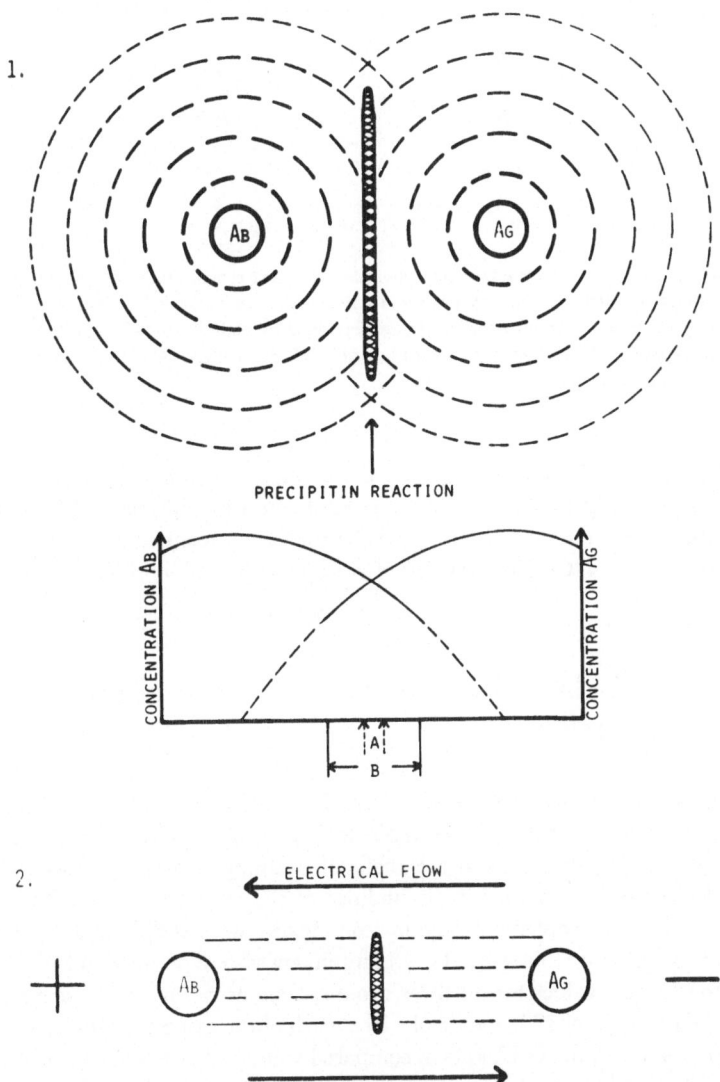

FIGURE 12. Principles of immunodiffusion and countercurrent electrophoresis. (1) Immunodiffusion. At the top is a schematic representation of diffusion areas generated in a standard immunodiffusion plate. The decreasing concentrations of antibody (AB) and antigen (AG) as they approach the zone of equivalence (B) are shown below. A precipitin reaction (A) occurs when the reactants reach precipitation equilibrium in the gel. (2) Countercurrent electrophoresis. The diagram represents electrophoretically forced diffusion of AG toward the anode (+) by electrical flow and AB toward the cathode (−) by endosmotic flow. The latter is caused by a backflow of positively charged ions.

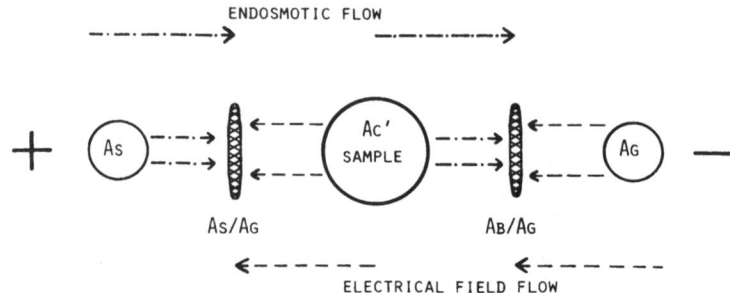

FIGURE 13. Double countercurrent immunoelectrophoresis. Schematic representation of a double countercurrent system to simultaneously identify antibody (AB) and antigen (AG) in an isolated, dissociated (AC') immune complex. Dissociated antibody–antigen complexes are separated by endosmotic flow and electrical field flow, respectively. The separated AB and AG are allowed to react with test antigen (AG) or antiserum As) by simultaneous countercurrent electrophoresis.

lated complexes, which have been typed by immunofluorescence, are placed in the anodal wells and isolated antigens and tumor fractions in the cathodal wells. Electrophoresis is allowed to proceed for another 30 min, and the interacted reagents are allowed to diffuse and react overnight at 4°C. The presence of precipitin lines is considered positive.

5. Analysis of Isolated Immune Complexes in Human Malignant Melanoma

Throughout this study, the melanoma patients were categorized into three groups according to the stage of their disease: those with a primary lesion, those with localized disease that had not spread beyond the regional draining nodes, and those with widely disseminated disease. We compared the findings of the classic C'1q and Raji-cell assays (which measure total complement-binding complexes) with the total complex detection phase of the Georgetown University (G.U.) multiassay system outlined in Fig. 5. The C'1q assay gave the highest values for all three groups, demonstrating the presence of immune complexes in 6 of 57, 65 of 173, and 78 of 110 of each of the respective three patient groups. The Raji-cell assay and the G.U. system compared well, with average values of 3 of 57, 42 of 173, and 70 of 110 by the Raji-cell assay and 3 of 57, 40 of 173, and 69 of 110 by the G.U. system. These results are given in Table III. However, when the analytical aspect of the G.U. system was applied to the positive samples from each group, there was an overall reduction in the number of complexes that possessed components associated with either the patients' autologous tumor cells or their immunological reactivity against the growing tumor.

Analyzed for tumor-associated antibody, the primary-tumor group showed that all the 3 of 57 complex-positive samples contained tumor-directed antibody. The localized group showed a reduction from the initial 40 of 173 to 37 of 173 samples positive for tumor-associated antibody, while the widespread-tumor group dropped from 69 of 110 positive samples to 14 of 110 positive for tumor-associated antibody. Analysis for tumor-associated antigen in these groups revealed that the 3 of 57 in the primary group remained unchanged, while the 40 of 173 in the localized group dropped to 30 of 173. The widespread group also dropped, from 69 of 110 to 10 of 110 containing detectable tumor-associated antigen. Table IV summarizes these findings.

Further analysis by immunofluorescent localization of the isolated complex antibodies showed that 3 of 3 of the primary group all contained antibodies directed against the plasma membranes of the autologous tumor cells. The localized group demonstrated the presence of 23 of 37 samples containing membrane-directed antibodies and 14 of 37 containing antibodies directed against components of the tumor-cell cytoplasm. The widespread group showed a swing toward the cytoplasmic antigens, with only 2 of 14 of the complexed antibodies being directed against the membranes, while 12 of 14 were directed against the cytoplasmic antigens. Table V presents these findings.

Analysis of the antigens from the isolated complexes showed a lower number than those containing antibody, perhaps due to our inability to isolate and detect antigens or because some of the complexed antibodies were directed against tumor-cell materials that are either altered and shed or are by-products that we are unable to extract. In the primary group, 3 of 3 of the positive samples correlated well with the antibody findings in that they all contained antigens related to the tumor-cell membranes. The localized group showed a lower level of detectable tumor-associated complexed antigen, but appeared to stay in reasonable correlation with the antibody findings. There were 21 of 30 samples positive for membrane-associated antigen and 9 of 30 positive for cytoplasmic antigens. The widespread group demonstrated 2 of 10 positive for membrane-associated antigens, which correlated

TABLE III

Detection of Total Circulating Immune Complexes in Human Malignant Melanoma by Three Techniques

Tumor stage	C'1q assay	Raji-cell assay	G.U. system[a]
Primary	6/57 (11)	3/57 (5%)	3/57 (5%)
Localized	65/173 (38%)	42/173 (24%)	40/173 (23%)
Widespread	78/110 (71%)	70/110 (64%)	69/110 (63%)

[a]The G.U. system denotes PEG precipitation–sedimentation, affinity chromatography, and sucrose-density-gradient isolation.

TABLE IV

Analysis of Tumor-Associated Material in Immune Complexes Isolated from Patients with Malignant Melanoma by the Georgetown University System

Tumor stage	Antibody	Antigen
Primary	3/57 (5%)	3/57 (5%)
Localized	37/173 (21%)	30/173 (17%)
Widespread	14/110 (13%)	10/110 (9%)

TABLE V

Analysis of the Specificity of the Tumor-Directed Antibodies Isolated from Immune Complexes in Human Malignant Melanoma

Tumor stage	Membrane-directed	Cytoplasma-directed
Primary	3/3 (100%)	0/3
Localized	23/37 (62%)	14/37 (38%)
Widespread	2/14 (14%)	12/14 (86%)

TABLE VI

Analysis of the Tumor-Associated Antigens Isolated from the Immune Complexes of Patients with Malignant Melanoma

Tumor stage	Membrane-associated	Cytoplasma-associated
Primary	3/3 (100%)	0/3
Localized	21/30 (70%)	9/30 (30%)
Widespread	2/10 (20%)	8/10 (80%)

with the membrane-directed antibody findings, and 8 of 10 positive for cytoplasma-associated antigens. In all cases, these samples were the same as those in which positive tumor-directed antibodies had been demonstrated. Table VI shows the distribution of these antigens throughout the three patient groups.

6. Presence of Antiimmunoglobulin Complexes

During this study, it was noted that several patients demonstrated the presence of heavy-zone immune complexes on the PEG gradients and that these complexes appeared to be in the sedimentation range of 36–50 S. Some of these complexes proved to be of high affinity and difficult to disrupt, acid treatment being the only technique that produced results. Once dissociated, they also demonstrated the presence of antibody without any indication of the presence of antigen. Further analysis showed that some of these complexes were aggregates of the same immunoglobulin, while others appeared to contain immunoglobulins of either different classes or subclasses of the same immunoglobulin. The complete analysis of these complexes is still under way, but it appears that three main types of antiimmunoglobulin activity could be demonstrated within the components of these complexes (Fig. 14): (1) anti-Fc or rheumatoid factor; (2) anti-$F(ab')_2$ or anti-hinge region; and (3) a blocking antiimmunoglobulin that appears to be reactive against the membrane-directed antibody, neutralizing its localization on the autologous tumor-cell membrane (Table VII). This later antiimmunoglobulin appeared to fit most of the criteria for an autoantiidiotype.

The separation of antibody–antibody complexes was difficult, and neither the conventional agarose block nor the TLC technique used for ordinary immune complexes appeared to work. The antibodies carried the same net charges and therefore migrated in a similar fashion. However, these antiimmunoglobulins were either of different immunoglobulin classes or of different subclasses and could be isolated by polyacrylamide-gel electrophoresis and agarose-gel electrophoresis at right angles to the polyacrylamide run.

The separated antibodies were recovered by cutting the opaque spots from the gel, following screening with a long-wavelength UV lamp, and allowing the antibodies to diffuse into a small volume or buffer. The antibodies were concentrated to 50 $\mu g/ml$ by negative-pressure dialysis and tested by latex flocculation for activity against isolated human Fc and $F(ab')_2$ fragments absorbed onto latex beads.

During this investigation, isolated immunoglobulins were tested against the autologous tumor cells by indirect immunofluorescence and their types and subclasses tested by immunodiffusion in agarose against monospecific typing antisera raised in rabbits and goats. It was found that some complexes contained IgG antibodies that were reactive against the autologous tumor cells and another IgG, of a different subclass, that was not reactive with the tumor cells but appeared to be complexed with the antitumor antibody. These immunoglobulins were also negative in both the latex flocculation assays. Further experimenta-

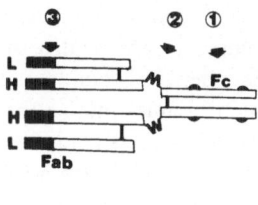

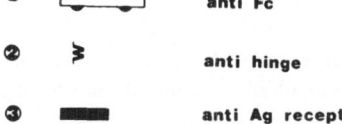

FIGURE 14. Different types of antiimmunoglobulins. Diagram indicating the three main antigenic determinants on the IgG molecule recognized by antiimmunoglobulins.

TABLE VII

Analysis of Antiimmunoglobulin Complexes Isolated from Patients with Malignant Melanoma

Tumor stage	Type of antiimmunoglobulin		
	Anti-Fc	Anti-$F(ab')_2$	Antireceptor
Primary	0/57	2/57 (4%)	0/57
Localized	47/173 (27%)	57/173 (33%)	35/173 (20%)
Widespread	4/110 (4%)	19/110 (17%)	28/110 (25%)

tion revealed that the action of the antitumor antibody could be abolished by prior incubation with the other immunoglobulin, isolated from the same complex. These antiimmunoglobulins appeared to be specific for their target antibodies and did not react with other antibodies from other complexes. Although it is ambitious to call human antibodies idiotypic in their mode of specificity, this criterion was indicated when it was shown that target antitumor antibodies appeared to be reactive only in the autologous situation, were cytotoxic, and were directed against markers on the autologous tumor-cell membrane. Further experimentation is required to fully explain the significance of these findings, but it is not unreasonable to hypothesize that such antiimmunoglobulins may be responsible for the abolition of the membrane-directed host antibody attack. This may be caused by their action against the cell clone responsible for the production of the antitumor antibody or the antitumor antibody itself, or both. Such an action would be the network theory of Jerne (1973) in practice.

7. Conclusions

The detection of circulating immune complexes is possible in most diseases, but not all the complexes are related to the disease process. The standard assay systems do not differentiate between complexes that arise due to a secondary immunological process, proceeding at the same time as the disease in question, and the immunological parameters related to the disease. In our studies, we found that the complement-binding-immune-complex detection systems such as Raji and the C'1q assays often gave a high degree of false positives. These appeared to be caused by secondary immunological reactions taking place at the same time. The multiassay system outlined in this chapter allows the different complexes present to be isolated and recovered for analysis. The different systems also allow each individual complex to be classified according to its immunoglobulin class, antigen type, complement-fixing ability, and size. The result of this analysis is that a clearer picture of the available complexes may be gained and their relationship to both the extent and stage of the disease may be assessed.

The immunofluorescent and immunodiffusion studies on the isolated antibodies and antigens revealed that not all the tumor-associated material could be easily typed. There was clearly other tumor-associated material available that could not be localized by immunofluorescence but appeared to be tumor-associated due to its presence in the serum of the tumor-bearing host. However, such a system of complex analysis yields only minute amounts of material for analysis. There is, however, an answer to this problem—plasmapheresis (Hersey *et al.*, 1976, 1978), which is a system whereby vast quantities of serum may be removed and the complexes isolated in quantity. We have begun to study plasmapheresis samples from melanoma patients (Phillips *et al.*, 1980) with a view to isolating reasonable quantities of immune complexes for use either in immunodiagnosis or as reagents for the production of monoclonal antibodies (L. M. Jerry, personal communication) raised against antigens defined by the human host. Such reagents would greatly increase the specificity of human diagnostic research and would help to define all the types of antigens present on tumor cells. The autologous system would also be useful for studying circulating antigen by affinity methods or for the refinement of a radioimmunoassay. We feel that the system for the isolation and analysis of circulating immune complexes outlined herein is not perfect, but it does yield data on the individuality of the complexes and is often able to detect other disease processes that are underlying the neoplasm. Many tumor-bearing hosts also have low levels of autoantibodies (Ziegler, 1973) that reflect a type of immune derangement or breakdown of immunological control. The nature of these autoantibodies is also an indication of the degree of tissue damage caused by the neoplastic growth. These autoantibodies rarely become involved in the formation of immune complexes, but do reflect simultaneous pathological phenomena in the patient.

The formation of antibody–antibody complexes is another indication of immune-control malfunction. The function of such complexes may only be guessed at—a clearance system for the removal of complexes and damaged immunoglobulin or a potentiation system mediated through macrophage processing. The processing of immunoglobulin complexes, such as rheumatoid factor and a tumor-directed antibody, may result in the macrophage's recognizing the antigen receptor or hypervariable region of the antitumor antibody as a antigenic site, and through lymphocyte interaction an antiimmunoglobulin is produced against that antibody. The resulting antiimmunoglobulin would have a restricted specificity and would meet many of the requirements of an antiidiotype.

The net result would be the neutralization of the antitumor antibody and even its shutdown at the clonal level. This action would produce both an escape system for the tumor to grow and metastasize and large immune complexes through which the production of the antiimmunoglobulin could be perpetuated.

Great interest is centered around circulating immune complexes, but until better technology is developed and it is understood that the composition and physicochemical nature of the complexes are important, the field will not advance. The materials contained in the complexes may prove to be a valuable source of reagents for the study of the interactions between the host's immune system and the growing neoplasm. Coupled with the hybridoma technology, these materials may provide some of the most unique reagents available to the human and experimental tumor immunologist.

ACKNOWLEDGMENTS. The authors wish to acknowledge the technical assistance of Mrs. P. Satchithanandam, the photographic expertise of Mr. N. More, and the typing skills and editorial help of Mrs. E. A. Phillips. Finally, thanks to all the patients who helped to make this study possible.

References

Ann, T., 1980, Binding of soluble immune complex to Fc receptors on human neutrophils—Detection by double coating indirect rosette formation, *Int. Arch. Allergy Appl. Immunol.* **61**:1980.

Aoki, T., Walling, M. J., Bushar, G. S., Liu, M., and Hsu, K. C., 1976, Natural antibodies in sera from healthy humans on surfaces of type C RNA viruses and cells from primates, *Proc. Natl. Acad. Sci. U.S.A.* **73**:2491.

Avrameas, S., and Ternynck, T., 1976, Use of iodide salts in the isolation of antibodies and their dissolution of specific immune precipitates, *Biochem. J.* **102**:37c.

Baldwin, R. W., and Robbins, R. A., 1976, Factors interfering with immunological rejection of tumours, *Br. Med. Bull.* **32**:118.

Baldwin, R. W., Price, M. R., and Robbins, R. A., 1972, Blocking of lymphocyte-mediated cytoxicity for rat hepatoma cells by tumour specific antigen antibody complexes, *Nature (London) New Biol.* **238**:185.

Bartfield, H., 1969, Distribution of rheumatoid factor activity in non-rheumatoid states, *Ann. N. Y. Acad. Sci.* **168**:126.

Baum, J., Stastny, P., and Ziff, M., 1964, Effects of the rheumatoid factor and antigen/antibody complexes on the vessels of the rat mesentery, *J. Immunol.* **93**:985.

Bodurtha, A. J., Chee, D. O., Laucius, J. F., Mastrangelo, M. J., and Prehn, R. T., 1975, Clinical and immunological significance of human melanoma cytotoxic antibody, *Cancer Res.* **35**:189.

Canevari, S., Fossati, G., Della Porta, G., and Balzarini, G. P., 1975, Humoral cytotoxicity in melanoma patients and its correlation with the extent and course of the disease, *Int. J. Cancer* **16**:722.

Creighton, W. D., Lambert, P. H., and Meischer, F. A., 1975, Detection of antibodies and soluble antigen/antibody complexes by precipitation with polyethylene glycol, *J. Immunol.* **2**:1219.

Dandliker, W. B., Alonso, R., de Sausserre, V. A., Kierszenbaum, F., Levison, S. A., and Shapiro, H. C., 1967, The effect of chaotropic ions on the dissociation of antigen antibody complexes, *Biochemistry* **6**:1460.

De Vries, J. E., Cornain, S., and Rumke, P., 1975, Humoral and cellular immunity in melanoma patients, *Behring Inst. Mitt.* **56**:148.

Feltkamp, T. E. W., and Boode, J. H., 1971, Elution of antibodies from biopsy tissue, *J. Clin. Pathol.* **23**:629.

Foidart, J. B., Salmon, J. P., Berthoux, F. J., and Mathieu, P., 1979, Binding of soluble immune complexes to human glomerular complement receptors, *Kidney Int.* **15**:303.

Gilboa, N., Durante, D., Guggenheim, S., and Lacher, J, 1979, Immune deposit nephritis and single component cryoglobulinemia associated with chronic lymphocytic leukemia: Evidence for a role of circulating IgG–anti-IgG immune complexes in the pathogenesis of the renal lesion, *Nephron* **24**:223.

Golbus, S. M., and Wilson, C. B., 1979, Experimental glomerulonephritis induced by *in-situ* formation of immune complexes in glomerular capillary wall, *Kidney Int.* **16**:148.

Hartmann, D. P., 1976, The identification and role of anti-immunoglobulins in human malignancy, Ph.D. thesis, McGill University, Montreal, Canada.

Haskova, V., Kaslik, J., Riha, I., Matl, I., and Rovensky, J., 1978, Simple method of circulating immune complex detection in human sera by polyethylene glycol precipitation, *Z. Immunol. Immunobiol.* **54**:399.

Heidelberger, M., 1956, *Lectures in Immunochemistry,* Academic Press, New York.

Hellström, I., and Hellström, K. E., 1970, Colony inhibition studies on blocking and non-blocking serum effects on cellular immunity to Maloney sarcomas, *Int. J. Cancer* **5**:195.

Hellström, I., Hellström, K. E., Evans, C. A., Heppner, G. H., Pierce, G. E., and Yang, J. P., 1969, Serum-mediated protection of neoplastic cells from inhibition by lymphocytes immune to their tumour-specific antigens, *Proc. Natl. Acad. Sci. U.S.A.* **62**:362.

Hersey, P., Edwards, A., Adams, E., Ibister, J. P., Murray, E., Biggs, J. C., and Milton, G. W., 1976, Antibody-dependant cell-mediated cytotoxicity against melanoma cells induced by plasmapheresis, *Lancet* **1**:825.

Hersey, P., Murray, E., Ruygrok, S., Edwards, A., and Milton, G. W., 1978, Blocking factors against melanoma line-dependant antibody relationship to disease activity in melanoma patients, *Aust. N. Z. J. Surg.* **48**:26.

Heusser, C., Boesman, M., Nordin, J. H., and Isliker, H., 1973, Effect of chemical and enzymatic radioionation on *in vitro* human C1q activities, *J. Immunol.* **110**:820.

Inman, J. K., and Dintzis, H. M., 1969, The derivatizion of cross-linked polyacrylamide beads, controlled introduction of functional groups for the preparation of special biochemical absorbents, *Biochemistry* **8**:4074.

Jerne, N. K., 1973, The immune system, *Sci. Am.* **229**:52.

Kabat, E. A., and Mayer, M. M., 1971, *Experimental Immunochemistry,* 2nd ed., pp. 22–96, Charles C. Thomas, Springfield, Illinois.

King, T. E., Schwarz, M. I., Dreisin, R. E., Pratt, D. S., and Theofilopoulos, A. N., 1979, Circulating immune complexes in pulmonary eosinophilic granuloma, *Ann. Intern. Med* **91**:397.

Klein, G., 1975, Immunological surveillance against tumours, in: *Immunological Aspects of Neoplasia,* 26th Ann. Symp. Cancer. Res., pp. 21–57, Williams and Wilkins, Baltimore.

Kleinschmidt, W. J., and Boyer, P. D., 1972, Interaction of protein antigens and antibodies. I. Inhibition studies with the egg albumin anti-egg albumin system, *Biochim. Biophys. Acta* **263**:245.

Lewis, M. G., Loughridge, L. W., and Phillips, T. M., 1971a, Immunological studies on a patient with the nephrotic syndrome associated with malignancy of non-renal origin, *Lancet* **2**:134.

Lewis, M. G., Phillips, T. M., Cook, K. B., and Blake, J., 1971b, Possible explanation for the loss of detectable antibody in patients with disseminated melanoma, *Nature (London)* **232**:52.

Lewis, M. G., Avis, P. J. G., Phillips, T. M., and Sheikh, K. M. A., 1973, Tumour associated antigens in human malignant melanoma, *Yale J. Biol. Med.* **46**:661.

Lewis, M. G., Hartmann, D., and Jerry, L. M., 1976, Antibodies and anti-antibodies in human malignancy: An expression of deranged immune regulation, *Ann. N. Y. Acad. Sci.* **276**:316.

Lewis, M. G., Phillips, T. M., and Rowden, G., 1978a, Beneficial and detrimental effects of humoral immunity in malignancy, *Pathobiol. Ann.* **8**:217.

Lewis, M. G., Phillips, T. M., Rowden, G., and Jerry, L. M., 1978b, Humoral immune reactions in cancer patients, in: *The Handbook of Cancer Immunology*, Vol. 3 (H. Waters, ed.), p. 159, Garland STPM Press, New York.

Lewis, M. G., Phillips, T. M., Rowden, G., and Jerry, L. M., 1978c, Humoral immune factors in metastasis in human cancer, *Prog. Cancer Res. Ther.* **5**:245.

Lewis, M. G., Phillips, T. M., and Rowden, G., 1980, Serological Identification of tumour antigens in human malignant melanoma, in: *Serologic Analysis of Human Cancer Antigens* (S. A. Rosenberg, ed.) p. 385, Academic Press, New York.

MacFadden, D. K., 1976, Immunological characteristics of clonal differentiation and metastatic spread of a murine mammary tumour, Ph.D. thesis, McGill University, Montreal, Quebec, Canada.

Mantovani, B., Rabinovitch, M., and Nussenzweig, V., 1972, Phagocytosis of immune complexes by macrophages: Different roles of the macrophage receptor sites for complement, C3, and for immunoglobulin, IgG, *J. Exp. Med.* **135**:780.

Mastrangelo, M. J., Laucius, J. F., and Outzen, H. C., 1974, Fundamental concepts in tumour immunology: A brief review, *Semin. Oncol.* **1**:291.

Morton, D. L., Malmgren, R. A., Holmes, E. C., and Ketchman, A. S., 1968, Demonstration of antibodies against human malignant melanomas by immunofluorescence, *Surgery* **65**:233.

Movat, H. Z., 1979, Tissue injury and inflammation induced by immune complexes: The critical role of the neutrophil leukocyte, *Exp. Mol. Pathol.* **31**:201.

Nussenzweig, V., 1974, Receptors for immune complexes on lymphocytes, *Adv. Immunol.* **19**:217.

Old, L. J., Boyse, E. A., Geering, G., and Oettgen, H. F., 1968, Serologic approaches to the study of cancer in animals and man, *Cancer Res.* **28**:1288.

Olsen, J. L., Phillips, T. M., Lewis, M. G. And Solez, K. 1979, Malignant melanoma with renal deposits containing tumour antigens, *Clin. Nephrol.* **12**:74.

O'Neill, G., 1976, Control of an EL4 lymphoma in nude mice by passively administered antibody, *Eur. J. Cancer* **12**:749.

Pesce, A. J., Phillips, T. M., Ooi, B. S., Evans, A., Shank, R. A., and Lewis, M. G., 1980, Immune complexes in transitional cell carcinoma, *J. Urol.* **123**:486.

Phillips, T. M., and Draper, C. C., 1975, The detection of circulating immune complexes in patients with *Schistosoma mansoni, Br. Med. J.* **2**:476.

Phillips, T. M. and Lewis, M. G., 1970, A system of immunofluoresence in the study of tumour cells, *Rev. Eur. Etud. Clin. Ciol.* **15**:1016.

Phillips, T. M., and Lewis, M. G., 1980, Detection of circulating immune complexes by polyethylene glycol sedimentation and double counter-current immunoelectrophoresis, in: *Serologic Analysis of Human Cancer Antigens* (S. A. Rosenberg, ed.) p. 701, Academic Press, New York.

Phillips, T. M., McDonald, J. S., Smith, F. P., Queen, W. D., Lewis, M. G. and Israel, L., 1980, Aggressive plasmapheresis in patients with metastatic cancer: Its effect on circulating immune complexes, in: *New Trends in Human Immunology and Metastatic Cancer: Its Effect on Circulating Cancer Immunotherapy* (B. Serrou and C. Rosenfeld, eds.) p. 521, Doin/Saunders, Paris, France.

Poskitt, P. K. F., Poskitt, T. R., and Wallace, J. H., 1974, Renal deposition of soluble immune complexes in mice bearing B-16 melanoma, *J. Exp. Med.* **140**:410.

Pyrhonen, S., Timonen, T., Heikkinen, A., Penttinen, K., Alftan, O., Saksda, E., and Wagen, O., 1976, Rheumatoid factor as an indicator of serum blocking activity and tumour recurrence in bladder tumours, *Eur. J. Cancer* **12**:87.

Ruoslahti, E., 1976, Antigen–antibody interaction, antibody affinity and dissociation of immune complexes, in: *Immunoadsorbents in Protein Purification* (E. Ruoslahti, ed.), pp. 3–7, University Park Press, Baltimore.

Sacher, R. A., Phillips, T. M., Shashaty, G. G., Jacobson, R. J., Rath, C. E. and Lewis, M. G., 1980, The demonstration of immune complexes in thrombotic thrombocytopenic purpura and the effects of exchange transfusion, Scand. J. Haematol. **24**:373.

Sinclair, N. R. St. C., 1978, Immunoregulation by antibody and antigen–antibody complexes, *Transplant. Proc.* **10**(2):349.

Sjögren, H. O., Hellström, I., and Bansal, S. C., 1971, Suggestive evidence that blocking antibodies of tumour bearing individuals may be anti-antibody complexes, *Proc. Natl. Acad. Sci. U.S.A.* **68**:1372.

Steensgard, J., and Jacobsen, C., 1979, A new gradient former and simplified procedure for zonal centrifugation of immune complexes, *J. Immunol. Methods* **29**:173.

Sutherland, J. C., Markham, R. V., and Mardiney, M. R., 1974, Subclinical immune complex in the glomeruli of kidneys post-mortem, *Am. J. Med.* **57**:536.

Theofilopoulos, A. N., Wilson, C. B., and Dixon, F. J., 1976, The Raji cell radioimmune assay for detecting immune complexes in human sera, *J. Clin. Invest.* **57**:169.

Uhr, J. W., and Phillips, J. M., 1966, *In vitro* sensitization of phagocytes and lymphocytes by antigen–antibody complexes, *Ann. N. Y. Acad. Sci.* **129**:793.

Vansnick, J. L., Vanroost, E., Markowitz, B., Cambiaso, C. L., and Masson, P. L., 1978, Enhancement by IgM rheumatoid factor of *in-vitro* ingestion by macrophages and *in-vivo* clearance of aggregated IgG or antigen/antibody complexes, *Eur. J. Immunol.* **8**:279.

Waaler, E., 1940, On occurrence of factor in human serum activating specific agglutination of sheep blood corpuscles, *Acta Pathol. Microbiol. Scand.* **17**:172.

Waller, M., Curry, S., and Richard, A., 1968, Serological specificity of IgG and IgM anti-globulin antibodies in anti G(ma) antisera, *Exp. Immunol.* **3**:631.

Whitehouse, J. M. A., 1973, Circulating antibodies in human malignant disease, *Br. J. Cancer* **28**:170.

Yoshida, T. O., and Andersson, B., 1972, Evidence for a receptor recognizing antigen complexes immunoglobulin on the surface of activated mouse thymus lymphocytes, *Scand. J. Immunol.* **1**:401.

Ziegler, J. L., 1973, Cryoglobulinaemia in tropical splenomegaly syndrome, *Clin. Exp. Immunol.* **15**:65.

Zubler, R. H., Lange, G., Lambert, P. H., and Miescher, P. A., 1976, Detection of immune complexes in unheated sera by modified ^{125}I-C1q binding test: Effect of heating on the binding of C1q by immune complexes and application of the test to systemic lupus erythematosus, *J. Immunol.* **116**:232.

17

Molecular and Immunological Characterization of Human Melanoma-Associated Antigens

R. A. REISFELD, D. R. GALLOWAY, R. P. McCABE, AND ALTON C. MORGAN, JR.

1. Introduction

During the last decade, there has been an increasing amount of evidence indicating that the neoplastic state is characterized by cell-surface changes, and this development has led to a concerted effort by many investigators to characterize cell-surface markers associated with human tumor cells. This research effort was further stimulated by the anticipation that the thorough characterization of human tumor markers may aid in the delineation of neoplastic transformation and advance the development of immunological approaches for diagnosis, prognosis, and thereapy of cancer. In this regard, the finding of antigens that are shed into the extracellular environment of tumor cells has received considerable attention (Grimm *et al.,* 1976; Bystryn, 1977; McCabe *et al.,* 1978; Gupta *et al.,* 1979; Galloway *et al.,* 1981a), since it may further aid in the development of approaches designed to improve detection and therapy of cancer.

No effort is made herein to review the extensive literature dealing with the characterization of human tumor-associated antigens, and only a few selected references were chosen as background for reviewing our findings dealing with human melanoma-associated antigens (MAAs) delineated in this chapter. The key to our successful approach in character-

R. A. REISFELD, D. R. GALLOWAY, R. P. McCABE, AND ALTON C. MORGAN, JR. • Department of Molecular Immunology, Scripps Clinic and Research Foundation, La Jolla, California 92037.

izing these antigens present in spent culture media and extracts derived from cultured human melanoma cells was the development of a sensitive radioimmunometric antibody-binding assay for the evaluation of specific xenoantisera produced against these tumor markers (McCabe *et al.*, 1978, 1979a). This assay, initially utilizing cultured melanoma cells and later spent culture medium of such cells as targets together with radiolabeled protein A to quantitate antibody binding, made it possible for us to select a highly useful xenoantiserum directed to MAAs. This antiserum 6522, produced by injecting a rabbit with cultured human melanoma cells (M21), recognized two MAAs following suitable absorption with human red blood cells and lymphoblastoid cells. Specifically, one antibody population reacted only with melanoma cells, while the other was reactive with various tumor cells of nonlymphoid origin and some fetal cells (McCabe *et al.*, 1979a). In addition, both antibody populations reacted with freshly explanted melanoma cells, since absorption of xenoantiserum 6522 with surgically removed melanoma tissue abolished its reactivity with cultured M21 melanoma cells (Galloway *et al.*, 1981a).

Our next efforts were then directed toward the development of antimelanoma xenoantisera specifically directed against each of the two antigens recognized by xenoantiserum 6522 in order to elucidate the molecular profile of MAAs shed into the culture medium of human melanoma cells.

2. Characterization of Antimelanoma Xenoantisera

Cultured melanoma cells (2×10^7) intrinsically labeled with [^{3}H]valine were extracted with either 3 M KCl (Reisfeld *et al.*, 1971) or 4 M urea (Galloway *et al.*, 1981a). Chromatography on gelatin–Sepharose 4B quantitatively removed fibronectin from the antigen extracts and thus prevented antigenic competition from this highly immunogenic molecule. A xenoantiserum (8995) was produced by injecting rabbits with the 3 M KCl extract from cultured human melanoma cells (M21) that had been depleted of HLA-A, B, and HLA-DR antigens by KBr flotation. This extract was reacted with lentil lectin, covalently coupled to CNBr-activated Sepharose 4B, and then injected with this carrier into rabbits. Another xenoantiserum (9446) was prepared from the spent medium of M14 melanoma cells, grown under serum-free conditions (Chee *et al.*, 1976). This spent culture medium, following concentration by Amicon filtration, was subjected to KBr flotation (McCabe *et al.*, 1978) to remove histocompatibility antigens that are associated with high-density lipoproteins (HDL). Further purification of the fraction devoid of HDL was achieved by ion-exchange chromatography on a carboxymethyl cellulose (CMC) column. Proteins passing through this column were reacted with *Ricinus communis* lectin, covalently coupled to CNBr-activated Sepharose 4B, and injected as such into rabbits to produce antimelanoma antiserum 9446.

Radioimmunometric antibody-binding assays indicated that antiserum 9446 recognized antigenic structures present on both melanoma and carcinoma cells, but did not react with either human lymphoid cells or fibroblasts. Antiserum 8995, on the other hand, appeared to react only with melanoma cells (Galloway *et al.*, 1981a). A typical binding profile of these two antisera is shown in Fig. 1.

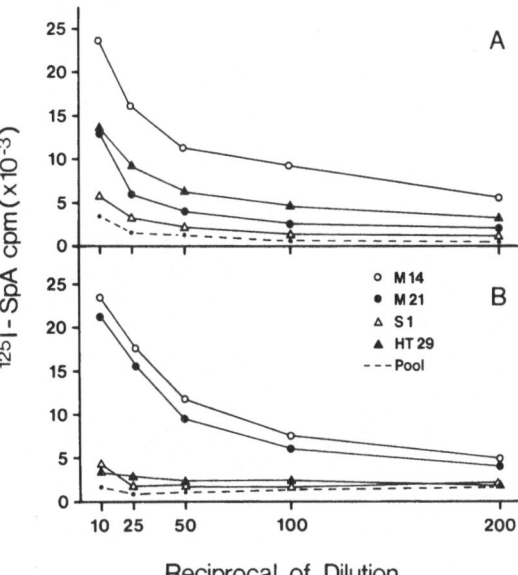

FIGURE 1. Specificity of two xenoantisera to cell-surface MAAs following absorption with human erythrocytes and pooled cultured lymphoblasts as determined with a radioimmunometric [^{125}I] *Staphylococcus aureus* protein A ([^{125}I]-SpA) antibody-binding assay 2-fold serial dilutions of the xenoantiserum (50 : 1) were reacted against 5×10^5 M21 (●) and M14 melanoma cells (○), HT29 colon-carcinoma cells (▲), S1 sarcoma cells (△), and pooled lymphoblastoid cells (----). (A) Specificity of anti-94K xenoantiserum 9466; (B) specificity of anti-240K xenoantiserum 8995.

3. Purification of Melanoma-Associated Antigens

The use of cellulose cation-exchange chromatography and specific antibody-affinity chromatography greatly increased the efficiency of MAA purifications. A number of results obtained with this purification scheme are illustrated in Fig. 2, which depicts sodium dodecyl sulfate–polyacrylamide gel electrophoretic (SDS-PAGE) analyses of crude spent medium from melanoma cells (Fig. 2A) and of this same material following the various purification steps (Fig. 2B–E). One key element of our strategy to purify MAAs from spent culture media of melanoma cells was the use of gelatin–Sepharose chromatography to quantitatively remove fibronectin. The removal of this, the most prominent among the components in spent media, aided our purification effort. In addition, it removed at the same time one of the most immunogenic components, thus eliminating some of the antigenic competition during the production of antimelanoma antisera. Another important step in our purification scheme was CMC ion-exchange chromatography at pH 5.7 in 0.01 M phosphate buffer, since it effectively separated the MAAs with molecular weights of 94,000 (94K) and 240,000 (240K) (Fig. 2B, C). The 94K antigen passes through the CMC column, while the 240K antigen binds to it and can be subsequently eluted with 0.5 N NaC1 in 0.01 M phoshate buffer, pH 5.7. As a final purification step, the two fractions separated by CMC chromatography were passed over affinity columns consisting of anti-MAA xenoantisera 8995 and 9446, respectively, coupled to protein A–Sepharose. The molecular profiles of the acid eluates (0.01 M phosphoric acid, pH 3) from these immunoadsorbents are indicated by the SDS-PAGE profiles depicted in Figs. 2D and E. It is quite evident from these data that it is feasible to purify the 240K and 94K MAAs from spent culture media using a combination of cation-exchange and antibody-affinity chromatography.

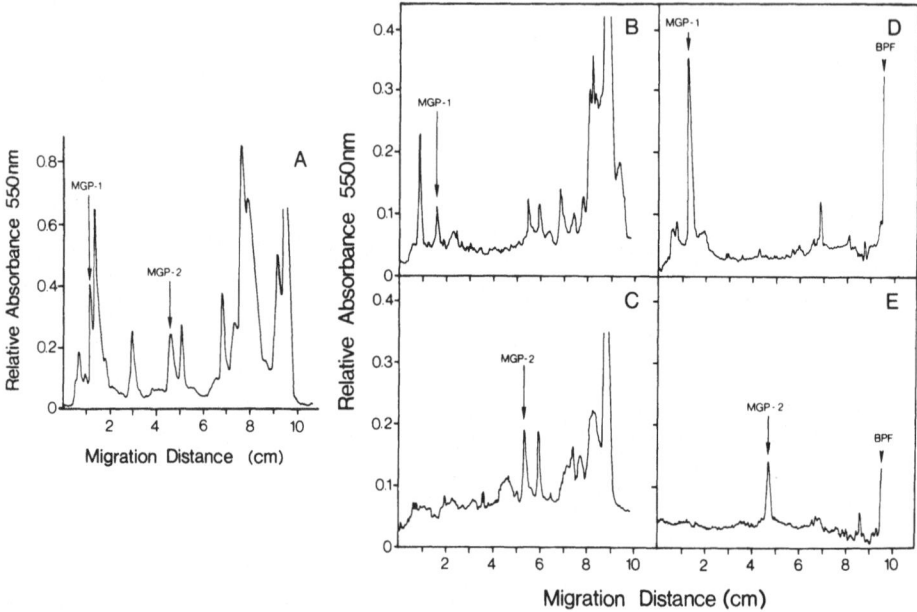

FIGURE 2. 5% SDS-PAGE analysis of [³H]valine-labeled spent culture media from M14 melanoma cells. (A) Unfractionated spent media; (B) CMC eluate (CM-2) fraction; (C) CMC effluent (CM-1) fraction; (D) antibody-affinity column eluate of CM-2 fraction; (E) antibody-affinity column eluate of CM-1 fraction. (MGP) melanoma glycoprotein; (BPF) bromphenol blue front.

4. Molecular Profile of Melanoma-Associated Antigens

4.1. Delineation with Polyclonal Xenoantisera

The antimelanoma xenoantisera 6522, 8995, and 9446 facilitated analysis of the molecular profiles of intrinsically radiolabeled antigens expressed or shed or both by cultured melanoma and carcinoma cells. The immunoprecipitates obtained with these antisera were routinely analyzed by SDS-PAGE and visualized by autoradiography following fluorographic processing (Galloway *et al.*, 1981a). A typical profile resulting from the analysis of several human tumor cell lines is shown in Fig. 3. It is evident from these data that xenoantiserum 6522 recognized in spent culture media two antigens that are consistently associated with all human melanoma cell lines tested thus far; these antigens were differentiated by their respective molecular weights of 240,000 and 94,000. Additional analyses indicated that the 94K antigen was also shed from human carcinoma cell lines, whereas neither of the two antigens appeared present on human fibroblasts or B lymphoblasts. The 240K antigen appears unique to human melanoma cells.

The difference in reactivity among the three antimelanoma xenoantisera, i.e., 6522, 9446, and 8995, became even more evident from SDS-PAGE analyses of indirect immunoprecipitates obtained by reacting spent culture media from [³H]valine labeled cultured melanoma cells (M21) with these three xenoantisera. As indicated by the SDS-PAGE profiles shown in Fig. 4, it is clearly evident that xenoantiserum 6522 is reactive with both

240K and 94K MAAs, whereas antisera 9446 and 8995 react in a specific fashion with the 94K and 240K antigens, respectively. Table I summarizes the results of a number of different experiments and illustrates the distribution of 94K and 240K antigens on cultured tumor cells, lymphoblasts, fibroblasts, and their spent culture media. These data were obtained by using either cells or their spent culture media that had not been immunodepleted with other antisera prior to any reaction with unabsorbed anti-MAA xenoantisera.

The specificity of the xenoantisera used for characterization of MAAs by indirect immunoprecipitation was further substantiated by immunodepletion experiments. For example, spent culture medium from intrinsically labeled melanoma cells was immunodepleted by an immunoadsorbent, i.e., anti-human lymphocyte xenoantiserum (ALS) coupled to protein A–Sepharose, prior to subsequent analysis by indirect immunoprecipitation using either unabsorbed antimelanoma xenoantisera or normal rabbit sera. A typical result of such an immunodepletion experiment is illustrated in Fig. 5.

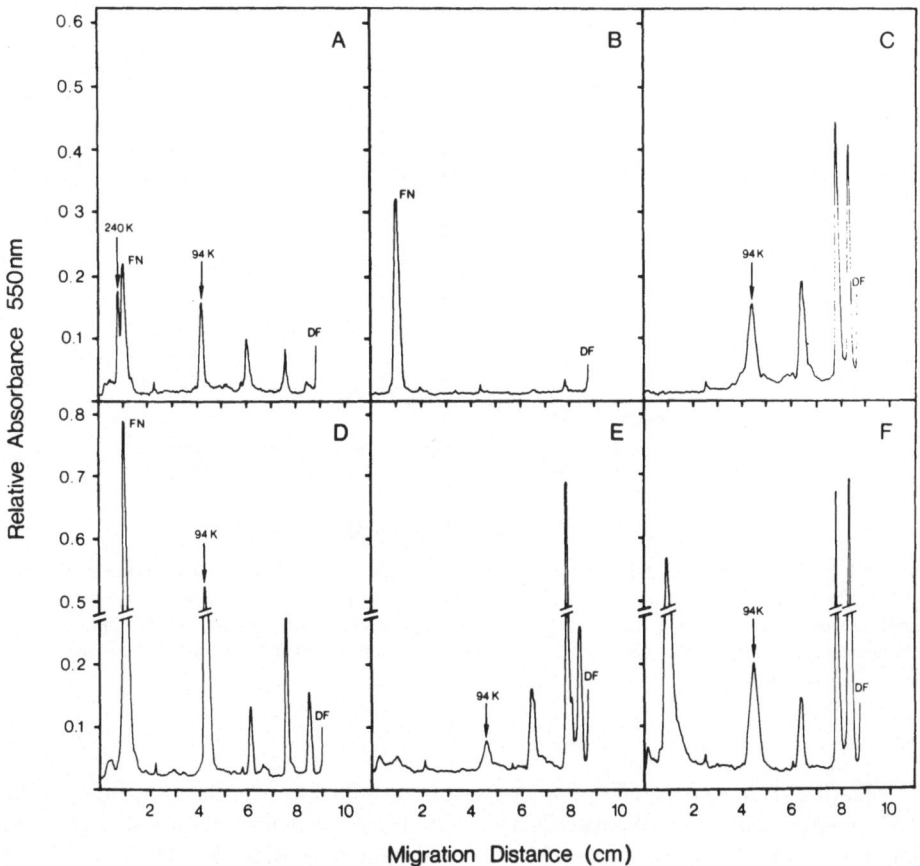

FIGURE 3. SDS-PAGE molecular profiles of indirect immunoprecipitates obtained by reacting intrinsically labeled ([³H]valine) spent culture medium from various tumor lines with anti-MAA xenoantiserum 6522. (A) M14 melanoma; (B) HAM-SK fibroblasts; (C) HT29 colon carcinoma; (D) T24 bladder carcinoma; (E) D-98 HeLa cells; (F) MANO carcinoma. (FN) Fibronectin; (DF) dye front.

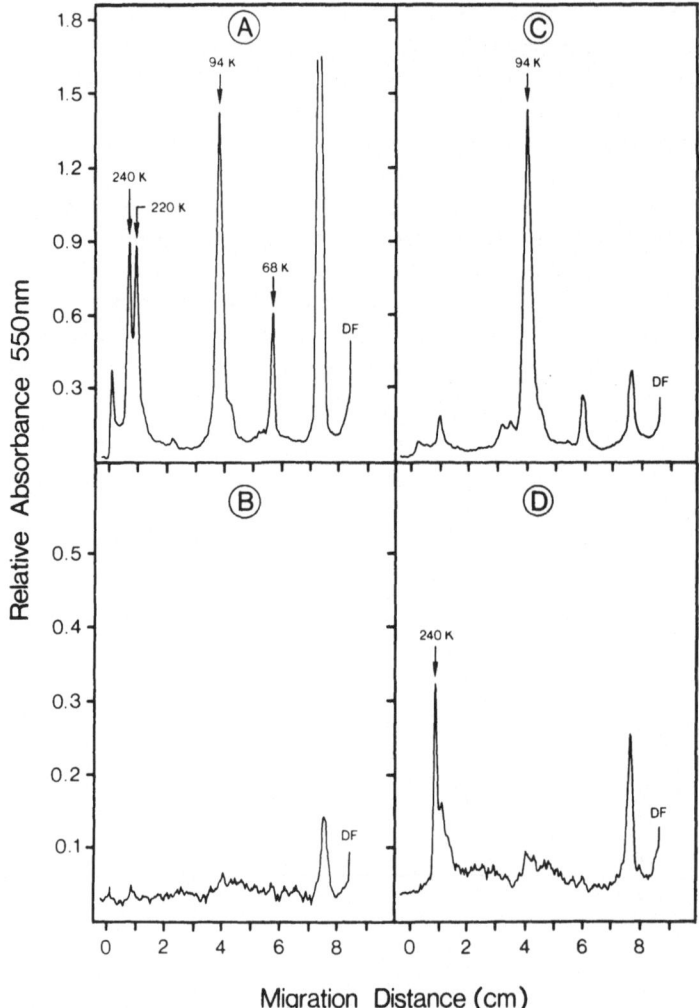

FIGURE 4. SDS-PAGE profiles of indirect immunoprecipitates obtained by reacting spent culture media from intrinsically labeled [³H]valine cultured human melanoma cells (M21) with immunoadsorbents prepared from specific xenoantisera. The resulting fluorographs of 5% acrylamide gels were scanned at 500 nm. (A) Anti-melanoma xenoantiserum 6522; (B) ALS; (C) anti-94K xenoantiserum 9446; (D) anti-240K xenoantiserum 8995. (DF) dye front.

During these same studies, fibronectin was identified as a major component of the shed proteins from all melanoma cells and most of the carcinoma cell lines studied (Figs. 3 and 5). A specific human fibronectin antiserum (kindly provided by Dr. E. Ruoslahti) was used to identify fibronectin that could also be specifically removed by passing spent culture media through a gelatin–Sepharose column (Engvall and Ruoslahti, 1977). The efficiency of fibronectin removal by this method is illustrated in Fig. 5, which also depicts the position identification of fibronectin in the spent culture medium of melanoma cells.

TABLE I
Distribution of Melanoma-Associated Antigens on Cultured Cells

Type	Histological derivation	Cell line	MAA 94K	MAA 240K
Melanoma	Dermal	FO	+	+
	Dermal	BW V	+	+
	Dermal	SH No. 1	+	+
	Dermal	CAR No. 1	+	+
	Dermal	CAR No. 2	+	− [a]
	Dermal	SH No. 3	+	+
	Dermal	SH No. 5	+	+
	Dermal	M 10	+	+
	Dermal	M 14	+	+
	Dermal	M 21	+	+
	Dermal	M 51	+	+
	Dermal	BE	+	+
	Uveal	LIN	+	+
Carcinoma	Breast	MDA-MB231	+	−
	Breast	MDA-MB468	+	−
	Breast	MDA-MB4355	+	−
	Breast	MDA-MB361	+	−
	Bladder	MANO	+	−
	Bladder	T24	+	−
	Vulva	Colo 16	+	−
	Vulva	A 431	+	−
	Colon	HT-29	+	−
	Cervix	HeLa D-98	+	−
Lymphoblast	B-cell	Raji	−	−
	B-cell	FO LCL	−	−
	B-cell	Victor	−	−
	B-cell	RPMI 4098	−	−
	B-cell	WI-L2	−	−
	B-cell	Daudi	−	−
	T-cell	1301	−	−
	T-cell	MOLT-4	−	−
Fibroblast	Adult skin	HAM-SK	−	−
	Fetal skin	79-4	−	−
	Fetal skin	Flow 2000	−	−
	Fetal lung	MRC-5	−	−
	Fetal lung	IMR-90	−	−
Miscellaneous	Fetal brain	Flow 3000	+	−
	Fetal uveal melanocytes	FeMEL 78-3B	+	−
	Teratocarcinoma	PA No. 1	−	−

[a] Expressed on the cell surface, but shedding is not detectable in spent culture medium.

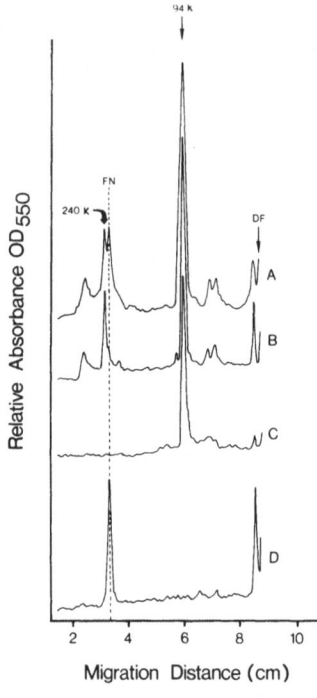

FIGURE 5. SDS-PAGE profiles on 5% acrylamide gels of indirect immuno-precipitates obtained by reacting immunodepleted (ALS–*Staphylococcus aureus* Cowan I) and non immunodepleted spent culture medium from intrinsically labeled ([³H]valine) 21 SCRF cells with various xenoantisera. (A) Anti-MAA xenoantiserum 6522 reacted with M21 spent medium; (B) anti-MAA xenoantiserum 6522 reacted with ALS-depleted M21 spend medium; (C) anti-94K xenoantiserum 9446 reacted with ALS-depleted M21 spent medium; (D) xenoantiserum to human fibronectin (FN) reacted with M21 spent medium. (DF) dye front.

4.2. Monoclonal Antibody as a Molecular Probe for Melanoma-Associated Antigens

Monoclonal antibody 165 developed in our laboratory against 94K MAA (Imai *et al.*, 1981) proved to be an excellent probe to dissect the molecular profile of this tumor marker. Results from an initial comparative immunochemical analysis of the reactivities of mono-clonal antibody 165 and polyclonal antiserum 6522 with spent medium from cultured mel-anoma cells (M14) demonstrated that these two antisera detected similar antigenic struc-tures. This was evident, since immunodepletion of the spent culture medium with polyclonal antiserum 6522 removed all antigenic structures reactive in indirect immuno-precipitation with monoclonal antibody 165 (Fig. 6B). Conversely, an initial immunode-pletion of the spent culture medium with monoclonal antibody 165 removed all 94K mol-ecules reactive with the polyclonal xenoantiserum 6522 without affecting any of the other proteins immunoprecipitated by this antiserum (Fig. 6C). The data shown in Fig. 6D–F, which depict results from a number of control experiments, also point to the high specificity of the monoclonal antibody, which clearly reacts only with the 94K antigen molecule (Gal-loway *et al.*, 1981b).

Two-dimensional gel electrophoresis of the 94K antigens immunoprecipitated with monoclonal antibody 165 from spent media of melanoma (M14) and carcinoma (T24) cell lines indicated that the 94K MAAs in the spent media of the two different cell lines were not only very similar but also homogeneous, i.e., lacking any detectable size or charge microheterogeneity. The relative isoelectric points are practically identical, i.e., pI 6.2 for the 94K antigen from melanoma and pI 6.3 for the antigen from carcinoma cell lines. These data also reveal the absence of any structural polymorphism of the 94K MAA detectable by the high-resolution two-dimensional gel analysis (Galloway *et al.*, 1981b).

A comparison between the tryptic peptide maps of the 94K antigens associated with melanoma and carcinoma cell lines, made by high-pressure liquid chromatographic analysis, clearly indicated that these molecules are practically identical. The tryptic peptides of both antigens separated into 9–10 major components with identical retention times. The peptide maps of both antigens reveal components with retention times of 20, 28, 34, 41, 71, 79, 84, and 109 min. The data from two-dimensional gel electrophoresis and from tryptic peptide maps clearly demonstrated the similarity in polypeptide structure of the 94K molecules found in the spent media of melanoma and carcinoma cells (Fig. 7).

To assess whether structural integrity of the 94K MAA was required for its interaction with monoclonal antibody 165, the 94K molecules found in the spent culture media of melanoma cells were subjected to enzymatic degradation. As depicted in Fig. 8, chymotrypsin treatment of the 94K antigen resulted in the cleavage of two antigen fragments of molecular weight 66K and approximately 15K that were recognized by monoclonal antibody 165 as shown by SDS-PAGE analysis of indirect immunoprecipitates. It is apparent from the data shown in Fig. 8 that a relatively small amount of the 94K molecule was not digested by chromotrypsin under the conditions used. These data suggest that integrity of the 94K molecule is not required for interaction with the monoclonal antibody in indirect immunoprecipitation. It can be concluded from the identification of at least two chymo-

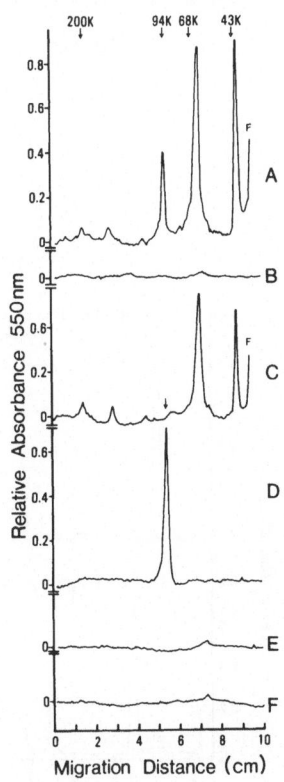

FIGURE 6. Comparison between reactivities of polyclonal antimelanoma antiserum 6522 and monoclonal anti-94K antibody 165 with spent culture fluid of intrinsically labeled ([³H]valine) melanoma cells (M14) by SDS-PAGE (5% gel) analysis following selective immunodepletion. Each immunodepletion of spent culture media with antiserum was repeated three times, and the remaining supernate was then reacted with a specific antiserum. (A) Immunoprecipitation with polyclonal antiserum 6522; (B) immunodepletion with the same antiserum; (C) immunodepletion with monoclonal antibody 165 followed by immunoprecipitation with antiserum 6522; (D) immunoprecipitation with monoclonal antibody 165; (E) immunodepletion with antibody 165 followed by immunoprecipitation with the same monoclonal antibody; (F) immunodepletion with antiserum 6522 followed by immunoprecipitation with monoclonal antibody 165. Molecular-weight markers: myosin (200,000), phosphorylase B (94,000), bovine serum albumin (68,000), and ovalbumin (43,000). (FN) Fibronection.

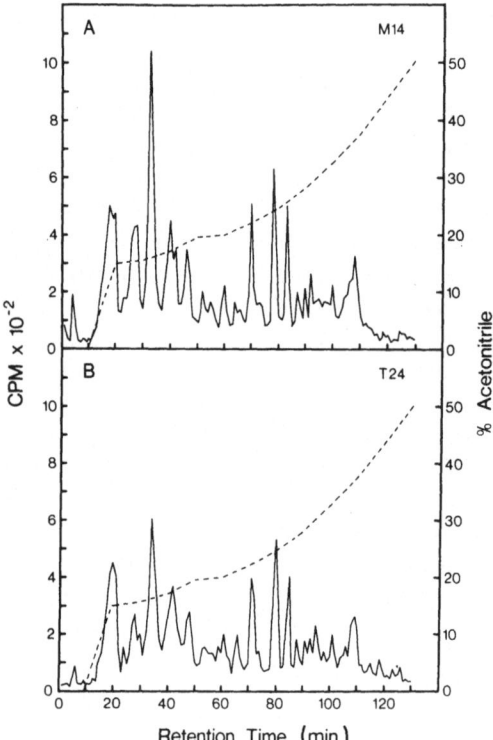

FIGURE 7. Tryptic peptide maps of 94K antigens isolated by indirect immunoprecipitation with monoclonal anti-94K antibody 165. (A) Peptide profile of 94K antigen isolated from spent culture media of melanoma cells (M14); (B) peptide profile of 94K antigen isolated from spent culture media of bladder-carcinoma cells (T24).

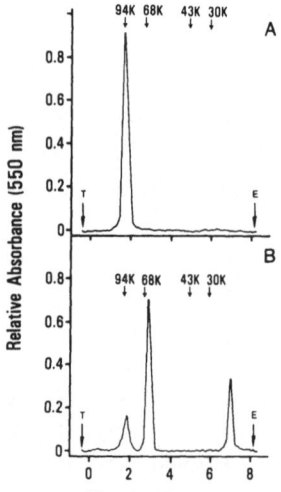

FIGURE 8. Limited chymotrypsin digestion of 94K antigens present in the spent culture media of intrinsically labeled ([^{3}H]valine) melanoma cells (M14). (A) SDS-PAGE (10% gel) profile of an indirect immunoprecipitate obtained with monoclonal anti-94K antibody 165; (B) SDS-PAGE (10 % gel) profile of an indirect immunoprecipitate obtained with the same antibody following chymotrypsin digestion. Molecular-weight markers phosphorylase B (94,000), bovine serum albumin (68,000), ovalbumin (43,000), and carbonic anhydrase (30,000). (T) top of gel scan; (E) end of gel scan.

tryptic peptides that the monoclonal antibody likely detects common antigenic determinants on the 94K molecule.

4.3. Subunit Composition of 94K and 240K Melanoma-Associated Antigens

Some investigators suggested that tumor-associated antigens may be modulated histocompatibility antigens and thus consist of a similar two-chain structure in which one polypeptide is noncovalently associated with β_2-microglobulin (β_2m) (for a review, see Curry et al., 1979a). When we tested this supposition in human melanoma by the use of serological and immunochemical techniques, we found that serologically detectable MAAs are not associated with β_2m on the surface of cultured human melanoma cells (M51). Thus, coating of M51 cells with cow anti-human β_2m antiserum did not affect MAA reactivity with anti-MAA xenoantisera in a sensitive indirect rosette microassay. An accompanying positive control experiment indicated a significant reduction in the reactivity of two anti-HLA xenoantisera with the M51 cells coated with the cow anti-human β_2m antiseraum (McCabe et al., 1980).

These observations strongly suggested the lack of a close spatial relationship between MAAs and β_2m on the surface of cultured human melanoma cells. Although these data appeared clear-cut, we wanted to rule out that (1) MAAs are associated with β_2m in such a configuration as to make β_2m inaccessible to anti β_2m antiserum on the cell surface or (2) MAAs shed from the cell surface associated with β_2m in the spent medium because of an affinity between these two molecules. In this regard, reaction of MAAs with an anti-β_2m immunoadsorbent indicated that no detectable amounts of MAAs were removed, although this same adsorbent did bind significant amounts of β_2m in a control experiment. Conversely, an anti-MAA immunoadsorbent did bind significant amounts of MAAs without removing any β_2m (McCabe et al., 1980). The lack of any association between β_2m and MAAs determined by serological methods was corroborated by immunochemical analyses. Specifically, indirect immunoprecipitation experiments analyzed by SDS-PAGE revealed that anti-MAA xenoantiserum 6522 precipitated 94K and 240K MAA but failed to coprecipitate β_2m. On the other hand, a rabbit anti-human β_2m antiserum did immunoprecipitate β_2m from the spent medium of melanoma cells without coprecipitating 94K or 240K MAA. All these data led us to stipulate that MAAs are distinct from β_2m, a conclusion that was corroborated by the findings of several other investigators (Carey et al., 1979; Woodbury et al., 1980; Brown et al., 1980), who similarly could not find any association between β_2m and MAAs using both polyclonal and monoclonal antisera. The lack of any significant association between human MAAs and β_2m fails to support the notion that MAAs are modified human histocompatibility antigens. Further lack of support for this contention is also confirmed from our previous findings that indicated that MAAs segregate independently of HLA-A,B antigens on somatic-cell hybrids derived from the fusion of murine fibroblasts with human melanoma cells (Curry et al., 1979b).

The possible subunit composition of 94K and 240K MAAs was indicated by SDS-PAGE analysis under both reducing and nonreducing conditions of their immunoprecipitates obtained with both polyclonal and monoclonal anti-MAA antibodies. Results from such analyses suggested that the 94K MAA consists of a single polypeptide claim, whereas the 240K molecule may be part of a larger molecular complex (Galloway et al., 1981b).

5. Role of Carbohydrate in Shedding and Cell-Surface Expression of Melanoma-Associated Antigens

It became of considerable interest to study the mode of antigen shedding from cultured melanoma cells since we (McCabe *et al.*, 1978, 1979a,b; Galloway *et al.*, 1981a,b) as well as several other investigators (Grimm *et al.*, 1976; Stuhlmiller *et al.*, 1979; Bystryn, 1977; Gupta *et al.*, 1979) had repeatedly observed this phenomenon. Data obtained by us indicating affinity of the 94K and 240K MAAs for specific plant lectins (McCabe *et al.*, 1979a,b) and metabolic radiolabeling with sugars (Morgan *et al.*, 1981a) strongly suggested that they were glycoproteins. These observations together with data obtained by a number of investigators suggesting that addition of carbohydrate plays a key role in secretion and membrane intercalations of several proteins (Pouyssegur and Pastan, 1977; Hughes *et al.*, 1977; Hickman and Kornfield, 1978; Olden *et al.*, 1978) provided the rationale to investigate the role of carbohydrate in shedding and cell-surface expression of MAAs.

Our approach was to intrinsically radiolabel cultured melanoma cells with amino acids or sugars or both and then to test the effect of various inhibitors of glycosylation on the incorporation of these labels into proteins. Specifically, [^{3}H]valine incorporation was used to determine the levels of total protein, while [^{3}H]glucosamine, [^{3}H]-1-mannose and [^{3}H]-2-mannose were utilized to measure carbohydrate associated with protein. These incorporated labels were measured either by trichloroacetic acid (TCA) precipitation or as label associated with specific immunoprecipitated proteins to establish protein levels and the extent of glycosylation. The inhibition of shedding of 240K and 94K MAAs and fibronectin and the effect of inhibitors of glycosylation on synthesis and glycosylation were determined by scanning autoradiographs of SDS-PAGE profiles of indirect immunoprecipitates of either spent media or lysates of cultured melanoma cells obtained with specific antimelanoma xenoantisera. Initial experiments established dose levels of inhibitor and incubation conditions that resulted in at least 2-fold greater inhibition of carbohydrate incorporation than amino acid label into TCA-precipitable material.

Exposure of melanoma cells for 3 days to 2-deoxyglucose (0.01 mM), an inhibitor of lipid-linked glycosylation, resulted in 70% inhibition of valine incorporation into TCA-precipitable proteins. SDS-PAGE profiles of immunoprecipitated spent medium revealed the absence not only of 240K and 94K MAAs but also of other glycoproteins with molecular weights of 185K, 120K, and 65K. In contrast, shedding of fibronectin was not at all affected by 0.01 mM 2-deoxyglucose. Glucosamine proved not useful for our studies, since it inhibited protein synthesis and shedding at least 34% more than it did glycosylation. Cytochalasin B, an inhibitor of glucose transport (Bissell, 1976; Tannenbaum *et al.*, 1977; Rampal *et al.*, 1980), markedly inhibited shedding of fibronectin without affecting release of MAAs, suggesting that shedding of 94K and 240K MAAs is inhibited by agents capable of abolishing lipid-linked glycosylation and not by those abrogating glucose transport (Morgan *et al.*, 1981a). This notion was strongly supported by our results achieved wth tunicamycin, which had been shown by several investigators to be a specific inhibitor of dolichol-dependent, *N*-asparagine-linked glycosylation (Tkacz and Lampen, 1975; Keller *et al.*, 1979; Olden *et al.*, 1979).

After establishing conditions under which any effects of tunicamycin could be ascribed solely to this antibiotic's effect on glycosylation and not to its toxic effects, we found that the shedding of 240K and 94K MAAs was selectively inhibited by this drug. Thus, the level of inhibition of glycosylation at graded doses of tunicamycin correlated with the level of inhibition of shedding of 240K and 94K MAAs. Also, the time–course of reduction in glycosylation of MAAs correlated with the time–course of reduction in shedding of MAAs (Fig. 9). Furthermore, removal of tunicamycin resulted in the resumption of glycosylation and release of only glycosylated 240K ad 94K MAAs. Inhibition of shedding of MAAs by tunicamycin could be reversed by addition of *N*-acetyl glucosamine, but not by glucose.

In marked contrast to shedding, cell-surface expression of 240K and 94K MAAs remained unaffected by tunicamycin treatment despite the demonstrated lack of glycosylation of cell-surface MAAs. Thus, melanoma cells exposed to tunicamycin (0.5 μg/ml) did not shed MAAs, but bound monoclonal antibody to 94K MAA in amounts similar to untreated cells (Fig. 10). In addition, immunoprecipitation of cell lysates from control and melanoma cells adapted to grow in the presence of tunicamycin, labeled with [3H]valine and [3H]glucosamine, showed that amino-acid-labeled 240K and 94K MAAs were present in equal amounts; however, there was a lack of detectable glucosamine label associated with these molecules as well as a slight decrease in mobility of 240K and 94K MAAs and fibronectin in 5% polyacrylamide gels (Morgan *et al.*, 1981a). These data clearly indicated that the low dose levels of tunicamycin used in our experiments affect only shedding of and neither synthesis nor intracellular transport or intercalation into the plasma membrane of 240K and 94K MAAs. A similar inability of tunicamycin to affect these processes was reported for fibronectin (Olden *et al.*, 1978), influenza viral proteins (Nakamura and Compani, 1978), procollagen (Duskin and Bornstein, 1978), and HLA-A,B antigens (Krangel *et al.*, 1979).

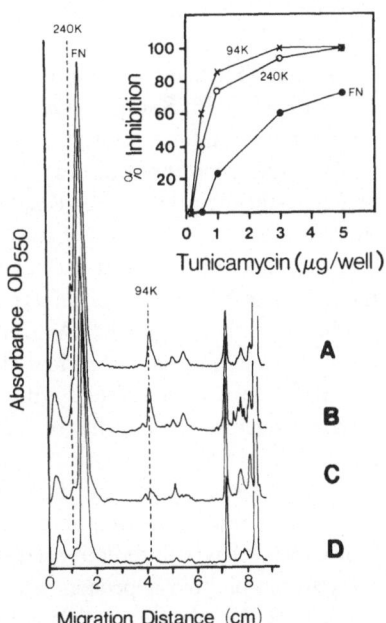

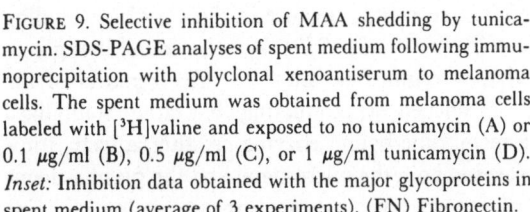

FIGURE 9. Selective inhibition of MAA shedding by tunicamycin. SDS-PAGE analyses of spent medium following immunoprecipitation with polyclonal xenoantiserum to melanoma cells. The spent medium was obtained from melanoma cells labeled with [3H]valine and exposed to no tunicamycin (A) or 0.1 μg/ml (B), 0.5 μg/ml (C), or 1 μg/ml tunicamycin (D). *Inset:* Inhibition data obtained with the major glycoproteins in spent medium (average of 3 experiments). (FN) Fibronectin.

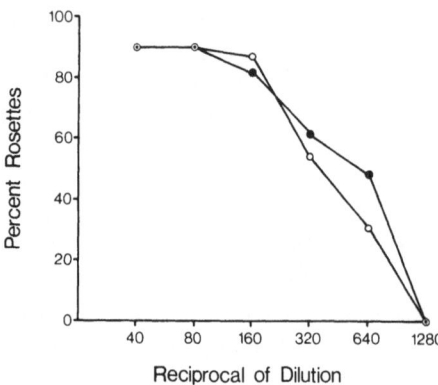

FIGURE 10. Effect of tunicamycin on cell-surface expression of MAAs. Control (●) or melanoma cells adapted to grow in 0.5 μg/ml tunicamycin and that did not shed MAAs (○) were tested for binding of monoclonal antibody (165) to 94K MAA. The percentage of melanoma cells binding antibody at each dilution was enumerated with anti-mouse-IgG-coated sheep erythrocytes.

5.1. Mechanism of Shedding of Melanoma-Associated Antigens

As far as an explanation for the inhibition of shedding of MAAs by tunicamycin is concerned, it appears that glycoproteins deficient in carbohydrate may become more hydrophobic and retreat into the lipid matrix of the plasma membrane. Thus, these molecules may behave more like intrinsic membrane components that are not shed to any degree from melanoma cells. This notion is supported at least in part by findings of others (Pouyssegur and Pastan, 1977) indicating that antibody binding to a 92K glucose-regulated protein on a glycosylation-deficient murine fibroblast cell strain was not affected in the mutant strain, although exposure of the molecule on the cell surface was reduced. Our data with inhibitors of lipid-linked glycosylation, i.e., 2-deoxyglucose and tunicamycin, certainly support the idea that lipid-linked glycosylation is the effective mechanism involved in the inhibition of shedding of 240K and 94K MAAs. This conclusion is supported by our finding that cytochalasin B, which is known to alter cytoskeletal structure (Wessels *et al.*, 1971) and inhibit pinocytosis (Heiniger and Marshall, 1979) and glucose transport (Tannenbaum *et al.*, 1977; Bissell, 1978; Rampal *et al.*, 1980), was ineffective in inhibiting shedding of MAAs, although it did inhibit incorporation of glucosamine into these molecules.

Further concerns regarding the actual mechanism of tunicamycin-induced inhibition of MAA shedding led us to reexamine whether our findings support the postulate that tunicamycin acts at the level of the microsomal membrane *N*-acetyl glucosamine transferase. Actually, our data were inconsistent with the notion that the microsomal membrane is the site where tunicamycin affects glycosylation of MAAs. Thus, tunicamycin-induced inhibition of shedding of MAAs from melanoma cells was specifically reversed by exogenous *N*-acetyl glucosamine. These data, suggesting a low-affinity binding of tunicamycin to transferase, are inconsistent with a recent report indicating that the binding of tunicamycin to microsomal transferase is in effect irreversible because of the very high binding affinity of the drug for specific transferase (Keller *et al.*, 1979). We also found that glycosylation and subsequent shedding of MAAs resumed within 2 hr after removal of the antibiotic. These conflicting data can be reconciled by postulating that either solubilized transferase behaves differently than the membrane-bound enzyme or, alternatively, tunicamycin acts on lipid-dependent transferases at both the microsomal and the plasma-membrane level. In this regard, a number of reports have indicated an association of lipid-dependent transferase activity with plasma membranes (Waechter and Lennarz, 1976).

Although reports in the literature indicate that in cell lysates tunicamycin acts at the level of the endoplasmic reticulum (Tkacz and Lampen, 1975; Keller et al., 1979; Datama and Schwartz, 1979; Rampal et al., 1980), there is no rigorous proof that the drug acts solely at this level when used with intact cells. While it is admittedly highly speculative at this time to postulate interactions with plasma-membrane transferase, it may nevertheless help to explain the mechanism of the selective inhibition of MAA shedding induced by tunicamycin. According to this speculation, MAAs, unlike other glycoproteins found on the cell surface of melanoma cells, would be inserted into the plasma membrane in nonglycosylated form. Glycosylation by enzymes in the plasma membrane would then render the proteins more hydrophilic and facilitate their processing into the extracellular matrix and subsequent shedding into spent medium. In accordance with this postulate, low concentrations of tunicamycin would be selectively taken up by plasma-membrane enzyme, while higher levels would result in saturation of plasma-membrane enzyme, intracellular entry of the antibiotic, and resultant action of the drug on microsomal transferase. Thus, MAAs representing a minority of proteins glycosylated after insertion into the plasma membrane would be selectively inhibited by limiting levels of tunicamycin. It is quite clear that additional experiments are definitely required to determine whether this speculation regarding the mode of glycosylation is warranted and whether it is characteristic for tumor-specific markers of malignant transformation.

6. Functional Properties of 94K and 240K Melanoma-Associated Antigens

The derivation of a melanin-producing cell strain from human fetal uvea (FeMEL 78-3B) made it possible for us to ascertain whether either of the two MAAs was an oncofetal antigen. Analysis of spent culture medium and detergent [0.50% Nonidet P-40 (NP-40)] lysates of the fetal melanocytes, intrinsically labeled with [^{3}H]valine and [^{3}H]glucosamine, with polyclonal anti-MAA 6522 and monoclonal anti-94K antibody indicated that indirect immunoprecipitates contained mainly components with molecular weights of 200K and 90K (Fig. 11). The 200K component was identified as fibronectin with antifibronectin antiserum and migrated more rapidly than fibronectin (220K) detected in the spent medium of melanoma cells. Both components were shown to be glycoproteins, since they readily incorporated [^{3}H]-6-glucosamine. The same 90K glycoprotein present in spent medium of the fetal melanocytes was also detected in the NP-40 extracts of these cells that had been intrinsically labeled with [^{3}H]glucosamine. Indirect immunoprecipitation of this NP-40 extract with monoclonal antibody to the 94K glycoprotein of melanoma cells confirmed the immunological identity of the 90K and 94K glycoproteins. In contrast to the shedding of the 90K glycoprotein, the 240K MAA was not detected in spent culture medium of fetal melanocytes (Morgan et al., 1981b).

The tissue distribution of the 94K MAA was further evaluated by reacting spent culture media of a variety of cell lines with polyclonal anti-MAA directed to intact human melanoma cells (Fig. 12). An evaluation of the indirect immunoprecipitates by SDS-PAGE analysis was made of spent culture medium of melanoma cells (Fig. 12A) intrinsically radiolabeled under the same conditions as fetal melanocytes (Fig. 12B), fetal fibroblasts (Fig. 12C), teratocarcinoma cells (Fig. 12D), and adult skin fibroblasts (Fig. 12E). It is

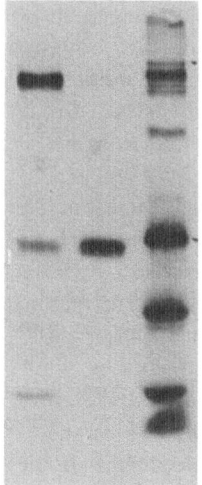

FIGURE 11. Size of MAAs shed by human fetal melanocytes. SDS-PAGE autoradiograph of [³H]valine-labeled spent culture medium from fetal melanocytes (1, 2) and melanoma cells (3) immunoprecipitated with antimelanoma serum 6522 (1, 3) and monoclonal anti-94K antibody (2). Molecular-weight markers: human plasma fibronectin (220,000), β-galactosidase (130,000), phosphorylase B (94,000), and human serum albumin (68,000).

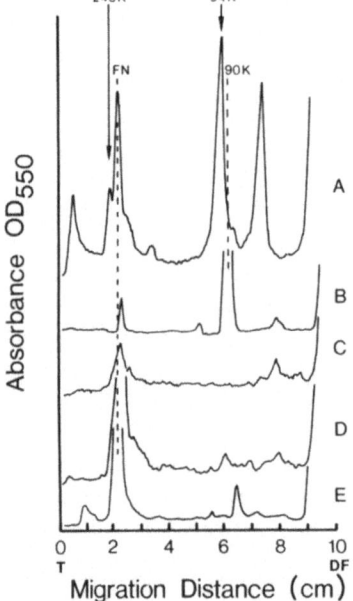

FIGURE 12. Lack of MAA shedding by adult or fetal cells of mesodermal origin. SDS-PAGE profiles of spent culture medium from M21 melanoma cells (A), FeMEL 78-3B (B), FeSKIN 78 (C), PA No. 1 teratocarcinoma cells (D), and HAM-SK adult skin fibroblasts (E, end of gel scan) immunoprecipitated with antiserum 6522. (T) top of gel scan; (DF) dye front.

apparent from the data depicted in Fig. 12 that all cell lines analyzed shed fibronectin; however, only the fetal melanocytes shed a 90K glycoprotein that is immunologically identical to the 94K molecule shed from cultured melanoma cells.

An effort was made to induce the 240K MAA, shed by malignant melanocytes of both epidermal and uveal origin, by viral [simian virus 40 (SV_{40})] transformation of fetal melanocytes. Interestingly enough, the SV_{40}-transformed fetal melanocytes failed to shed the 240K MAA as detected by monospecific and polyspecific polyclonal antimelanoma antisera.

The failure of viral transformation to induce the expression of 240K MAA on fetal melanocytes may be explained by considering that SV_{40} transformation may be equivalent to initiation without conferring tumorigenicity.

Most remarkably, however, following SV_{40} transformation, both fibronectin and 94K MAA found in the spent medium of the transformed melanocytes showed the same molecular weights as their counterparts detected in the spent medium of cultured melanoma cells (Morgan et al., 1981a). This finding was in direct contrast to that obtained with nontransformed fetal melanocytes. These differences in molecular weight observed among fibronectin and MAAs shed from transformed and nontransformed fetal melanocytes may reflect the degree of glycosylation of these molecules, a supposition supported by the observation that fibronectin and MAAs shed from fetal melanocytes actually showed an increase in molecular weight after transformation over these same components shed from nontransformed fetal melanocytes. One explanation for this phenomenon may be that the well-known increase in glucose uptake, resulting in enhanced intracellular glucose concentration, may increase glycosylation and thus shedding of MAAs. This notion is strengthened by our previous observation that excellular glucose concentration actually did regulate glycosolation and subsequent shedding of MAAs (Morgan and Reisfeld, 1981; Morgan et al., 1981a). The apparent increase in molecular weight of 94K MAA and fibronectin as evidenced by increased mobility on SDS-PAGE may actually be the consequence of alterations in oligosaccharide chains or addition of carbohydrate to additional asparagine residues that are normally not glycosylated.

All the data we have obtained thus far support the notion that the 94K MAA is an oncofetal antigen expressed on cells of ectodermal and endodermal but not mesodermal origin. Thus, 94K was absent from fetal cells of mesodermal origin (fetal fibroblasts, teratocarcinoma cells) and present on fetal melanocytes. It may be that 94K molecules are present on fetal melanocytes because they are dividing cells, since fetal-antigen expression has been commonly observed on terminally differentiated cells that are undergoing multiplication (Jerry et al., 1976). Although there are exceptions to the rule that equates fetal-antigen expression with proliferation (Granatek et al., 1979), most observations support the contention that tumor cells, i.e., retrodifferentiated normal cells, share some differentiation products with fetal cells of the same tissue origin.

To determine the relationship of expression and shedding of MAAs to transformation and differentiation, we analyzed the effect of tumor promoters on the shedding of glycoproteins from melanoma cells into their spent culture medium. Our model system for these studies consisted of two melanoma cell lines, CAR No. 1 and CAR No. 2, derived from the same patient at different stages of tumor progression. The profile of antigens in the spent media of these two cell lines is almost identical with the exception that the 240K MAA is absent from the CAR No. 2 line. Treatment of this cell line with a phorbol ester, i.e., 12-O-tetradecanoyl phorbol-13 acetate (TPA) (0.01–0.01 μg/ml), or with phorbol, its non-promoter analogue, results in the appearance of the 240K MAA in the spent culture medium of the formerly deficient CAR No. 2 cells after exposure to TPA for 24 hr. In contrast, phorbol did not induce shedding of the 240K molecule (Fig. 13). Shedding of a 180K molecule, always detectable in the spent culture medium of untreated CAR No. 2 cells, was inhibited in TFA-treated cultures.

Treatment of melanoma cells with phorbol ester caused differentiation with development of neuritelike processes and enhanced production of melanin. Exposure of normal

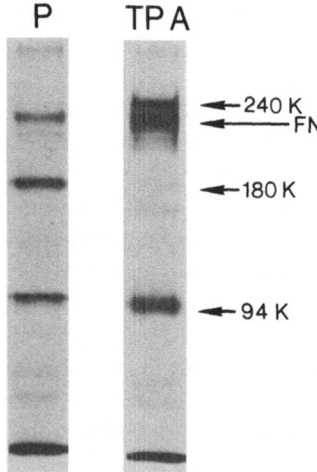

P   TPA

←240 K
←——FN

←180 K

←94 K

FIGURE 13. SDS-PAGE profile illustrating the induction of 240K MAA on CAR No. 2 melanoma cells following treatment with phorbol ester. Cells were treated with either phorbol (P) or phorbol ester (TPA), 0.05 μg/ml. Melanoma cells were intrinsically labeled with [^{3}H]leucine after 24 hr of exposure to P or TPA, and their spent culture medium was harvested after an additional 2 days of exposure. Indirect immunoprecipitation of components in the spent culture media was achieved with polyclonal xenoantiserum 6522. (FN) Fibronectin.

fetal melanocytes to TPA (0.005–0.2 μg/ml) resulted in biphasic changes that were not observed with phorbol treatment. At low doses of TPA, neuritelike processes were formed and melanin production increased; at higher dose levels of TPA, there was a lack of this differentiation, but cells became more retractable and changed to a more epithelial morphology. Fibronectin shedding was also increased by TPA treatment of fetal melanocytes. However, there was no detection of any shedding of the 240K MAA, although the evidence cited above suggested a transformed phenotype. In additional experiments, SV$_{40}$-transformed fetal melanocytes, transformed more than 12 times after lytic crisis, synthesized and shed molecules immunologically similar to the 240K MAA (Morgan and Reisfeld, 1981).

These data, taken together, suggest that the 240K MAA shed by melanoma cells may be a marker of tumorigenicity. It appears that this particular marker is synthesized by "initiated" cells like the CAR No. 2 cells or the SV$_{40}$-transformed fetal melanocytes. On the other hand, it seems that "promotion" without initiation is not sufficient to induce synthesis of the 240K MAA.

In summary, our studies suggest an important role of the 240K and 94K MAAs in the elicitation of host immune responses and point to changes in expression and glycosylation of these tumor markers that may be associated with transformation events. It appears likely that these two immunochemically defined MAAs may eventually be of some practical use for the detection of melanoma and other forms of malignancies.

7. Conclusions

Approaches designed to characterize human MAAs by molecular and immunological means proved successful. The keys to this success were (1) the development of a sensitive radioimmunometric antibody-binding assay for the evaluation of specific xenoantisera to MAAs; (2) the production of polyclonal and monoclonal antibody specifically reactive with MAAs; and (3) the effective purification of two MAAs with molecular weights of 94,000

(94K) and 240,000 (240K) by ion-exchange chromatography coupled with lectin and antibody-affinity chromatography. Another key factor that aided the purification and characterization of the 94K and 240K glycoprotein tumor markers was the availability of these antigens in shed form in serum-free spent media of intrinsically radiolabeled melanoma cells.

The characterization of the two MAAs clearly indicated that the 94K marker is an oncofetal antigen present on tumor cells of different histological origin, whereas the 240K molecule appears to be a specific marker of tumorogenicity on melanoma cells. These two human tumor markers are certainly unique when compared with other glycoproteins found on the surface of tumor cells in that their shedding into spent culture media is dependent on their degree of glycosylation. Interestingly enough, glycosylation appears not necessary for recognition of these antigens on the cell surface by specific monoclonal antibody.

The results from our studies point to an important role of the 240K and 94K MAAs in the elicitation of host immune responses. It also seems likely that changes in expression and glycosylation of these two tumor markers may be associated with cell transformation. It is anticipated that these two human MAAs will eventually prove useful for the diagnosis and prognosis of malignant melanoma.

ACKNOWLEDGMENTS. The authors' research cited herein was supported by Grant CA 28420 from the National Institutes of Health and Grant IM-218 from the American Cancer Society. This chapter is Publication No. 2415 from the Department of Molecular Immunology, Scripps Clinic and Research Foundation.

References

Bissell, M. J., 1978, Transport as a rate limiting step in glucose metabolism in virus-transformed cells: Studies with cytochalasin B, *J. Cell Physiol.* **89**:701.

Brown, J. P., Wright, P. W., Hart, C. E., Hellström, K. E., and Hellström, I., 1980, Protein antigens of normal and malignant human cells identified by immunoprecipitation with monoclonal antibodies, *J. Biol. Chem.* **255**:4980.

Bystryn, J. C., 1977, Release of cell surface tumor-associated antigens by viable melanoma cells from humans, *J. Natl. Cancer Inst.* **59**:325.

Carey, T. E., Lloyd, K. O., and Takahashi, T., 1979, Cell surface antigen of human malignant melanoma: Solubilization and partial characterization, *Proc. Natl. Acad. Sci. U.S.A.* **76**:2898.

Chee, D. O., Boddie, A. W., Jr., Roth, J. A., and Morton, D. L., 1976, Production of melanoma-associated antigens by a defined malignant melanoma cell strain grown in chemically defined medium, *Cancer Res.* **36**:1503.

Curry, R. A., Quaranta, V., Wilson, B. S., McCabe, R. P., Natali, P. G., Pellegrino, M. A., and Ferrone, S., 1979a, Expression of HLA antigens on cultured human melanoma cells: Lack of association with melanoma associated antigens, in: *Current Trends in Tumor Immunology* (S. Ferrone, C. Gorini, R. B. Herberman, and R. A. Reisfeld, eds.), pp. 347–376, Garland STPM Press, New York.

Curry, R. A., Quaranta, V., Pellegrino, M. A., and Ferrone, S., 1979b, Serologically detectable human melanoma associated antigens are not genetically linked to HLA-A and B antigens, *J. Immunol.* **123**:2630.

Datama, R., and Schwartz, R. T., 1979, Interference with glycosylation of glycoproteins: Inhibition of formation of lipid linked oligosaccharides *in vivo*, *J. Biochem.* **184**:113.

Duskin, D., and Bornstein, P., 1978, Impaired conversion of procollagen to collagen by fibroblasts and bone treated with tunicamycin, an inhibitor of protein glycosylation, *J. Biol. Chem.* **252**:955.

Engvall, E., and Ruoslahti, E., 1977, Binding of soluble form of fibroblast surface protein, fibronectin, to collagen, *Int. J. Cancer* **20**:1.

Galloway, D. R., McCabe, R. P., Pellegrino, M. A., Ferrone, S., and Reisfeld, R. A., 1981a, Tumor associated antigens in spent medium of human melanoma cells: Immunochemical characterization with xenoantisera, *J. Immunol.* **162**:62.

Galloway, D. R., Imai, K., Ferrone, S., and Reisfeld, R. A., 1981b, Molecular profiles of human melanoma-associated antigens, *Fed. Proc. Fed. Am. Soc. Exp. Biol.* **40**:59.

Granatek, C. H., Scheinberg, B. M., and Cory, P. M., 1979, Unmasking of fetal determinants on adult bone marrow cells, *Nature (London)* **281**:484.

Grimm, E. A., Silver, H. K. B., Roth, J. A., and Morton, D. L., 1976, Detection of tumor-associated antigen in human melanoma cell line supernatants, *Int. J. Cancer* **17**:559.

Gupta, R. K., Irie, R. F., Chee, D. O, and Morton, D. L., 1979, Demonstration of two distinct antigens in spent tissue culture medium of human malignant melanoma cell line, *J. Natl. Cancer Inst.* **63**:347.

Heiniger, H. J., and Marshall, J. D., 1979, Pinocytosis in L cells: Its dependence on membrane sterol and the cytoskeleton, *Cell Biol. Int. Rep.* **3**:409.

Hickman, S., and Kornfield, S., 1978, Effect of tunicamycin on IgM, IgA, and IgG secretion by mouse plasmacytoma cells, *J. Immunol.* **121**:990.

Hughes, R. C., Meager, A., and Nair, R., 1977, Effect of 2-deoxy D-glucose on the cell-surface glycoproteins of hamster fibroblasts, *Eur. J. Biochem.* **72**:265.

Imai, K., Ng, A. K., and Ferrone, S., 1981, Characterization of monoclonal antibodies to melanoma-associated antigens, *J. Natl. Cancer Inst.* **66**:489.

Jerry, L. M., Lewis, M. G., and Ronden, G., 1976, Fetal antigens in non-neoplastic conditions, *Cancer Res.* **36**:3446.

Keller, P. K., Boon, D. Y., and Crum, F. C., 1979, N-Acetyl glucosamine-1-phosphate transferase from hen oviduct: Solubilization, characterization, and inhibition by tunicamycin, *Biochemistry* **18**:3946.

Krangel, M. S., Orr, H. T., and Strominger, J. L., 1979, Assembly and maturation of HLA-A and HLA-B antigens *in vivo*, *Cell* **18**:979.

Lever, J. E., 1979, Modulation of glucose uptake in animal cells, *J. Biol. Chem.* **254**:2961.

McCabe, R. P., Ferrone, S., Pellegrino, M. A., Kern, D. H., Holmes, E. C., and Reisfeld, R. A., 1978, Isolation and immunochemical evaluation of human melanoma-associated antigens, *J. Natl. Cancer Inst.* **60**:773.

McCabe, R. P., Quaranta, V., Frugis, L., Ferrone, S., and Reisfeld, R. A., 1979a, A radioimmunometric antibody binding assay for the evaluation of xenoantisera to melanoma associated antigens, *J. Natl. Cancer Inst.* **62**:455.

McCabe, R. P., Galloway, D. R., Ferrone, S., and Reisfeld, R. A., 1979b, Human melanoma associated antigens (MAA): Serological and structural characteristics, in: *Current Trends in Tumor Immunology* (S. Ferrone, L. Gorini, R. B. Herberman, and R. A. Reisfeld, eds.), pp. 269–286, Garland STPM Press, New York.

McCabe, R. P., Indiveri, F., Galloway, D. R., Ferrone, S., and Reisfeld, R. A., 1980, Lack of association of serologically detectable human melanoma-associated antigens with β_2-microglobulin: Serological and immunochemical evidence, *J. Natl. Cancer Inst.* **68**:703.

Morgan, A. C., and Reisfeld, R. A., 1982, Biological significance of human melanoma associated antigens defined by xenoantisera, *Adv. Immunopathol.* (in press).

Morgan, A. C., Galloway, D. R., Imai, K., and Reisfeld, R. A., 1981, Human melanoma-associated antigenic role of carbohydrate in shedding and cell surface expression, *J. Immunol.* **126**:365.

Morgan, A. C., Galloway, D. R., Jensen, F. C., Giovanella, B. C., and Reisfeld, R. A., 1981a, Immunochemical delineation of an oncofetal antigen on cultured human fetal melanocytes, *Proc. Natl. Acad. Sci. U.S.A.* **78**:3834.

Nakamura, K., and Compani, R. W., 1978, Effects of glucosamine, 2-deoxyglucose and tunicamycin on glycosylation, sulfation, and assembly of influenza viral proteins, *Virology* **84**:303.

Olden, K., Pratt, R. M., and Yamada, K. M., 1978, Role of carbohydrates in protein secretion and turnover: Effects of tunicamycin on the major cell surface glycoprotein of chick embryo fibroblasts, *Cell* **13**:461.

Olden, K., Pratt, R. M., Jaworski, C., and Yamada, K. M., 1979, Evidence for role of glycoprotein carbohydrates in membrane transport: Specific inhibition by tunicamycin, *Proc. Natl. Acad. Sci. U.S.A.* **76**:791.

Pouyssegur, J. M., and Pastan, I., 1977, Mutants of mouse fibroblasts altered in the synthesis of cell surface glycoproteins, *J. Biol. Chem.* **252**:1639.

Rampa. A. L., Pinkofsky, H. B., and Jung, C. Y., 1980, Structure of cytochalasins and cytochalasin B binding sites in human erythrocyte membranes, *Biochemistry* **19**:679.

Reisfeld, R. A., Pellegrino, M. A., and Kahan, B. D., 1971, Salt extraction of soluble HLA antigens, *Science* **172**:1134.

Stuhlmiller, G. M., Green, R. W., and Seigler, H. F., 1978, Solubilization and partial isolation of human melanoma tumor-associated antigens, *J. Natl. Cancer Inst.* **61**:61.

Tannenbaum, J., Tannenbaum, S. W., and Godman, G. C., 1977, The binding sites of cytochalasin D. II. Their relationship to hexose transport and to cytochalasin B, *J. Cell Physiol.* **91**:239.

Tkacz, J. S., and Lampen, J. O., 1975, Tunicamycin inhibition of polyisoprenyl-*N*-acetylglucosaminyl pyrophosphate formation in calf liver microsomes, *Biochem. Biophys. Res. Commun.* **65**:248.

Waechter, C. J., and Lennarz, W. J., 1976, The role of polyprenol-linked sugars in glycoprotein synthesis, *Annu. Rev. Biochem.* **45**:95.

Wessels, N. K., Spooner, B. S., and Ash, J. F., 1971, Microfilaments in cellular and developmental processes: Contractile microfilament machinery of many types is reversibly inhibited by cytochalasin B, *Science* **171**:135.

Woodbury, R. C., Brown, J. P., Yeh, M. Y., Hellström, I., and Hellström, K. E., 1980, Identification of a cell surface protein, p 97, in human melanomas and certain other neoplasma, *Proc. Natl. Acad. Sci. U.S.A.* **77**:2183.

18

Cell-Surface Structure and State of Malignancy in Human Malignant Melanoma

CLEMENS SORG, JOSEF BRÜGGEN, DOROTHEA TERBRACK,
FEREYDOUN VAKILZADEH, LUDWIG SUTER, AND
EGON MACHER

1. Introduction

Human malignant melanoma is a spontaneous tumor that progresses from the initial pre-malignant lesions to highly metastatic forms. Clinical and histological observations of this process and some recent knowledge gained on experimental tumor models suggest that tumor progression is a complex multistage process. In the course of this process, several distinct properties have to be aquired by the tumor cells either sequentially or in parallel (Poste and Fidler, 1980; Nicolson *et al.*, 1977). Properties of prime importance are believed to be invasiveness, neovascularization, resistance to rejection mechanisms, and adaptation to and growth in a different organ or tissue. It has been shown in animal tumor models that the capacity to metastasize is a phenotypically expressed property of a tumor cell; moreover, even the target organ seems to be predetermined by the phenotype (Dexter *et al.*, 1978; Hart and Fidler, 1980; Nicolson and Winkelhake, 1975; Nicolson *et al.*, 1978; Nowell, 1976; Schirrmacher *et al.*, 1979a; Susuki *et al.*, 1978). The mechanisms by which primary tumors develop highly malignant variants have been circumscribed by the term retrodifferentiation and are unknown (Coggin and Anderson, 1974; Renselaer Potter, 1978; Uriel, 1979). That the process of retrodifferentiation might also be reversed is indi-

CLEMENS SORG, JOSEF BRÜGGEN, DOROTHEA TERBRACK, FEREYDOUN VAKILZADEH, LUDWIG SUTER, AND EGON MACHER • Department of Experimental Dermatology, Universitäts-Hautklinik, 4400 Münster, West Germany.

cated in experiments wherein nonmetastasizing variants were isolated from metastases (Tao and Burger, 1977). It is logical to assume that phenotypic changes that are associated with the expression of different biochemical and biological properties are also associated with changes in the cell surface, which in fact has been demonstrated in several instances (Fogel *et al.*, 1979; Killion and Kollmorgen, 1976; Nicolson and Winkelhake, 1975; Poste, 1977; Schirrmacher *et al.*, 1979b; Sorg *et al.*, 1978; Yogeeswaran *et al.*, 1978, 1979). Correlation of changes in malignant properties with changes in cell-surface constituents seems to be possible and might lead ultimately to serological typing of malignancy on single cells or tumor tissue. The development of variants with different biological and biochemical properties would also challenge the notion that tumors express specific antigens that are specific not only for the neoplastic state but also for a histological type of tumor. In this chapter, we will review our serological studies on melanoma-associated antigens and our attempts to relate the expression of cell-surface antigens to a certain state of malignancy.

2. Melanoma-Associated Antigens

2.1. Failure to Detect Melanoma-Specific Antigens

Human malignant melanoma shows the phenomenon of spontaneous regression at a relatively high rate (Bowden, 1968; Happle *et al.*, 1975). Even though the mechanisms involved in spontaneous regression of human melanoma remain undetermined, an immunological mechanism is suspected by virtue of the observation of a mononuclear-cell infiltrate at the regression site (Berg, 1959; Happle *et al.*, 1975). A prerequisite for immunological control of a tumor is the expression of surface structures on tumor cells that are antigenic for the immune system and thus may function as rejection antigens. It is clear that tumor cells express on their cell surfaces different structural and functional elements from their normal counterparts. With regard to human malignant melanoma, considerable effort has been devoted to the question as to whether these surface structures represent tumor-specific antigens (Houghton *et al.*, 1980) and whether they are functional in immunological (Hellström *et al.*, 1973; Herbermann, 1973) or nonimmunological rejection mechanisms (Hibbs, 1974). The reports on the existence of melanoma antigens with respect to tumor specificity and common cross-reactivity are inconsistent (Morton *et al.*, 1968; Oettgen, 1974; Cornain *et al.*, 1975; The *et al.*, 1975; Viza and Phillips, 1975; Lewis and Philipps, 1972). In a previous study, we therefore investigated whether serological reactions against cultured melanoma cells could be found in melanoma patients (Seibert *et al.*, 1977). A considerable proportion of positively reacting sera were found not only in melanoma patients but also in patients with tumors other than melanoma and in healthy control persons. No evidence was found for antibodies against common cross-reacting or individual specific melanoma antigens. An analysis of specificity revealed that besides some reactivity against blood-group and histocompatibility antigens, the reactivity was directed mainly against tumor-associated fetal antigens.

Similar results were obtained with xenogeneic antisera raised in nonhuman primates against cultured human melanoma cells (Brüggen *et al.*, 1978). After exhaustive absorption with AB Rh$^+$ red blood cells and pooled platelets from about 200 donors, the sera were still reactive to various degrees in the microimmune-adherence test with other melanoma lines, with embryonic fibroblasts and with nonmelanoma lines. As proven by absorption experiments, the main specificity of the antisera was not directed against components of the fetal calf serum used for cell culture or against mycoplasma grown from commercial fetal calf serum. In addition, no cross-reactivity was observed with bacillus Calmette Guérin (Minden *et al.*, 1974), and in blocking experiments no reactivity against extracts of common bacterial antigens or mixed molds was detected. Absorption with embryonic fibroblasts or embryonic tissue showed that the reactivity of most antisera was directed against melanoma-associated antigens expressed also on fetal tissue. It was not possible to determine whether the remaining reactivity on some cell lines was melanoma-specific or directed against fetal antigens not contained in the fetal material used for absorption. Extending our study to various nonmelanoma cell lines, we found that the 10 monkey antisera tested reacted with 4–43% of 46 nonmelanoma lines compared to 62–100% of 16 melanoma lines. This indicates a preferential reactivity of sera with melanoma lines. Apart from this preference of sera for melanoma cell lines, there was no indication of a melanoma-specific antigen.

2.2. Heterogeneity of Melanoma-Cell Populations

One of the general assumptions in tumor immunology is that tumor-associated or tumor-specific surface antigens are expressed by the tumor cell in a constant and uniform manner. As shown for the expression of histocompatibility antigens on human lymphoblastoid cells (Pellegrino *et al.*, 1972; Ferrone *et al.*, 1973; Everson *et al.*, 1974) and human fibroblasts (Brautbar *et al.*, 1973), the expression of human leukocyte antigen (*HLA*) complex antigens remains constant over extended culture periods. In another report (Goldstein and Singal, 1972), the expression of HLA antigens on fibroblasts was found to disappear with increasing age. Recently, it was shown that various tumor cells may express histocompatibility antigens different from those of the parental line (Schirrmacher *et al.*, 1980). While the expression of histocompatibility antigens that generally are not believed to belong to the class of so-called differentiation antigens appears to remain, by and large, rather constant during culture, antigens that are associated with a neoplastic state seem to be subject to greater fluctuations.

During our own extensive serological studies on membrane-associated antigens of cultured melanoma cells (Seibert *et al.*, 1977), we were unable to fully reproduce our results obtained several months before on cell lines that had been kept in culture continuously. Since technical errors could be excluded, it was assumed that the cell lines might have altered their pattern of surface antigens. Several questions relate directly to this phenomenon, such as: (1) Is the antigen pattern of a cell line at a given moment representative for a tumor, and consequently (2) is an immunological reaction *in vitro* a valid correlate to the *in vivo* situation? (3) Does a tumor *in vivo* also change its surface structure? (4) Could the change in surface antigens be the basis for an efficient immunological escape mechanism? In a subsequent study, we investigated conditions that might lead to an alteration of cell-surface structure (Sorg *et al.*, 1978). Established melanoma cell lines were cultured for one passage (approximately 1 week) in different lots of fetal calf and newborn calf sera and then tested against a panel of previously positively reacting sera from melanoma patients and other human sera. Investigated with the indirect immunofluorescence test, the cells showed varying degrees of reactivity ranging from positive to negative reactions depending on the supplementing serum in the culture medium. When standardized culture conditions were used and the cells were tested by immune adherence at intervals of several weeks against panels of sera from melanoma patients, from tumor patients other than melanoma, from pregnant women, and from normal donors, most of the sera reacted identically, but some sera had changed not only quantitatively but also qualitatively from a negative to a positive reaction and vice versa, indicating a shift in the spectrum of expressed antigens. When single cell clones from a cell line were isolated and tested against a panel of antisera, striking differences in reactivity were observed, suggesting that the shift in the spectrum of expressed antigens was due to the outgrowth of dominating subclones with antigen pattern different from the previously dominating subclones. This conclusion was further supported by experiments in which a weakly positively reacting serum was employed to separate a cell line into positively and negatively reacting sublines. Unit-gravity sedimentation and density-gradient sedimentation was used to separate rosetted from nonrosetted tumor cells that had been prepared by immune adherence. From these results, it was concluded that cultured cell lines are in a dynamic state and that differentiation that may be induced by various environmental signals (Brunner, 1977) is one of the major mechanisms accounting for a change in antigen expression.

The critical question now is whether similar events take place *in vivo*. Clinical and histological observations provide evidence that this in fact may be so. At present, we have four well-documented cases of malignant melanoma in our clinic in which the primary tumor had completely regressed while a metastasis was growing in the draining lymph node. If we assume that the regression phenomenon was induced by a specific immunological reaction and if we assume that the reaction was directed against a melanoma-specific antigen on the cell surface, the question remains to be answered why some tumor cells escaped rejection and could settle in the lymph node. Considering our *in vitro* data, another explanation seems to be more likely, *viz.*, that variant tumor cells with a different antigen pattern on the surface that could escape a hypothetical immune reaction against the primary tumor or local growth-control mechanisms (Brunner, 1977). This interpretation is supported by a series of findings in experimental tumor systems (Fidler, 1978; Fogel *et al.*, 1979; Miller and Heppner, 1979; Tao and Burger, 1977). From the histology, we know that melanomas are morphologically heterogeneous. This is documented by Fig. 1, which shows the rare situation in which two morphologically distinct clones of melanoma cells are growing in close proximity, yet separated from each other by a strip of connective tissue.

2.3. Melanoma-Associated Antigens and Their Relationship to Parameters of Malignancy

As a consequence of the observations discussed above, it is logical to assume that tumor progression involves the appearance and disappearance of tumor-cell variants with different biochemical and biological properties that might also be reflected on the cell surface. In this section, we describe our attempts to correlate patterns of cell-surface antigens with certain parameters of malignancy (Brüggen *et al.*, 1981). As one parameter of malignancy, we studied the production of plasminogen activator, which is widely considered to correlate

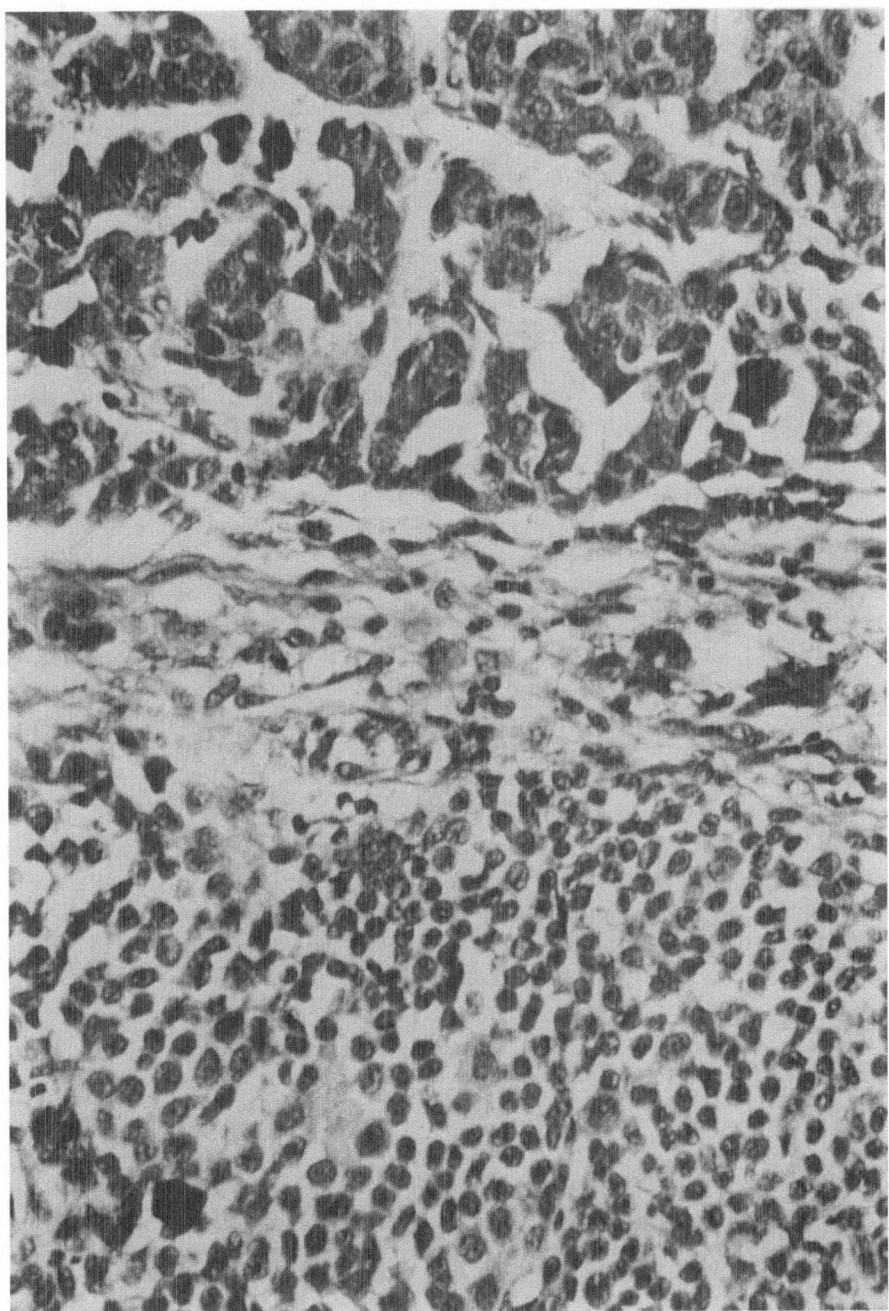

FIGURE 1. Two morphologically distinct clones of melanoma cells in a superficial spreading melanoma that are separated by a strip of connective tissue.

with invasive growth of normal (Beers et al., 1975; Buonassisi and Venter, 1976; Laug et al., 1975; Ossowski et al., 1979; Rifkin et al., 1974; Strickland et al., 1976; Unkeless et al., 1974) and neoplastic cells (Christman et al., 1975; Newcomb et al., 1978; Reich, 1975; Silagi, 1976) and which has been found to correlate by and large with tumorigenicity (Goldberg, 1974; Jones et al., 1975; Mak et al., 1976; Nagy et al., 1977); yet, examples with no correlation have also been reported (Montesano et al., 1977; Mott et al., 1974; Nicolson and Winkelhake, 1975; San et al., 1977; Wilson and Reich, 1979). As a further parameter of malignancy, growth in the athymic nude mouse was studied (Fogh et al., 1977; Giovanella et al., 1978; Gershwin et al., 1977). It has been shown that growth in the nude mouse clearly distinguishes malignant from normal tissue, yet not all tumors grow and those that grow are different with respect to the latency period or the amount of cells needed to induce a tumor. It was noted by Gershwin et al. (1977) that the growth patterns of tumors of various histological types do not correlate with their basic biological aggressiveness observed clinically.

For the plasminogen-activator assay, melanoma cell lines were cultured for 48 hr in serum-free medium, and the supernatants were assayed to lyse ^{125}I-fibrogen in the presence or absence of bovine plasminogen. As shown in Table I, the plasminogen-dependent lysis of fibrinogen is different in supernatants of various melanoma cell lines, ranging from a high activity in those of Mel A-375 to no detectable activity in those of SK-Mel 25. Growth of melanoma cell lines in the nude mouse was assayed by subcutaneous injection of cells into dorsal sites. The results obtained are also summarized in Table I. The cell lines displayed remarkable differences in their capacity to produce tumors. Six of seven melanoma lines tested were positive, whereas the line SK-Mel 25 was negative. Within the group of growing cells, quantitative differences were observed with respect to the latency period or the tumor mass developed after 40 days, respectively. The data on plasminogen-activator production and growth in the nude mouse were further compared with the reactivity of cell lines with xenogeneic sera raised in monkeys against Mel A-375 and SK-Mel 25, which had been characterized extensively before (Brüggen et al., 1978). The cell lines are listed from left to right according to their decreasing capacity to grow in the nude mouse. As can be seen, the production of plasminogen activator and the serological reactivity of cell lines correlates remarkably well with tumor growth in the nude mouse. While the reactivity with

TABLE I

Biological Properties and Cell-Surface Antigens of Human Melanoma Lines

	Cell Lines						
Property	Mel A-375	Mel 57	MeWo	Mel 2a	Mel 67	RPMI 5966	SK-Mel 25
Fibrinolytic activity[a]	1234.0 ± 40.4	540.6 ± 21.2	204.5 ± 12.4	85.6 ± 4.2	150.1 ± 4.2	81.7 ± 6.2	0
Tumor growth in the nude mouse after 40 days (mm^3)[b]	700 (660–720)	200 (180–210)	250 (250–260)	160 (145–175)	40 (34–46)	25 (21–29)	0
Monkey antisera[c]							
Anti-375	80	40	40	40	40	20	<10
Anti-SK 25	0	10	20	20	20	20	40

[a]Expressed as mIU urokinase per 2×10^5 cells; 100 mIU causes 100% lysis.
[b]The number of cells implanted was 5×10^6; 6 mice per group. The ranges of growth are shown in parentheses.
[c]Immune adherence test; reciprocal titer of end-point reaction.

TABLE II

Growth in the Nude Mouse and Plasminogen-Activator Production by Sublines of SK-Mel 25

Sublines of SK-Mel 25	Number of mice that developed tumors/ number of injected animals	Fibrinolytic activity[a]		Tumor growth after 40 days (mm³)[b]
		Plasminogen-dependent	Plasminogen-independent	
S 3	0/6	0	0	—
S 4	0/6	0	0	—
S 5	2/4	187.6 ± 12.0	0	370 (335–405)
S 6	0/6	0	0	—
S 7	0/6	0	0	—
S 9	0/6	75.3 ± 8.6	0	—
S 13	2/4	62.0 ± 4.1	0	51 (45–57)

[a,b] See Table I footnotes.

the autologous line is highest, there is little or no cross-reactivity between Mel A-375 and SK-Mel 25. The other cell lines, which are arranged to form a continuum between the two lines with respect to their biological properties, show intermediate reactivities with both antisera. Surface iodination and fractionation on sodium dodecyl sulfate–polyacrylamide gels also revealed striking differences in patterns between the two lines.

In a previous study, described in Section 2.2, we have shown that one may isolate from an established cell line single cell clones that are distinct with regard to their surface antigens (Sorg *et al.*, 1978). Here, we isolated single cell clones from the line SK-Mel 25 according to differences in growth patterns and morphology. The clones were grown to sublines, and their supernatants were tested for plasminogen-dependent or -independent fibrinolytic activity. Furthermore, the cells were also injected into the nude mouse. The combined results are shown in Table II. Of the seven clones tested, only three showed a moderate plasminogen-dependent fibrinolytic activity in contrast to the parental line. Quite remarkably, subclone S 5, which released the highest amounts of plasminogen activator, also grew in the nude mouse, whereas S 13 was borderline and S 9 did not grow at all.

From these results, the question arose whether the subclones with an apparently higher malignancy potential displayed differences in the expression of cell-surface antigens. And further, had the sublines with a higher malignancy potential shifted their spectrum of expressed antigens into the direction of the spectrum expressed by Mel A-375? Antisera were therefore raised in rhesus monkeys against sublines S 5, S 7, and S 9. After absorption with AB Rh⁺ red blood cells and pooled platelets of more than 200 donors, the reactivity against the sublines and the melanoma lines SK-Mel 25, Mel-57, and Mel A-375 was compared. All antisera against sublines reacted with the parental line SK-Mel 25; however, differences in reactivity of antisera against sublines with the parental line and other sublines could be observed (data not shown). Anti-serum anti-S 5 reacted strongly with the autologous subline S 13 and to a lesser degree with the parental line SK-Mel 25 and its subline S 7, yet was clearly positive on Mel 57 in contrast to anti-serum anti-S 7. On the other hand, anti-57 did not react with SK-Mel 25 and its sublines S 7 and S 9, but was positive on subline S 5. Since the titers of antisera were low and differences in reactivity among sublines were small, the conclusion that melanoma cells may change their malignancy potential and that these changes may also be reflected in changes of membrane constituents could not be drawn unequivocally from these experiments. The resolving power of xenoantisera had also been pushed to its limits during these experiments. To detect clonal markers on melanoma sublines, a more sophisticated immunochemical approach would have been necessary. The advent of the hybridoma technique (Köhler and Milstein, 1975) for production of monoclonal antibodies therefore opened new dimensions for the analysis of melanoma-associated antigens (Carrel *et al.*, 1980; Imai *et al.*, 1980; Herlyn *et al.*, 1980; Yeh *et al.*, 1979).

2.4. Immunohistological Studies

2.4.1. Generation of Hybridoma Antibodies

BALB/c mice were immunized with cultured melanoma cells, and the spleen cells were fused with the line P3-X63-AG8-653 using polyethyleneglycol. The hybridoma supernatants were screened for antibodies using an enzyme-linked immunosorbent assay (ELISA), which has been described in detail elsewhere (Suter *et al.*, 1980). The following scheme was used: In the first stage, supernatants were tested on pooled leukocytes and platelets. Positively reacting antibodies were discarded. The negative ones were tested in a second-stage screening on various melanoma lines. Thereafter, negative supernatants were discarded. Positive supernatants were tested in a third-stage screening on purified pooled monocytes of at least 46 donors and several B-lymphoblastoid cell lines. The few remaining negative supernatants were then screened for their fine specificity on various melanoma lines and their variant sublines as well as on several nonmelanoma lines.

Monoclonal antibodies of the A and S series were prepared against Mel A-375 or SK-Mel 25, respectively. The two monoclonal antibodies M 5 and M 14 were generated and characterized in detail by Carrel *et al.* (1980). The reactivity of antibodies with a wide variety of melanoma and nonmelanoma lines is shown in Table III. Antibodies of the A series react strongly with A-375 and not with other melanoma lines. There is only a weak reactivity of A.1.27 with the colon carcinoma HT-29 and with embryonic skin fibroblasts (E.FIB). On the other hand, monoclonals of the S series display a wide and highly interesting spectrum of reactivity. The antibodies show a clear-cut preference for melanoma lines and do not react with nonmelanoma lines so far. Of particular interest are S 15 and S 16, which distinguish among various sublines of SK-Mel 25. M-5 and M-14 also show a clear-cut preference for melanoma lines, yet some minor cross-reactivity with nonmelanoma lines also became evident. The results demonstrate that clonal antigens do exist and can be detected with monoclonal antibodies. So far, our studies had been limited to specificity testing on cultured cell lines. We then asked the questions whether our monoclonal antibodies and monkey antisera can also distinguish melanoma cells from normal tissue in cryostat sections and, further, whether the antibodies distinguish clonal variants within a tumor and whether clonal antigens or patterns thereof can be correlated to the malignancy state of a clonal variant. If the latter were possible, antisera and monoclonal antibodies would be immediately applicable in diagnosis and prognosis of malignant melanoma.

In the following section, we will give a brief account of the current state of our work along these lines.

TABLE III
Reactivity of Monoclonal Antibodies with Human Cell Lines[a]

Cell lines tested	Monoclonal antibodies								
	A.1.6[b]	A.1.19[b]	A.1.27[b]	A.1.43[b]	S.14[c]	S.15[c]	S.16[c]	M-5[d]	M-14[d]
Melanoma									
A-375	5.3	6.0	6.3	4.3	6.4	−	−	−	3.1
SK-Mel 25	−	−	−	−	7.1	3.8	5.6	2.8	2.9
Sublines:									
S-3	−	−	−	−	6.5	−	3.3	−	−
S-5-M	−	−	−	−	6.5	4.4	3.3	−	−
S-7	−	−	−	−	6.3	4.5	4.0	−	−
S-9-M	−	−	−	−	6.8	−	−	−	−
S-13	−	−	−	−	6.5	4.2	2.5	2.4	−
Mel 57	−	−	−	−	−	−	3.0	−	2.7
MeWo	−	−	−	−	5.0	−	−	2.6	2.4
Mel 67	−	−	−	−	3.0	−	--	2.4	−
Mel 2a	−	−	−	−	2.4	−	2.3	−	−
RPMI 4454	−	−	−	−	2.3	−	−	5.2	4.6
SK-Mel 7	−	−	−	−	5.0	−	−	−	−
Nonmelanoma:									
TERA I	−	−	−	−	−	−	−	−	−
TERA II	−	−	−	−	−	−	−	−	2.3
HELA	−	−	−	−	−	−	−	−	−
HT-29	−	−	2.3	−	−	−	−	3.2	−
A.FIB	−	−	−	−	−	−	−	2.7	−
E.FIB	−	−	2.5	−	−	−	−	2.7	−
Lymphocytes (46 donors)	−	−	−	−	−	−	−	−	−

[a]Screening was performed by an ELISA as described by Suter et al. (1980). A test/control ratio of greater than 2.0 was considered positive. For the origin of cell lines, see Brüggen et al. (1978).
[b]Raised against Mel A-375.   [c]Raised against SK-Mel 25.   [d]Provided by S. Carrel (see Carrel et al., 1980).

2.4.2. Reactivity of Xenogeneic Antisera and Monoclonal Antibodies on Cryostat Sections of Various Melanoma Tissues

Cryostat sections of biopsies from various stages of melanoma as well as nevus-cell nevi and basal-cell carcinoma were reacted first with monkey antisera or monoclonal antibodies and in a second step with an enchancing antiserum. In a third step, fluorescein-conjugated antibody was added. For evaluation, the reaction strength was scored on a + to + + + basis. The average reactivity of an antiserum was expressed by a reaction index that is the arithmetic mean of all scores gained on a particular tumor stage. Table IV illustrates the reactivity of melanoma antisera and monoclonal antibodies with nevus-cell nevi. The five nevus-cell nevi have been further differentiated into dermal, quiescent, papillomatous, compound, and active or junction nevus. Even though the reactivity of antibodies in some instances is quite strong, the reactivity index is generally low for monkey antisera and low for monoclonal antibodies. Table V shows the results obtained with monkey antisera on nevus-cell nevi, basal-cell epithelioma, and various stages of malignant melanoma. In the course of this study, it was found that some monkey antisera reacted with a

TABLE IV

Reactivity of Antisera and Monoclonal Antibodies against Melanoma Cell Lines with Human Nevus-Cell Nevus

Nevus-cell nevus[a]	Monkey antisera[b]							Monoclonal antibodies					
	a-375	a-57	a-67	a-144	a-S-5	a-S-7	a-SK-25	M-14	M-15	A.1.5	A.1.19	A.1.20	A.1.27
Dermal	0	0	+	0	+	+ +	+	0	0	0	0	+	0
Quiescent	0	0	0	+ + +	+ +	+ + +	+	0	0	0	0	+	+
Papillomatous	+	0	0	+ +	+ +	+	+	+	+	+	0	+	0
Compound	+ +	0	+	0	+ +	+ +	+	0	0	0	0	+	+
Active (junction)	+ +	+	0	0	+	+	+ +	0	0	0	0	+	+
Index of reactivity[c]	1.0	0.2	0.4	1.0	1.6	2.0	1.2	0.2	0.2	0.2	0.0	1.0	0.6

[a]Cryostat sections.   [b]Tested by indirect immunofluorescence.   [c]Arithmetic mean of reactions.

TABLE V

Reactivity of Monkey Antisera with Cryostat Sections of Malignant Melanoma

Type of tissue[a]	Total number tested	Monkey antisera[b]						
		a-375	a-57	a-67	a-144	a-SK-25	a-S-5	a-S-7
Nevus-cell nevus	5	1.0	0.2	0.4	1.0	1.2	1.6	1.2
Basal-cell epithelioma	5	1.2	0.2	0.2	0.4	0.8	0.6	0.2
LMM level IV	2	2.5	0.5	0.5	0.5	1.5	3.0	2.5
SSM level III	2	2.0	1.5	0.0	1.0	0.5	2.5	2.5
SSM level IV	5	2.2	0.8	0.0	2.0	1.0	3.0	1.8
NMM level III	2	3.0	3.0	0.5	0.0	2.5	2.5	2.5
MM								
skin metastases	8	2.0	1.5	1.4	1.0	2.1	2.5	1.4
Lymph node metastases	2	2.5	0.5	0.5	0.5	3.0	2.5	2.0

[a](LMM) Lymph-node metastatic malignant melonoma; (SSM) superficial spreading melanoma.
(NMM) nodular malignant melanoma; (MM) malignant melanoma.
[b]Tested by indirect immunofluorescence. Results are reaction indexes.

TABLE VI

Reactivity of Monoclonal Antibodies with Cryostat Sections of Malignant Melanoma

Type of tissue[a]	Total number tested	Monoclonal antibodies[b]								
		M-14	M-5	A.1.5	A.1.6	A.1.18	A.1.19	A.1.20	A.1.27	A.1.43
Nevus-cell nevus	5	0.2	0.2	0.2	0.8	0.4	0	1.0	0.6	0.6
Basal-cell epithelioma	5	0.4	0.8	0	0.2	0.2	0	0.4	1.0	0.8
LMM level IV	2	0.0	0.5	1.5	1.0	1.0	1.0	1.5	1.0	1.0
SSM level III	2	1.0	1.0	0.5	2.0	1.5	0.5	0.5	0.5	1.0
SSM level IV	5	1.4	1.2	1.6	1.0	0.6	1.2	2.2	2.4	1.2
NMM level III	2	0.0	0.0	2.5	2.0	1.0	1.0	1.5	2.5	1.0
MM										
Skin metastases	8	0.6	0.9	0.6	1.5	0.2	0.6	1.4	1.1	0.3
Lymph node metastases	2	0.0	0.0	1.5	1.0	1.0	0.0	2.5	0.5	0

[a,b]See Table V footnotes.

wide variety of skin cells, particularly with basal and epidermal cells, and therefore were excluded from further studies. The sera listed in Table V showed a high selectivity for melanoma cells and even differentiated between these stages of melanoma. Serum a-375, which reacted most strongly with nodular melanoma, was less reactive with basal-cell epithelioma and nevus-cell nevi. Anti-serum anti-57 showed a pronounced reactivity with nodular melanoma and was not reactive or only weakly reactive with melanoma of other stages. Similarly, anti-serum anti-67 was negative or showed only background reactivity on most melanoma stages, but was clearly positive on skin metastasis.

Similar patterns of reactivity were found with monoclonal antibodies as shown in Table VI. M-14 and M-5 were found positive on SSM level III and IV, but negative on lymph-node metastasis as well as nodular melanoma level III. Similarly, A.1.27 shows a clear-cut preference for SSM level IV and NMM level III, but no reactivity or minor reactivity with lymph-node metastases.

The evaluation of fluorescence reactions in the form of a reaction index poses some problems, because it does not give a differentiated description of the true situation. Sometimes a reaction had to be scored as weakly positive because only a clone of cells within a large population of tumor cells was brightly stained. This is illustrated in Fig. 2, which

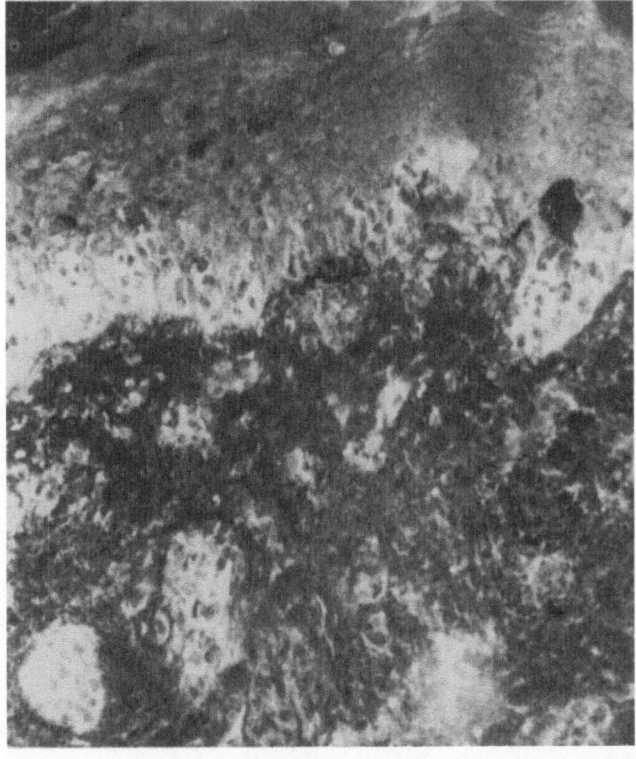

FIGURE 2. Indirect fluorescent staining with monoclonal antibody A.1.27 of a cryostat section of SSM level IV.

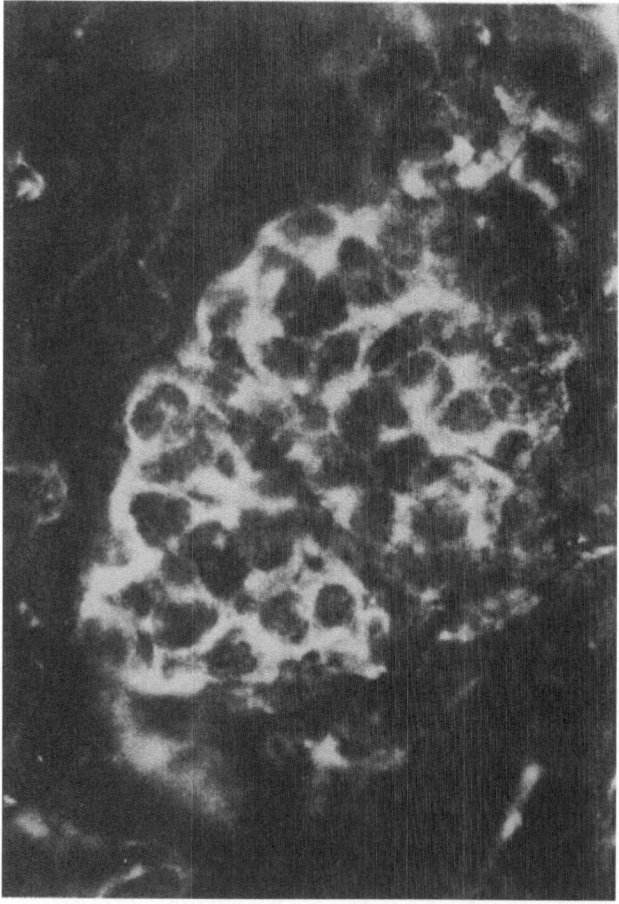

FIGURE 3. Indirect fluorescent staining with monkey antiserum anti-375 of a cryostat section of SSM level IV.

shows a section through an SSM level IV. As one can see, positively stained cells are found along the basal-cell layer. A large accumulation of cells that stained brightly was also found in the corium. Yet, as became evident from a neighboring section that was stained with hematoxylin–eosin, other tumor-cell clusters that were in the vicinity were negative. Figure 3 demonstrates this more clearly. It shows a tumor-cell cluster within an SSM level IV that stained brightly positive while the surrounding tumor tissue was negative.

3. Concluding Remarks

In the course of our studies, we were unable to detect melanoma-specific antigens either with melanoma patients sera or with xenogeneic antisera or monoclonal antibodies.

We could detect only antigens or patterns of antigens that were preferentially expressed on melanoma cells. The various melanoma cell lines were found to be different in their biological and biochemical properties. This was also true for the expression of surface antigens. Furthermore, it was found not only that various tumor cell lines were different from each other but also that melanoma lines were heterogeneous and consisted of variant sublines that distinguished themselves from the parental line by their biological, biochemical, and antigenic properties. Monkey antisera and monoclonal antibodies that were tested on cryostat sections of various stages of melanoma showed a clear-cut preference for melanoma cells and even further distinguished clonal variants within the tumor. Our data so far do not allow definition of antigenic markers for a particular stage of a tumor. Larger numbers of tumors have to be tested to obtain an accurate frequency distribution of antigens over the various tumor stages. This task is complicated by the fact that clonal variants may be formed in a primary tumor, which may emigrate and form metastases. For our future work, the critical question is whether we produce monoclonal antibodies with specificities that cover the whole spectrum of clonal variants within the melanoma lineage. So far, we have used only cultured cell lines for immunization and specificity screening. There is a tendency apparent in Table VI and less pronounced also in Table V that our antibodies and antisera preferentially react with the SSM type and less so with metastases. This raises the suspicion that the phenotype that adapts to the artificial culture conditions and proliferates is of the SSM type, even though most of the cell lines used were derived from metastatic melanoma. Whether or not this interpretation is correct, further studies should also include biopsy material of various metastases for immunization and specificity screening.

References

Beers, W. H., Strickland, S., and Reich, E., 1975, Ovarian plasminogen activator: Relationship to ovulation and hormonal regulation, *Cell* 6:387.

Berg, J. W., 1959, Histological aspects of the relation between gastric adenomatous polyps and gastric cancer, *Cancer* 11:1149.

Bowden, L., 1968, Spontaneous regression of malignant melanoma, in: *XIII Congressus Internationalis Dermatologiae,* München 1967, Vol. 2 (W. Jadassohn and C. G. Schirren, eds.), pp. 915–925, Springer-Verlag, Berlin, Heidelberg, and New York.

Brautbar, C., Pellegrino, N. A., Ferrone, S., Reisfeld, R. A., Payne, R., and Hayflick, L., 1973, Fate of HL-A antigens in aging cultured human dioploid cell strains. II. Quantiative absorption studies, *Exp. Cell Res.* 78:367.

Brüggen, J., Sorg, C., and Macher, E., 1978, Membrane associated antigens of human malignant melanoma, V. Serological typing of cell lines using antisera from non-human primates, *Cancer Immunol. Immunother.* 5:53.

Brüggen, J., Macher, E., and Sorg, C., 1981, Expression of surface antigens and its relation to parameters of malignancy in human malignant melanoma, *Cancer Immunol. Immunother.* 10:121.

Brunner, G., 1977, Membrane impression and gene expression: Towards a theory of cytodifferentiation, *Differentiation* 8:123.

Buonassisi, V., and Venter, J. C., 1976, Hormone and neurotransmitter receptors in an established vascular endothelial cell line, *Proc. Natl. Acad. Sci. U.S.A.* 73:1612.

Carrel, S., Accolla, R. S., Carmagnola, A. L., and Mach, J. -P., 1980, Common human melanoma-associated antigen(s) detected by monoclonal antibodies, *Cancer Res.* 40:2523.

Christman, J. K., Acs, G., Silagi, S., and Silverstein, S. C., 1975, Plasminogen activator: Biochemical characterization and correlation with tumorigenicity, in: *Proteases and Biological Control* (E. Reich, D. B. Rifkin, and E. Shaw, eds.), pp. 827–839, Cold Spring Harbor Laboratory, Cold Spring Harbor, New York.

Coggin, J. H., Jr., and Anderson, N. G., 1974, Cancer, differentiation and embryonic antigens: Some central problems, *Adv. Cancer Res.* **19**:105.

Cornain, S., de Vries, J. E., Collard, J., Vennegoor, C., van Wingerden, I., and Rümke, P., 1975, Antibodies and antigen expression in human melanoma detected by the immune adherence test, *Int. J. Cancer* **16**:981.

Dexter, D. L., Kowalski, H. M., Blazar, B. A., Fligiel, Z., Vogel, R., and Heppner, G. H., 1978, Heterogeneity of tumor cells from a single mouse mammary tumor, *Cancer Res.* **38**:3174.

Everson, L. K., Polcinik, B. A., and Rogentine, G. N., 1974, HL-A expression on the G_1, S and G_2 cell cycle stages of human lymphoid cells, *J. Natl. Cancer Inst.* **53**:913.

Ferrone, S., Cooper, N. R., Pellegrino, N. A., and Reisfeld, R. A., 1973, Interaction of histocompatibility (HL-A) antibodies and complement with synchronized human lymphoid cells in continuous culture, *J. Exp. Med.* **137**:55.

Fidler, I. J., 1978, Tumor heterogeneity and the biology of cancer invasion and metastasis, *Cancer Res.* **38**:2651.

Fogel, M., Gorelik, E., Segal, S., and Feldman, M., 1979, Differences in cell surface antigens of tumor metastases and those of the local tumor, *J. Natl. Cancer Inst.* **62**:585.

Fogh, J., Fogh, J. N., and Orfeo, T., 1977, One hundred and twenty-seven cultured human tumor cell lines producing tumors in nude mice, *J. Natl. Cancer Inst.* **59**:221.

Gershwin, N. E., Ikeda, R. N., Kawakami, T. G., and Owens, R. P., 1977, Immunobiology of heterotransplanted human tumors in nude mice, *J. Natl. Cancer Inst.* **58**:1455.

Giovanella, B. C., Stehlin, J. S., and Williams, L. J., 1972 Development of invasive tumors in the nude mouse after injection of cultured human melanoma cells, *J. Natl. Cancer Inst.* **48**:1531.

Giovanella, B. C., Stehlin, J. S., Williams, L. J., Lee, S. S., and Shepard, R. C., 1978, Heterotransplantation of human cancers into nude mice: A model system for human cancer chemotherapy, *Cancer* **42**:2269.

Goldberg, A., 1974, Increased protease levels in transformed cells: A casein overlay assay for the detection of plasminogen activator production, *Cell* **2**:95.

Goldstein, S., and Singal, D. P., 1972, Loss of reactivity of HL-A antigens in clonal populations of cultured human fibroblasts during aging *in vitro*, *Exp. Cell Res.* **75**:278.

Happle, R., Schotola, I., and Macher, E., 1975, Spontanremission und Leukodern bei malignem Melanom, *Hautarzt* **26**:120.

Hart, I. R., and Fidler, I. J., 1980, Role or organ selectivity in the determination of metastatic patterns of B16 melanoma, *Cancer Res.* **40**:2281.

Hellström, I., Warner, G. A., Hellström, K. E., and Sjögren, H. O., 1973, Sequential studies on cell-mediated tumor immunity and blocking serum activity in ten patients with malignant melanoma, *Int. J. Cancer* **11**:280.

Herlyn, M., Clark, W. H., Jr., Mastrangelo, M. J., Guerry, D., IV, Elder, D. E., LaRossa, D., Hamilton, R., Bondi, E., Tuthill, R., Steplewski, Z., and Koprowski, H., 1980, Specific immunoreactivity of hybridoma-secreted monoclonal anti-melanoma antibodies to cultured cells and freshly derived human cells, *Cancer Res.* **40**:3602.

Herbermann, R. B., 1973, Cellular immunity to human tumor-associated antigens, *Isr. J. Med. Sci.* **9**:300.

Hibbs, J. B., Jr., 1974, Discrimination between neoplastic and non-neoplastic cells *in vitro* by activated macrophages, *J. Natl. Cancer Inst.* **53**:1487.

Houghton, A. N., Taormina, M. C., Ikeda, H., Watanabe, T., Oettgen, H. F., and Old, L. J., 1980, Serological survey of normal humans for natural antibody to cell surface antigens of melanoma, *Proc. Natl. Acad. Sci. U.S.A.* **77**:4260.

Imai, K., Molinaro, G. A., and Ferrone, S., 1980, Monoclonal antibodies to human melanoma-associated antigens, *Transplant. Proc.* **12**:380.

Jones, P. A., Laug, W. E., and Benedict, W. F., 1975, Fibrinolytic activity in a human fibrosarcoma cell line and evidence for the induction of plasminogen activator secretion during tumor formation, *Cell* **6**:245.

Killion, J. J., and Kollmorgen, G. M., 1976, Isolation of immunogenic tumor cells by affinity chromatography, *Nature (London)* **259**:674.

Köhler, G., and Milstein, C., 1975, Continuous cultures of fused cells secreting antibody of predefined specificity, *Nature (London)* **256**:495.

Laug, W. E., Jones, P. A., and Benedict, W. F., 1975, Relationship between fibrinolysis of cultured cells and malignancy, *J. Natl. Cancer Inst.* **54**:173.

Lewis, M. G., and Philipps, T. M., 1972, Separation of two distinct tumor-associated antibodies in the serum of melanoma patients, *J. Natl. Cancer Inst.* **49**:915.

Mak, T. W., Rutledge, G., and Sutherland, D. J. A., 1976, Androgen-dependent fibrinolytic activity in a murine mammary carcinoma (Shionogi SC 115 cells) *in vitro, Cell* **7**:223.

Miller, F. R., and Heppner, G. H., 1979, Immunologic heterogeneity of tumor cell subpopulations from a single mouse mammary tumor, *J. Natl. Cancer Inst.* **63**:1457.

Minden, P., McClatchy, J. K., Wainberg, M., and Weiss, D. W., 1974, Shared antigens between *Mycobacterium bovis* (BCG) and neoplastic cells, *J. Natl. Cancer Inst.* **53**:1325.

Montesano. R., Drevon, C., Kuroki, T., Saint Vincent, L., Handleman, S., Sanford, K. K., DeFeo, D., and Weinstein, I. B., 1977, Test for malignant transformation of rat liver cells in culture: Cytology, growth in soft agar and production of plasminogen activator, *J. Natl. Cancer Inst.* **59**:1651.

Morton, D. L., Malmgren, R. A., Homes, E. C., and Ketcham, A. S., 1968, Demonstration of antibodies against human malignant melanoma by immunofluorescence, *Surgery* **64**:233.

Mott, D. N., Fabisch, P. H., Sani, B. P., and Sorof, S., 1974, Lack of correlation between fibrinolysis and the transformed state of cultured mammalian cells, *Biochem. Biophys. Res. Commun.* **61**:621.

Nagy, B., Ban, J., and Brdar, B., 1977, Fibrinolysis associated with human neoplasia: Production of plasminogen activator by human tumors, *Int. J. Cancer* **19**:614.

Newcomb, E. W., Silverstein, S. C., and Silagi, S., 1978, Malignant mouse melanoma cells do not form tumors when mixed with cells of a non-malignant subclone: Relationships between plasminogen activator expression by the tumor cells and the host's immune response, *J. Cell Physiol.* **95**:169.

Nicolson, G. L., and Winkelhake, J. L., 1975, Organ specificity of blood borne tumor metastasis determined by cell adhesion?, *Nature (London)* **255**:230.

Nicolson, G. L., Birdwell, C. R., Brunson, K. W., Robbins, J. C., Beattie, L., and Fidler, I. J., 1977, Cell interactions in the metastatic process: Some cell surface properties associated with successful blood borne tumor spread, in: *Cell and Tissue Interactions* (J. W. Lash and M. M. Burger, eds.), pp. 225–241, Raven Press, New York.

Nicolson, G. L., Brunson, K. W., and Fidler, I. J., 1978, Specificity of arrest, survival, and growth of selected metastatic variant cell lines, *Cancer Res.* **38**:4105.

Nowell, P. C., 1976, The clonal evolution of tumor cell populations, *Science* **194**:23.

Oettgen, H. F., 1974, Serology of cancer, in: *Clinical Immunobiology,* Vol. 2 (F. H. Bach and R. A. Good, eds.), pp. 206–231, Academic Press, New York and London.

Ossowski, L., Biegel, D., and Reich, E., 1979, Mammary plasminogen activator: Correlation with involution, hormonal modulation and comparison between normal and neoplastic tissue, *Cell* **16**:929.

Pellegrino, M. A., Ferrone, S., Nathalie, P. G., Pellegrino, A., and Reisfeld, R. A., 1972, Expression of HL-A antigens in synchronized cultures of human lymphocytes, *J. Immunol.* **108**:573.

Poste, G., 1977, The cell surface and metastasis, in: *Cancer Invasion and Metastasis: Biologic Mechanisms and Therapy* (S. B. Day, ed.), pp. 19–47, Raven Press, New York.

Poste, G., and Fidler, I. J., 1980, The pathogenesis of cancer metastasis, *Nature (London)* **283**:139.

Reich, E., 1975, Plasminogen activator: Secretion by neoplastic cells and macrophages, in: *Proteases and Biological Control* (E. Reich, D. B. Rifkin, and E. Shaw, eds.), pp. 333–341, Cold Spring Harbor Laboratory, Cold Spring Harbor, New York.

Renselaer Potter, V., 1978 Phenotypic diversity in experimental hepatomas: The concept of partially blocked ontogeny, *Br. J. Cancer* **38**:1.

Rifkin, D. B., Loeb, J. N., Moore, G., and Reich, E., 1974, Properties of plasminogen activators formed by neoplastic human cell cultures, *J. Exp. Med.* **139**:1317.

San, R. H. C., Rice, J. M., and Williams, G. N., 1977, Lack of correlation between plasminogen activating factor production and tumorigenicity in rat liver epithelial cells, *Cancer Lett.* **3**:242.

Schirrmacher, V., Bosslet, K., Shantz, G., Clauer, K., and Hübsch, D., 1979a, Tumor metastases and cell mediated immunity in a model system in DBA/2 mice. IV. Antigenic differences between a metastasizing variant and the parental tumor line revealed by cytotoxic T lymphocytes, *Int. J. Cancer* **23**:245.

Schirrmacher, V., Shantz, G., Clauer, K., Komitowski, D., Zimmermann, H.-P., and Lohmann-Matthes, M.-L., 1979b, Tumor metastases and cell mediated immunity in a model system in DBA/2 mice. I. Tumor invasiveness *in vitro* and metastasis formation *in vivo, Int. J. Cancer* **23**:233.

Schirrmacher, V., Hübsch, D., and Garrido, F., 1980, Syngeneic tumor cells can induce alloreactive T killer cells: A biological role for transplantation antigens, *Proc. Natl. Acad. Sci. U.S.A.* **77**:5409.

Seibert, E., Sorg, C., Happle, R., and Macher, E., 1977, Membrane associated antigens of human malignant melanoma. III. Specificity of human sera reacting with cultured melanoma cells, *Int. J. Cancer* **19**:172.

Silagi, S., 1976, Effects of 5-bromodeoxyuridine on tumorigenicity, immunogenicity, virus production, plasminogen activator, and melanogenesis of mouse melanoma cells, *Int. Rev. Cytol.* **45**:65.

Sorg, C., Brüggen, J., Seibert, E., and Macher, E., 1978, Membrane-associated antigens of human malignant melanoma. IV. Changes in expression of antigens on cultured melanoma cells, *Cancer Immunol. Immunother.* **3**:259.

Strickland, S., Reich, E., and Sherman, M. I., 1976, Plasminogen activator in early embryogenesis: Enzyme production by trophoblast and parietal endoderm, *Cell* **9**:231.

Susuki, N., Withers, R., and Koehler, M. W., 1978, Heterogeneity and variability of artificial lung colony-forming ability among clones from mouse fibrosarcoma, *Cancer Res.* **38**:3349.

Suter, L., Brüggen, J., and Sorg, C., 1980, Use of an enzyme-linked immunosorbent assay (ELISA) for screening of hybridoma antibodies against cell surface antigens, *J. Immunol. Methods* **39**:407.

Tao, T.-W., and Burger, M. M., 1977, Non-metastasizing variants selected from metastasizing melanoma cells, *Nature (London)* **270**:437.

The, T. H., Higes, H. A., Schaffrodt Koops, H., Lamberts, H. B., and Nieweg, H. O., 1975, Surface antigens on cultured malignant melanoma cells as detected by membrane immunofluorescence method with human sera: Lack of tumour-specific reactions on melanoma cell lines, *Ann. N. Y. Acad. Sci.* **254**:528.

Unkeless, J. C., Gordon, S., and Reich, E., 1974, Secretion of plasminogen activator by stimulated macrophages, *J. Exp. Med.* **139**:834.

Uriel, J., 1979, Retrodifferentiation and the fetal patterns of gene expression in cancer, *Adv. Cancer Res.* **29**:127.

Viza, D., and Phillips, J., 1975, Identification of an antigen associated with malignant melanoma, *Int. J. Cancer* **16**:312.

Wilson, E. L., and Reich, E., 1979, Modulation of plasminogen activator synthesis and chick embryo fibroblasts by cyclic nucleotides and phorbol myristate acetate, *Cancer Res.* **39**:1579.

Yeh, M.-Y., Hellström, I., Brown, J. P., Warner, G. A., Hansen, J. A., and Hellström, K. E., 1979, Cell surface antigens of human melanoma identified by monoclonal antibody, *Proc. Natl. Acad. Sci. U.S.A.* **76**:2927.

Yogeeswaran, G., Stein, B. S., and Sebastian, H., 1978, Altered cell surface organisation of gangliosides and sialylglycoproteins of mouse metastatic melanoma variant lines selected *in vivo* for enhanced lung implantation, *Cancer Res.* **38**:1336.

Yogeeswaran, G., Sebastian, H., and Stein, B. S., 1979, Cell surface sialylation of glycoproteins and glycosphingolipids in cultured metastatic variant RNA-virus transformed non-producer BALB/c 3T3 cell lines, *Int. J. Cancer* **24**:193.

19

Immunotherapy of Melanoma

LYNN E. SPITLER AND CHARLES SCOTT

1. Introduction

Are there tumor-associated transplantation antigens (TATAs) on human tumor cells? If there are, are human subjects capable of mounting an immune response to those TATAs? Does clinical malignancy develop because of a failure of the normal immunological response to the tumor? The answers to these very basic questions of tumor immunology are unknown at present, and it seems unlikely that they will be answered in the near future.

To design a truly rational approach to tumor immunotherapy, it is essential to have answers to these questions. For example, if a patient with malignancy lacks the immune-response gene to respond to that tumor, immunopotentiator therapy would never be effective. In this circumstance, the appropriate immunotherapeutic approach might be to modify the presentation of the TATA so that the host could recognize and respond to it. This might be accomplished by coupling it to an immunogenic carrier.

Given these unknowns, we are left with the choice of either not attempting immunotherapy until more information is available or designing protocols that seem most rational, with the data at hand. It is not too surprising, therefore, that the trials that have been performed to date have not been more successful. Nonetheless, information is being generated that should lead to improvement in our immunotherapy attempts in the future.

2. Malignant Melanoma

Patients with malignant melanoma seem to be ideal subjects for immunotherapy trials. There are several lines of evidence suggesting that immune responses may be important in the control of the growth of melanoma. A vigorous host response is often seen in the primary lesion. The incidence of partial regression of primary malignant melanoma has been esti-

LYNN E. SPITLER AND CHARLES SCOTT • Paul M. Aggeler Memorial Laboratory, Department of Medicine, Children's Hospital, University of California Medical Center, San Francisco, California 94118.

mated to be as high as 15% (Little, 1971; McGovern, 1972). The occurence of halo nevi and vitiligo in patients with melanoma further suggests an immune response to melanocytes. Patients may undergo a prolonged remission following excision of the primary lesion only to have a metastasis appear many years later, suggesting that tumor cells had been present and held in check by the immune response during this period. Finally, regression of widespread metastases may occasionally occur, suggesting an immune mechanism.

The intradermal location of melanoma is ideal for the induction of cellular immune reactivity, which could be enhanced by immunotherapy. There is an adequate period before the appearance of recurrent disease to allow time for immunotherapy to act. Since adjuvant chemotherapy has not been effective, one would not be withholding effective chemotherapy to conduct an immunotherapy trial.

3. Bacillus Calmette Guérin

The rationale of bacillus Calmette Guérin (BCG) therapy is shown in Table I. There is no doubt that intratumoral injection of BCG can result in regression of the injected lesions in immunocompetent patients (Morton, 1974; Bast et al., 1974). Complications following intratumoral administration of BCG are common (Bast et al., 1974) and may be severe (McKahn et al., 1975). These lesions could often be treated in other ways such as surgery, heated perfusion, or chemotherapy. It was hoped, however, that local administration of BCG would enhance tumor-specific immune responses and prevent further recurrences. Thus, intratumoral administration of BCG might offer additional benefits not provided by more standard means of therapy. Unfortunately, there have not been any studies to date documenting a decreased recurrence rate or increased survival following intratumoral BCG, so that continued use of this form of therapy is probably not indicated in view of the associated side effects and the efficacy of other forms of therapy.

Systemic administration of BCG has been given to patients with melanoma both for nonspecific immunopotentiation and for specific enhancement of reactivity to melanoma antigens, sinc it was reported that there is cross-reactivity between antigens on the surface of BCG and melanoma cells (Bucana and Hanna, 1974). There was considerable enthusiasm for this approach several years ago. It was reported that chemoimmunotherapy with dimethyl triazeno imidazole carboxamide (DTIC) and BCG was superior to DTIC alone

TABLE I

Rationale of Bacillus Calmette Guérin Therapy[a]

1. Intratumoral injection of BCG may cause production of a delayed hypersensitivity reaction to the BCG that could destroy tumor cells nonspecifically as "innocent bystanders."
2. Intratumoral injection of BCG might cause stimulation of tumor-specific immunity by reacting with tumor antigens, producing an adjuvant like effect.
3. Systemic administration of BCG might cause nonspecific stimulation of the immune response.
4. Systemic administration of BCG might cause specific stimulation of antitumor immunity because of antigens in BCG that cross-react with melanoma antigens.

[a] Reproduced with permission from Spitler et al. (1980).

in therapy of patients with disseminated melanoma (Gutterman *et al.*, 1974). It was also reported that BCG was effective as surgical adjuvant therapy in patients with recurrent melanoma (Gutterman *et al.*, 1978). Both these studies have been criticized because of the use of historic controls. Eilber *et al.* (1976) also reported that BCG was effective as surgical adjuvant therapy in patients with lymph-node metastases of melanoma. This study has been criticized because the control group was not randomized. More recently, five studies have been reported in which patients with melanoma were randomized to receive BCG or standard therapy (controls) (Pinsky *et al.*, 1976; Beretta, 1980; Cunningham *et al.*, 1980; Morton, 1980; Terry *et al.*, 1980). These studies have shown that BCG does not lessen the recurrence rate or improve survival in these patients. One of these studies (Cunningham *et al.*, 1980) involved evaluation of 700 patients. The results of these studies seem to provide overwhelming evidence that BCG is not effective as surgical adjuvant therapy in melanoma.

Despite the negative results with trials of BCG in melanoma, there are reports that local administration of BCG may be effective in the therapy of other tumors. The most encouraging of these was in the treatment of superficial bladder cancer. Three separate groups have reported decreased frequency of recurrences in these patients following intravesical administration of BCG (Morales and Ersil, 1980; Lamm *et al.*, 1980; Camacho *et al.*, 1980). The efficacy of intrapleural administration of BCG in patients with lung cancer is still under evaluation, since one randomized trial showed clinical benefit to the patients receiving BCG (McKneally *et al.*, 1976), whereas another randomized trial showed no benefit (Lowe *et al.*, 1980).

4. Levamisole

Levamisole has been reported to enhance cell-mediated immunity in animals (Renoux and Renoux, 1972) and man (Tripodi *et al.*, 1973). Administration of levamisole has been reported to result in a prolonged disease-free interval and in increased survival in patients with unresectable carcinoma of the breast. (Rojas *et al.*, 1976). Recently, there have been preliminary reports that administration of levamisole is of clinical benefit to patients with colorectal cancer (Verhaegen *et al.*, 1980; Borden *et al.*, 1980) or multiple myeloma (Salmon *et al.*, 1980).

We completed a randomized trial of levamisole vs. placebo as surgical adjuvant therapy in patients with malignant melanoma. Patients eligible for the study were those judged to be at high risk for recurrence of melanoma. This included patients with high-risk primary melanoma or with cutaneous, subcutaneous, or lymph-node recurrence of melanoma. Patients were treated with surgery as appropriate. At entry into the study, patients were judged to be tumor-free by clinical and laboratory examination. Patients randomized to receive levamisole took 150 mg for 3 days each fortnight. Patients randomized to receive placebo took tablets identical in appearance on the same schedule. Administration continued for 2 years to cover the most likely time for recurrence.

A total of 203 patients were randomized. The distribution of prognostic variables was similar in both groups, supporting the efficacy of the randomization. These variables included age, sex, stage of disease, level and thickness of the primary, location of the primary, and number of lymph nodes involved (for patients with Stage II disease).

Patients were considered evaluable if they took the protocol medication for 3 months. There were 90 evaluable patients in each group. Follow-up data were available on all patients, and the median follow-up period was 3½ years.

Three end points were analyzed: time to first recurrence, time to first visceral recurrence,·and survival. Overall, there were no significant differences between the groups

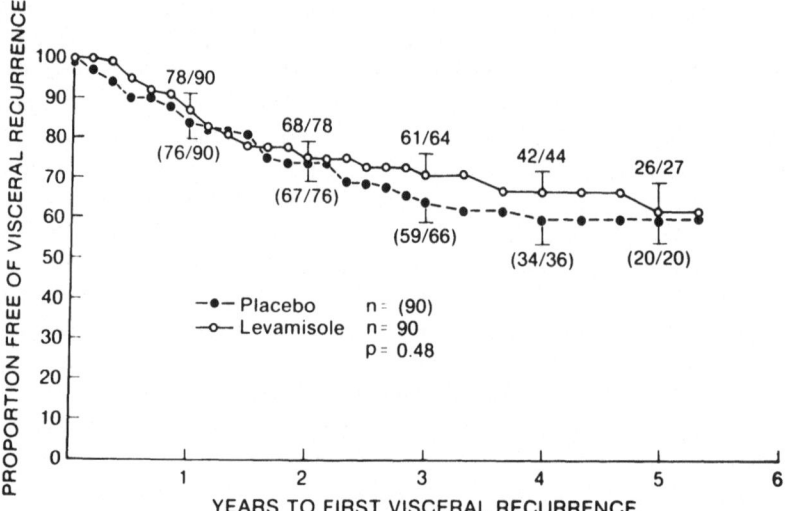

FIGURE 1. Time to first visceral recurrence in patients with malignant melanoma treated with levamisole or placebo. Numbers represent number of patients free of viseral recurrence during interval/number of patients entering each interval. Φ Standard errors of the mean. Reprinted with permission from Spitler and Sagebiel *et al.* (1980).

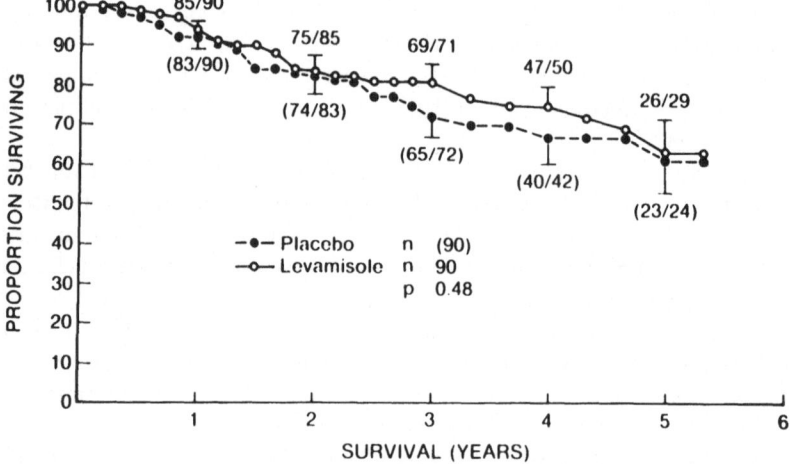

FIGURE 2. Survival in patients with malignant melanoma treated with levamisole or placebo. Numbers represent number of patients surviving during interval/number of patients entering each interval. Φ Standard errors of the mean. Reprinted with permission from Spitler and Sagebiel *et al.* (1980).

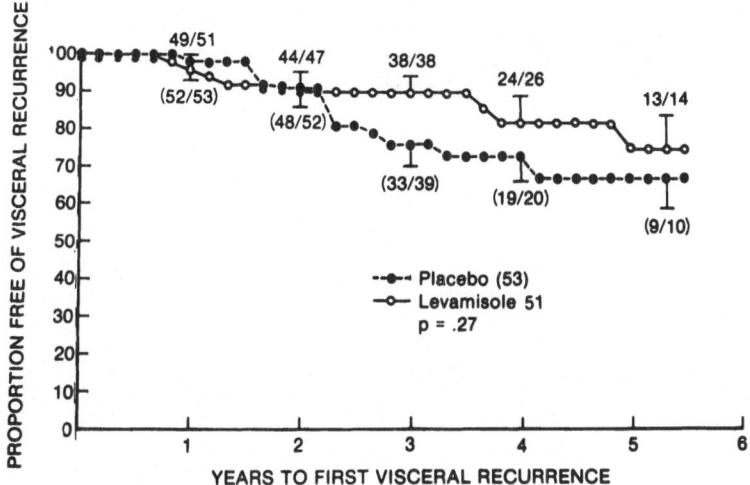

FIGURE 3. Time to first visceral recurrence in patients with Stage I malignant melanoma treated with levamisole or placebo. Numbers represent number of patients free of visceral recurrence during interval/number of patients entering each interval. Φ Standard errors of the mean. Reprinted with permission from Spitler and Sagebiel *et al.* (1980).

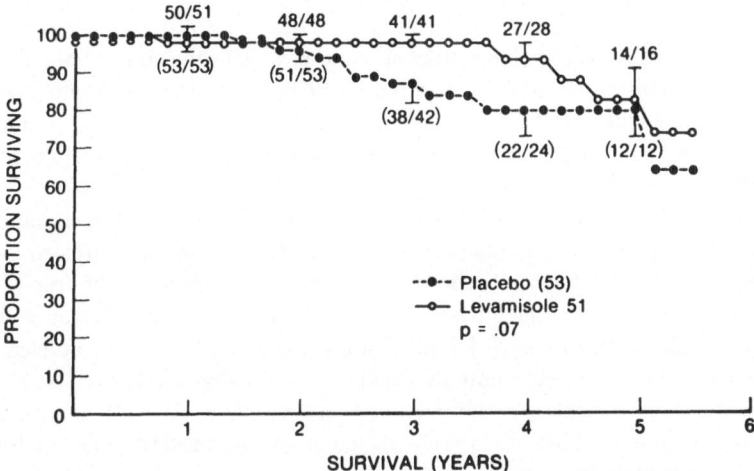

FIGURE 4. Survival in patients with Stage I melanoma treated with levamisole or placebo. Numbers represent number of patients surviving during interval/number of patients entering each interval. Φ Standard errors of the mean. Reprinted with permission from Spitler and Sagebiel *et al.* (1980).

receiving levamisole and placebo (Figs. 1 and 2). In patients with Stage I disease, there was a trend in favor of levamisole with regard to time of first visceral recurrence and survival (Figs. 3 and 4). For survival, the two-tailed p value was 0.07, thus approaching statistical significance. To determine the efficacy of levamisole in patients with Stage I melanoma, a new study specifically designed for that purpose would be required. Such a study appears warranted.

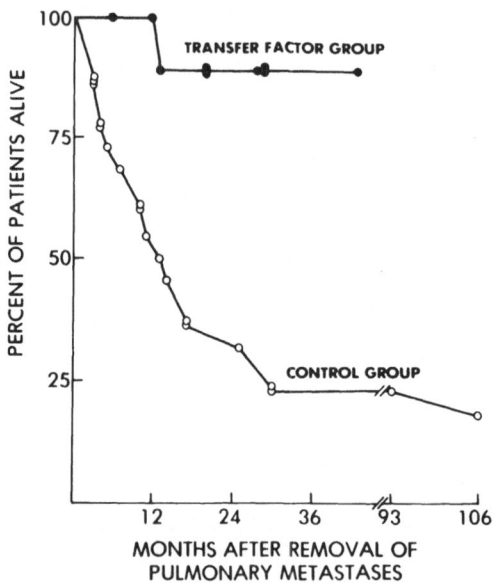

FIGURE 5. Cumulative survival rates following thoracotomy. Reprinted with permission from Gonzales *et al.* (1980).

5. Transfer Factor

Transfer factor is a dialyzable extract of leukocytes that can cause enhanced delayed-hypersensitivity skin-test reactivity. (Lawrence, 1955). Encouraging results have been reported in therapy with transfer-factor patients with primary or secondary immunological deficiency disease, infectious disease, diseases of unknown etiology, and malignancy (Spitler, 1978).

We evaluated the results of transfer-factor therapy in patients with metastatic malignant melanoma. Patients with pulmonary metastases of melanoma were treated with surgery followed by transfer factor. To be eligible, they were required to be free of known residual disease by clinical and laboratory parameters following thoracotomy. Patients received subcutaneous injections of 1 unit of transfer factor (the amount derived from 5×10^8 lymphcytes) every 3 weeks until they had been tumor-free for 2 years. At 12 months after thoracotomy, all patients were alive. After a median follow-up of 20 months, only one patient had died (Fig. 5). Historic controls treated at another medical center with surgery alone had a significantly lower survival rate. These results suggest that transfer factor may prolong survival in patients with Stage II melanoma and a small residual tumor burden. These results are similar to those obtained previously in patients with osteogenic sarcoma (Levin *et al.*, 1975). These encouraging results are being pursued in a randomized trial of transfer factor vs. placebo in patients with high-risk primary or recurrent melanoma similar in design to the randomized levamisole trial described in Section 4.

6. The Future

The field of immunotherapy is in its infancy, comparable to the stage of development of chemotherapy 20 years ago. There is no immunotherapeautic agent that has definitely been shown to be effective in cancer therapy, but some encouraging results are emerging. Numerous new immunopotentiating agents are becoming available. A few of these that have already entered clinical trials in man are listed in Table II. Some of these, such as Krestin, levaisole, and isoprinosine, are already commercially available in other countries, such as Japan and European countries, but so far are not commercially available in the United States.

7. Summary

Several trials of immunotherapy have been conducted in patients with malignant melanoma. Intratumoral administration of BCG carries the possibility of serious side effects and has not been shown to be more effective than other forms of treatment in preventing recurrence. Systemic administration of BCG as surgical adjuvant therapy has been shown to be ineffective. The results with levamisole show possible efficacy in patients with Stage 1 disease and warrant further evaluation. It is too early to judge what the efficacy of transfer factor will prove to be, but a randomized trial to ascertain its efficacy has been initiated. New, more potent agents may provide more benefit to patients in the future. Further, new approaches or combinations of immunotherapies or both may be more effective than the therapies available at present.

TABLE II

Immunopotentiators Undergoing Trials in Man

Bacterial preparations
  Bacillus Calmette Guefin (BCG)
  Methanol-extraction residue of BCG (MER)
  Muramyl dipeptide (MDP)
  Corynebacterium parvum
Transfer factor
Levamisole
Lymphokine
Isoprinosine
Polysaccharides
  Lentinan
  Schizophyllan
  Glucan
  Krestin
Thymic factors
  Thymosin
  TP-1
  Serum thymic factors (FTS)
  Thymopoietin
Inducer of serum thymic factors: cyclomunine
Interferon
Interferon inducers
  Poly 1C
  Poly AU

References

Bast, R. C., Jr., Zbar, B., Borsos, T., and Rapp, H. J., 1974, BCG and cancer (second of two parts), *N. Engl. J. Med.* **290**:1458-1469.

Beretta, G., 1980, Randomized study of prolonged chemotherapy, immunotherapy, and chemoimmunotherapy as an adjuvant for Stage I and II malignant melama (trial 6), Presented at the Second International Conference on the Immunotherapy of Cancer: Present Status of Trials in Man, Bethesda, Maryland, April 28-30.

Borden, E. C., Crowley, J., Davis, T. E., and Wolberg, W. H., 1980, Levamisole: Effects in primary and recurrent colorectal carcinoma, Presented at the Second International Conference on the Immunotherapy of Cancer: Present Status of Trials in Man, Bethesda, Maryland, April 28-30.

Bucana, C., and Hanna, M. G., Jr., 1974, Immunoelectronmicroscopic analysis of surface antigens common to *Mycobacterium bovis* (BCG) and tumor cells, *J. Natl. Cancer Inst.* **53**:1313-1323.

Camacho, F., Pinsky, C., Kerr, D., Whitmore, W., and Oettgen, H., 1980, Treatment of superficial bladder cancer with intravesical BCG, Presented at the Second International Conference on the Immunotherapy of Cancer: Present Status of Trials in Man, Bethesda, Maryland, April 28-30.

Cunningham, T. J., Schoenfeld, D., Nathanson, L., Wolter, J., Patterson, W. B., and Borden, E., 1980, A controlled ECOG study of adjuvant therapy (BCG, BCG-DTIC) in patients with stage I and II malignant melanoma, Presented at the Second International Conference on the Immunotherapy of Cancer; Present Status of Trials in Man, Bethesda, Maryland, April 28-30.

Eilber, R. F., Morton, D. L. Holmes, E. C., Sparks, F. C., and Ramming, K. P., 1976, Adjuvant immunotherapy with BCG in treatment of regional-lymph node metastases from malignant melanoma, *N. Engl. J. Med.* **294**:237-240.

Gonzales, R. L., Wong, P., and Spitler, L. E., 1980, Adjuvant immunotherapy with transfer factor in patients with melanoma metastatic to lung, *Cancer* **45**:57-63.

Gutterman, J. U., Mavligit, G., Gottlieb, J. A., Burgess, M. A., McBride, C. E., Einhorn, L., Freireich, E. J., and Hersh, E. M., 1974, Chemoimmunotherapy of disseminated malignant melanoma with dimethyl triazeno imidazole carboxamide and bacillus Calmette-Guerin, *N. Engl. J. Med.* **291**:592-595.

Gutterman, J. U., Mavligit, G. M., McBride, C. M., Richman, S. P., Burgess, M. A., and Hersh, E. M., 1978, Postoperative immunotherapy for recurrent malignant melanoma: An updated report, in: *Immunotherapy of Cancer: Present Status of Trials in Man* (W. D. Terry and D. Windhorst, eds.), pp. 35-55, Raven Press, New York.

Lamm, D. L., Thor, D. E., Harris, S. C., Stogdill, V. D., and Radwin, H. M., 1980, Intravesical and percutaneous BCG immunotherapy of recurrent superficial bladder cancer, Presented at the Second International Conference on the Immunotherapy of Cancer: Present Status of Trials in Man, Bethesda, Maryland, April 28-30.

Lawrence, H. S., 1980, The transfer in humans of delayed skin sensitivity to streptococcal M substance and to tuberculin with disrupted leukocytes, *J. Clin. Invest.* **34**:219-230.

Levin, A. S., Byers, V. S., Fudenberg, H. H., Wybran, J., Hackett, A. J., Johnston, J. O., and Spitler, L. E., 1975, Osteogenic sarcoma: Immunologic parameters before and during immunotherapy with tumor-specific transfer factor, *J. Clin. Invest.* **55**:487-499.

Little, J. H., 1971, Partial regression in primary cutaneous malignant melanoma, *Pathology* **3**:62.

Lowe, J., Iles, P. B., Shore, D. F., Langman, M. J. S., and Baldwin, R. W., 1980, Intrapleural BCG in operable lung cancer, *Lancet* **2**:11-14.

McGovern, V. J., 1972, Melanoma: Growth patterns, multiplicity and regression, in: *Melanoma and Skin Cancer* (W. H. McCarthy, ed.), pp. 95-106, VCN Blight, Government Printer, Sydney, Australia.

McKahn, C. F., Hendrickson, C. G., Spitler, L. E., Gunnarsson, A., Banerjee, D., and Nelson, W. R., 1975, Immunotherapy of melanoma with BCG: Two fatalities following intralesional injection, *Cancer* **35**:514-520.

McKneally, M. F., Maver, C., and Kausel, H. W., 1976, Regional immunotherapy of lung cancer with intrapleural B.C.G., *Lancet* **2**:377-379.

Morales, A., and Ersil, A., 1980, Prophylaxis and treatment of non-infiltrating bladder cancer with BCG, Presented at the Second International Conference on the Immunotherapy Cancer: Present Status of Trials in Man, Bethesda, Maryland, April 28-30.

Morton, D. L., 1974, BCG immunotherapy of malignant melanoma: Summary of a seven-year experience, *Surgery* **180**:635–643.

Morton, D. L., 1980, Adjuvant immunotherapy of malignant melanoma: Results of a randomized trial, Presented at the Second International Conference on the Immunotherapy of Cancer: Present Status of Trials in Man, Bethesda, Maryland, April 28–30.

Pinsky, C. M., Hirshaut, Y., and Wanebo, H. J., 1976, Randomized trial of bacillus Calmette-Guérin (percutaneous administration) as surgical adjuvant immunotherapy for patients with Stage II melanoma, *Ann. N.Y. Acad. Sci.* **277**:187–192.

Renoux, G., and Renoux, M., 1972, Action immunostimulante de derives du phenylimidothiazide sur les cellules spleniques formatrices d'anticorps, *C. R. Acad. Sci. Ser. D* **274**:756–757.

Rojas, A. F., Mickiewicz, E., Feierstein, J. N., Glait, H., and Olivari, A. J., 1976, Levamisole in advanced human breast cancer, *Lancet* **1**:211–215.

Salmon, S. E., Alexanian, R., and Dixon, D., 1980, Chemoimmunotherapy for multiple myeloma: Effect of levamisole, Presented at the Second International Conference on the Immunotherapy of Cancer: Present Status of Trials in Man, Bethesda, Maryland, April 28–30.

Spitler, L. E., 1978, Transfer factor, in: *Handbook Series in Clinical Laboratory Science*, Section F: *Immunology*, Vol. 1, Part 1 (A. Baumgarten and F. F. Richards, eds.), pp. 87–106, CRC Press, West Palm Beach, Floria.

Spitler, L. E., 1980, BCG, levamisole, and transfer factor in the treatment of cancer, *Prog. Exp. Tumor Res.* **25**:178–192.

Spitler, L. E., and Sagebiel, R., 1980, A randomized trial of levamisole versus placebo as adjuvant therapy in malignant melanoma, *N. Engl. J. Med.* **303**:1143–1147.

Terry, W. D., Hodes, R. J., and Rosenberg, S. A., 1980, Treatment of stage I and II malignant melanoma with adjuvant immunotherapy or chemotherapy: Preliminary anylysis of a prospective, randomized trial, Presented at the Second International Conference on the Immunotherapy of Cancer: Present Status of Trials in Man, Bethesda, Maryland, April 28–30.

Tripodi, D., Parks, L. C., and Brugmans, J., 1973, Drug-induced restoration of cutaneous delayed hypersensitivity in anergic patients with cancer, *N. Engl. J. Med.* **289**:354–357.

Verhaegen, H., DeCree, J., DeCock, W., and Verhaegen-Declercq, M. L., 1980, Levamisole therapy in patients with colorectal cancer, Presented at the Second International Conference on the Immunotherapy of Cancer: Present Status of Trials in Man, Bethesda, Maryland, April 28–30.

20

Biological Studies of Antimelanoma Monoclonal Antibodies

ZENON STEPLEWSKI, KENNETH F. MITCHELL, AND
HILARY KOPROWSKI

1. Introduction

The notion that tumors may bear antigens that do not exist on other cells of the host organism was originally inferred from the remissions that are occasionally seen in cancer and that were thought to occur because of an immune response to the tumor. The lymphocytic infiltration of the tumor bed in tumors such as melanoma also supports this hypothesis. All ideas on the diagnosis and immunotherapy of cancer are based on the assumption that such antigens exist. However, despite a great deal of work, experimental evidence for the existence of such tumor-specific or tumor-associated antigens remains scanty. Nevertheless, the necessary fundamental molecular basis that must underlie the expression of such antigens can be defined, and a rational approach to their study can be undertaken.

Conceptually, "new antigens" could arise from point mutations in genes the products of which are normal constituents of the cell surface. Alternatively, oncodevelopmental antigens expressed during ontogeny and on tumor cells may appear as tumor antigens. Differentiation antigens and normal antigens that are overexpressed on tumor cells may also appear as tumor-associated antigens. The general phenomenon in these cases is the inappropriate expression of normal antigens. A final possibility is that tumor antigens may come from an exogenous source of genetic information, as is the case for antigens of viral origin. Thus, surface changes that appear to be an expression of tumor antigens may be either qualitative or quantitative in nature and of a variety of different kinds.

The availability of monoclonal antibodies has circumvented one major problem associated with the characterization of tumor-cell antigens, i.e., the heterogeneity of antibodies present in antisera. A second problem, the low avidity of antibody, is avoided through two

ZENON STEPLEWSKI, KENNETH F. MITCHELL, AND HILARY KOPROWSKI • The Wistar Institute of Anatomy and Biology, Philadelphia, Pennsylvania 19104 circumstances: (1) the large amounts of antibody present in tissue-culture fluids from hybridomas and (2) the selection procedure, which tends to eliminate those clones that secrete only small amounts of antibody of low affinity.

The production of hybrid cells has already been described in detail (Koprowski *et al.*, 1978). The general procedure we have used is the fusion of spleen and myeloma cells with the aid of polyethylene glycol. Hybrid cells are selected by hypoxanthine, aminopterin, and thymidine (HAT) medium, which prevents the growth of parental myeloma cells deficient in hypoxanthine-guanine phosphoribosyl transferase (HGPRT). Spleen cells do not have the ability to grow in tissue culture and survive for only a short time; however, they contribute the enzyme that the myeloma cells lack and thus contribute to the successful survival of the hybrid.

Microscopic colonies of growing cells can usually be detected in hybrid cultures by days 7–10 after fusion. These colonies are placed in fresh culture vessels and their progeny subsequently cloned to ensure that the antibodies produced are truly monoclonal in origin.

The general strategy for the identification of melanoma-specific monoclonal antibodies is as follows: Initially, all hybrid cell line supernatants are tested for the presence of mouse immunoglobulin. The binding of these antibodies to human tissue-culture melanoma cells is simultaneously assessed by indirect radioimmunoassay (RIA). Culture supernatants that show binding to target cells are tested on larger panels of cells to determine whether the antigen exists on many types of human cells or is expressed only on melanoma tumor cells. At this point, somewhat arbitrary decisions are made based on the level of binding detected. The types of results obtained with various antibodies are described in detail below. Many antibodies with broad specificities for many types of human cells are usually discovered; for reasons of expediency, these are often eliminated from further consideration. Some antibodies with "interesting" ranges of activity, although not necessarily melanoma-specific, have been studied further. Antibodies with the desired specificity (usually those that bind to melanoma cells but that do not bind, or bind only minimally, to nonmelanoma cells) are subjected to further investigation in two general areas: biochemical studies are undertaken for the isolation and characterization of the target antigens, and biological studies are undertaken for determination of whether the antibodies can mediate immunological effector functions such as complement-mediated cytolysis or antibody-dependent cell-mediated cytolysis (ADCC). The principal technique we have used for the characterization of tumor antigens is immunoprecipitation of antigens from radiolabeled cells followed by sodium dodecyl sulfate–polyacrylamide gel electrophoresis (SDS-PAGE) for determination of the molecular weight of the isolated radioactive antigens.

2. Monoclonal-Antibody-Defined Melanoma Antigens

Characterization of the binding specificities of antigens isolated from the surfaces of iodinated melanoma cells has been undertaken with several antibodies. The results have been as described in the following sections.

FIGURES 1, 3–5, and 7–11. Diagrammatic representations of the binding of monoclonal antibodies as detected in RIA. (CPM) Specific binding after subtraction of control cpm. The control immunoglobulin source used was P3 × 63Ag8 supernatant. Control counts were usually 100–200 cpm.

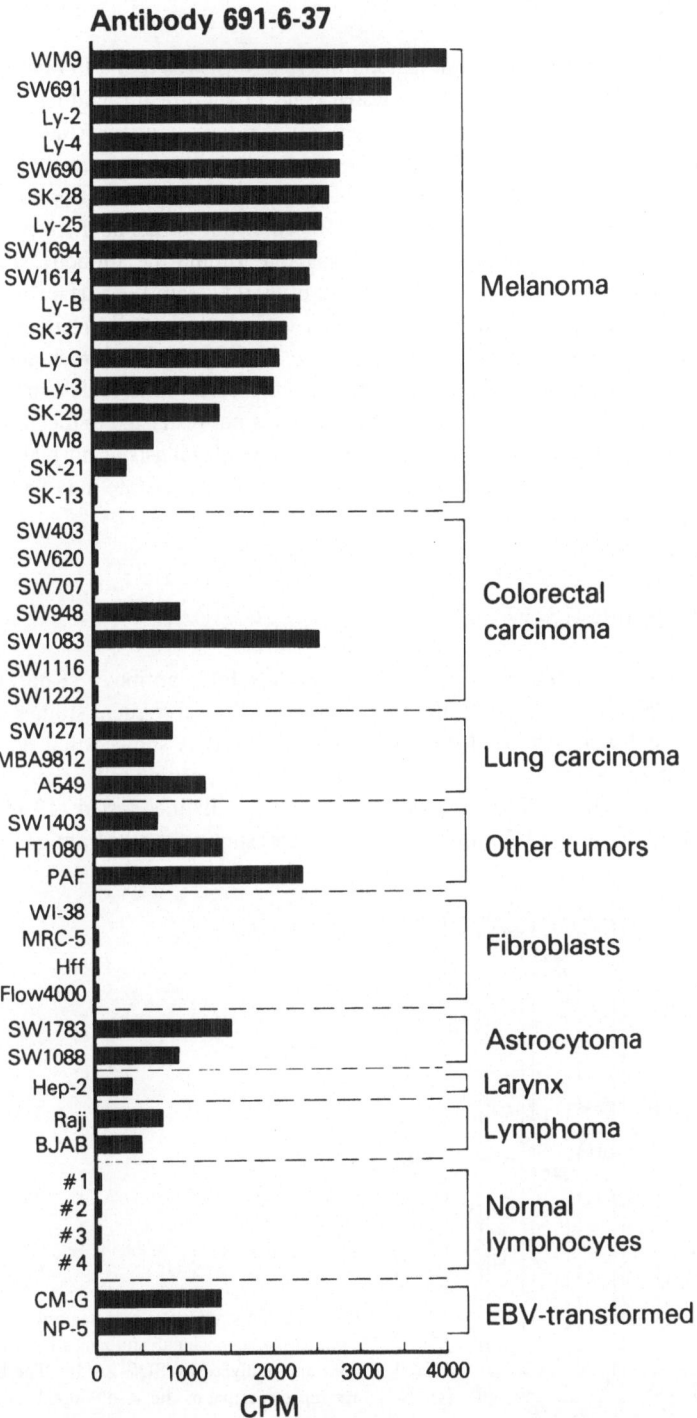

FIGURE 1

2.1. Antibody 691-6-37

This antibody, of isotype immunoglobulin G_1 (IgG_1), was found to bind in RIA to all but 1 (SK 13) of 17 melanoma cell lines tested (Fig. 1). Significant binding was also found to 2 of 7 colorectal-carcinoma cell lines tested, all 3 lung carcinomas tested, 1 breast carcinoma (SW 1403), 1 sarcoma (HT 1080), 1 simian-virus-40-transformed cell line (PAF), 2 astrocytomas, 1 laryngeal carcinoma (HEP-2), 2 lymphomas, and 2 Epstein–Barr-virus-transformed lymphoid cell lines. None of the 4 normal fibroblasts or the 4 preparations of normal peripheral-blood lymphocytes tested was able to bind the antibody. This antibody precipitates a molecule with a molecular weight of 80,000 from the surface-iodinated melanoma cells (Fig. 2). Quantitatively, the antigen varies substantially from cell line to cell line; the largest amount detected so far has been found on WM 9 melanoma cells. No differences in the molecular weight of the antigen have been found to date among different cell lines. The fact that the expression of the antigen is not restricted to melanoma cells but occurs on a variety of tumor cells, albeit not on cultured fibroblasts or normal lymphocytes, suggests that an event involving a change to a rapidly dividing state may be necessary for the expression of this molecule.

2.2. Antibody 691-13-17

Initial analysis of the binding properties of this IgG_1 antibody (Koprowski *et al.*, 1978) showed that it binds specifically to melanoma cells. Subsequent studies (M. Herlyn *et al.*, 1980; Steplewski, 1980) of binding as detected by RIA showed that not only melanoma cells, but also some astrocytomas and all HLA-DR-positive cells, express an antigen detected by this antibody. The majority of melanoma cell lines tested (19 of 25) bound antibody 691-13-17 (Fig. 3). Immunochemical studies showed that the antigen precipitated

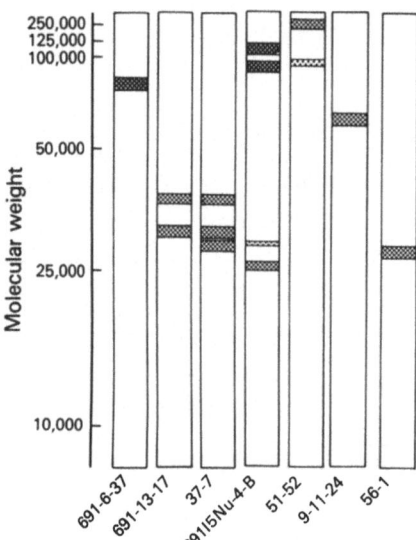

FIGURE 2. Diagrammatic representation of antigens precipitated by monoclonal antibodies from melanoma cell lines and analyzed by SDS-PAGE. The band positions are representative of the results obtained by use of the Laemmli gel system with a 10% acrylamide-bisacrylamide concentration at a ratio of 38:1.

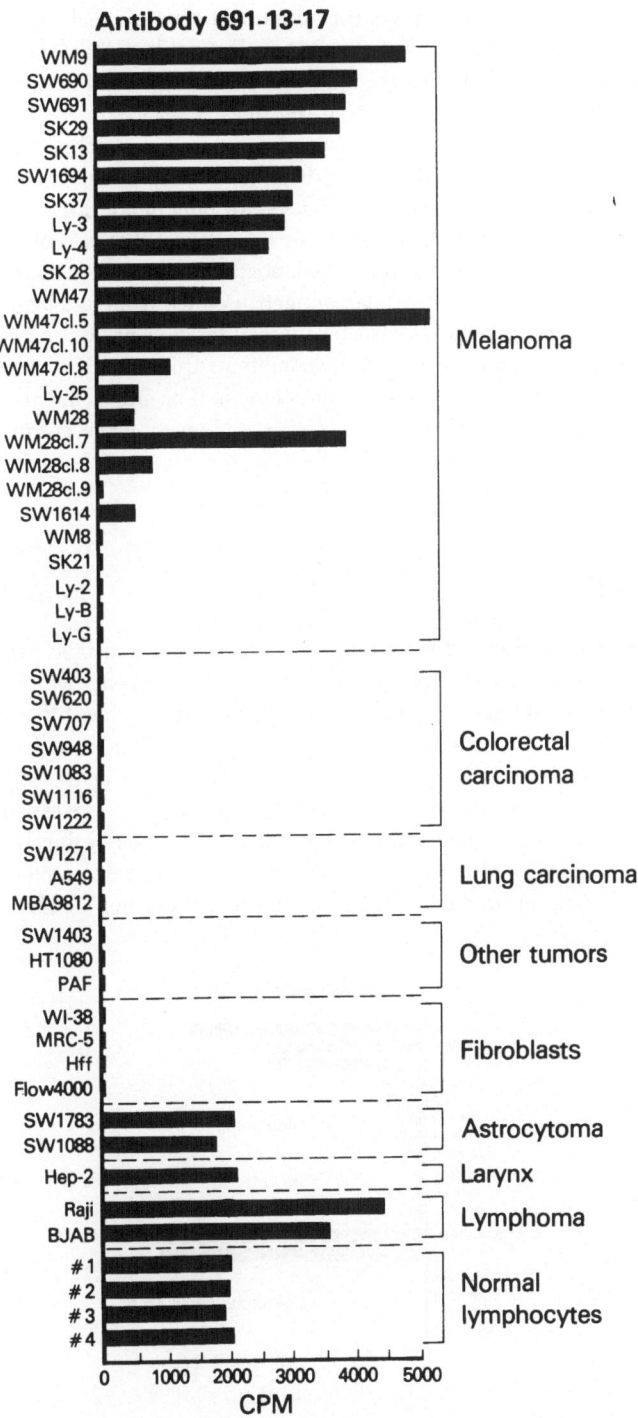

FIGURE 3

by this antibody has the characteristics of the human antigens encoded by the *HLA-D* locus
[D-related (DR) antigens] (Mitchell *et al.*, 1981a). The antibody has, to date, reacted with
all DR-bearing cells tested, including the majority of melanomas, all peripheral-blood lymphocytes, and a variety of cultured lymphoid cell lines. The precipitated molecules consist
of two polypeptide chains with molecular weights of approximately 38,000 and 31,000.
These peptides, designated α and β, are not disulfide-bonded to one another in the native
state. Proteins from different melanoma cell lines show only minor differences in migration
patterns, which differences are best explained by the allelism that is known to occur at the
DR locus. Antigens isolated from cultured melanoma cells have been found to be slightly
different in molecular weight from similar antigens isolated from autologous lymphocytes
(Fuhrer *et al.*, 1982). The structural basis for these differences has yet to be elucidated, but
may arise during adaptation to tissue-culture conditions from a variety of causes involving
the protein or carbohydrate components of the antigen. The site of the antigenic determinant with which antibody 691-13-17 reacts is as yet unknown; however, it is clear that this
antigenic determinant could reside on either the α or β chain or be a conformational determinant requiring a contribution from both chains.

2.3. Antibody 37-7

Results of RIA show that this antibody has a pattern of reactivity similar to that of
691-13-17 on a panel of different cell types (Fig. 4). The antibody, which is of the IgG_{2a}
isotype, precipitates an antigen from melanoma cell line SK 37 that differs from that precipitated by 691-13-17. An additional protein component with a molecular weight of
approximately 28,000 is also precipitated by antibody 37-7 (see Fig. 2). Sequential precipitation has shown that both antibody 691-13-17 and antibody 37-7 are capable of removing
all DR antigens detectable by the reciprocal antibody. The relationship between the first
two bands and the additional protein precipitated by 37-7 remains unknown. It may be
speculated that binding of antibody 37-7 stabilizes the interaction of DR with a weakly

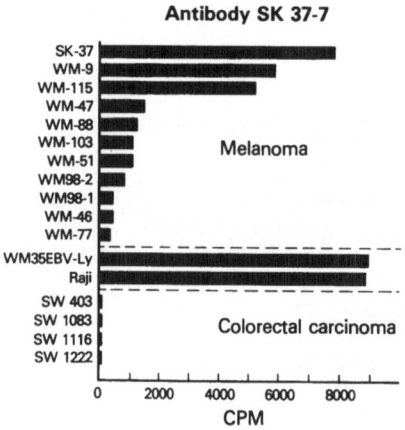

FIGURE 4

bound surface component, thus facilitating its coprecipitation. However, a clear-cut resolution of this problem has yet to be reached. The differences between this antibody and 691-13-17 make for several comparisons. The difference in isotype, IgG_{2a} vs. IgG_1, will make studies on the biological properties of these two molecules doubly interesting. Similarly, the slight differences between the antigens precipitated by the two antibodies suggest that the target determinant may be different, even though the antigen on which the determinant resides appears to be the same.

2.4. Antibody 69115Nu-4B

The production of hybridoma 691I5Nu-4B involved several unconventional features because mice were immunized with cells of a somatic-cell hybrid. Hybrid line 691-I-5, which was formed from the fusion of human melanoma line SW 691 and mouse fibroblast line IT-22, retains the tumorigenic property of its human parent when injected into nude mice. Hybrid cell line 691I5Nu, derived from nude mouse tumor produced by 691-I-5, was karyotyped and found to contain human chromosomes 14, 17, and 21 only. This melanoma hybrid line was used to immunize mice for the production of hybridoma 691I5Nu-4B. Spleen cells from these mice were fused with myeloma cells in the usual way. One of the hybridomas resulting from these experiments secretes an antibody of isotype IgG_{2a} that binds to every melanoma tested so far (Koprowski et al., 1978; M. Herlyn et al., 1980). Tests for the binding of this antibody to tissue samples from patients show positive results for in vivo melanoma cells (Steplewski et al., 1979; Steplewski, 1980). The only other tumor cells found to bind this antibody are two astrocytoma cell lines. Although a low level of binding in RIA was detected with some human embryonal fibroblasts, quantitative adsorption experiments (M. Herlyn et al., 1980) did not remove this binding, while adsorption to astrocytoma and melanoma cells easily did.

The binding specificity of antibody 691I5Nu-4B in RIA is presented in Fig. 5. The antigen with which this antibody reacts appears to have the characteristics of a tumor-specific antigen, since it was found on all melanomas tested but, with the exception of only two astrocytomas, on no other cell lines. The Nu4B antigen consists of four distinct polypeptide chains with molecular weights of 116,000, 95,000, 29,000, and 26,000 (Figs. 2 and 6). The chain of molecular weight 116,000 and the two smaller polypeptide chains show disulfide bonding in the native state, forming a trimolecular complex with an apparent molecular weight of 133,000. The 95,000 protein is noncovalently attached to this complex, as demonstrated by the fact that all four chains coelute from gel filtration columns with a K_{av} consistent with an approximate molecular weight of 250,000 (Mitchell et al., 1981b).

Studies performed to date indicate that the molecules isolated from different melanoma and astrocytoma cell lines have indistinguishable structures. This identicalness of structure, together with the fact that both melanocytes and astrocytes are derived from cells that migrate from the neural crest during embryogenesis, suggests that the Nu4B antigen may arise as a result of the reexpression of genes normally expressed in the fetus. If this hypothesis is true, the antigen is an oncofetal structure; however, its function with respect to fetal cells or melanoma cells remains unknown.

For a test of the expression of the Nu4B antigen in situ, specimens of melanomas, giant hairy nevi, familial premalignant lesions, and other pigmented tissues were obtained

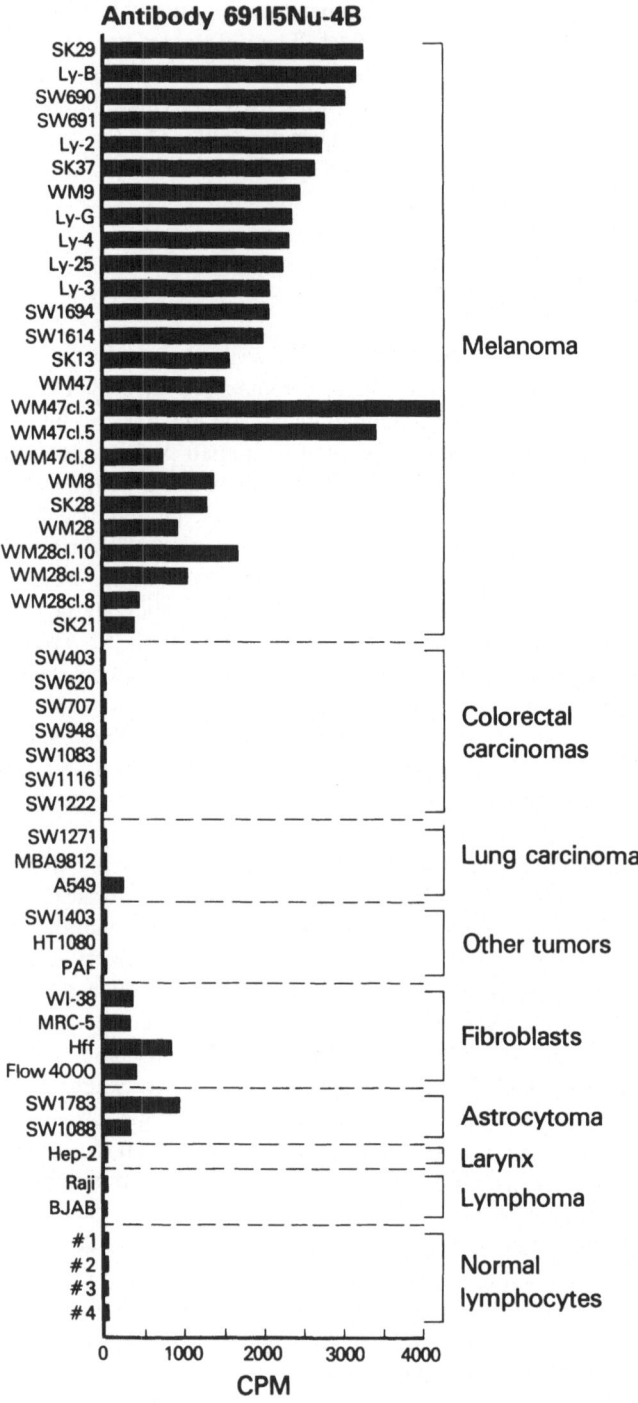

FIGURE 5

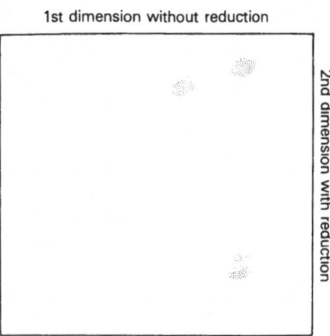

1st dimension without reduction

2nd dimension with reduction

FIGURE 6. Diagrammatic representation of the antigens precipitated from melanoma cells by antibody 691I5Nu-4B. Antigens were subjected to SDS-PAGE in a first dimension (horizontally right to left) without reduction. Subsequently, the gel strip was soaked in Laemmli sample buffer containing β-mercaptoethanol and then electrophoresed at right angles. The radioactive spots constituting the two low-molecular-weight polypeptides are found directly below the high (116,000)-molecular-weight protein, indicating that these three entities were disulfide-bound in the native state. The 95,000 entity migrates independently of the trimer in the first dimension.

from patients and tested by an indirect immunoperoxidase staining procedure (Thompson, personal communications). These studies have clearly shown that antibody 691I5Nu-4B binds to *in situ* melanoma cells, but not detectably to normal melanocytes in adjacent regions of the skin. Interestingly, melanocytes in nevi and other premalignant or nonmalignant lesions also do not bind the antibody; expression of the antigen therefore appears to accompany the transition to a "full-blown" malignant state.

2.5. Antibody 56-NS-1

For production of the hybridoma that secretes this IgG_1 antibody, BALB/c mice were immunized with a membrane preparation from melanoma cell line WM 56 (M. Herlyn *et al.*, 1980). Fusion was carried out between spleen cells from these immunized mice and a variant of P3 $\times$ 63Ag8 that does not secrete immunoglobulin, P3 $\times$ 63Ag8,653. The binding of antibody 56-NS-1 has been tested by RIA on melanoma cell lines; to date, the antibody has been found to have a specificity only for melanoma cells. However, not all melanoma cell lines bind the antibody as shown in Fig. 7. This antibody precipitates an antigen with a reduced molecular weight of 28,000 (see Fig. 2), as demonstrated by SDS-PAGE. The antigen migrates as a diffuse band, a property that is a characteristic of glycosylated proteins, and is clearly distinct from the DR and Nu4B molecules described above. No further information is available at present on the structure of this antigen.

2.6. Antibody 51-NS-52

This IgG_{2a} antibody was produced through the immunization of mice against a membrane preparation from the "familial melanoma" cell line WM 51. The myeloma parent of the hybrid was P3 $\times$ 63Ag8,653 as used for 56-NS-1 (see Section 2.5.). The antibody was found to bind to five of eight melanoma cell lines, but also to two astrocytomas and to one of two lung carcinomas. Raji cells also bound small amounts of this antibody (Fig. 8). This antibody reacts with a monomeric antigen the molecular weight of which is in the vicinity of 196,000 (see Fig. 2). The antibody also precipitates a small amount of an antigen with a molecular weight of approximately 94,000 (Fig. 2). The properties of this smaller

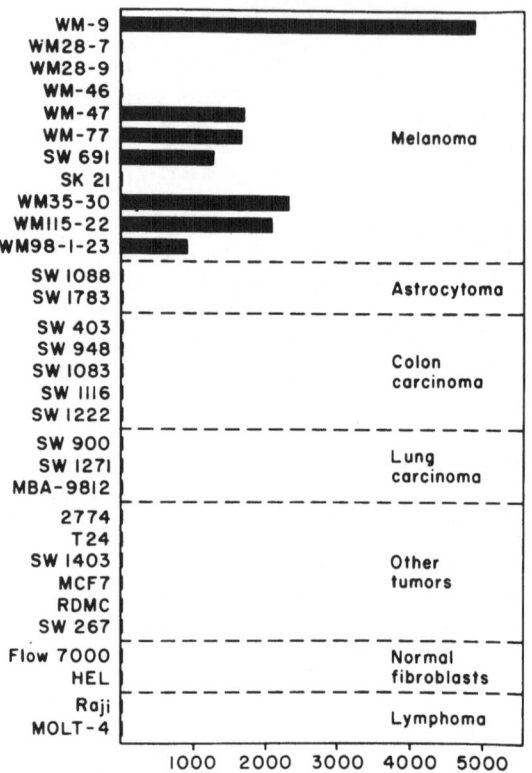

FIGURE 7

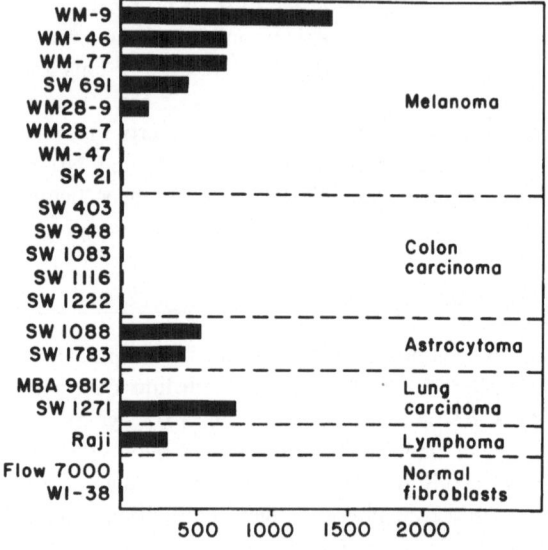

FIGURE 8

antigen are reminiscent of those described by Imai *et al.* (1980), who precipitated an antigen of molecular weight 94,000 from melanoma-cell tissue-culture supernatants and from carcinoma supernatants. However, the antibody kindly provided to us by this group precipitated an antigen of molecular weight 240,000 from melanoma-cell membranes; this is clearly distinct from the antigen precipitated by the antibody 51-NS-52.

2.7. Antibody 9-11-11

This hybridoma was established through the immunization of mice with a membrane preparation from melanoma cell line WM 9 (M. Herlyn *et al.*, 1980) and the subsequent fusion of spleen cells to P3 × 63Ag8. Binding analysis of this IgG$_1$ antibody by RIA (Fig. 9) has shown that besides binding to a majority of melanoma cell lines tested, the antibody binds to two astrocytomas, two of three lung carcinomas, and one breast carcinoma (SW 1403). Antibody 9-11-11, which is secreted by two identical clones (9-11-11 and 9-11-24), precipitated an antigen with a molecular weight of approximately 60,000; like the antigen precipitated by 56-NS-1, this antigen bands in a manner characteristic of glycosylated proteins (see Fig. 2). At present, no further information on the structure of this antigen is available.

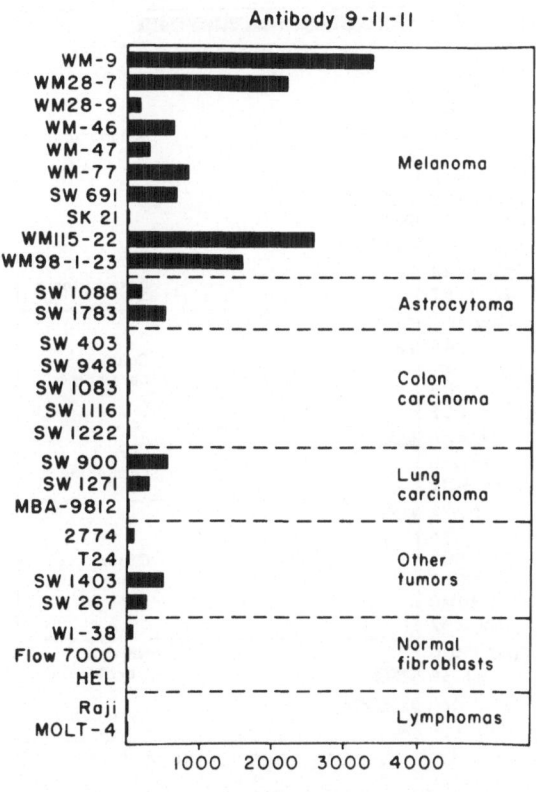

FIGURE 9

2.8. Antibody 9-19

This hybridoma was established from splenocytes from the same mouse as antibody 9-11-11 after the immunization with a membrane preparation from WM 9 cells. As shown in Fig. 10, the IgM antibody secreted by this hybridoma binds significantly to 6 of 11 melanomas tested and, to a lesser extent, to 1 colon carcinoma, 1 lung carcinoma, and 1 ovarian carcinoma (2774), to Raji and MOLT-4 cells, and to embryonal fibroblast cell line WI 38. The antigen detected by this antibody has not yet been identified.

2.9. Antibody 691-19-19

This IgG$_1$ antibody reacts with a majority of melanoma cells tested and, minimally, with astrocytomas; the results of RIA with all other tumors and normal cells tested were clearly negative (Fig. 11). Although we were unable to detect this antigen through immunoprecipitation, new evidence suggests that it may be a protein of high molecular weight (approximately 260,000).

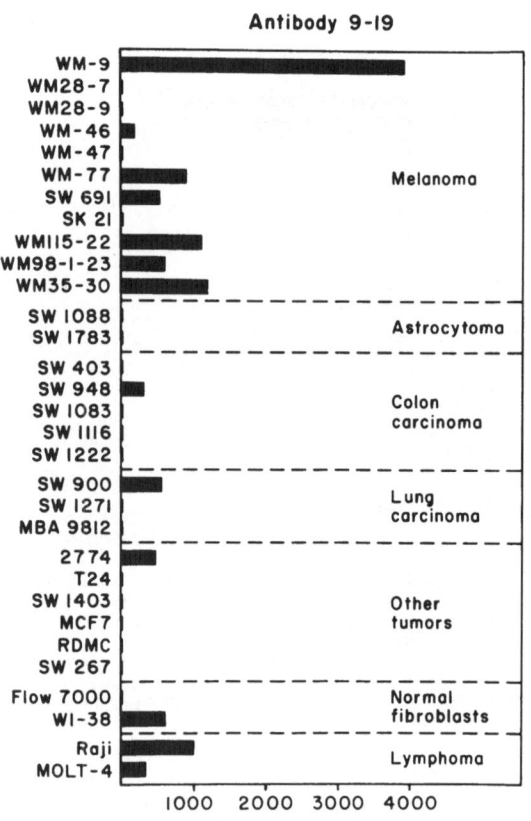

FIGURE 10

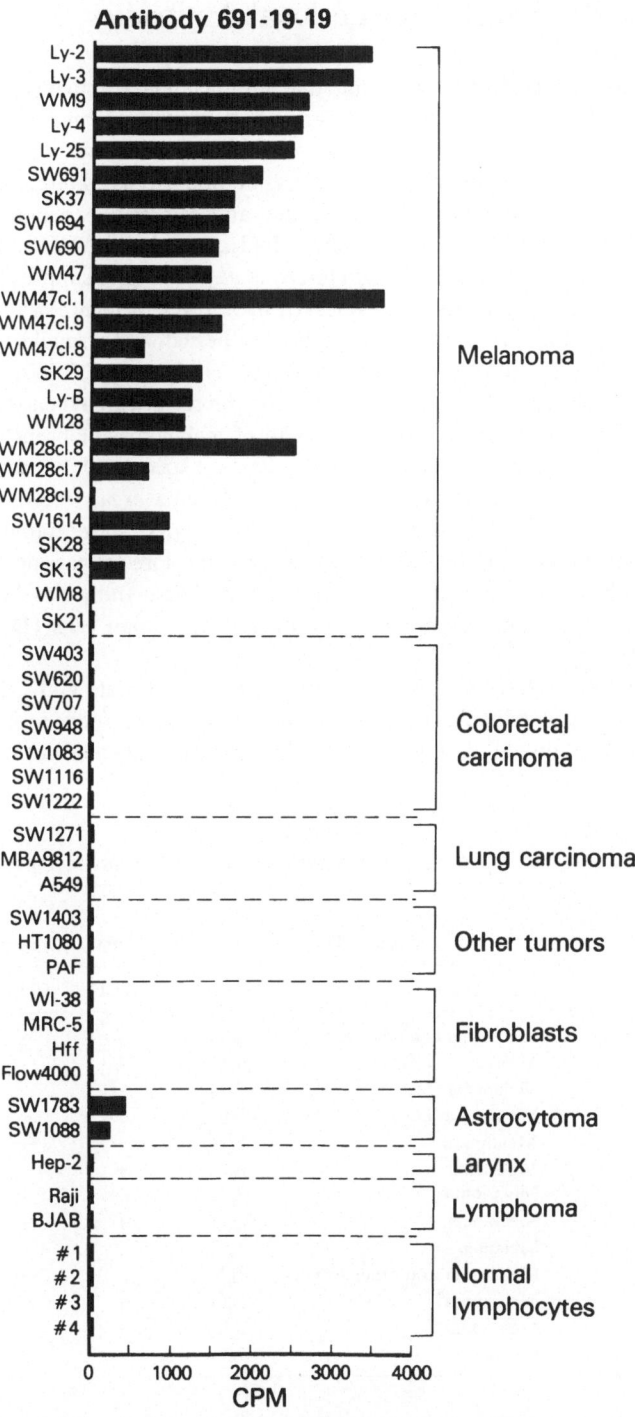

FIGURE 11

3. Biological Functions of Monoclonal Antibodies

In preliminary experiments, we found that antimelanoma antibodies produced by hybridoma mass culture 691-6 suppress the growth of human melanomas in nude mice (Koprowski *et al.*, 1978). However, the mechanism of tumor inhibition remains unclear, particularly since these antibodies do not lyse the same tumor cells *in vitro* in the presence of complement. In other experiments, we found that anti-colorectal carcinoma monoclonal antibody 1083-17-1A (17-1A), which is of isotype IgG_{2a}, is active in ADCC. This antibody is specific for colorectal-carcinoma cells (D. Herlyn *et al.*, 1979) and suppresses the growth of colorectal carcinoma in nude mice, as evidenced by a lower incidence of tumors in antibody-treated animals than in controls, a longer latency period, and a smaller volume of the few tumors that grow in antibody-treated animals (D. Herlyn *et al.*, 1980). The growth-inhibiting property of antibody 17-1A is specific for colorectal-carcinoma cells, as shown by the lack of effect of the antibody on the growth of melanomas or bronchogenic carcinomas. Since this antibody is active in ADCC *in vitro*, we speculated that the same mechanism is responsible for tumor regression *in vivo* (D. Herlyn *et al.*, 1980). Other monoclonal anticolorectal carcinoma antibodies of isotype IgM were found to mediate complement-dependent cytotoxicity (CDC) against human colorectal-carcinoma cells either grown in tissue culture or freshly obtained from patients. These antibodies do not lyse cells of normal colonic mucosa or other normal or malignant human cells (D. Herlyn and H. Koprowski, 1981).

Interestingly, anti-colorectal carcinoma antibodies that mediate CDC do not inhibit the growth of colorectal-carcinoma cells in nude mice. This lack of tumor-growth inhibition may be related to the antibody isotype, since all hybridoma antibodies in this group were of the IgM class.

TABLE I

Biological Functions of Antimelanoma Monoclonal Antibodies

Hybridoma	Antibody Specificity	Isotype	Cytotoxicity in: ADCC	CDC	Tumor-growth inhibition in nude mice?[a]
691-6 (mass culture)	Melanoma and other tumors	IgG_1	+	−	Yes
691-13-17	Melanoma (DR)	IgG_1	+	−	No
691-6-11	Melanoma (DR)	IgG_1	+	−	No
37-7	Melanoma (DR)	IgG_{2a}	+	−	NT
69I15Nu-4B	Melanoma	IgG_{2a}	+	−	No
51-NS-52	Melanoma	IgG_{2a}	+	−	NT
56-NS-1	Melanoma	IgG_1	+	−	NT
691-6-37	Melanoma	IgG_1	+	−	NT
9-11-11	Melanoma	IgG_1	+	−	No
9-19-26	Melanoma and other tumors	IgM	−	+	No
3723	Melanoma[b]	IgG_1	+	−	NT
3724	Melanoma[b]	IgG_{2a}	+	−	NT
3727	Melanoma[b]	IgG_1	+	−	NT

[a](NT) Not tested.
[b]Monoclonal antimelanoma antibodies kindly supplied by Dr. S. Ferrone of Scripps Clinic and Research Foundation. La Jolla, California.

3.1. Cytotoxic Activities of Monoclonal Antimelanoma Antibodies

All but one of the antimelanoma antibodies listed in Table I mediate ADCC *in vitro*. Included in this group are the three antibodies directed against the DR antigen. Two of these antibodies, 691-13-17 and 691-6-11, are of isotype IgG_1; the third, 37-7, is of isotype IgG_{2a}. In this group are also the antibodies directed against antigens expressed only by melanoma cells. Of these, two are isotype IgG_{2a} (691I5Nu-4B and 51-NS-52) and one is of isotype IgG_1 (56-NS-1). Three melanoma-specific antibodies produced by hybridomas established by Dr. S. Ferrone (Imai *et al.*, 1980) are also reactive in ADCC. These are antibody 3734, of isotype IgG_{2a}, and antibodies 3723 and 3727, both of isotype IgG_1. Finally, IgG_1 antibodies 691-6-37 and 9-11-11, both directed against antigens present not only on melanoma cells but also on other tumors, also mediate ADCC. The specific reactivities of these antibodies in ADCC closely follow their binding specificities as established by RIA and are totally removed by adsorption to melanoma cells. In contrast to their ability to mediate ADCC, of the panel of antibodies presented in Table I, only one, IgM antibody 9-19-26, mediates cytotoxicity in the presence of complement.

3.2. Inhibition of Growth of Melanomas in Nude Mice

We succeeded in suppressing colorectal-carcinoma growth in nude mice by use of anti-colorectal carcinoma antibody 1083-17-1A (D. Herlyn *et al.*, 1980), which is of isotype IgG_{2a}; in contrast, antibody 691I5Nu-4B, also of the IgG_{2a} isotype and specific for melanoma cells, did not suppress the growth of melanoma in nude mice. However, another IgG_{2a} antibody (37-7, Table 1) specifically inhibited growth of melanoma tumors in nude mice. Two IgG_1 antibodies directed against the DR antigen, 691-13-17 and 691-9-11, were unable to suppress the growth of melanoma in nude mice, even though the melanoma cell lines showed high binding of these antibodies in RIA. A third IgG_1 antibody, 9-11-11, which is active *in vitro* in ADCC, was also unable to inhibit tumor growth in nude mice. Finally, as in the case of anti-colorectal carcinoma antibodies of the IgM isotype, IgM antimelanoma antibody 9-19-26 did not inhibit tumor growth in nude mice, although *in vitro* it was active in CDC.

ACKNOWLEDGMENTS. The work reported herein was supported in part by Grants CA-10815, CA-21124, CA-25298, and CA-25874 from the National Cancer Institute, Grant RR-05540 from the Division of Research Resources, and funds from the Pew Memorial Trust.

References

Fuhrer, J. P., Ward, F. E., Mitchell, K. F., Steplewski, Z., and Koprowski, H., 1982, Structural variation in the DR antigens of human melanoma, *Hum. Immunol.* (in press).

Herlyn, D., and Koprowski, H., 1981, Monoclonal anticolon carcinoma antibodies in complement-dependent cytotoxicity, *Int. J. Cancer* **27**:769.

Herlyn, D., Herlyn, M., Steplewski, Z., and Koprowski, H., 1979, Monoclonal antibodies in cell-mediated cytotoxicity against human melanoma and colorectal carcinoma, *Eur. J. Immunol.* **9**:657.

Herlyn, D., Steplewski, Z., Herlyn, M., and Koprowski, H., 1980, Inhibition of growth of colorectal carcinoma in nude mice by monoclonal antibody, *Cancer Res.* **40**:717.

Herlyn, M., Clark, W. H., Jr., Mastrangelo, M. J., Guerry, D., IV, Elder, D. E., LaRossa, D., Hamilton, R., Bondi, E., Tuthill, R., Steplewski, Z., and Koprowski, H., 1980, Specific immunoreactivity of hybridoma-secreted monoclonal anti-melanoma antibodies to cultured cells and freshly derived human cells, *Cancer Res.* **40**:3602.

Imai, K., Molinaro, G. A., and Ferrone, S., 1980 Monoclonal antibodies to human melanoma-associated antigens, *Transplant. Proc.* **12**:380.

Koprowski, H., Steplewski, Z., Herlyn, D., and Herlyn, M., 1978, Study of antibodies against human melanoma produced by somatic cell hybrids, *Proc. Natl. Acad. Sci. U.S.A.* **75**:3405.

Mitchell, K. F., Fuhrer, J. P., Steplewski, Z., and Koprowski, H., 1981a, Biochemical characterization of human melanoma cell surfaces: dissection with monoclonal antibodies, *Proc. Natl. Acad. Sci. U.S.A.* **77**:7287.

Mitchell, K. F., Fuhrer, J. P., Steplewski, Z., and Koprowski, H., 1981b, Structural characterization of the "melanoma-specific" antigen detected by monoclonal antibody 691I5-Nu4B, *Mol. Immunol.* **18**:207.

Steplewski, Z., 1980, Monoclonal antibodies to human tumor antigens,*Transplant. Proc.* **12**:384.

Steplewski, Z., Herlyn, M., Herlyn, D., Clark, W. H., Jr., and Koprowski, H., Reactivity of monoclonal anti-melanoma antibodies with melanoma cells freshly isolated from primary and metastatic melanoma,*Eur. J. Immunol.* **9**:94.

21

The Features of Malignant Melanoma Organ-Specific Neoantigens Recognized by the Antitumor Immune Response of the Human Host

D. M. P. THOMSON

1. Introduction

Human histocompatibility antigens have been defined with alloantisera from immunized subjects. Alloantisera have proved invaluable in defining the polymorphism of these antigens and monitoring their purification. Xenoantibodies to the human leukocyte antigen (*HLA*) complex, even to purified HLA antigens in sharp contradistinction, have not been reagents of great value in revealing HLA allospecificity (Sanderson, 1977). Likewise, by immunizing xenogeneic animals with experimental or human tumor materials, few, if any, tumor-antigen epitopes have been identified to which the tumor-bearing hosts respond. Cancer antigens to which the human responds, accordingly, may never be defined by immunizing xenogeneic animals with a hodgepodge of tumor materials.

In experimental tumor models, the existence of tumor-specific transplantation antigens was established on the basis of the rejection of transplantable tumors in previously immunized syngeneic recipients. *In vitro* assays of cell-mediated and humoral responses have been used to monitor the isolation of tumor-specific antigens (TSAs) involved in the response (Baldwin and Glaves, 1972; Thomson *et al.*, 1973). In fact, we found that a chem-

D. M. P. THOMSON • The Montreal General Hospital, The Montreal General Hospital Research Institute, Montreal, Quebec, Canada H3G 1A4.

ically induced TSA could be recognized with syngeneic tumor immune serum but not with xenogeneic antiserum (Thomson and Alexander, 1973), and the immunoglobulin G (IgG) from the syngeneic tumor-immune serum was used in affinity chromatography to isolate the papain-solubilized TSAs from tumor-cell membranes (Thomson et al., 1973).

The principal evidence that human tumors express neoantigens has come from in vitro assays of cell-mediated and humoral responses, but a great deal of skepticism was generated by the nonreproducibility of the microcytotoxicity assay (Baldwin, 1975; Herberman and Oldham, 1975). As a consequence, none of the available in vitro assay is widely accepted, and many disbelieve the existence of organ-specific neoantigens. Despite the doubts, since the 1960s, published studies have suggested that human neoplasms of the same organ and histogenesis share neoantigens (Shuster et al., 1978). In view of the skepticism, it is no wonder then that such assays have not been felt to be useful to monitor the isolation of the sensitizing antigen, a substance the very existence of which is questioned.

Halliday and Miller (1972), however, described a most promising in vitro assay of human antitumor immunity that is based on the phenomenon that leukocytes from patients with cancer, after being incubated with extracts of cancer of the same organ and histogenesis, lose their former ability to adhere to glass. A modified assay (Holan et al., 1974), called tube leukocyte-adherence inhibition (LAI) by Grosser and Thomson (1975), was adopted, and it was automated by computer-driven image analysis (Tataryn et al., 1978; Thomson et al., 1979a).

A distinct advantage of the LAI assay is that isolates of the tumor can be substituted for the phosphate-buffered saline (PBS) cancer extract to determine the molecule or molecules that carry the putative antigenic determinant. With a purified tumor antigen, there may be a greater chance of successfully producing in xenogeneic animals an antiserum that recognizes the same antigenic epitope as humans bearing the tumors, especially if hydridoma technology is used.

This review will not only describe the physicochemical features of the organ-specific neoantigens of malignant melanoma that have been delineated using the antitumor response of the human host, but also present unequivocal evidence for the specificity of the human antitumor immune response assayed by tube LAI.

2. Tube Leukocyte-Adherence-Inhibition Assay

The evidence that human cancers express neoantigens rests on the in vitro measurement of the host's antitumor immune response to tumor products: accordingly, it is important to describe briefly the assay used, so that the reader may assess the limits of the methodology.

Tumor extracts are prepared as previously described from metastatic deposits in the liver of autopsy specimens (Grosser and Thomson, 1975). For use in the assay, the stock extracts, stored in 0.3-ml volumes at $-70°C$, are rapidly thawed and diluted with Medium 199 to approximately 100 μg protein/0.1 ml. The samples are discarded after one use.

Venous blood samples from patients are collected in two heparinized, 10-ml Vacutainer® tubes and incubated vertically, at 37°C for 45 min. The leukocyte-rich fraction is aspirated and centrifuged at $200g$ for 5 min. The supernatant is discarded, and the pellet is resuspended in 3.5 ml ice-cold Tris-buffered NH_4Cl solution to lyse contaminating red blood cells. Then, after being washed with Medium 199, the leukocytes are suspended in medium at a concentration of 10^7 cells/ml.

The tube LAI assay is performed as we previously described (Grosser and Thomson, 1975) in 20-ml, 16 × 150 mm glass test tubes in triplicate for each antigen (Grosser and Thomson, 1975). To each tube is added 0.3 ml Medium 199, 0.1 ml tumor extract containing approximately 100 µg protein, and 0.1 ml of the suspended peripheral-blood leukocytes (PBI). Well agitated, the tubes are laid horizontally so that the contents cover four fifths of the length of the tube and are incubated at 37°C in a 5% CO_2, humidified atmosphere. Two hours later, the tubes are stood upright, and the contents at the bottom are gently agitated with a Pasteur pipette. A sample is then withdrawn and pipetted onto a hemocytometer with a surface marked only by a single square, outlining an area of 16 mm^2.

Within the square, the cells are counted automatically by a computerlinked image analyzer. The computer calculates the mean number on nonadherent cells, standard deviation, and coefficient of variation, and expresses the results as a nonadherance index (NAI):

$$NAI = \frac{A - B}{B} \times 100$$

where A equals a sample of the number of nonadherent cells incubated with the specific cancer extract and B equals a sample of the number of nonadherent cells incubated with the other unrelated, control cancer extract. In our studies, less than 5% of hospitalized patients with benign diseases or cancer of organs unrelated to the specific cancer extracts used have NAIs of 30 or greater; hence, NAIs of 30 or greater are accepted as positive (Grosser and Thompson, 1975; Marti and Thomson, 1976; Flores *et al.*, 1977; Lopez *et al.*, 1978; O'Connor *et al.*, 1978; Tataryn *et al.*, 1978, 1979; Ayeni *et al.*, 1980).

2.1. Validity of Leukocyte-Adherence Inhibition

Partly as the result of the difficulties experienced with the reproducibility of microcytotoxicity studies, doubt has been cast on the claims for existence of an antitumor response to human cancer. The following points, we believe, refute the misgivings:

1. Our initial results (Grosser and Thomson, 1975) in breast-cancer and control patients were confirmed by yet two other investigators and showed that about 80% of patients with early breast cancer and 5% of other patients tested before surgery had LAI reactivity (Flores *et al.*, 1977).

2. Another study of breast-cancer and other patients, in which the samples of leukocytes were coded and the analysis performed by still another two investigators, gave nearly identical results, in that about 80% of patients with early breast cancer and 3% of control patients tested before surgery had LAI reactivity (Lopez *et al.*, 1978; O'Connor *et al.*, 1978).

3. In two other studies, one in gastrointestinal cancer and another in various cancers, carried out by yet two more workers, the nonadherent cells were counted automatically by

image analysis. The results indicated that about 80% of patients with early cancer reacted specifically to their cancer, but fewer than 3% of other patients showed LAI reactivity (Tataryn *et al.*, 1978, 1979; Ayeni *et al.*, 1980).

4. Coded PBL from patients with epidermoid-lung cancer or inflammatory lung lesions were provided from another hospital. All patients were tested before the diagnoses were known and before any surgical procedure. The results of the individual assays, moreover, were reported the same day they were performed. About 80% of patients with early lung cancer were LAI$^+$, whereas patients with inflammatory lung disease seldom reacted (Thomson *et al.*, 1981a).

5. At the First LAI Workshop, Buffalo, New York, May 1978, the tube LAI assay was successfully demonstrated by R. Schwartz with samples of leukocytes coded by Drs. McCoy and Takasugi (Thomson, 1979). Maluish and Halliday (1979), too, demonstrated the hemocytometer assay, successfully.

6. Four human cancers of differing origins, grown in nude mice, were provided and coded by independent investigators. The tumors were extracted and then identified as to their site of origin by determining with which tumor extract known LAI$^+$ leukocytes reacted. Four of four coded transplanted human tumors were identified correctly (Thomson *et al.*, 1981b).

7. Dr. Lauerova, from the Research Institute of Clincal and Experimental Oncology, Brno, Czechoslovakia, who was sponsored by the International Union Against Cancer, spent about 4 weeks in our laboratory to determine why some laboratories have failed to confirm the sensitivity and specificity claimed for LAI. Using the same samples of leukocytes and cancer extracts, R. Schwartz and Dr. Lauerova compared their LAI results calculated by the computer-driven image analyzer. The LAI results of R. Schwartz in breast cancer were as previously published. The LAI results of Dr. Lauerova, on the other hand, showed much more variation. The level of acquired skill in the assay, we concluded, is the single most important variable in achieving valid results.

8. Other laboratories, needless to say, have confirmed the presence of an antitumor response to human organ-specific neoantigens by LAI (Sanner *et al.*, 1979; Shani *et al.*, 1978; Powell *et al.*, 1975; Russo *et al.*, 1978; Fujisawa *et al.*, 1977; Halliday *et al.*, 1975, 1977).

3. Blocking Tube Leukocyte-Adherence-Inhibition

When, in early experiments, serum was tested for blocking activity by adding it to the assay, we observed that it caused too many cells to be nonadherent (Grosser and Thomson, 1975). To avoid this problem, we decided to preincubate leukocytes with serum with the idea that the specific effect of the serum might be mediated during the incubative period. And by washing the cells free of excess serum, the nonspecific effect of serum in the assay would be eliminated while retaining the specific effect. In subsequent experiments, we found that preincubating leukocytes with differing tumor isolates was a valid approach for detecting tumor antigen (Marti *et al.*, 1976; Grosser and Thomson, 1976; Lopez and Thomson, 1977; Thomson *et al.*, 1978, 1979b).

3.1. Methodology

To detect the presence of specific antigen in a sample, an aliquot from the sample is brought to 0.5 ml with Medium 199 containing 20% fetal calf serum and then added to a minimum of 1.3×10^7 PBL, from patients previously shown to be LAI^+, suspended in 0.5 ml Medium 199. The mixture is incubated for 30 min at $37°C$ in a 5% CO_2, humidified atmosphere with frequent agitation of the tubes. Then the cells are spun down, washed with Medium 199, and plated in the direct tube LAI assay. All samples are coded and unknown to the experimenter testing the sample.

3.2. Specificity

When leukocytes from an LAI^+ melanoma patient are preincubated with a PBS extract of malignant melanoma or unrelated tumor, washed, and then placed in the regular tube LAI, the leukocytes preincubated with the melanoma-cancer extract now fail to react, but the same cells preincubated with other unrelated cancer extract respond positively in the LAI assay to the malignant-melanoma cancer extract (Fig. 1). Those samples that block the LAI response are then tested on LAI^+ leukocytes from patients with an unrelated cancer to prove that the blocking was indeed tumor-specific.

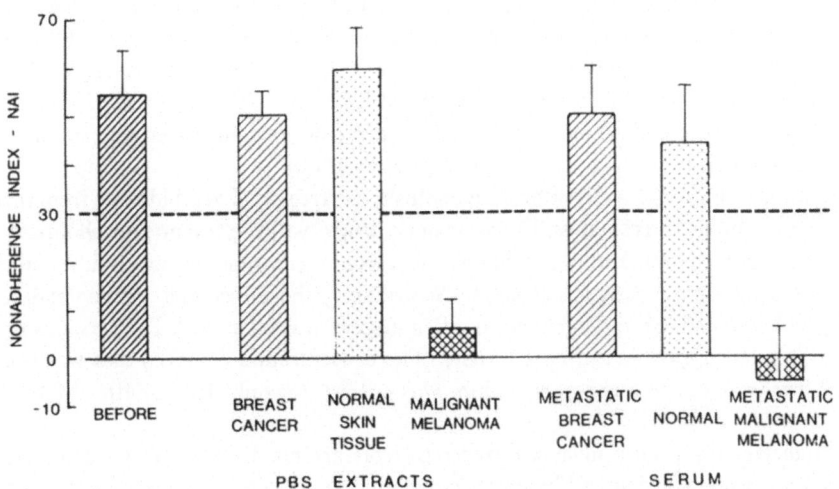

FIGURE 1. Nonadherence index (NAI) of leukocytes from patients with malignant melanoma before and after preincubation with different tumor extracts or sera. The LAI^+ response of melanoma patients is blocked by PBS extracts of malignant melanoma, but not of breast cancer or normal skin. Similarly, serum from patients with malignant melanoma, but not breast cancer or normal patients, negates the positive response. Specificity of the blocking is shown by incubating the substance with LAI^+ leukocytes from patients with a different cancer. Significance of NAI: positive, ≥ 30; negative, < 30.

As a means for detecting tumor antigen, the blocking tube LAI assay has several advantages over the regular tube LAI assay. First, lesser protein concentrations of the isolates can be tested, unlike the regular assay, in which 100 μg protein is essential so that the number of nonadherent cells is optimal for counting. Second, it is not essential to pair and titrate the isolates because when they are used as a blocking antigen, the isolates are removed once they have had an opportunity to either react or not react with the cells; the cells are then incubated with the well-titrated and standardized crude extracts. Third, because there are no constraints on the quantity of material used in the blocking assay, it is possible to determine the minimum quantity of each sample that blocks the LAI response, and this allows the enrichment of the specific activity of the isolate to be calculated after each step of purification.

The blocking tube LAI assay also has disadvantages; more PBL are required, preincubation by adding one more step leads to more technical errors or artifacts. Consequently, only assayers with skill and experience in the regular LAI assay can reliably test materials.

3.3. Mechanism Mediating the Leukocyte-Adherence-Inhibition Phenomenon and Blocking

3.3.1. Prostaglandins

Leukocytes from LAI^+ patients, for 1–2 weeks after surgery, cease to react (Grosser and Thomson, 1975; Marti and Thomson, 1976). In studying the possible mechanism(s) of the immunosuppression, corticosteroids were implicated as being important: corticosteroid levels rose during surgery and remained elevated for some days (Flores et al., 1976), corticosteroids added in vitro to the assay inhibited LAI activity (Flores et al., 1976; Grosser et al., 1980), and LAI^+ leukocytes were inhibited from reacting when the patients had received corticosteroids shortly before (Grosser et al., 1980).

A key step in the synthesis of prostaglandins is the freeing of arachidonate from membrane phospholipids. Steroidal antiinflammatory drugs, which prevent phospholipase A_2 activation, inhibit the removal of arachidonic acid from membrane phospholipids, and this blocks the synthesis of products from it. Accordingly, the effect that prostaglandin E_2 (PGE_2) had when added to the leukocytes after surgery was examined. PGE_2 reversed the surgical immunosuppression of LAI activity. The concentration of PGE_2 that was preincubated briefly with the leukocytes in vitro was critical, for only 10^{-5} to 10^{-6} M had an effect.

Leukocytes from most advanced-cancer patients are not LAI^+, and it was hypothesized that the defect was induced by excess circulating tumor antigen covering all the active binding sites of the reactive cells (Grosser and Thomson, 1976). It seemed appropriate, nonetheless, to determine what effect PGE_2 might have on these nonreactive leukocytes.

PGE_2 converted the negative response of advanced-cancer patients to positive (Kaneti et al., 1981). The change in response was dependent on the same critical concentration of PGE_2, and it happened quickly. PGE_2, it is known, stimulates adenylate cyclase to raise intracellular levels of cyclic AMP (cAMP). In fact, the leukocytes' intracellular cAMP was elevated 4- to 5-fold immediately after incubation with PGE_2. Other substances that elevate intracellular cAMP or inhibit its degradation also heightened the LAI response.

When LAI^+ leukocytes were incubated with indomethacin, the LAI^+ response was not impaired; if anything, the highest concentrations of indomethacin enhanced the response. So it seems reasonable to conclude that PGE_2 can affect the leukocytes' LAI response by modulating the levels of intracellular cAMP. But if these levels are adequate, the biochemical and physiological changes in response to an antigenic stimulus can take place in the absence of arachidonic acid metabolism to PGE_2.

3.3.2. Calcium Ion

Calcium-ion influx is a critical link between a specific stimulus and the resultant physiological response. Stimulation of the cell increases either the influx of Ca^{2+} or the release of Ca^{2+} from the cell membrane. The transient increase of free Ca^{2+} in the cytosol triggers biochemical reactions, culminating in physiological responses (Cheung, 1980). Calcium ionophore increases the permeability of cell membranes to calcium, and calcium thus flows down a concentration gradient. When Ca ionophore at 10^{-6} M is admixed with one of the two antigens, then the ionophore causes increased leukocyte nonadherence and a positive LAI response of normal leukocytes to the mixture of antigen and ionophore. LAI^+ leukocytes preincubated with the ionophore, on the other hand, no longer show a positive response.

Ouabain, too, inhibited an LAI^+ response, and when it was admixed with one antigen at 10^{-6} M and incubated with normal leukocytes, the leukocytes responded to the antigen and ouabain mixture as though the cells were incubated with a sensitizing antigen. Ouabain inhibits the sodium-potassium ATPase; this reduces the sodium concentration gradient across the cell membrane, in turn reducing the magnitude of exchange-coupled calcium. The overall effect is to increase the net intracellular calcium concentration.

Lidocaine, when admixed with one antigen and incubated with normal leukocytes, had no effect on the glass-adherence properties. But if LAI^+ leukocytes are briefly preincubated with lidocaine, they no longer exhibit reactivity. Lidocaine becomes incorporated into biological membranes and affects many cellular functions dependent on calcium permeability by preventing calcium uptake; the LAI phenomenon is negated in its presence because the binding of tumor antigen does not now result in an influx of calcium to initiate the biochemical reactions and physiological changes.

There is the possibility that the calcium gating mechanism or mechanisms are influenced either by arachidonate metabolites of the lipoxygenase pathway or by protein carboxymethylation or by both. And in recent experiments, we have found that inhibitors of the lipoxygenase pathway also negate the LAI^+ response. Arachidonate products of the lipoxygenase pathway, so it seems, have an important role in the phenomenon of LAI, whatever the mechanism.

3.3.3. Other Factors

The LAI^+ cells need energy to react, for inhibitors of metabolism block the response. Further, the microfilaments of the cell must also function, for substances such as cytochalasin B and colchicine, which disrupt the action of microfilaments, also negate the LAI^+ response.

3.3.4. Interrelationship of LAI-Reactive Cells, Tumor Antigen, and Mediators

Analogous to other leukocytes, in particular the mast cell (Foreman and Lichenstein, 1980), it seems probable that the cytophilic antitumor antibody on the membrane of monocytes is cross-linked by tumor antigen that is transduced into information useful to the cell (Grosser *et al.*, 1976; Marti *et al.*, 1976). The transduction is believed to involve the opening of calcium channels in the cell membrane, allowing calcium to enter the cell; this affects the polarization of the cell, and a rise in free calcium concentration within the cell brings about biochemical reactions, culminating in a physiological response (Cheung, 1980).

The control of the biochemical reactions activated by calcium entry seems to involve intracellular cyclic nucleotide levels, for intracellular cAMP is thought to regulate the calcium gate mechanism(s). And intracellular cAMP, raised by PGE_2 stimulation *in vitro*, would stimulate a protein kinase to phosphorylate the channels to inhibit calcium entry; equally important, other proteins would be phosphorylated, thus reversing the biochemical and physiological events initiated originally by the binding of tumor antigen.

When the cancer is not advanced, the host bearing the tumor reacts briskly against the tumor *in vitro* (Grosser and Thomson, 1975) and *in vivo* (Leveson *et al.*, 1977). So it seems likely that leukocytes from patients with advanced cancer, having repeatedly encountered tumor antigen *in vivo*, have already undergone a series of biochemical and physiological changes, which explains why they fail to respond in the LAI assay. This situation, in fact, can be reproduced *in vivo*: LAI^+ leukocytes, when preincubated with antigen, do not react in the tube LAI assay (Grosser and Thomson, 1976), but if after the preincubation with soluble antigen they are briefly exposed to PGE_2, the leukocytes regain their reactivity.

In short, leukocytes encountering tumor antigen in the preincubation step of the blocking assay are delivered a stimulus that induces the specialized cells to express their program. Until the leukocytes recover from the physiological event induced by the soluble antigen, any subsequent encounter, for instance, with tumor antigen in the standard tube LAI, is unlikely to evoke the programmed biochemical changes and the physiological response that leads to the phenomenon of LAI.

4. Organ-Specific Neoantigens of Human Cancer

Human cancers, arising in an organ and of similar histogenesis, express a cell-surface molecule with a common antigenic determinant to which only patients with a like cancer react; the organ-specific neoantigens are recognized by allogeneic or autochthonous leukocytes from patients with the same cancers (Grosser and Thomson, 1975; Halliday *et al.*, 1975, 1977; Fujisawa *et al.*, 1977; Rutherford *et al.*, 1977; Russo *et al.*, 1978; Shani *et al.*, 1978).

Leukocytes from patients with cancer react positively with unrelated cancer extracts so seldom that when it does occur, we are never certain whether it represents an example of more than one neoantigen being expressed by the principal cancer or an antigenic stimulus from a dysplastic lesion or early cancer of the other organ.

Yet Rudczynski *et al.* (1978) showed that human cancer can share a common neoantigen. Breast-cancer patients, they reported, showed a specific LAI response to tissue-culture lines of breast and throat adenocarcinoma. Sanner *et al.* (1980), too, recently reported that tissue-culture lines of breast and lung adenocarcinoma shared neoantigens, for lung-cancer patients reacted to extracts from tissue-culture lines of breast and lung cancer. Also, using leukocyte-migration-inhibition assays, other investigators have reported that tumors from different organs may share tumor antigens.

Still, we, with the standard tube LAI, have not observed that cancer patients exhibit an immune response against tumor neoantigens from two different organs. Notwithstanding that, the LAI response of breast-cancer patients, stimulated by PGE_2, showed reactivity to both breast- and lung-cancer extracts, though the response to the lung cancer was much less. And the LAI response of lung-cancer patients, stimulated by PGE_2, while high against the lung-cancer extracts, also revealed reactivity, though much less, against the breast-cancer extract. So far, PGE_2-stimulated leukocytes from other cancer patients have not exhibited reactivity to more than one organ-specific neoantigen.

A number of possibilities can be envisaged to account for cross-reacting tumor antigens. Some cancers could express multiple organ-specific neoantigens. Alternatively, some cancers may express a common tumor antigen that has no relationship to the origin of the cancer. A third possibility that appeals to us, especially in the instance of the breast and lung cancer, is that the structure of the organ-specific neoantigen determinants may be nearly alike. Thus, the binding site of leukocytes from breast-cancer patients, while binding strongly to the breast cancer neoantigen, also fit, though less well, the lung-cancer antigenic determinant; in this latter circumstance, the imperfect fit of tumor antigen and binding site on the antigen-sensitive cells would not be expected to generate as strong a signal to initiate the programmed cell functions that in turn result in the altered glass-adherence properties of the leukocytes. The weak LAI response of lung-cancer patients to the breast-cancer antigen can be similarly explained.

4.1. Expression by Premalignant Lesions

In most tissues, the development of a neoplasm is a gradual process involving a series of sequential alterations during preneoplastic and premalignant phases (Foulds, 1975). The ultimate cancer phenotype is associated with the loss of some specialized functions and with the appearance of proteins that are usually present either at an earlier stage in development or in a different tissue (Potter, 1978). Consequently, many types of human and experimental malignant neoplasms are associated with phenotypic characteristics of embryonal, fetal, or regenerating cells or tissues (Weinhouse and Ono, 1972). Some markers, in fact, appear early in the cancer process and long before the appearance of overt cancer (Farber *et al.*, 1979; Ogawa *et al.*, 1979). Indeed, the phenotypic cancer markers are often considered to be the result of altered gene control and expression and seemingly are intimately associated with the malignant behavior (Holliday, 1979).

Potter (1978) makes the point that a fetal organ consists of a cell population that participates in an organized series of changes resulting in a functional organ. A clonal neoplasm, to the contrary, will not recall the total program, although it may have much of the phenotypic variation seen in a population of normal cells from the same organ. The neoplastic cells, unlike the normal, have a block in their differentiation, called either "blocked ontogeny" or "partially blocked ontogeny" (Potter, 1978).

Stem cells of an organ presumably at some point during their differentiation express organ-specific neoantigens, but the final adult cells of the organ do not. Yet, when cells become dysplastic or cancerous, they express, once again, the organ-specific neoantigen; their differentiation is blocked, so it seems, before the point where the organ-specific neoantigens are no longer expressed. Even though the organ-specific neoantigens are yet another cancer phenotype, the unique characteristic of these antigens is their immunogenicity in humans, for none of the phenotypic cancer markers described so far shares this feature.

Yet some investigators have concluded—on the basis of their results with *in vitro* assays—that cancer patients are sensitized to normal tissue antigens of the organ. But as far as we can tell, leukocytes of most cancer patients are not sensitized to normal tissue antigens: first, leukocytes from LAI^+ patients do not react to extracts of the normal organ; second, patients with severe inflammatory organ disease, as a rule, are not LAI^+. Even so, there are patients without cancer but with dysplastic lesions who do react specifically to the cancer extracts (Flores *et al.*, 1977; O'Connor *et al.*, 1978; Tataryn *et al.*, 1979; Sanner *et al.*, 1979; Fritze *et al.*, 1979). These positive responses seem to happen because these noncancerous but probably premalignant lesions express organ-specific neoantigens due to the the fact that their differentiation is blocked like a cancer arising from the same organ.

4.2. Coisolation with β_2-Microglobulin

The putative tumor antigen in the PBS extracts elutes in the void volume of a molecular-sieve column of Sepharose 4B (Grosser and Thomson, 1975), indicating that it either has a high molecular weight or is particulate, such as part of a membrane. When, in fact, the surface membranes of the cancer cells are separated from the cell sap, the putative tumor-antigen activity is recovered mostly with the cell-membrane fraction.

4.2.1. Ultracentrifugal Flotation of Lipoproteins

McCabe *et al.* (1978) reported the isolation of melanoma-associated antigens (MAAs) from cultured human melanoma cells. They used ultracentrifugal flotation on KBr to separate MAA; and HLA antigens. HLA antigens, associated with high-density lipoproteins, were found in the upper fraction, and the MAAs remained below. MAAs isolated in this manner retained their immunological functions, as evidenced by their ability to produce hypersensitivity reactions in 70% of melanoma patients and 20% of controls and to specifically combine with an antimelanoma xenoantiserum.

The LAI-active material, in sharp contradistinction, was recovered in the upper fraction that contains the HLA antigens. As described in more detail elsewhere by Khosravi *et al.* (1982), they supplied us with coded samples of KBr-separated tumor materials from malignant-melanoma and colon-cancer cells that had been grown in tissue culture. For both cancer specimens, the LAI-active material was in the upper fraction, which was also enriched for HLA antigens and β_2-microglobulin (β_2m).

These results are not surprising, since histocompatibility antigens of normal tissues and the TSAs of many chemically induced animal tumors are an integral part of the cell membrane, and their isolation depends on making them water-soluble. Limited papain digestion of purified cell membranes was the method originally used to isolate HLA antigens; this method of digestion was also chosen to solubilize human cancer antigens. In addition, this was the approach used for solubilizing TSAs of chemically induced tumors (Baldwin and Glaves, 1972; Thomson and Alexander, 1973).

When the papain-solubilized putative tumor antigen was chromatographed on a calibrated Sephadex G150 column, the activity was found in all the molecular-weight ranges assayed, but the principal activity eluted consistently at a molecular weight of 100,000 or so (Fig. 2). This material, analyzed by sodium dodecyl sulfate (SDS) gel electrophoreis, was composed of smaller subunits, and a band at a molecular weight of 12,000 was outstanding. This suggested that the putative tumor antigen might contain β_2m. At that time, we had found, too, that the isolated TSA of a chemically induced tumor was composed of smaller subunits of which one had a molecular weight of about 12,000 (Thomson et al., 1976).

Intrigued by the possibility that the neoantigens of human tumors and of chemically induced tumors might be similar to histocompatibility antigens in structure and in linkage to β_2m, we passed the human material with putative tumor-antigen activity through an affinity column of horse anti-human β_2m. Retained by the affinity column, the putative tumor antigen was eluted with the chaotropic agent KSCN (Thomson et al., 1976)(Fig. 2). The tumor antigen seems to bind to the affinity column specifically: the putative tumor antigen does not bind to an immunoadsorbent column of normal IgG (Thomson et al., 1978), nor does the putative antigen bind to an affinity column of antiserum raised to the material that had not bound to the anti-β_2m affinity column (Thomson et al., 1980a). Doubtless, the putative tumor antigen copurifies with β_2m. Confirming our studies, Malley et al. (1979) reported that the malignant-melanoma tumor antigen as assayed by LAI copurifies with β_2m. Using antisera raised in monkeys to MAAs, Khosravi et al., (1980) found that both MAA and HLA activity were enriched in the upper KBr fraction. Moreover, they applied shed material from melanoma cultures to a Sepharose 4B rabbit anti-human β_2m IgG affinity column, eluted the bound material with 3 M KSCN, and found that β_2m, HLA, and MAAs had bound to the affinity column. These findings lend further support to our original report on the association of β_2m with one type of MAA.

The tumor antigens, isolated from the anti-β_2m affinity column, have three principal bands when analyzed by SDS gel electrophoresis: at molecular weights of about 12,000, 25,000, and 40,000 (Thomson et al., 1976, 1978). Nonetheless, the molecular weight of the polypeptide chain carrying the organ-specific neoantigen determinant is not yet known.

Originally, the HLA large component and no other membrane components were reported to be bound to β_2m (Robb et al., 1976; Nakamuro et al., 1977). Recent studies indicate that β_2m does bind certain membrane components that are the same in molecular size as the HLA large components but are different antigenically from the HLA large components (Tada et al., 1978). For that matter, the T/a and Qa-2 antigens in the mouse, it is reported, are linked to β_2m (Ostberg et al., 1975; Michailson et al., 1977). Besides, the male specific antigen (H-Y) is associated with β_2m, though coded for by the Y chromosome (Fellous et al., 1978). Membrane proteins, associated with β_2m, may possibly have a regulatory role during cell differentiation, so the expression of a β_2m-linked cell-surface protein with organ specificity would be in keeping with the concept that β_2m associates with cell-surface proteins that, somehow, play a role in cell differentiation.

Histocompatibility antigens seem to be markers of self-recognition (Zinkernagel and Doherty, 1974). The T cell recognizes an "altered-self" antigen formed by an interaction between H-2-coded structures at the D and K regions of the major histocompatibility complex (MHC) and the "inducing" antigen (Doherty et al., 1976). The mechanism by which antigen associates with MHC-coded gene products is not yet clear, but the two concepts that are favored are the "altered-self" and "dual-recognition" models (Shearer et al., 1975; Schrader and Edelman, 1976).

Because the organ-specific neoantigen coisolates with β_2m and when analyzed on SDS gel electrophoresis resembles the pattern of histocompatibility antigens, we suggested that the organ-specific neoantigen may well be part of an "altered-self" histocompatibility antigen (Thomson et al., 1976). Other possibilities include: HLA molecules act as adapters that combine with the antigenic molecule to form hybrid antigens, containing elements of self and nonself, or the organ-specific neoantigens could be expressed separately on the cell surface, but share many of the structural and antigenic features of the HLA antigens (Thomson et al., 1978).

The *HLA* complex consists of a set of genes on chromosome 6 that controls polymorphic cell-surface antigens that provoke graft rejection. The known loci span sufficient DNA to code for about 2000 average proteins, but at present much of the DNA has no defined function. So yet another possibility is that the organ-specific neoantigens are like embryonic analogues of the adult HLA antigens, each system operating as mediator of cell–cell recognition, the former functioning only in the embryo and the latter both in the fetus and in the adult. With the development of a neoplasm, cell differentiation is blocked, and the embryonic analogues of the MHC are expressed. But why the organ-specific neoantigens should be immunogenic in the adult host if they are coded for by a normal gene locus is not understood.

4.3. Isolation from Serum

As the tumor grows, tumor antigen is shed from the cell surface membranes into the local milieu, and eventaully, when the tumor mass has grown larger, antigen escapes into the systemic circulation. Some of the organ-specific neoantigens are eliminated by kidney filtration after being degraded to a molecular weight of 48,000 from their high-molecular-weight form (Lopez and Thomson, 1977).

Sera from patients with advanced malignant melanoma when incubated with LAI$^+$ leukocytes from patients with malignant melanoma block the response in an immunologically specific manner (Fig. 1). On a molecular-sieve column, the putative antigen elutes in the molecular-weight range of 80,000–150,000 or more (Lopez and Thomson, 1977; Thomson et al., 1980b); like HLA antigens, it is precipitated by polyanions and coisolates with the high-density lipoprotein (HDL) fraction of serum (Allison et al., 1977; Lopez and Thomson, 1977). The HDL fraction of serum elutes in a broad peak in the excluded and included volumes of a Sephadex G150 column; tumor antigen activity is found in this peak. Also, a small protein peak that has antigen activity is often observed at a molecular

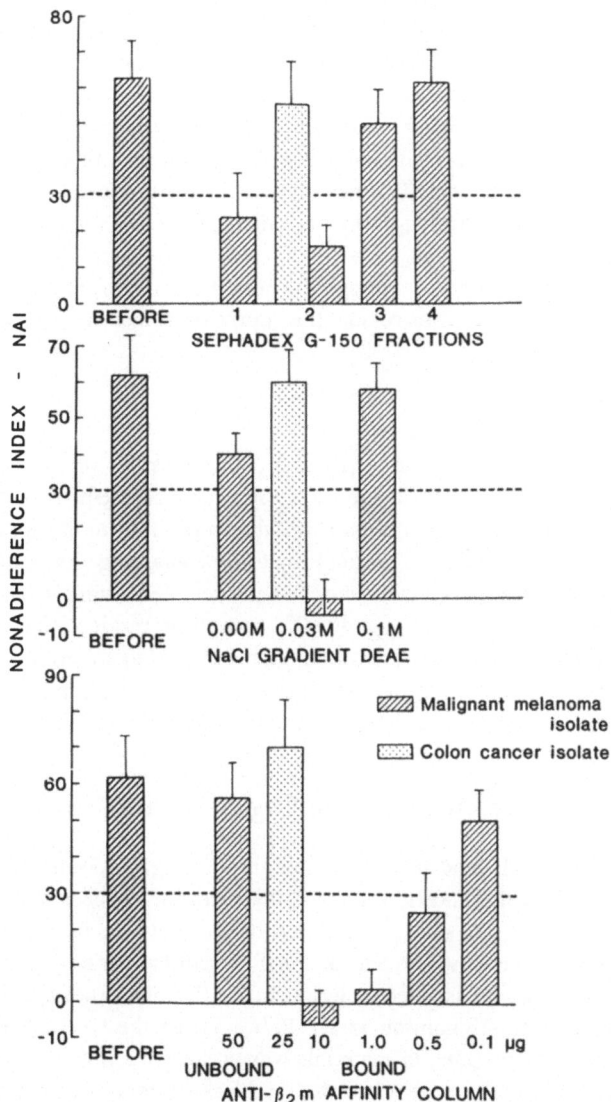

FIGURE 2. Results of testing of isolates for tumor-antigen activity by their ability to negate the LAI[+] response of leukocytes from melanoma patients. *Top:* NAI of leukocytes before and after incubation with papain-solubilized melanoma membrane materials isolated from a Sephadex G150 column. Fraction 2, material eluting from 80,000 to 150,000, negates the LAI response, but similarly prepared colon material does not. Though not observed with this sample, antigen activity is often noted in other fractions. *Middle:* The results show that the papain-soluble antigen elutes from a DEAE ion-exchange column at a low salt concentration. *Bottom:* The results show that the papin-soluble melanoma antigen, applied to an anti-human β_2m affinity column, is in the fraction that is retained and then eluted by 3.0 M KSCN. Those fractions that negate LAI activity are then tested on LAI+ leukocytes from patients with a different cancer to prove that the blocking is specific.

weight of about 48,000. The fact that the serum-derived cell-surface components such as HLA antigen and the organ-specific neoantigen coisolate with HDL material is consistent with the proposed nature of integral membrane proteins. Singer and Nicholson (1972) have proposed that these molecules are relatively hydrophobic and embedded in the lipid bilayer of the plasma membrane. Organ-specific neoantigens and HLA antigens found in serum are likely in a relatively native configuration and are present as discrete molecular entities associated with lipids and lipoproteins similar to those present in their native environment on the cell surface. Moreover, these findings suggest that the organ-specific neoantigens are secreted from the cell surface during normal cell metabolism and not released primarily as a result of cell death.

When we tried to purify the organ-specific neoantigens from serum, their lipoprotein structure created difficulties; for this reason, this source for tumor antigens was abandoned.

4.4. Isolation from Urine

The tumor antigens from urine of patients with metastatic breast and colon cancer were partially purified by a combination of physicochemical methods and affinity chromatography using IgG from the sera of patients who were LAI^+ to the appropriate cancer antigen (Thomson et al., 1980a). The final material, containing the putative breast- or colon-cancer tumor antigen, was greatly enriched and revealed a unique band on SDS gels at a molecular weight of about 38,000–40,000, as well as residual fine bands at about 25,000–30,000, which, seemingly, were contaminants. The β_2m subunit, though observed, was lost in the latter isolation steps (Thomson et al., 1980a). In a similar manner, organ-specific neoantigens of malignant melanoma have been partially purified.

4.5. Recent Progress in Purification of Organ-Specific Neoantigens

Though we have had some success in isolating the organ-specific neoantigens from various sources and differing cancers, as yet no tumor antigen has been purified sufficiently for sequencing. Until now, the slow progress has been largely the fault of the LAI assay. Initially, tumor isolates were substituted for the PBS cancer extracts, consuming considerable quantities of the scarce, isolated materials in the titration process and leaving insufficient material to continue (Thomson et al., 1976). When the blocking LAI assay was introduced, excessive consumption of materials was no longer a problem, and enrichment of antigen activity could be calculated because the blocking assay was not affected by the protein concentration of the isolates. Then, the limiting factor became an adequate supply of LAI^+ leukocytes, for these came from patients with small cancers before surgery. Obviously, these patients were not plentiful. Supplies of LAI^+ leukocytes became ample with the discovery that PGE_2-stimulated leukocytes from advanced cancer patients now responded positively. Now, the greater availability of reactive cells means that new approaches can be tried, and more fractions can be prepared and tested from each isolation step. By pooling only those fractions with LAI activity, more impurities can be eliminated at each isolation step. Thus, we have recently turned our attention to examining what additional steps could be used to yield a pure tumor antigen.

The principal problem associated with using the anti-β_2m affinity-column step is that light and heavy chains of γ-gobulin bleed from the column and contaminate the bound and eluted isolate. When we tried to purify the organ-specific neoantigen without the affinity column by a combination of diethylaminoethyl (DEAE) ion-exchange chromatography, preparative isoelectric focusing, and molecular-sieve chromatography, the final active isolate still contained too many components as determined by SDS and two-dimensional (2-D) gel electrophoresis. To the contrary, material isolated by the anti-β_2m affinity chromatography contains about 3 heavy bands and some minor components by SDS gel electrophoresis and from 10 to 30 discrete spots by 2-D gel electrophoresis. What we believe to be a major contaminant, at least in part, is a component with a molecular weight of 28,000 or so and with a heterogeneous charge, for it runs across the whole 2-D gel, from acidic to alkaline ends; seemingly, at least some of this protein is light chain.

To separate the putative tumor antigen isolated from the anti-β_2m affinity column from the contaminants, we examined preparative isoelectric focusing. The LAI-active material was found in the pI range of 5.5–6.0, but it still contained some of the 28,000-molecular-weight polypeptides. Agarose-gel electrophoresis did not adequately separate the LAI-active material from the 28,000-molecular-weight polypeptides or other minor contaminants. The best method investigated so far seems to be hydroxyapatite chromatography, for it separates most of the light chains, as determined by double-antibody precipitation, and other contaminants from the organ-specific neoantigen, yet achieves good recovery of the antigen.

Another promising separation technique that we have used only a few times and that needs to be examined further is high-performance liquid chromatography (HPLC)–steric exclusion and ion exchange. On steric-exclusion HPLC, the material with putative tumor antigen activity—papain-solubilized from tumor-cell membranes and separated by DEAE ion-exchange chromatography before being isolated by anti-B$_2$m affinity chromatography—showed discrete protein peaks at molecular weights of about 160,000, 38,000, 28,000, and 12,000. The 38,000, 28,000, and 12,000 protein peaks contained LAI-active material; the lower-molecular-weight products seem to be fragments of the whole molecule on which the putative antigenic site is situated. Presumably, the higher-molecular-weight forms of the molecule, often noted when the antigen was isolated first by molecular-sieve chromatography (Thomson et al., 1976), represent dimerized polypeptide chains that are disrupted by eluting the antigens from the affinity column with 3 M KSCN.

Urine from patients with metastatic cancer is a plentiful source of organ-specific neoantigen. But when we tried to expand the scale of isolation by affinity chromatography with γ-globulin from LAI$^+$ patients, the quantity of contaminants, presumably light chain bleeding from the affinity columns, became a serious drawback for this method; consequently, we turned to using physiocochemical separation methods.

The first problem in isolating a sufficient quantity of tumor antigen from urine is the large volumes of fluid that have to be concentrated. The 2-liter Amicon® stirred cell works well in concentrating 50–200 liters of urine. DEAE ion-exchange chromatography, using a shallow, stepwise salt gradient, rapidly separates tumor antigen from most urinary protein. Blue-Sepharose CL-4B® affinity chromatography removes albumin. And an anti-human light chain affinity column is essential to remove the abundant light chains that because of their heterogeneous charge and dimerization are difficult to separate completely from the tumor antigens. Steric-exclusion chromatography, Sephadex G-75® superfine, separated low- and high-molecular-weight contaminants from the tumor antigen. Still other

contaminants were removed by hydroxyapatite chromatography. This approach to puri-
fying the tumor antigen yields about 2 mg of material from 100-liters of urine that is markedly enriched for LAI activity. The material seems to contain tumor antigen of different
molecular weights, with some of the higher-molecular-weight material being aggregates.
Analyzed by SDS gel electrophoresis, the material has major polypeptide chains at molecular weights of about 38,000, 28,000, and 12,000.

Although the organ-specific neoantigens elute at similar points on molecular-sieve,
ion-exchange, and hydroxyapatite chromatography, we have noticed slight but consistent
differences in their behavior when they are isolated by these physicochemical techniques.
The variations in their behavior on physicochemical separation may originate from the
different amino acid residues that create each organ-specific antigenic epitope.

As yet, no xenogeneic animal immunized with isolated material containing the organ-
specific neoantigen has produced an antiserum with unmistakable specificity for the organ-
specific neoantigen epitope. Still, the antisera seem to be able to bind the organ-specific
neoantigens, probably through the recognition of a common determinant that is defined by
the framework structure of a heavy chain. Table I summarizes the features of the organ-
specific neoantigen of malignant melanoma.

TABLE I

*Summary of the Features of the Organ-Specific Neoantigen of Malignant Melanoma Recognized
by the Tumor-Bearing Host's Response*

Procedure	Source		
	Solid tumor (papain-solubilized)	Serum[a]	Urine[a]
Steric-exclusion chromatography, Sephadex G150	$\approx$ 80,000–150,000 mol. wt.	80,000 to >150,000 mol. wt.	$\approx$ 40,000 mol. wt.
DEAE ion-exchange chromatography	Eluted with low salt molarity	N.D.	Eluted with low salt molarity
Preparative isoelectric focusing (pI)	$\approx$ 5.5–6.1	N.D.	$\approx$ 5.6–6.1
Hydroxyapatite chromatography	Eluted with low phosphate molarity		Eluted with low phosphate molarity
Affinity chromatography, anti-human β_2m	Binds specifically	N.D.	N.D.
IgG from LAI$^+$ patients	Binds specifically	Binds specifically	Binds specifically
HPLC, steric exclusion	β_2m isolate: peaks at 160,000, 38,000, 28,000, 12,000 mol. wt.	N.D.	Peaks at 38,000, 28,000 mol. wt.
SDS gel electrophoresis	β_2m isolate: bands at 12,000, 25,000, 40,000 mol. wt.		IgG isolate: bands at 25,000, 30,000, 38,000 mol. wt.
Xenogeneic antisera to tumor-antigen epitope	None	None	None

[a](N.D.) Not determined.

5. Summary

The organ-specific neoantigen exhibited by malignant melanoma is physicochemically similar to other neoantigens expressed by cancers arising in other organs. Nonetheless, subtle differences exist in the organ-specific neoantigens, for those of each organ are recognized separately by the tumor-bearing host's immune response. The difference in the organ-specific neoantigens from one organ to another is probably no greater than are the allotypes of HLA antigens from each other. No doubt, the antigenic determinant on the polypeptide chain that is responsible for organ specificity will reside in a small number of amino acid residues located on the surface of the molecule. The organ-specific antigenic determinant of the protein is probably dependent on the conformation of the native molecule, so it is not essential for the amino acid residues of an antigenic determinant to be sequentially adjacent in the primary structure of the molecule. The folding of a polypeptide chain into a compact globular-shaped protein will bring some sequentially distant amino acid residues into spatial proximity; thus, the amino acid residues of an antigenic determinant can be sequentially distant but spatially adjacent in the secondary structure. In this event, the antigenic determinant depends strongly on the native configuration of the molecule. Further, it might be expected that all organ-specific neoantigens will have a similar framework structure or common portion, which may even be identical to proteins expressed on fully differentiated cells of the same organ, and it will be a hypervariable region that bestows organ specificity.

The significance of the organ-specific neoantigens in ontogeny is unknown, but clearly each cancer cell, no matter how undifferentiated it appears morphologically, expresses this cell-surface protein. Seemingly, the organ-specific neoantigen is coded for by the cell genome, and so it is not a new, unique antigen like tumor-specific transplantation antigens of chemically induced animal tumors. If this is a molecule that is normally expressed by stem cells, it is indeed curious how this antigen has not induced self-tolerance during fetal development. When this antigen is purified and sequenced, not only should it prove possible to develop new, simple immunodiagnostic assays, but also, given knowledge of the structure of the tumor antigen, possibly its relationship to other cell-surface proteins and its biological significance in the neoplastic process might then be better understood.

ACKNOWLEDGMENTS. The author's research cited herein was supported by grants from the Medical Research Council of Canada, The National Cancer Institute of Canada, and The Cancer Research Society, Inc., of Montreal.

References

Allison, J. P., Pellegrino, M. A., Ferrone, S., Callahan G. N., and Reisfeld, R. A., 1977, Biologic and chemical characterization of HLA antigens in human serum, *J. Immunol.* **118**:1004.

Ayeni, R. O., MacFarlane, J. K., and Thomson, D. M. P., 1980, A computerized tube leukocyte adherence inhibition assay to detect antitumor immunity in early human cancer: A review of two years' experience, *Surgery* **87**:380.

Baldwin, R. W., 1975, *In vitro* assays of cell-mediated immunity to human solid tumors: Problems of quantitation, specificity and interpretation, *J. Natl. Cancer Inst.* **55**:745.

Baldwin, R. W., and Glaves, D., 1972, Solubilization of tumor-specific antigen from plasma membrane of an aminoazo dye-induced rat hepatoma, *Clin. Exp. Immunol.* **11**:51.

Cheung, W. Y., 1980, Calmodulin plays a pivotal role in cellular regulation, *Science* **207**:19.

Doherty, P. C., Blanden, R. V., and Zinkernagel, R. M., 1976, Specificity of virus immune effector T cells for H-2K or H-2D compatible interactions: Implications for H-antigen diversity, *Transplant. Rev.* **29**:8.

Farber, E., Cameron, R. G., and Laishes, B. A., 1979, Physiological and molecular markers during carcinogenesis, in: *Carcinogens: Identification and Mechanisms of Action*, p. 319, Raven Press, New York.

Fellous, M., Gunther, E., Kemler, R., Wiels, J., Berger, R., Guenet, J. L., Jakob, H., and Jacob, F., 1978, Association of the H-Y male antigen with β_2-microglobulin on human lymphoid and differentiated mouse teratocarcinoma cell lines, *J. Exp. Med.* **148**:58.

Flores, M., Thomson, D. M. P., and MacFarlane, J. K., 1976, Effect of surgery on antitumor immunity measured by tube leukocyte adherence inhibition assay in breast cancer, *Surg. Forum* **27**:91.

Flores, M., Marti, J. H., Grosser, N., MacFarlane, J. K., and Thomson, D. M. P., 1977, An overview: Antitumor immunity in breast cancer assayed by tube leukocyte adherence inhibition, *Cancer* **39**:494.

Foreman, J. C., and Lichtenstein, L. M., 1980, Clinical pharmacology of acute allergic disorders, *Annu. Rev. Med.* **31**:181.

Foulds, L., 1975, Neoplastic Development, in: *Neoplastic Development*, Vol. 2 (L. Foulds, ed.), pp. 549–636, Academic Press, New York.

Fritze, D., Schulte-Uentrop, C., and Kaufmann, M., 1979, Leukocyte adherence inhibition (LAI) tests in patients clinically suspected of having breast cancer using a panel of breast carcinoma extracts, *Eur. J. Cancer* **15**:1491.

Fujisawa, T., Waldman, S. R., and Yonemoto, R. H., 1977, Leukocyte adherence inhibition by soluble tumor antigens in breast cancer patients, *Cancer* **39**:506.

Grosser, N., and Thomson, D. M. P., 1975, Cell-mediated immunity in breast cancer patients evaluated by antigen-induced leukocyte adherence inhibition in test tubes, *Cancer Res.* **35**:2571.

Grosser, N., and Thomson, D. M. P., 1976, Tube leukocyte (monocyte) adherence inhibition assay for the detecting of anti-tumour immunity. III. "Blockade" of monocyte reactivity by excess free antigen and immune complexes in advanced cancer patients, *Int. J. Cancer* **18**:58.

Grosser, N., Marti, J. H., Proctor, J. W., and Thomson, D. M. P., 1976, Tube leukocyte adherence inhibition assay for the detection of anti-tumour immunity. I. Monocyte is the reactive cell, *Int. J. Cancer* **18**:39.

Grosser, N., Thomson, D. M. P., Flores, M., and MacFarlane, J. K., 1980, A mechanism of suppression of anti-tumor immunity (LAI reactivity) by surgery, *Cancer Immunol. Immunother.* **7**:263.

Halliday, W. J., and Miller, S., 1972, Leukocyte adherence inhibition: A simple test for cell-mediated tumor immunity and serum blocking factors, *Int. J. Cancer* **9**:477.

Halliday, W. J., Maluish, A. E., Little, J. H., and Davis, N. L., 1975, Leukocyte adherence inhibition and specific immunoreactivity in malignant melanoma, *Int. J. Cancer* **16**:645.

Halliday, W. J., Maluish, A. E., and Stephenson, P. M., 1977, An evaluation of leukocyte adherence inhibition in the immunodiagnosis of colorectal cancer, *Cancer Res.* **37**:1962.

Herberman, R. B., and Oldham, R. K., 1975, Problems associated with study of cell-mediated immunity to human tumors by microcytotoxicity assays, *J. Natl. Cancer Inst.* **55**:749.

Holan, V., Hasek, M., Bubenik, J., and Jitka, C. H., 1974, Antigen-mediated macrophage adherence inhibition, *Cell. Immunol.* **13**:107.

Holliday, R., 1979, A new theory of carcinogenesis. *Br. J. Cancer* **40**:513.

Kaneti, J., Thomson, D. M. P., and Reid, E. C., 1981, Prostaglandin E_2 affects the tumor immune response in prostatic carcinoma, *J. Urol.* **126**:65.

Khosravi, M., Liao, S. K., and Dent, P. B., 1980, Relationship of melanoma associated antigens to histocompatibility antigen and β-2 microglobulin in material spontaneously shed by cultured human melanoma cells, Presented at the *XIth International Pigment Cell Conference*, Sendai, Japan, October 1980.

Khosravi, M., Liao, S. K., Thomson, D. M. P., and Dent, P. B., 1982, Relationship of melanoma-associated antigens to histocompatibility antigen and β_2 microglobulin in material spontaneously shed by cultured human melanoma cells (submitted).

Levenson, S. H., Howell, J. H., Holyoke, E. D., and Goldrosen, M. H., 1977, Leukocyte adherence inhibition:

an automated microassay demonstrating specific antigen recognition and ablocking activity in two-murine tumor systems, *J. Immunol. Meth.* **17**:153.

Lopez, M. J., and Thomson, D. M. P., 1977, Isolation of breast cancer tumour antigen from serum and urine. *Int. J. Cancer* **20**:834–848.

Lopez, M., O'connor, R., MacFarlane, J. K., and Thomson, D. M. P., 1978, The natural history of antitumour immunity in human breast cancer assayed by tube leucocyte adherence inhibition, *Br. J. Cancer* **38**:660.

Malley, A., Burger, D. R., Vandenbark, A. A., Frikke, M., Finke, P., Begley, D., Acott, K., Black, J., and Vetto, R. M., 1979, Association of melanoma tumor antigen activity with β_2-microglobulin, *Cancer Res.* **39**:619.

Maluish, A. E., and Halliday, W. J., 1979, Hemocytometer leukocyte adherence inhibition technique, *Cancer Res.* **39**:625.

Marti, J., and Thomson, D. M. P., 1976, Anti-tumour immunity in malignant melanoma assay by tube leucocyte-adherence inhibition, *Br. J. Cancer* **34**:116.

Marti, J. H., Grosser, N., and Thomson, D. M. P., 1976, Tube leukocyte adherence inhibition assay for the detection of anti-tumour immunity. II. Monocyte reacts with tumour antigen via cytophilic antitumour antibody, *Int. J. Cancer* **18**:48.

McCabe, A., Ferrone, S., Pellegrino, M. A., Kern, D. H., Holmes, E. C., and Reisfeld, R. A., 1978, Purification and immunologic evaluation of human melanoma-associated antigens, *J. Natl. Cancer Inst.* **60**:773.

Michailson, J., Flaherty, L., Vitetta, E., and Poulik, M. D., 1977, Molecular similarities between the Qa2 alloantigen and and other gene products of the 17th chromosome of the mouse, *J. Exp. Med.* **145**:1066.

Nakamuro, K., Tanigaki, N., and Pressman, D., 1977, Common antigenic structures of HLA antigens. VII. Selective combination binding of β_2-microglobulin with HLA large component in cultured human cell lines, *Immunology* **32**:139.

O'Connor, R., MacFarlane, J. K., Murray, D., and Thomson, D. M. P., 1978, A study of false positive and negative responses in the tube leucocyte adherence inhibition (tube LAI) assay, *Br. J. Cancer* **38**:674.

Ogawa, K., Medline, A., and Farber, E., 1979, Sequential analysis of hepatic carcinogenesis: The comparative architecture of preneoplastic, malignant, prenatal, postnatal and regenerating liver, *Br. J. Cancer* **40**:782.

Ostberg, L., Rask, L., Wigzell, H., and Peterson, P. A., 1975, Thymus leukaemia antigen contains β_2-microglobulin, *Nature (London)* **253**:735–737.

Potter, V. R., 1978, Phenotypic diversity in experimental hepatomas: The concept of partially blocked ontogeny, *Br. J. Cancer* **38**:1.

Powell, A. E., Sloss, A. M., Smith, R. N., Makley, J. T., and Hubay, C. E., 1975, Specific responsiveness of leukocytes to soluble extracts of human tumors, *Int. J. Cancer* **16**:905.

Robb, R. J., Strominger, J. L., and Mann, D. L., 1976, Rapid purification of detergent-solubilized HLA antigens by affinity chromatography employing anti-β_2-microglobulin serum, *J. Biol. Chem.* **251**:5427.

Rudczynski, A. B., Dyer, C. A., and Mortensen, R. F., 1978, Detection of cell-mediated immune reactivity of breast cancer patients by the leukocyte adherence inhibition response to MCF-7 extracts, *Cancer Res.* **38**:3590.

Russo, A. J., Douglass, H. O., Jr., Leveson, S. H., Howell, J. H., Holyoke, E. D., Harvey, S. R., Chu, T. M., and Goldrosen, M. H., 1978, Evaluation of the microleukocyte adherence inhibition assay as an immunodiagnostic test for pancreatic cancer, *Cancer Res.* **38**:2023.

Rutherford, J. C., Walters, B. A. J., Cavage, G., and Halliday, W. J. 1977, A modified leukocyte adherence inhibition test in the laboratory investigation of gastrointestinal cancer, *Int. J. Cancer* **19**:43.

Sanderson, A. R., 1977, HLA "help" for human β_2-microglobulin across species barriers, *Nature, (London)* **269**:414.

Sanner, T., Brennhovd, I., Christensen, I., Jorgensen, O., and Kvaloy, S., 1979, Cellular antitumor immune response in women with risk factors for breast cancer, *Cancer Res.* **39**:654.

Sanner, T., Kotlar, H. K., and Eker, P., 1980, Immune response in lung cancer patients measured by a modified leukocyte adherence inhibition test using serum, *Cancer Lett.* **8**:283.

Schrader, J. W., and Edelman, G. M., 1976, Participation of the H-2 antigens of tumor cells in their lysis by syngeneic T cells, *J. Exp. Med.* **143**:601.

Shani, A., Ritts, R. E., Jr., and Thynne, G. S., 1978, A prospective evaluation of the leukocyte adherence inhibition test in colorectal cancer and its correlation with carcinoembryonic antigen levels, *Int. J. Cancer* **22**:113.

Shearer, G. M. Rehn, T. G., and Garbarino, C. A., 1975, Cell mediated lympholysis of trinitrophenyl-modified autologous lynphocytes: Effector cell specificity to modified cell surface components by the H-2K and H-2D serological regions of the murine major histocompatibility complex, *J. Exp. Med.* **141**:1348.

Shuster, J., Thomson, D. M. P., and Gold, P., 1978, Immunodiagnosis, in: *Immunological Aspects of Cancer* (J. E. Castro, ed.), Chapt. 12, pp. 283–312, M.T.P. Press, Lancaster, England.

Singer, S. J., and Nicholson, G. L., 1972, The fluid mosaic model of the structure of cell membranes; cell membranes are viewed as two-dimensional solutions of oriented gobular proteins and lipids, *Science* **175**:720.

Tada, N., Tanigaki, N., and Pressman, D., 1978, Human cell membrane components bound to β_2-microglobulin in T cell-type lines, *J. Immunol.* **120**:513.

Tataryn, D. N., MacFarlane, J. K., and Thomson, D. M. P., 1978, Leucocyte adherence inhibition for detecting specific tumour immunity in early pancreatic cancer, *Lancet* **1**:1020.

Tataryn, D. N., MacFarlane, J. K., Murray, D., and Thomson, D. M. P., 1979, Tube leukocyte adherence inhibition (LAI) assay in gastrointestinal (GIT) cancer, *Cancer* **43**:898.

Thomson, D. M. P., 1979, Demonstration of tube leukocyte adherence inhibition assay with coded samples of blood, *Cancer Res.* **39**:627.

Thomson, D. M. P., and Alexander, P., 1973, A cross-reacting embryonic antigen in the membrane of rat sarcoma cells which is immunogenic in the syngeneic host, *Br. J. Cancer* **27**:35.

Thomson, D. M. P., Eccles, S., and Alexander, P., 1973, Antibodies and soluble tumour-specific antigens in blood and lymph of rats with chemically induced sarcomata, *Br. J. Cancer* **28**:6.

Thomson, D. M. P., Gold, P., Freedman, S. O., and Shuster, J., 1976, The isolation and characterization of tumor-specific antigens of rodent and human tumors, *Cancer Res.* **36**:3518.

Thomson, D. M. P., Rauch, J. E., Weatherhead, J. C., Friedlander, P., O'Connor, R., Grosser, N., Shuster, J., and Gold, P., 1978, Isolation of human tumour-specific antigens associated with β_2-microglobulin, *Br. J. Cancer* **37**:753.

Thomson, D. M. P., Tataryn, D. N., Lopez, M., Schwartz, R., and MacFarlane, J. K., 1979a, Human tumor-specific immunity assayed by a computerized tube leukocyte adherence inhibition, *Cancer Res.* **39**:638.

Thomson, D. M. P., Tataryn, D. N., O'Connor, R., Rauch, J., Friedlander, P., Gold, P., and Shuster, J., 1979b, Evidence for the expression of human tumor-specific antigens associated with β_2-microglobulin in human cancer and in some colon adenomas and benign breast lesions, *Cancer Res.* **39**:604.

Thomson, D. M. P., Tataryn, D. N., and Schwartz, R., 1980a, Partial purification of organ-specific neoantigens from human colon and breast cancer by affinity chromatography with human toumour-specific γ globulin, *Br. J. Cancer* **41**:86.

Thomson, D. M. P., Tataryn, D. N., Weatherhead, J. C., Friedlander, P., Rauch, J., Schwartz, R., Gold, P., and Shuster, J., 1980b, A human colon tumour antigen associated with β_2-microglobulin and isolated from solid tumour, serum and urine is unrelated to carcinoembryonic antigen, *Eur. J. Cancer* **16**:539.

Thomson, D. M. P., Ayeni, R. O., MacFarlane, J. K., Tataryn, D. N., Terrin, M., Schraufnagel, D., Wilson, J., and Mulder, D. S., 1981a, A coded study of anti-tumor immunity to human lung cancer assayed by tube leukocyte adherence inhibition, *Ann. Thorac. Surg.* **31**:314.

Thomson, D. M. P., Neville, A. M., Phelan, K., Schwartz-Scanzano, R., and Vandevoorde, J. P., 1981b, Human cancers transplanted in nude mice retain the expression of their organ-specific neoantigens, *Eur. J. Cancer Clin.Oncol.* **17**:1191.

Weinhouse, S., and Ono, T., 1972, *Isozymes and Enzyme Regulation in Cancer,* University Park Press, Baltimore.

Zinkernagel, R. M., and Doherty, P. C., 1974, Immunological surveillance against altered self components by sensitized T lymphocytes in lymphocytic choriomeningitis, *Nature (London)* **251**:547.

22

Immunochemical Analysis of the Antigenic Profile of Human Melanoma Cells with Monoclonal Antibodies

Barry S. Wilson, Kohzoh Imai, Pier-Giorgio Natali, Neil E. Kay, Renato Cavaliere, Michele A. Pellegrino, and Soldano Ferrone

1. Introduction

Tumor immunologists have been investigating the antigenic profile of cancer cells in order to define cellular changes induced by malignant transformation. Characterization of these changes may aid our understanding of the interaction between tumor cells and the host's immune system, may identify markers to determine the molecular basis of malignant transformation, and may provide unique antigenic determinants to apply immunological approaches for diagnosis and therapy of tumors. We have focused our efforts on melanoma, since this tumor represents a type of human cancer in which the immune response is believed to participate in its pathogenicity and may affect its clinical course. This belief is supported by clinical evidence and by the detection of cellular and humoral immunity to tumor-associated antigens in melanoma patients. Interested readers may refer to recent reviews on these topics (Hellström and Hellström, 1974; Ferrone and Pellegrino, 1978, 1979; Mastrangelo *et al.*, 1979). We have investigated the expression of cytoplasmic and

Barry S. Wilson, Kohzoh Imai, Neil E. Kay, Michele A. Pellegrino, and Soldano Ferrone • Department of Molecular Immunology, Scripps Clinic and Research Foundation, La Jolla, California 92037. Pier-Giorgio Natali and Renato Cavaliere • Istituto Regina Elena, 00161 Rome, Italy. Present Address for Dr. Wilson: Department of Pathology, University of Michigan Medical School, Ann Arbor, Michigan 48109.

plasma-membrane-bound tumor-associated antigens as well as of histocompatibility antigens on human melanoma cells. The latter antigens have been included in our studies because of their role as informational molecules in the immune response (Benacerraf and McDevitt, 1972) and because of their functional and structural relationships with tumor-associated antigens in certain tumor systems (Callahan et al., 1978; Curry et al., 1979).

In this chapter, we will first examine melanoma cells for the presence of alien histocompatibility antigens, which will then be analyzed for structural and functional properties; we will then outline our serological and immunochemical approaches to identify tumor-associated antigens with monoclonal xenoantibodies and describe the characteristics of three types of these antigens. We use the term tumor-associated antigens to describe antigens other than histocompatibility antigens that are present in tumors but absent from their non malignant counterparts. This category may also include differentiation antigens. Finally, we will discuss the biological relevance and the clinical implications of our results.

2. Expression of Histocompatibility Antigens on Human Melanoma Cells

In several animal systems, malignant transformation of cells is associated with changes in the quantity of histocompatibility antigens detectable on the cell membrane (for reviews, see Cikes and Friberg, 1977; Callahan et al., 1978; Curry et al., 1979) and/or with the appearance of histocompatibility alloantigens alien to the phenotype of the host from which the tumor was derived (for reviews, see Callahan et al., 1978; Parmiani et al., 1979). Alien histocompatibility antigens may differ structurally from their normally expressed counterparts. For example, murine alien H-2 alloantigens have been reported to differ from their normally expressed H-2 alloantigens in susceptibility to papain digestion, behavior during gel filtration, and affinity for β_2-microglobulin (Rogers et al., 1979). The biological relevance of alien histocompatibility antigens is suggested by the well-tested theory that gene products of the major histocompatibility complex play a decisive role in cell–cell interactions (for reviews, see Eichmann, 1980; Thorsby et al., 1981) and by the report that alien histocompatibility antigens may either influence or be a target for the host's antitumor immune response (for reviews, see Fujiwara et al., 1978; Martin and Imamura, 1980).

The existence of alien histocompatibility antigens on human tumor cells is suggested by the observations that some human tumor cells react abnormally with HLA-A and B alloantisera in the cytotoxic test (Takasugi and Terasaki, 1972) and that HLA-B5-negative fibroblasts may acquire the ability to absorb HLA-B5 alloantisera after transformation with simian virus 40 (Pellegrino et al., 1976). We have tested human melanoma cells for their HLA-A, B antigenic profile in order to detect the appearance of genetically inappropriate HLA-A, B allospecificities. In addition, we have tested melanoma cells for the expression of Ia-like antigens, a type of histocompatibility antigen that is not expressed on normal melanocytes (Natali et al., 1981). The Ia-like antigens, which include the HLA-DR antigens, are a highly polymorphic series of molecules restricted in tissue distribution and central to cell–cell communications within the immune system (for a review, see Ferrone et al., 1978).

2.1. HLA-A, B Antigens

The HLA-A,B antigenic profile of 20 cultured human melanoma cell lines was determined in a quantitative adsorption assay (Pellegrino *et al.*, 1972) designed to avoid spurious reactions caused by the abnormal susceptibility of melanoma cells to complement-dependent lysis (Ferrone and Pellegrino, 1977) and/or by the interference of contaminating antibodies that are usually present in operationally specific HLA-A,B alloantisera. Although more accurate than direct typing, this approach restricts the number of HLA-A, B alloantigens that can be analyzed, since the majority of HLA alloantisera available in our laboratory contain low-titer and low-affinity antibodies, making them unsuitable for the adsorption assay. The results of testing 20 cultured human melanoma cell lines for their ability to adsorb alloantisera to HLA-A1, A2, A3, A9, A10, B5, B7, B8, B12, and B17 revealed three cases in which more than two allospecificities could be detected at one of the *HLA-A, B* loci: cell lines M4 and MF4 expressed specificities 2, 3, and 9 at locus *A* and both cell lines HS 597 T and HS 695 T expressed specificities 5, 12, and 17 at locus *B* (Pellegrino *et al.*, 1981). However, in each instance, this extra allospecificity could be explained by serological cross-reactivity within the *HLA* system. Representative results are shown in Table I.

Comparison of the amounts and the phenotypes of the HLA-A, B antigens of cultured melanoma cells with that of autologous fibroblasts or cultured B-lymphoid cells showed no quantitative or qualitative differences in the majority of the cases studied (Pellegrino *et al.*, 1977, 1981); however, in one case, the melanoma cells expressed a lower level of HLA-A, B alloantigens compared to the autologous B-lymphoid cells, while in another case, some allospecificities absent from the autologous fibroblasts were expressed by the melanoma cells only during the early passage levels in culture. Unfortunately, peripheral-blood lymphocytes (PBL) from the donor of the latter melanoma cell line were unavailable for HLA-

TABLE I

Expression of HLA-A, B Antigens on Autologous Human Melanoma Cells, Fibroblasts, and Lymphoblasts

Cell line		HLA-A[a]					HLA-B[a]				
Code	Derivation	1	2	3	9	10	5	7	8	12	17
M4	Tumor	—	7	8	8	—	3	—	—	15	—
MF4	Skin	—	4	6	8	—	3	—	—	15	—
M10	Tumor	—	—	15	6	—	8	—	—	—	—
ML10	PBL	—	—	14	12	—	6	—	—	—	—
MF10	Skin	—	—	10	8	—	11	—	—	—	—
M15	Tumor	—	—	—	130	—	65	—	—	—	—
ML15	PBL	—	—	—	5	—	5	—	—	—	—
HS 600 T	Tumor	—	20	—	20	—	20	—	—	80	—
HS 600 SK	Skin	—	20	—	20	—	70	—	—	—	—
HS 695 T	Tumor	—	20	250	—	—	20	—	—	20	80
HS 695 SK	Skin	—	20	3	—	—	—	—	—	—	—

[a]Figures are AD_{50} ($\times$ 10^{-2}) values, namely, the number of cells necessary to reduce the cytolytic activity of alloantisera in an antigen-binding inhibition assay by 50%. — Indicates AD_{50} values higher than 500×10^2.

A, B typing, making it impossible to establish whether this transient expression of HLA-A, B allospecificities reflected appearance of genetically inappropriate alloantigens on the tumor cells or loss of alloantigens from the autologous fibroblasts (Table I).

Thus, although differences in the levels of HLA-A, B antigens were noted between melanoma and autologous lymphoblasts and/or fibroblasts, we have not detected any alien HLA-A, B allospecificities on human melanoma cells (Pellegrino *et al.*, 1977, 1981). A similar conclusion has been reached by Pollack *et al.* (1980a, b), who have analyzed the HLA-A, B antigenic profile of cultured melanoma cells.

2.2. Ia-Like Antigens

Testing of cultured melanoma cells with polyclonal and monoclonal xenoantibodies to framework determinants of human Ia-like antigens in serological assays has revealed positive reactions with the majority of melanoma cell lines (Winchester *et al.*, 1978; B. S. Wilson *et al.*, 1979; Herlyn *et al.*, 1980; Howe *et al.*, 1981; Pellegrino *et al.*, 1981) (see also Chapter 4). This unexpected detection of Ia-like antigens on melanoma cells has raised intriguing questions about the functional and structural properties of melanoma-derived Ia-like antigens as well as their clinical significance, especially since it has been reported that the expression of Ia-like antigens on guinea pig leukemic cells is required for immunogenicity of leukemia-specific antigens (Forni *et al.*, 1975) and that the immune response to tumor-associated antigens may influence the clinical course of melanoma (for reviews, see Ferrone and Pellegrino, 1978; Mastrangelo *et al.*, 1979). The evidence that melanoma-derived Ia-like antigens are immunologically functional includes their aforementioned reactivity with xenoantibodies to framework determinants of Ia-like antigens and their binding with antibodies specific for allotypic determinants that define the conventional serological polymorphism of the Ia-like antigenic system (Pollack *et al.*, 1980a, b and unpublished observations). Furthermore, melanoma-derived Ia-like antigens are immunogenic in xenogeneic combinations (B. S. Wilson *et al.*, 1979; Herlyn *et al.*, 1980). However, conflicting results have been reported about the stimulatory activity of melanoma cells in mixed-lymphocyte reactions. According to Pollack *et al.* (1980b), melanoma cells have no stimulatory activity in the primary mixed-lymphocyte reaction, while similar experiments performed in collaboration with Dr. E. Thorsby show that melanoma cells can stimulate to a limited but significant extent in this assay. Finally, studies in collaboration with Dr. Fritz Bach at the University of Minnesota have shown that melanoma cells can stimulate allogeneic lymphocytes in primed lymphocyte typing assays (unpublished results).

The level of Ia-like antigens on melanoma cells is quite variable (Fig. 1), and on cells where the level of Ia-like antigens is low, this occurs probably because of a reduced synthesis rather than an increased shedding of this antigen (B. S. Wilson *et al.*, 1980). The level of Ia-like antigen expression is not changed on melanoma cells incubated *in vitro* with interferon, although the level of HLA-A, B, C antigens and of β_2-microglobulin is significantly increased (Imai *et al.*, 1981c), similar to what was previously found for B-lymphoid cells (Heron *et al.*, 1978; Fellous *et al.*, 1979; Imai *et al.*, 1981d). These data suggest that Ia-like antigen expression is regulated differently from HLA-A, B, C antigen expression and that melanoma cells show no alterations in this regard.

Melanoma-derived Ia-like antigens, like their counterparts synthesized by B-lym-

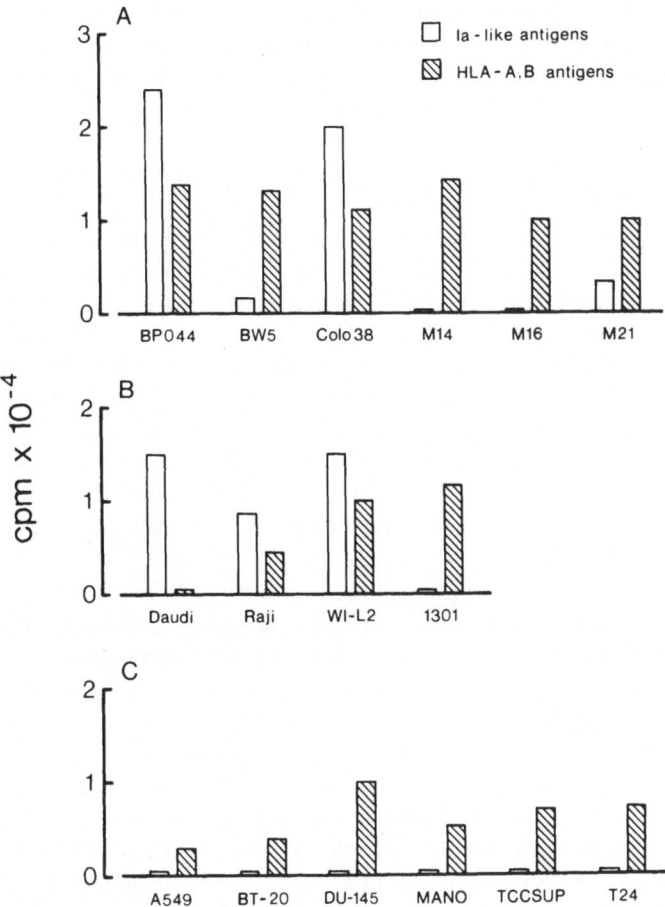

FIGURE 1. Level of expression of histocompatibility antigens on cultured melanoma cell lines (A) in comparison with that on lymphoblastoid cell lines (B) and carcinoma cell lines (C). Cultured cells (2×10^5) were treated with a saturating dose of monoclonal antibody Q5/13 to Ia-like antigens (Quaranta *et al.*, 1980) or Q1/28 to HLA-A,B antigens (Quaranta *et al.*, 1981b) for 1 hr at 4°C. The cells were then incubated with 10^5 cpm [^{125}I]protein A for 30 min, washed, and counted in a gamma counter.

phoid cells, are composed of two noncovalently associated glycopolypeptides (B. S. Wilson *et al.*, 1980). The larger α chain has an approximate molecular weight of 34,000, while the smaller β chain has an approximate molecular weight of 29,000. The β chain of melanoma cells exhibits increased electrophoretic mobility in sodium dodecyl sulfate–polyacrylamide gel electrophoresis (SDS-PAGE) under nonreducing conditions (B. S. Wilson *et al.*, 1980) similar to that for the β chain of B-lymphoid-cell-derived Ia-like antigens (Allison *et al.*, 1978; Ferrone *et al.*, 1978). The peptide maps and the N-terminal amino acid sequences of the Ia-like antigen α and β chains from a melanoma cell line and an autologous B-lymphoid cell line show a high degree of similarity (Alexander *et al.*, 1982). On the other hand, the degree of glycosylation of melanoma-derived Ia-like antigens may differ from that of B-lymphoid-cell derived Ia-like antigens; thus, a cultured melanoma cell line (M10) incorporated more [³H]glucosamine into the α chain relative to the β chain than did the autologous B-lymphoid cell line L10 (Fig. 2), although the two cell lines are similar in the incorporation of [³⁵S]methionine into the two subunits of these antigens (Fig. 3 and Table II). It is not known whether these differences in glycosylation affect the antigenicity of Ia-like antigens; however, this possibility should be considered in light of our recent finding that the carbohydrate moiety can influence the conformation of HLA antigens (B. S. Wilson et al., 1981b).

Ia-like antigens are expressed on freshly explanted melanoma lesions (Herlyn et al., 1980; Natali et al., 1981), indicating that the detection of these antigens on cultured melanoma cells is not an in vitro artifact. Within each lesion, melanoma cells are heterogeneous with respect to the expression of Ia-like antigens, since a variable percentage of tumor cells do not react with antibodies to Ia-like antigens (Natali et al., 1981). This subpopulation may comprise cells that are unable to synthesize these antigens and/or are in a phase of their growth cycle associated with a reduced expression of Ia-like antigens. In addition, the percentage of Ia-like-antigen-bearing melanoma cells within a lesion does not correlate with the primary, recurrent, and metastatic nature of the tumor or with the synthesis of melanin (Natali et al., 1981), but is inversely related to the degree of invasiveness of primary melanoma lesions.

Three lines of evidence suggest that the expression of Ia-like antigens on cells of the melanocyte lineage is restricted to those cells that have undergone malignant transformation: (1) Reaction of a fetal melanocyte cell line with monoclonal and polyclonal xenoantibodies to human Ia-like antigens has yielded negative results in serological assays and in indirect immuneprecipitation studies. (2) Indirect immunofluorescence of biopsies of normal skin and of nevi with monoclonal and polyclonal xenoantibodies to Ia-like antigens has not revealed any staining of melanocytes or of nevic cells. Even melanocytes activated by exposure to UV light or physiologically concentrated at body sites, i.e., breast areola, do not appear to express detectable amounts of Ia-like antigens. (3) Indirect immunofluorescence of premalignant senile freckle lesions with monoclonal antibodies to Ia-like antigens showed staining of those proliferating cells having the morphological characteristic of malignant transformation. These results strongly suggest that testing skin lesions for the expression of Ia-like antigens may help solve controversial diagnoses of melanoma, which occur in about 10% of cases (Truax et al., 1966).

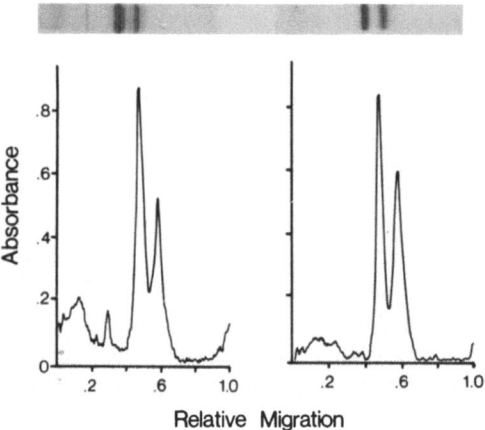

FIGURE 2. Differences in the degree of glycosylation of Ia-like antigens synthesized by autologous melanoma (M10) and B-lymphoid cell lines (L10). The cultured cells were intrinsically labeled with [³H]glucosamine and solubilized with Nonidet P-40 (NP-40), and the Ia-like antigens were immunoprecipitated with monoclonal antibody Q5/13. The α and β subunits of Ia-like antigens were separated by electrophoresis under reducing conditions in a 10% polyacrylamide SDS slab gel. The fluorographs for L10 cells (left) and M10 cells (right) are shown by densitometric tracing at 550 nm. The apparent molecular weights of the α and β chains are approximately 34,000 and 29,000, respectively.

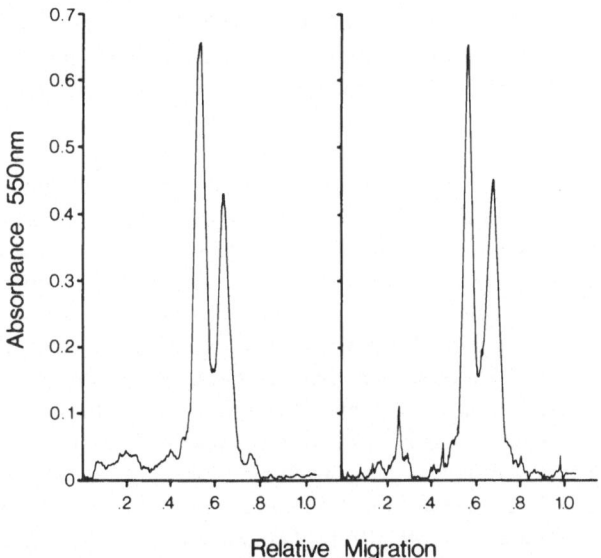

Relative Migration

FIGURE 3. Incorporation of [^{35}S]methionine into Ia-like antigens synthesized by autologous cultured melanoma (M10) and B-lymphoid cells (L10). The cultured cells were intrinsically labeled with [^{35}S]methionine and solubilized with NP-40, and the Ia-like antigens were immunoprecipitated with monoclonal antibody Q5/13. The α and β subunits of Ia-like antigens were separated by electrophoresis under reducing conditions in a 10% polyacrylamide SDS slab gel. The fluorographs for L10 cells *(left)* and M10 cells *(right)* are shown by densitometric tracing at 550 nm. The apparent molecular weights of the α and β chains are approximately 34,000 and 29,000, respectively.

TABLE II

Radioactivity Ratio between α and β Subunits of Ia-Like Antigens Synthesized by Cultured Melanoma (M10) and Autologous B-Lymphoid (L10) Cells

| | α/β Radioactivity ratio | | Ratio |
Radiolabel	L10 cells	M10 cells	difference
[^{3}H]Glucosamine	1.70	1.52	0.28
[^{35}S]Methionine	1.52	1.44	0.08

3. Approaches for Defining Tumor-Associated Antigens with Monoclonal Antibodies

3.1. Serological Approach

This approach was chosen over tests of cell-mediated immunity, since the former is more suited for rapid screening and is not dependent on patient availability. More important, the serological approach generates antibody reagents that greatly facilitate molecular characterization of the target antigens (discussed in detail in the next section), whereas analysis of the molecular profile of antigens detected by cell-mediated-immunity assays requires laborious biochemical procedures. There is at present no proof that these two assays recognize the same or different classes of antigens. In our studies, we employ both cultured melanoma cells and surgically removed melanoma tissues. Melanoma cells in long-term culture are free of other contaminating cell types and can be rapidly expanded to supply a large quantity of a relatively homogeneous tumor-cell population. In addition, analysis of the spent media from cultured cell lines can provide insight into which antigens may be shed into body fluids in quantities suitable for examination by radioimmunoassay. However, relating results with cultured cells to the *in vivo* situation can be misleading and requires that surgically removed melanoma lesions be analyzed before the clinical significance of an antigenic structure identified by a monoclonal antibody can be assessed.

All our studies have been performed with xenoantibodies rather than alloantibodies, because we have analyzed sera from more than 500 melanoma patients and have not found any suitable in titer and affinity for immunochemical analysis. In our early studies, we have used xenoantisera elicited with whole human melanoma cells, human melanoma–murine fibroblast hybrid cells, or soluble antigens isolated from melanoma cells or from their spent culture medium (McCabe *et al.*, 1978, 1979a; Ferrone *et al.*, 1980; Imai and Ferrone, 1980; Imai *et al.*, 1981a; Galloway *et al.*, 1981). However, we now prefer the hybridoma technique for producing xenoantibodies, since their monoclonal nature overcomes the many limitations imposed by conventional xenoantisera (B. S.Wilson *et al.*, 1981a). The procedure we use (Imai *et al.*, 1980, 1981b) is essentially the same as described by Köhler and Milstein (1975). Basically, splenocytes from mice immunized weekly with cultured melanoma cells are isolated 3 days following the last booster and fused with murine myeloma cells in the presence of 30% polyethylene glycol 1000. After an initial 24-hr culture period, the cells are placed in selective medium and then cultured in 96-well microtiter plates.

We use a three-step procedure to select growing hybridomas producing monoclonal antibodies specific for tumor-associated antigens. In the first step, supernatant fluids are tested for reactivity with a small panel of cultured normal and tumor cell lines. This is a conventional way to select antibodies showing promise of tumor-cell specificity. In the second step, these antibodies are sent to many different laboratories to have them independently evaluated for their reativity with normal and malignant cultured human cells; in this way, the number of cell lines used for testing can be greatly enlarged and, more important, the specificity of monoclonal antibodies for tumor-associated antigens can be established for general acceptance by the scientific community. The third step involves testing the antibodies against a large panel of surgically removed normal and malignant tissues so that those antibodies having application for immunotherapy or radioimaging of tumors may be identified.

For detecting the reaction of antibodies with cells, binding assays are preferred over lytic assays because the former are more sensitive and because the latter are complicated by the differential susceptibility of target cells to complement-dependent lysis. We routinely employ a radioimmunometric assay (McCabe *et al.*, 1979b), a rosette assay (Indiveri *et al.*, 1979), and an indirect immunofluorescence test, all of which measure the presence of antibodies on target cells by the uptake of an indirect reagent such as protein A of *Staphylococcus aureus* or an antiimmunoglobulin antibody. The indirect immunofluorescence assay is performed on viable or fixed cultured cells and on cryostat thin sections of fixed human tissues. The use of fixed cultured cells allows the antibody to penetrate the cell plasma membrane and exhibit fluorescent staining of the cytoplasm if detectable levels of antigen are present. We routinely employ acetone as the fixative because it retains the most detail after staining. The combination of immunofluorescent staining of tissue sections with traditional histological analysis is a necessary step to assess the dignostic potential of a monoclonal antibody.

The radioimmunometric assay and the rosette assay are comparable in sensitivity and have both been adapted for use in microtiter plates (Ferrone *et al.,* 1980). In the former assay, the indirect reagents are labeled with ^{125}I and are counted in an automated gamma counter, while in the latter assay, the indirect reagents are coupled to sheep erythrocytes and rosettes are scored by microscopic examination. Thus, the radioimmunometric assay is useful for quantitating the level of antigen expressed by cells, while the rosette assay can determine whether some or all of the target cells are reacting with the antibodies. In addition, the indirect rosette assay is also useful for fractionating heterogeneous populations of cells by separating rosetted from nonrosetted cells on a Ficoll-Hypaque density gradient and may be modified into an inhibition assay for comparing the specificity of different antibodies as well as for determining spatial and structural relationships among different membrane antigens on the cell surface.

3.2. Immunochemical Approach

To define the molecular characteristics of tumor-associated antigens, we have used immunochemical rather than classic biochemical approaches because the former can rapidly isolate small amounts of antigens from complex sources such as cellular extracts or spent culture media. An additional advantage of the immunochemical approach is that it allows the definition of antigenic relationships among structures with the same or similar molecular size, and it enables one to identify molecular heterogeneity within a given antigen through differential expression of antigenic determinants detectable with monoclonal antibodies. The usefulness of the latter approach has recently been demonstrated in the human Ia-like antigenic system (Quaranta *et al.,* 1981a). Finally, the immunochemical approach allows the elucidation of the biosynthetic sequence whereby antigens are processed, transported to the membrane, and then eventually released by cells.

Cells in long-term culture are extrinsically radiolabeled with ^{125}I by the Iodogen procedure (Salisbury and Graham, 1981) or grown in a medium containing either a radiolabeled carbohydrate or protein precursor; the labeled cells are then solubilized with an appropriate agent such as high or low salt concentration, chaotropes, or detergents. We routinely employ the nonionic detergent Nonidet P-40 (NP-40), since it is efficient for solubilizing both integral and peripheral membrane components. Immunoprecipitations are performed by first insolubilizing antibodies to either protein-A-bearing *Staphylococcus aureus* bacteria or protein-A-coupled Sepharose 4B. Murine immunoglobulin G_1 (IgG_1) antibodies that do not bind to protein A may be indirectly bound to protein A–Sepharose via a rabbit anti-mouse immunoglobulin antiserum or may be directly coupled to Sepharose through the CNBr reaction. The radiolabeled antigens isolated on immunoadsorbents are analyzed for molecular weight and subunit structure by SDS-PAGE (Laemmli, 1970). We prefer slab gels over tube gels, since the mobilities of many samples can be accurately compared within a single gel. Antigens labeled with ^{35}S or ^3H are readily detected with fluorographic enhancing techniques (Bonner and Laskey, 1974).

4. Detection and Characterization of Melanoma-Associated Antigens Using Monoclonal Antibodies

4.1. A High-Molecular-Weight Plasma-Membrane Antigen

Monoclonal antibodies 138.13, 225.28S, 473.54S, 653.40S, and 763.24T react in radioimmunometric assays with all cultured melanoma cell lines of our panel, but do not react with carcinoma and B-lymphoid cell lines (Table III); the extent of binding varied for the different melanoma targets. Analysis of viable and acetone-fixed melanoma cell lines by indirect immunofluorescence with the monoclonal antibodies showed smooth staining of the plasma membrane and no staining of the cytoplasm (Fig. 4 and Table IV). In binding assays performed with ^{125}I-radiolabeled antibodies, melanoma M21 cells coated with unlabeled monoclonal antibody 138.13, 225.28S, or 653.40S significantly inhibited the binding of either ^{125}I-labeled antibody. In contrast, monoclonal antibody 138.13, 225.28S, or 653.40S could inhibit the binding of ^{125}I-labeled 763.24T monoclonal antibody. These data suggest that monoclonal antibodies 138.13, 225.28S, and 653.40S identify the same or a closely associated antigenic determinant that is different from the one detected by monoclonal antibody 763.24T.

Three of the five monoclonal antibodies were tested by a number of different investigators for their reactivity in binding assays with a large panel of cultured normal and tumor cell lines (Fig. 5). Their results, in agreement with our own data, show conclusively that the antibodies react strongly with melanoma cell lines but not with the other types of cultured cells. In addition, Carrel (Switzerland) and Seeger (United States) found that the monoclonal antibodies react with glioma cell lines. That we detect 100% of our melanoma

TABLE III
Reactivity of a Panel of Human Cell Lines in an ^{125}I
Radioimmunometric Binding Assay with Monoclonal Antibodies to
Human Melanoma Cell Lines

	[^{125}I]S. aureus protein A bound (cpm)		
Cell line	465.12	225.28S	376.96
Melanoma			
BwV	<100	3,300	5,000
Colo 38	2,300	33,000	2,200
M14	1,800	16,400	9,500
M21	4,300	41,000	2,300
Carcinoma			
Mano	<100	<500	8,280
T24	<100	<500	4,200
Lymphoid			
			<10
Raji	<100	<500	0
			<10
WI-L2	<100	<500	0

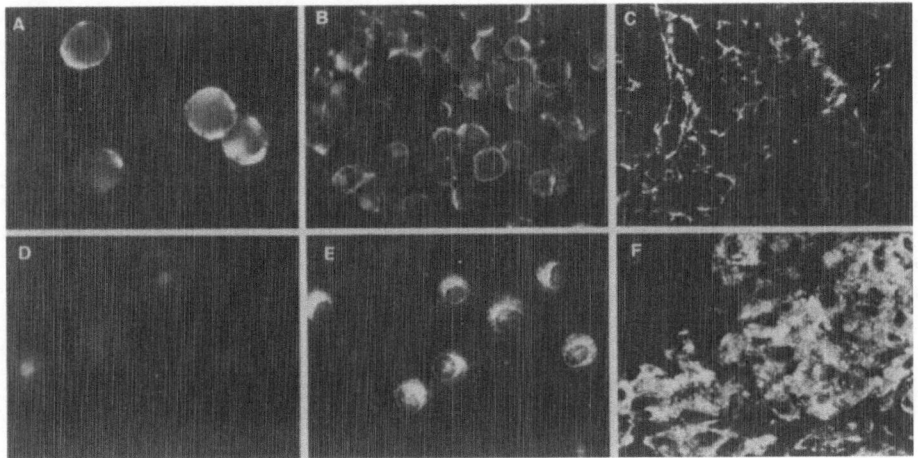

FIGURE 4. Indirect immunofluorescence staining of cultured melanoma cells (M21) and a surgically removed melanoma lesion with monoclonal antibodies 225.28S (A-C) and 465.12 (D-F). Staining was on viable cultured cells (A, D), cytocentrifuged and acetone-fixed cultured cells (B, E), and adjacent cryostat thin sections of a melanoma lesion that had been fixed witb acetone (C, F).

TABLE IV

Immunofluoresence Staining of Cultured Melanoma Cells with Monoclonal Antibodies 465.12 and 225.28S

Cell line	Plasma membrane staining[a]		Cytoplasmic staining[b]	
	465.12	225.28S	465.12	225.28S
BwV	±	+ +	+ +	−
M14	±	+ + +	+	−
M16	−	+ +	+ + +	−
M21	+	+ + +	+ + +	−

[a]Membrane staining of viable cells.
[b]Cytoplasmic staining was performed on cells after acetone fixation.

cell lines as positive in the binding assay while the summary results of the other investigators show only 80% as positive may be due to either technical differences (e.g., sensitivity of assays or criteria of positivity) or differences in the cell lines. In the latter case, either masking of the relevant antigen or polymorphism may be involved.

In an indirect immunofluorescence assay, monoclonal antibodies 225.28S and 653.40S stained 100% of the malignant-melanoma biopsies, which included primary, recurrent, and metastatic lesions of the melanotic and amelanotic type (results for 225.28S only in Table V). The staining was confined to the cell plasma membrane, was generally more intense at the periphery of the tumor cell nests, and varied in intensity among the cells of each

Table V

Indirect Immunofluorescence Staining of Cells of the Melanocyte Lineage with Monoclonal Antibodies to Ia-Like Antigens and to Tumor-Associated Antigens

	Anti Ia-like antigens Q5/13	Anti-alenoma-associated antigens	
Specimen		225.28S	465.12
Normal skin	Negative[a]	Negative	Negative[b]
Pigmented normal skin	Negative	Negative	Negative
Intradermal and compound nevi[c]	0/17	17/17	11/17
Primary, recurrent, and metastatic melanomas[c]	32/41	59/59	58/59

[a]Langerhans cells are positive.
[b]With the exception of sebaceous-gland cells, which are weakly stained.
[c]Number positive/number tested.

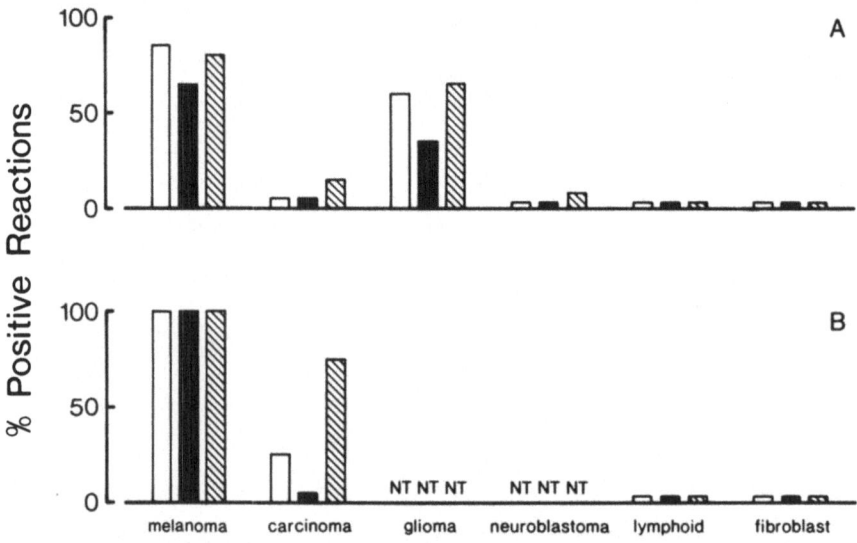

Figure 5. Independent evaluation of the specificity of monoclonal antibodies 225.28T (□), 473.54S (■), and 653.40S (□) for a panel of a cultured human cell lines. (A) Summary of the results of several different laboratories, including Burchiel (United States), Carrel (Switzerland), Herlyn (United States), Hersey (Australia), Seeger (United States), and Perlmann (Sweden) [reported in detail in Imai *et al.* (1981f)]; (B) summary of our own results. (% Positive Reactions) percentage of cell lines judged as reactive with the antibody; (NT) not tested.

tumor (see Fig. 4). It is not known whether the differential reactivity of the melanoma cells within a lesion reflects a stable hetereogeneous trait or results from differences in cell cycle. In addition, both monoclonal antibodies reacted with all cases of intradermal and compound nevi and with some basal-cell (4 of 6) and squamous-cell carcinomas (2 of 5). On the other hand, the monoclonal antibodies failed to react with normal melanocytes from either adult normal or pigmented skin or skin that had been irradiated with UV light (Table V) or

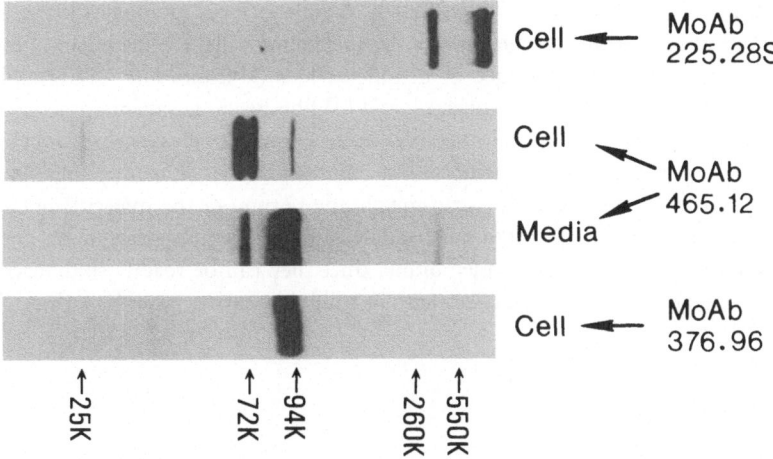

FIGURE 6. Molecular profile of tumor-associated antigens immunoprecipitated with monoclonal antibodies to melanoma cells. [^{3}H]Glucosamine-labeled melanoma-cell detergent extracts or radiolabeled spent culture medium from BwV cells were immunoprecipitated with the monoclonal antibodies and then electrophoresed on a 5–12.5% polyacrylamide gradient SDS-PAGE slab gel. The gel was processed by fluorography prior to exposure to Kodak XRP-1 film. Molecular-weight markers: nonreduced melanoma fibronectin (550,000); reduced melanoma fibronectin (260,000); phosphorylase a (94,000).

with 6 cases of benign pigmented skin lesions of nonmelanocyte origin (Table V). Furthermore, the monoclonal antibodies were unreactive with a large variety of normal and fetal cells of ectodermal, entodermal, or mesodermal–mesenchymal origin, as well as with carcinomas from several anatomical sites and with several types of brain tumors including four gliomas. The difference in reactivity of cultured vs. surgically removed gliomas with the monoclonal antibodies may reflect (1) the sensitivity of the assays used, (2) the expansion of a subpopulation of tumor cells bearing the antigen through passage in culture, (3) an increase in the level of expression of the antigen on tissue culture, or least likely (4) polymorphism of the antigenic determinants. In any case, the number of different tissues examined provides compelling evidence in support of the high degree of specificity exhibited by these monoclonal antibodies for proliferating cells of the melanocyte lineage.

Immunochemical studies with the five monoclonal antibodies (138.13, 225.28S, 473.54S, 653.40S, and 763.74T) identified two very high-molecular-weight components from either [^{3}H]glucosamine-, [^{35}S]methionine-, or [^{3}H]phenylalanine-labeled melanoma cells, indicating that both structures consist of protein as well as carbohydrate (representative results in Fig. 6). It is not yet known whether one or both chains carry the antigenic determinants detected by the monoclonal antibodies or whether the two chains are associated noncovalently. The larger component, which barely penetrates the 5% end of the gel, exhibited a much higher apparent molecular weight than our largest standard at 440,000, while the smaller component has an apparent molecular weight of 280,000. The size of the smaller component is similar to that of melanoma fibronectin, which has recently been shown to be 260,000 (Wilson et al., 1981c); however, no relationship exists between these two molecules, since: (1) two xenoantisera and a monoclonal antibody to fibronectin do not react with the 280,000 structure, while four of the monoclonal antibodies to the 280,000 molecule fail to react with fibronectin shed by melanoma cells; (2) melanoma fibronectin exists as a dimer of 560,000 bridged by disulfied bonds (Wilson *et al.,* 1981c), while the 280,000 component is not disulfide-bridged; and (3) fibronectin is shed in large amounts in the medium, while the 280,000 structure is not. Although most of the cell-membrane antigens reported so far are integral membrane structures that can be readily solubilized only by either proteolytic removal of the transmembrane portion of the molecule or detergent treatment (Singer, 1974), the high-molecular-weight antigens appear to be peripheral rather than integral to the plasma membrane, since they can be readily solubilized in the absence of detergent or by low-ionic-strength or mild denaturing conditions (Fig. 7). Also,

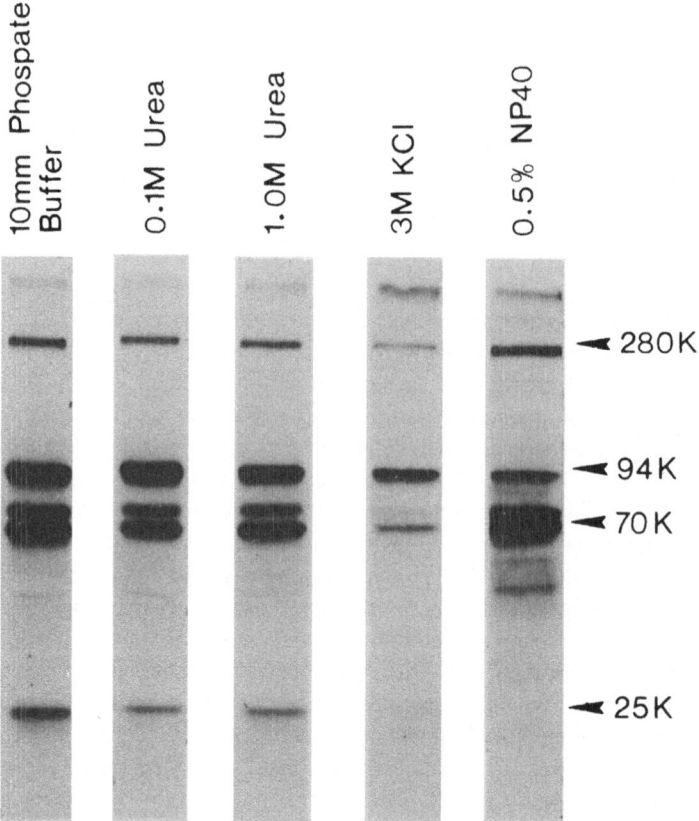

FIGURE 7. Solubilization of cytoplasmic and high-molecular-weight plasma-membrane tumor-associated antigens with various dissociating agents. [³H]Glucosamine-labeled BwV melanoma cells were extracted with various agents for 1 hr at 4°C. The extracts containing urea or KCl were dialyzed overnight against phosphate buffer. The various extracts were immunoprecipitated separately with monoclonal antibodies 225.28S and 465.12, and for convenience, the immunoprecipitates were combined and electrophoresed in a 5–12.5% polyacrylamide gradient SDS-slab gel. The gel was processed by fluorography prior to exposure to Kodak XRP-1 film. Molecular-weight markers: reduced melanoma fibronectin (280,000); phosphorylase a (94,000).

the structures of the two chains seen by SDS-PAGE are identical whether solubilized by detergent or by low-ionic-strength buffers. The high-molecular-weight antigens detected by the various monoclonal antibodies are apparently not shed to any great extent, since they are detectable in the spent culture medium of either [³H]phenylalanine- or [³H]glucosamine-labeled melanoma cell lines only when large amounts of labeled material are used and the time of exposure to X-ray film is vastly increased.

4.2. A 94,000 Plasma-Membrane Antigen

We have recently isolated a monoclonal antibody 376.96S that in binding assays reacts similarly with melanoma and carcinoma cells, but fails to react with B- and T-lymphoblast cell lines (see Table III). In indirect immunofluorescence, the antibody stains the plasma membrane of cultured melanoma cells, but the intensity of the stain is much less than is seen with any other of our monoclonal antibodies that react with the high-molecular-weight plasma-membrane antigen. The lower level of staining achieved with monoclonal antibody 376.96S is probably due to the level of antigen expressed by melanoma cells rather than to the affinity of the antibody, since the same level of staining is achieved over a wide range of antibody concentrations.

Indirect immunofluoresence analysis with cells of the melanocyte lineage showed that monoclonal antibody 376.96S reacts with 83% (15 of 18 cases) of primary melanoma lesions arising from superficial spreading, malignant lentigo or nodular type and with 65% (13 of 20 cases) of metastatic melanoma. The staining of melanoma lesions varied for cells within a tumor and did not correlate with the content of melanin. The antibody failed to stain any structures from normal skin except for limited areas of the basal layer and did not react with benign pigmented skin lesions (warts and angiomas), but it did stain 40% of nevi (8 of 20 cases of intradermal and compound) and 50% of skin carcinomas (6 of 12 basal-cell and squamous-cell).

When tested against a large variety of normal human tissues other than those from skin, the antibody showed only faint staining of stomach epithelium. Furthermore, the antibody did not react with tumors derived from gastrointestional tract, brain, urogenital, lung, thyroid–parotid, liver–gallbladder, and muscle, but it stained 22% (10 of 45 cases) of breast carcinomas that included infiltrating ductal, medullary, and lobular type.

Immunoprecipitation and SDS-PAGE analysis of [³H]glucosamine-labeled melanoma cells (BwV, Colo38) with monoclonal antibody 376.96S showed a single component with a molecular weight of 94,000 (see Fig. 6). A 94,000 structure could also be immunoprecipitated from ¹²⁵I-labeled melanoma NP-40 cell extracts, and this molecule did not increase in apparent molecular weight when SDS-PAGE was performed under nonreducing conditions, indicating that the 94,000 molecule is a glycoprotein and is not disulfide-bridged to any other components. Like the high-molecular-weight plasma-membrane antigen described in the last section, the 94,000 glycoprotein is peripheral rather than integral to the plasma membrane, since it is readily solubilized in the absence of detergents and by mild denaturing conditions (hypotonic salt extraction or 0.1 M urea). The 94,000 molecule detected by monoclonal antibody 376.96S is different from the one detected by monoclonal antibody 465.12, which will be described in the next section, since: (1) in sequential immunodepletion experiments, each of the antibodies was unable to deplete the 94,000 structure detected by the other antibody (Wilson *et al.,* 1982); and (2) the 94,000 molecule detected by monoclonal antibody 465.12 is readily shed into the tissue culture medium, while the one detected by monoclonal antibody 376.96S is not.

4.3. A Cytoplasmic Antigen

Monoclonal antibody 465.12 in [^{125}I]protein-A-binding assays against a panel of cultured human cell lines reacted weakly with melanoma cells, but did not react with carcinoma or B-lymphoid cells (see Table III). In indirect immunofluorescence, monoclonal antibody 465.12 showed a strong granular staining of the cytoplasm of virtually our entire cultured cell panel and a weak staining of the plasma membrane of some viable and acetone-fixed melanoma cell lines (see Fig. 4 and Table IV). In general, the intensity and frequency of cytoplasmic staining were greater in cultured melanoma than in carcinoma or cultured B-lymphoid cell lines (Raji and WI-L2). This antibody has not been sent to other laboratories for independent evaluation of its reactivity for cultured cells because its low level of binding to cell surfaces is unsuitable for detection by most assays currently in use.

Monoclonal antibody 465.12 reacted with all but one case of surgically removed melanomas tested including primary, recurrent, and metastatic lesions (see Table V). The staining was restricted mainly to the cytoplasm and exhibited the granular type of fluorescence similar to that seen in cultured melanoma cells (see Fig. 4). Variations in staining intensity were observed among cells of a given tumor as well as among different tumors and were independent of melanin content. When tested against 17 cases of intradermal and compound nevi, monoclonal antibody 465.12 reacted with 65% of the lesions (Fig. 8 and Table V). Interestingly, dermal nevi showed a diffuse–weak cytoplasmic stain, and junctionally active nevi showed the intense granular stain characteristic of melanoma cells. The significance of this difference is unknown at present. The monoclonal antibody failed to react significantly with normal skin (scant staining was associated with cells from the sebaceous glands) (Table V) and with 6 cases of benign pigmented skin lesions of nonmelanocyte origin. On the other hand, the antibody reacted with 3 of 8 cases of pigmented skin carcinomas (see Table IX).

When examined with a large group of surgically removed normal adult tissues, monoclonal antibody 465.12 exhibited moderate staining of the epithelium of the gastrointestinal tract and weak staining of normal adult epithelial cells from the small intestine, parotid gland, breast, urinary bladder, testes, endometrium, and thyroid (Tables VI and VII). The staining was confined to the cytoplasm and showed a distinct granular pattern varying in intensity in cells of a given tissue. In general, the reactivity of monoclonal antibody 465.12 with fetal tissues was similar to that seen in adult tissues, but the staining was much less intense (Table VI). These results indicate that the antigenic structure detected by monoclonal antibody 465.12 is expressed in a wide range of normal tissues of different embryonic origin.

In the indirect immunofluorescence assay, monoclonal antibody 465.12 stained surgically removed tumors derived from normal tissues both reactive and nonreactive with this monoclonal antibody (Tables VIII and IX). The cytoplasm of the tumor cells showed the typical granular staining, but was more frequent and intense than in any of the corresponding normal adult cells reactive with the monoclonal antibody. Interestingly, not all cases of

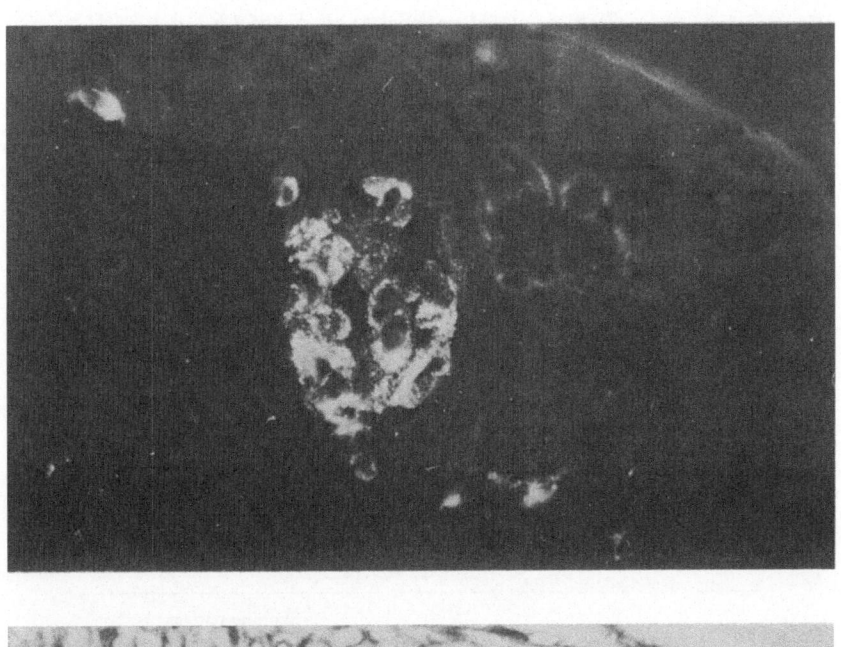

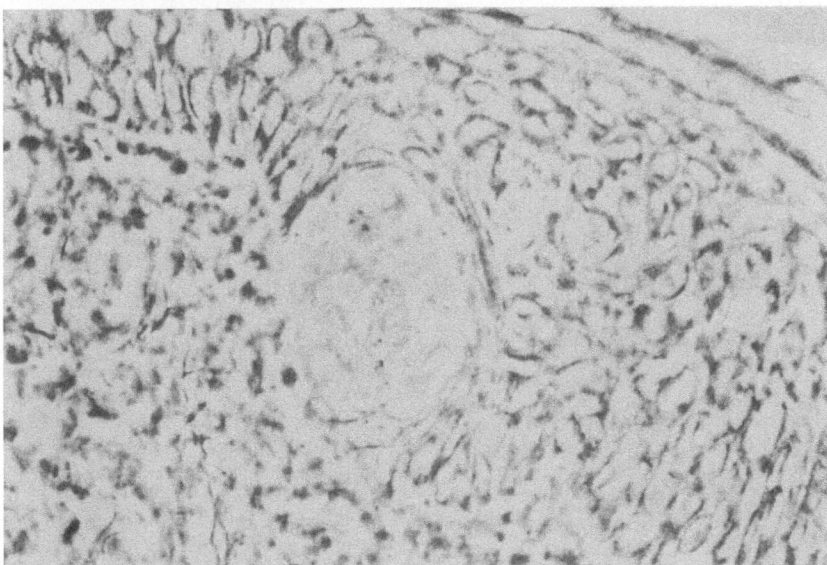

FIGURE 8. Indirect immunofluorescence staining of an acetone-fixed thin section of an intradermal nevus with monoclonal antibody 465.12. The section was treated with monoclonal antibody 465.12 for 30 min, then washed and stained with fluorescein-isothiocyanate-labeled rabbit anti-mouse IgG antibodies. The sections were observed by phase-contrast microscopy *(bottom)* and by fluorescence microscopy *(top)*. Note the granular staining of the cytoplasm of nevi cells.

TABLE VI

Reactivity of Normal Human Adult and Fetal
Tissues with Monoclonal Antibody 465.12

Tissues	Staining pattern[a]	
	Adult	Fetal
Colon–sigmoid	Strong	Weak
Rectum	Strong	Weak
Breast	Weak	NT
Endometrium	Weak	NT
Parotid	Weak	NT
Small intestine	Weak	Weak
Testes	Weak	NT
Thyroid	Weak	Negative
Urinary bladder	Weak	Negative

[a] Immunofluoresence. (NT) Not tested.

TABLE VII

Normal Human Adult and Fetal Tissues Nonreactive with Monoclonal
Antibody 465.12

Tissues	Staining pattern[a]	
	Adult	Fetal
Brain	Rare positive cell	Negative
Kidney	Rare positive cell	Negative
Ovary	Rare positive cell	NT
Liver	Negative	Negative
Lung	Negative	Negative
Pancreas	Negative	Negative
Peripheral blood	Negative	NT
Placenta	Negative	NT
Skin	Negative	Negative
Smooth and skeletal muscle	Negative	Negative
Spleen	Negative	Negative
Stomach	Negative	Negative
Sympathetic ganglia	Negative	NT
Thymus	Negative	NT
Tonsils	Negative	NT

[a] Indirect immunoflorescence assay performed on acetone-fixed tissue sections.
(NT) Not tested.

a given type of tumor reacted with the antibody. This disparity in the expression of the cytoplasmic antigen by tumor cells of a given type may result either from a lack of synthesis of the molecules or from the presence of a molecule that lacks the antigenic determinant detected by the monoclonal antibody. If the latter possibility is true, then the molecule would be polymorphic. At present, no histological or clinical features could be associated with the cytoplasmic-antigen-positive or -negative tumors; however, complete follow-ups on these patients will be necessary before any clinical associations can be drawn. Sarcoma was the only type of tumor that clearly did not react with monoclonal antibody 465.12 (Table IX); two other types of tumors that were unreactive (e.g., kidney clear-cell carcinoma and thymic carcinoma) included rare types, the numbers of which were too small to make any firm conclusions.

Immunoprecipitation of [^{3}H]glucosamine- and [^{3}H]phenylalanine-labeled melanoma (BwV, M21, and M10) and bladder-carcinoma cell lines (Mano and T24) with monoclonal antibody 465.12 revealed four glycopolypeptides with molecular weights of 94,000, 75,000, 70,000, and 25,000 (see Fig. 4). Electrophoresis of these four chains under non-reducing conditions did not reveal any higher-molecular-weight forms, indicating the absence of interchain disulfide bridges. The cytoplasmic antigen is also similar to the high-molelcular-weight components described in the previous section in that it can be readily solubilized under mild dissociating conditions (low ionic strength or 0.1 M urea) and in the absence of detergent (see Fig. 7). Thus, these molecules are also peripheral rather than integral proteins.

The four-chain subunit structure for the cytoplasmic antigen is unusual, and therefore we performed several experiments to exclude technical artifacts resulting from antibody

TABLE VIII

Reactivity of Monoclonal Antibody 465.12 with Various Human Tumors Derived from Normal Tissues Reactive with Monoclonal Antibody 465.12

Tumor biopsies	Number positive/number tested
Breast adenocarcinoma	22/34
Colon–sigmoid adenocarcinoma	5/6
Endometrial adenocarcinoma	3/7
Ovary adenocarcinoma	5/6
Parotid mixed-type tumors (Warthin's tumors)	2/6
Rectum adenocarcinoma	7/7
Thyroid goiter, adenocarcinoma	4/6
Urinary-bladder transitional-cell carcionoma	7/8

TABLE IX

Reactivity of Monoclonal Antibody 465.12 with Various Human Tumors Derived from Normal Tissues Nonreactive with Monoclonal Antibody 465.12

Tumor biopsies	Number positive/number tested
Brain	5/15
Esophagus epidermal carcinoma	1/2
Hydatiform mole	1/1
Kidney clear-cell carcinoma	0/1
Liver adenocarcinoma	1/2
Lung adenocarcinoma, squamous carcinoma	2/5
Pancreas adenocarcinoma	1/1
Sarcomas	0/7
Skin basal-cell and epidermal carcinoma	3/8
Stomach adenocarcinoma	2/7
Thymus carcinoma	0/1

contamination or proteolysis of the 94,000 component. First, to ensure that our antibody was truly monoclonal, we examined supernates from more than 20 clones derived from two separate subclonings of the original hybridoma and found that they all reproduced the same four-chain immunoprecipitation pattern (Fig. 9). Second, to exclude that the low-molecular-weight components are generated by proteolysis of the 94,000 component, the detergent extraction was routinely performed at 4°C and in the presence of the proteolytic inhibitor phenylmethylsulfonylfluoride (100 μM), and more than 10 experiments have reproduced the four-chain immunoprecipitation pattern; furthermore, in one experiment, the extraction procedure was performed at 37°C without the proteolytic inhibitor, and still the immunoprecipitation pattern was the same. We do not yet know whether one or all of the chains carry the antigenic determinant detected by monoclonal antibody 465.12; however, we favor the hypothesis that only some may carry the determinant, since it is sensitive to heat denaturation and therefore is probably protein rather than carbohydrate in nature.

Incorporation of different radiolabeled sugars into the four glycopolypeptides of the cytoplasmic antigen revealed that the 75,000 component is glycosylated differently from the other molecules (Table X). The 75,000 molecule incorporated [^{3}H]glucosamine and

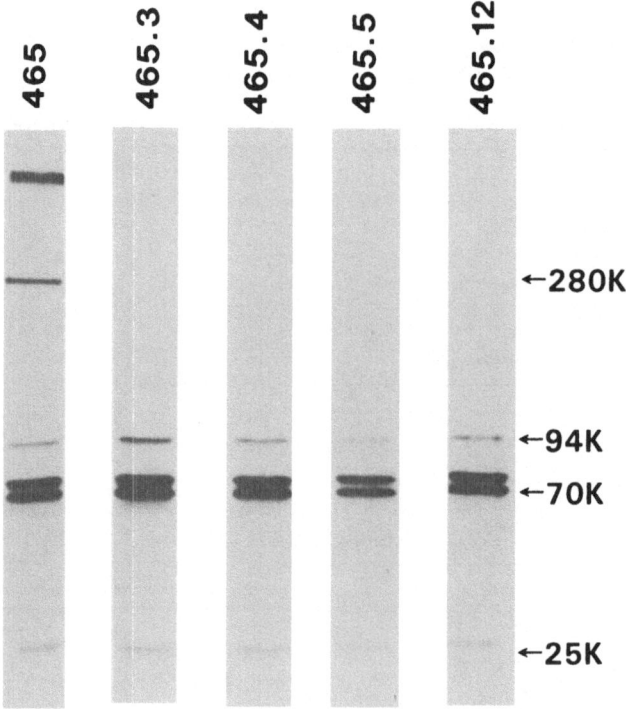

FIGURE 9. SDS-PAGE analysis of the tumor-associated antigenic structures immunoprecipitated by subclones of the 465 hybridoma, originally produced against cultured melanoma cells. The original hybridoma clone 465 and supernates from various subclones derived from this clone by limiting dilution were used to immunoprecipitate [^{3}H]glucosamine-labeled antigens from NP-40 detergent extracts of cultured BwV melanoma cells. Electrophoresis in a 5–12.5% polyacrylamide gradient SDS-slab gel and visualization by fluorography indicate that antibodies from all the 465 subclones identified the same four components. Molecular-weight markers: reduced melanoma fibronectin (280,000); phosporylase a (94,000).

Table X

Incorporation of Radiolabeled Sugars into the Glycopolypeptides Immunoprecipitated by Monoclonal Antibodies 465.12 and 225.28S

Monoclonal antibody	Glycopolypeptide[a]	D[6-³H]-Glucosamine	D[1-³H]-Galactose	L[6-³H]-Fucose	D[2-³H]-Mannose
465.12					
	94,000	+	+	+	+
	75,000	+	;	−	+
	70,000	+	+	+	+
	25,000	+	+	+	+
225.28S					
	>550,000	+	+	+	+
	280,000	+	+	+	+

[a]Glycopolypeptides are identified by their molecular weight in SDS-PAGE.

[³H]mannose, but failed to incorporate [³H]galactose or [³H]fucose. In addition, [³H]mannose incorporated more readily into the 75,000 structure than into the other glycopolypeptides immunoprecipitated by monoclonal antibody 465.12. Although there are examples of mature glycoproteins containing high-mannose neutral-oligosaccharide side chains (Robbins *et al.*, 1977; Hunt, 1979), the carbohydrate labeling characteristics and the following evidence support the possibility that the 75,000 glycopolypeptide represents an immature glycosylation step in the synthesis of a glycoprotein carrying *N*-asparagine-linked oligosaccharide (Robbins *et al.*, 1977; Hunt *et al.*, 1978; Tabas *et al.*, 1978): (1) Pulse-labeling studies using either a protein or a carbohydrate label show that the 75,000 molecule is synthesized prior to the other glycopolypeptides identified by monoclonal antibody 465.12. (2) SDS-PAGE analysis of the cytoplasmic antigen synthesized by B-lymphoblast cell lines (WI-L2, Raji) shows a slight reduction in the apparent molecular weights of the 94,000 and 70,000 molecules, but no difference in the molecular weight of the 75,000 molecule (Fig. 10). Glycosylation differences between the same molecules synthesized by different types of cells are more likely to occur at the last stage of glycoprotein maturation rather than at the immature high-mannose precursor step. (3) Treatment of melanoma cells with the antibiotic tunicamycin, an inhibitor of *N*-asparagine-linked oligosaccharide addition, results in the synthesis of two glycosylation precursors detectable with monoclonal antibody 465.12. One polypeptide of molecular weight 90,000 is the precursor to the 94,000 glycopolypeptide, while the other of molecular weight 60,000 appears to be a common precursor to the 75,000 and 70,000 glycopolypeptides (Fig. 11). The latter finding suggests that the differences between the 75,000 and 70,000 molecules lie in the carbohydrate side chains rather than in the polypeptide moiety. Pulse–chase experiments are in progress to prove that the 75,000 component is a precursor molecule and to define its relationship to the 94,000 and 25,000 components.

The large amount of antigen detectable by monoclonal antibody 465.12 in the cytoplasm as compared to that detectable on the cell surface suggested that this antigen may be rapidly released into the tissue-culture medium. Immunoprecipitation of the spent culture media of [³H]glucosamine- or [³H]-phenylalanine-labeled melanoma cells with monoclonal antibody 465.12 showed two chains with molecular weights of 94,000 and 72,000, with the

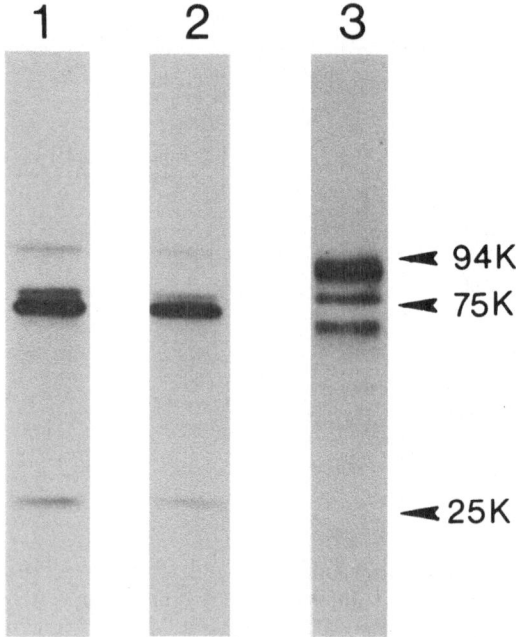

FIGURE 10. Comparison of the molecular weights of the cytoplasmic tumor-associated antigens immunoprecip-itated with monoclonal antibody 465.12 from different cultured cell lines. [³H]Glucosamine-labeled NP-40 detergent extracts of a melanoma cell line [BwV (1)], a carcinoma cell line [T24 (2)], and a B-lymphoblastoid cell line [WI-L2 (3)] were immunoprecipitated with monoclonal antibody 465.12 and then electrophoresed in a 5–12.5% polyacrylamide gradient SDS slab gel. The gel was processed by fluorography prior to exposure to Kodak XRP-1 film.

94,000 component in large excess over the 72,000 structure (see Fig. 6). The rapid secretion of the cytoplasmic antigen is evidenced by its presence in media 90 min after its synthesis. Electrophoresis of the two spent-media molecules under reducing and nonreducing condi-tions did not affect their mobility, showing that they are not disulfide-bridged. The 94,000 spent-media component is one of the major glycopolypeptides shed by melanoma cells and can be easily identified when unfractionated, labeled spent media are examined by SDS-PAGE. This 94,000 spent-media molecule is not the only molecule of this molecular weight shed by melanoma cells, since electrophoresis of labeled spent media reveals a second major component that increases in apparent molecular weight under nonreducing conditions. This latter 94,000 molecule is probably disulfide-bridged with another polypeptide in its native form. We do not as yet have any antibodies that react with the 94,000 spent-media molecule not detected by monoclonal antibody 465.12.

5. Discussion

Serological and immunochemical analysis of the antigenic profile of human melanoma cells has shown that they acquire Ia-like antigens and plasma-membrane-bound as well as cytoplasmic tumor-associated antigens. These markers appear at different stages of differ-

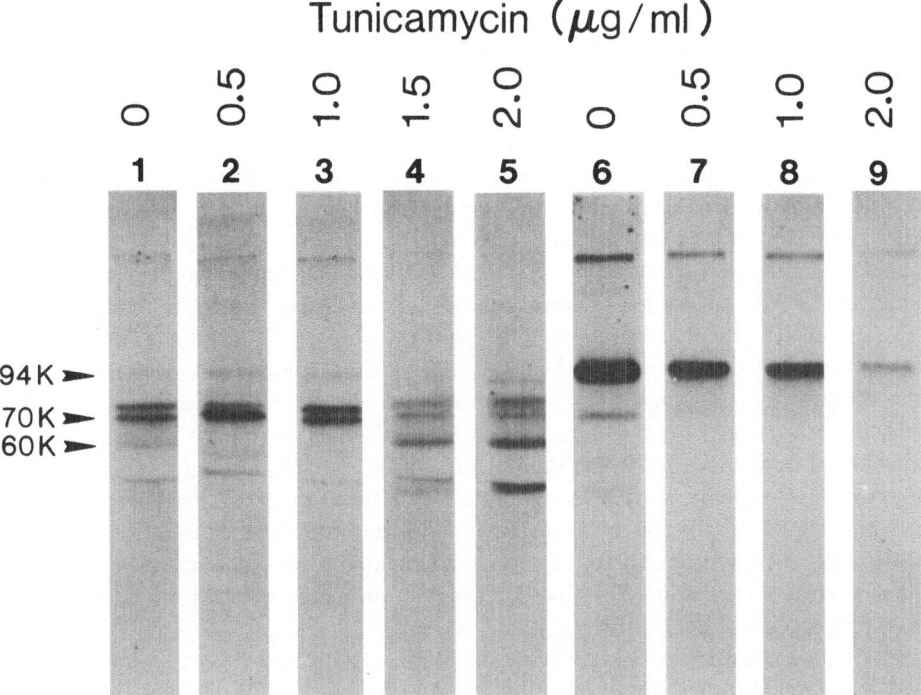

FIGURE 11. Effect of tunicamycin on the molecular weights of the cytoplasmic antigen detectable by monoclonal antibody 465.12. Melanoma cell line BwV was cultured for 18 hr with 100 μCi [³H]phenylalanine in the presence of various concentrations of the antibiotic tunicamycin. NP-40 detergent extracts of these cells (1–5) and the labeled spent culture medium (6–9) were immunoprecipitated with monoclonal antibody 465.12, and the labeled molecules were analyzed by electrophoresis in a 5–12.5% polyacrylamide gradient SDS slab gel. The gel was processed by fluorography prior to exposure to Kodak XRP-1 film.

TABLE XI

Differential Expression of Ia-Like Antigens and Tumor-Associated Antigens on Cells of the Melanocyte Lineage

| | | Melanoma-associated antigens | |
Cells	Ia-like antigens	Cytoplasmic (465.12)	Plasma-membrane (225.28S)
Melanocyte	−	−	−
Nevus	−	+(−)	+
Melanoma	+	+	+

entiation on cells of the melanocyte lineage (Table XI); thus, Ia-like antigens are not detectable on skin melanocytes or nevus cells, but are expressed by melanocytes that have undergone malignant transformation. The high-molecular-weight membrane-bound and the cytoplasmic tumor-associated antigens are absent from skin melanocytes, but are present on nevus and malignant-melanoma cells.

The unexpected appearance of Ia-like antigens on melanoma cells is not confined to this tumor, but may occur in other tumors of nonlymphoid origin (Fig. 12), although at a lower frequency. This phenomenon may be interpreted as an example of an alien histocompatibility antigen, and we now propose to broaden the definition of alien histocompatibility antigens to include both those alloantigens genetically foreign to the tumor host and those molecules absent from the nonmalignant counterpart of the tumor. Whether the mechanisms underlying these two phenomena are the same remains to be determined. Alien histocompatibility alloantigens that may appear on tumor cells have been reported to influence the nature, specificity, and regulation of the host's immune response (for a review, see Martin and Imamura, 1980). No data are available on the biological significance of Ia-like antigens on melanoma cells. It is conceivable that these antigens affect the interaction between melanoma cells and the host's immune system, since these molecules mediate and restrict cell–cell interactions required to generate immune responses. Furthermore, we have found decreased expression of Ia-like antigens on melanoma lesions from patients with massive spreading of the disease.

We have identified three types of tumor-associated antigens in human melanoma cells, two being membrane-bound and one cytoplasmic. The 280,000 and $> 550,000$ membrane-bound antigen is detectable only on melanoma, nevi, glioma, and some epidermal carcinomas, while the 94,000 membrane-bound antigen is present on a portion of melanomas, epidermal carcinomas, nevi, and some breast carcinomas. Both types of antigens are not detectable in normal tissues except for the presence of the 94,000 molecule in stomach epithelium and skin basal layer. The four-chain cytoplasmic antigen (94,000, 75,000, 70,000, and 25,000) is detectable in melanoma cells and in nevi cells as well as in a variety of normal tissues and tumors derived from normal tissues lacking this antigen. Furthermore, the cytoplasmic antigen is readily secreted by tumor cells into the culture medium.

Several types of tumor-associated antigens have been identified in the human melanoma system with conventional xenoantisera, monoclonal xenoantibodies, and sera from melanoma patients. The relationship between the cytoplasmic antigen described here and the antigens previously identified with melanoma-patient sera (Morton et al., 1968; Lewis and Phillips, 1972) cannot be determined because in the latter case no data are available on the structures of the antigens. Our cytoplasmic antigen is also clearly distinguishable from extensively investigated tumor-associated antigens such as α-fetoprotein or carcinoembryonic antigen, detectable with xenoantisera. The former is expressed in fetal liver rather than in the fetal gastrointestinal tract (Lee et al., 1979) and is a single molecule of molecular weight 70,000 (Ruoslahti et al., 1974), while the latter is a plasma-membrane component of molecular weight 200,000 (Kurpey et al., 1978). The 94,000 tumor-associated antigen that we previously identified with rabbit antisera in the spent medium of melanoma and carcinoma cell lines (Galloway et al., 1981) is the same 94,000 spent-media glycoprotein that we now detect with monoclonal antibody 465.12 to the cytoplasmic antigen (B. S. Wilson et al., 1982).

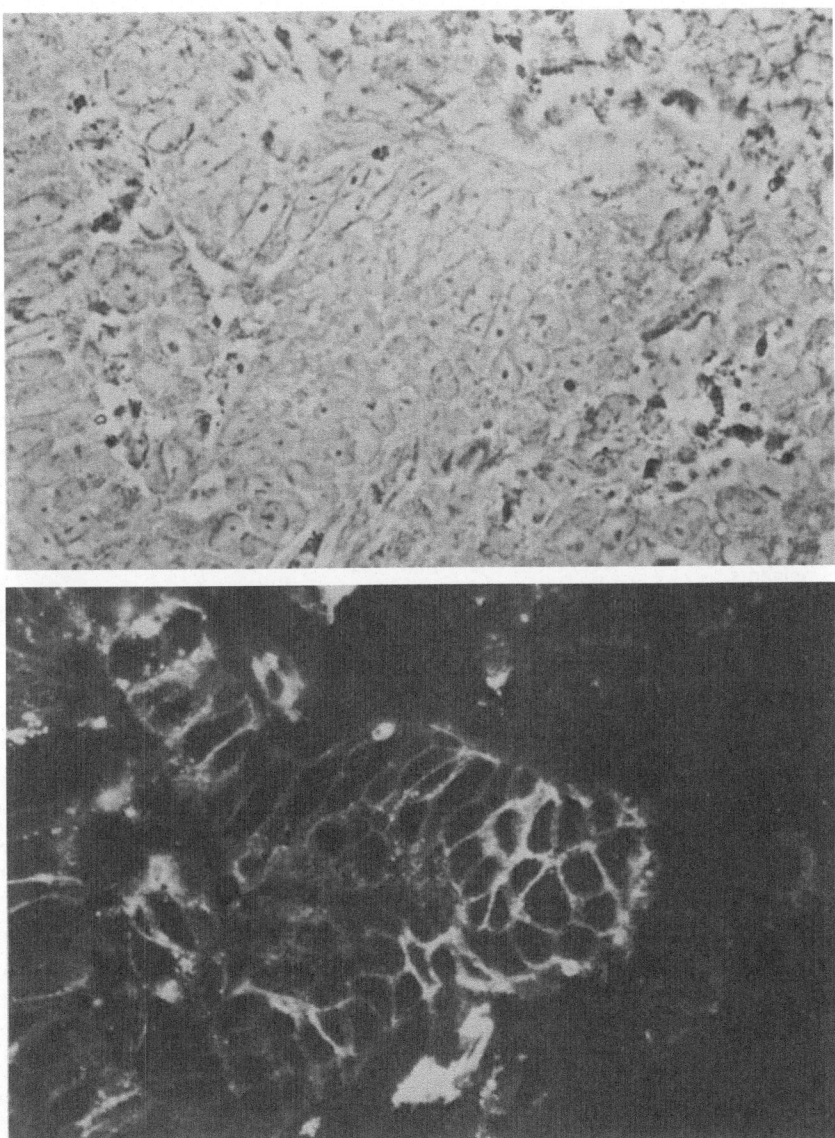

FIGURE 12. Indirect immunofuorescence staining of an acetone-fixed cryostat thin section of an adenocarcinoma of the rectum with monoclonal antibody Q5/13 to human Ia-like antigens. The section was incubated with the monoclonal antibody for 15 min, then washed and treated with fluorescein-isothiocyanate-labeled rabbit anti-mouse IgG antibody *(top)*. The same section was also examined by phase-contrast microscopy *(bottom)*.

What is the relationship between the plasma-membrane-bound tumor-associated antigens described here and those reported previously with xenoantibodies? The plasma-membrane antigen of molecular weight 94,000 that reacts with monoclonal antibody 376.96S appears to be similar in structure and tissue distribution to a 95,000 (Dippold *et al.*, 1980) and a 97,000 (Woodbury *et al.*, 1980) glycoprotein also identified with mono-clonal antibodies. We have received the anti-gp[95] monoclonal antibody from Dr. Dippold of Sloan–Kettering Institute, New York, and after performing immunodepletion studies in conjunction with our antibody, we conclude that these two antibodies react with antigeni-cally distinct structures (unpublished observations). The high-molecular-weight plasma-membrane antigen recognized by our monoclonal antibodies is different from any of the extensively characterized melanoma-associated antigens reported previously. Thus, the antigens defined with monoclonal antibodies by Herlyn *et al.* (1980) are absent from nevi and basal-cell carcinomas, the R24 antigen detected with a monoclonal antibody by Wood-bury *et al.* (1980) is glycolipid in nature, and the sizes of the components identified by monoclonal antibodies (Mitchell *et al.*, 1980) and by a chimpanzee antiserum (Stuhlmiller *et al.*, 1978) are much smaller than the components of the high-molecular-weight antigen. In addition, a 240,000 melanoma-associated antigen recently detected by xenoantisera in the spent culture media of melanoma cells (Galloway *et al.*, 1981) is antigenically unrelated to the large plasma-membrane antigen (B. S. Wilson *et al.*, 1982). Unfortunately, com-parison of our antibodies with other xenoantisera reported in the literature is not possible, since little or no information exists about the nature of the target antigens identified by the latter reagents.

An important question to be answered is whether the high-molecular-weight plasma-membrane antigen is related to those antigens identified with melanoma-patient sera, since the latter may have prognostic and therapeutic application (Werkmeister *et al.*, 1980). Ser-ological analysis of melanoma-patient sera has established the existence of autologous (Lewis and Phillips, 1972; Carey *et al.*, 1979) and common melanoma-associated antigens (Shiku *et al.*, 1976; Embleton *et al.*, 1980; Hersey *et al.*, 1979). Immunochemical studies with melanoma-patient sera show a glycoprotein of molecular weight 20,000–50,000 as an autologous melanoma antigen (Carey *et al.*, 1979) and a glycoprotein of molecular weight 15,000 as a common melanoma antigen (Hersey *et al.*, 1979), both of which are much smaller than our large plasma-membrane antigen. The relationship of our plasma-mem-brane antigens with the oncofetal antigens described for melanoma cells (Avis and Lewis, 1973; Irie *et al.*, 1976; Siebert *et al.*, 1977) will be known after we test our antibodies against fetal melanocytes. Thus, the question of whether the high-molecular-weight plasma-membrane antigen is immunogenic in melanoma patients cannot be answered with the present data. Our experience with patient sera suggests that these reagents will be of little value in solving this problem, and therefore we expect a solution only after human monoclonal antibodies to melanoma-associated antigens become available.

Finally, we would like to discuss the cross-reactivity of the monoclonal antibodies to the high-molecular-weight antigen with nevi, epidermal skin carcinomas, and gliomas. A sharing of antigenic determinants between nevi and melanoma has been shown previously with a monoclonal antibody to a 97,000 tumor-associated antigen (Brown *et al.*, 1981) and with cell-mediated immunity assays (N. I. Wilson, *et al.*, 1979). We are unaware of any reports describing antigens shared among the major epidermal skin malignancies, while cross-reactions between melanoma and glioma have been demonstrated with antibodies to melanoma-associated antigens (Herlyn et al., 1980) and with a monoclonal antibody and patient sera to glioma-associated antigens (for a review, see de Tribolet and Carrel, 1980). Further immunochemical studies will be necessary to determine whether the cross-reactive determinant is expressed on the same or different structures in these various types of cells.

6. Perspective

In this last section, we will briefly discuss the implications of our work and its future prospects for clinical and basic research. From a clinical viewpoint, double staining of pigmented skin lesions with monoclonal antibodies to Ia-lika antigens and to the high-molecular-weight plasma-membrane antigens may be useful to differentiate malignant from benign proliferating melanocytes. Also, the staining of lymph-node biopsies for the tumor-associated antigens may assist the identification and diagnosis of amelanotic metastatic lesions where histology and patient history are uncharacteristic of melanoma. The latter possibility is supported by a report describing the use of a chimpanzee antiserum (Stuhl-miller and Seigler, 1975) to melanoma antigens for the successful serological diagnosis of melanoma in three cases of metastatic lesions originally diagnosed as undifferentiated carcinoma by conventional pathological examination (Stuhlmiller et al., 1977). Indeed, up to 7% of melanoma diagnoses are uncertain (Truax et al., 1966) and would be benefited by an immunological approach, especially if it was applicable to formalin-fixed tissue sections routinely used by clinical pathologists.

The decreased levels of Ia-like antigens and of the tumor-associated antigens that we observed on massive spreading melanoma lesions compared with less malignant forms of melanoma suggest a correlation between expression of these antigens and clinical course of the disease. This hypothesis is consistent with the decreased levels of A, B, and H blood group isoantigens in carcinomas with poor prognoses (Davidsohn, 1972) and with a recent report describing prognostic relevance of a melanoma-associated antigen detected by melanoma-patient sera (Werkmeister et al., 1980). The levels of the cytoplasmic tumor-associated antigen present in patients' body fluids may also be of prognostic value for melanoma.

The monoclonal antibodies to plasma-membrane-bound tumor-associated antigens may be of value for radioimaging and for immunotherapy. Dr. Ghose (Dalhousie University, Halifax, Canada) has already injected five melanoma patients with radiolabeled antibodies reactive with the high-molecular-weight antigen and has succeeded in localizing metastasis in one of these patients (personal communication). Immunotherapy strategy with these antibodies must take into account their ability to lyse melanoma cells in conjunction with K cells, but not with human complement (Imai et al., 1981e). Thus, administration of these antibodies to melanoma patients may not necessarily affect the tumor, especially if the number and the activity of K cells are depressed. In fact, Dr. Roiston at the University of California, San Diego, and Dr. Natali from our group have injected melanoma patients with up to 10 mg of a monoclonal antibody to the high-molecular-weight antigen, but have not observed any effects on the tumor. Therefore, the most useful strategy for immunotherapy is to use the antibodies as a carrier to confer specificity to toxic substances (i.e., ricin lectin or radioisotopes) and to chemotherapeutic agents.

From a basic-science standpoint, we plan to use our library of monoclonal antibodies to further analyze the antigenic determinants of melanoma-derived Ia-like antigens and compare this with the profile of autologous B lymphocytes so that we may identify unique or aberrant determinants, especially in view of the abnormalities of glycosylation that may occur in tumor cells (for a review, see Hakomori, 1975) and of the influence carbohydrate side chains may have on the expression of protein antigenic determinants (B. S. Wilson *et al.*, 1981b). If such alien determinants are expressed, then one may ask whether a patient can mount an immune response against them and whether this response may influence the clinical course of the neoplasia. Studies are also in progress to determine whether the unexpected expression of Ia-like antigens on melanoma cells is limited to man or occurs in other animal species; if the latter is true, then animals will provide useful models to analyze the role of Ia-like antigens in the biology of the tumor.

Another area of study is the mechanism underlying the maturation and assembly of the various subunits comprising the tumor-associated antigens and the role of glycosylation in generating the overall structure of the molecule and in effecting its proper expression. Furthermore, information about the shedding of tumor-associated antigens from tumor cells may help to identify those antigens that are more likely to be elevated in body fluids of patients at certain times during the clinical course of the disease. Last, we plan to determine the relationship between the tumor-associated antigens detected by antibodies and those identified by cell-mediated immune reactions.

The various monoclonal antibodies we have described herein represent the beginning of our goal to exploit the hybridoma technique for developing a library of monoclonal antibodies to the many tumor-associated antigens of melanoma and to the various domains of each antigenic structure (i.e., individual, shared, and common, which may be the counterparts of private, public, and framework determinants of histocompatibility antigens). We believe that these antibodies will allow a more sophisticated classification of melanoma and allow the identification of antigens having diagnostic and prognostic value. In this regard, the expression of an antigenic determinant recognized by a monoclonal antibody on a Marek's-disease-virus-transformed, nonproducer lymphoma cell line is necessary, although not sufficient, for liver metastasis to occur (Shearman *et al.*, 1980). Furthermore, the various monoclonal antibodies will be used to determine whether the corresponding antigens have a homogeneous or heterogeneous distribution in a melanoma-cell population, since tumor-cell populations are heterogeneous with respect to various biological properties (Fidler *et al.*, 1978) and immunological pressures may modify the phenotype of susceptible cell populations (Boyse *et al.*, 1967). If indeed heterogeneity is found, then a cocktail of monoclonal antibodies to distinct tumor-associated antigens may be useful for radioimaging and immunotherapy. This approach will not only concentrate more antibody at the tumor cell surface but also limit the emergence of antigenic variants present in tumor populations. In the end, we may find that the best reagents are polyclonal, but this time they will consist of a known mixture of monoclonal antibodies with clearly defined specificity.

ACKNOWLEDGMENTS. The authors gratefully acknowledge the excellent secretarial assistance of Ms. Ellen Schmeding. This work was supported by National Institutes of Health Grants AI 19189, CA 32609, CA 32619, CA 32634, and CA 32635, and a special fellowship from the Leukemia Society of America (B. S. Wilson), a United States PHS Fogarty International Research Fellowship Award (5F05 TWO 2817-02) (K. Imai), a Research Career Development Award (M. A. Pellegrino), and an American Heart Association Established Investigatorship Award (S. Ferrone); and by Italian National Research Council Progetto Finalizzato "Controllo della Crescita Neoplastica: No. 80015996." K. Imai and N. E. Kay are visiting investigators from Sapporo Medical College (Japan) and the Veterans Administration Hospital (Minneapolis, Minnesota), respectively.

References

Alexander S., Lloyd, K. O., and Strominger, J. L., 1982, Characterization of the HLA-DR antigen of a continuous human melanoma cell line (submitted).

Allison, J. P., Walker, L. E., Russell, W. A., Pellegrino, M. A., Ferrone, S., Reisfeld, R. A., Frelinger, J. A., and Silver, J., 1978, Murine Ia and human DR antigens: Homology of amino terminal sequences, *Proc. Natl. Acad. Sci. U.S.A.* **75**:3953.

Avis, P., and Lewis, M. G., 1973, Tumor-associated fetal antigens in human tumors, *J. Natl. Cancer Inst.* **51**:1063.

Benacerraf, B., and McDevitt, H. O., 1972, Histocompatibility-linked immune response genes, *Science* **175**:273.

Bonner, W. M., and Laskey, R. A., 1974, A film detection method for tritium-labelled proteins and nucleic acids in polyacrylamide gels, *Eur. J. Biochem.* **46**:83.

Boyse, E. A., Stockert, E., and Old, L. J., 1967, Modification of the antigenic structure of the cell membrane by thymus-leukemia (TL) antigens, *Proc. Natl. Acad. Sci. U.S.A.* **58**:954.

Brown, J. P., Woodbury, R. G., Hart, C. E., Hellström, I., and Hellström, K. E., 1981, Quantitative analysis of melanoma-associated antigen p97 in normal and neoplastic tissues, *Proc. Natl. Acad. Sci. U.S.A.* **78**:539.

Callahan, G. N., Pellegrino, M. A., McCabe, R. P., Frugis, L., Allison, J. P., and Ferrone, S., 1978, Histocompatibility antigens on tumor cells: Spatial and structural relationship with tumor associated antigens, *Behring Inst. Mitt.* **62**:115.

Carey, T. E., Lloyd, K. O., Takahasi, T., Travassos, L. R., and Old, L. J., 1979, AU cell-surface antigen of human malignant melanoma: Solubilization and partial characterization, *Proc. Natl. Acad. Sci. U.S.A.* **76**:2898.

Cikes, M., and Friberg, S., 1977, Expression of cell surface antigens on cultured tumor cells, in: *Dynamic Aspects of Cell Surface Organization* (G. Poste and G. L. Nicolson, eds.), pp. 473–511, Elsevier/North-Holland, Amsterdam.

Curry, R., Quaranta, V., Wilson, B. S., McCabe, R. P., Natali, P. G., Pellegrino, M. A., and Ferrone, S., 1979, Expression of HLA antigens on cultured human melanoma cells: Lack of association with melanoma associated antigens, in: *Current Trends in Tumor Immunology* (S. Ferrone, S. Gorini, R. B. Herberman, and R. A. Reisfeld, eds.), pp. 347–366, Garland STPM Press, New York.

Davidsohn, I., 1972, Early immunologic diagnosis and prognosis of carcinoma, *Am. J. Clin. Pathol.* **57**:715.

De Tribolet, N., and Carrel, S., 1980, Human glioma tumor-associated antigens, *Cancer Immunol. Immunother.* **9**:207.

Dippold, W. G., Lloyd, K. O., Li, L. T. C., Ikeda, H., Oettgen, H. F., and Old, L. J., 1980, Cell surface antigens of human malignant melanoma: Definition of six antigenic systems with mouse monoclonal antibodies, *Proc. Natl. Acad. Sci. U.S.A.* **77**:6114.

Eichmann, K., 1980, Conclusion: A simple, conservative model for antigen-specificity and MHC-restriction in lymphocyte communication, *Springer Semin. Immunopathol.* **3**:277.

Embleton, M. J., Price, M. R., and Baldwin, R. W., 1980, Demonstration and partial purification of common melanoma-associated antigen(s), *Eur. J. Cancer.* **16**:575.

Fellous, M., Komoun, M., Gresser, I., and Bono, R., 1979, Enhanced expression of HLA antigens and β_2-microglobulin on inteferon-treated human lymphoid cells, Eur. J. Immunol. 9:446.

Ferrone, S., and Pellegrino, M. A., 1977, Cytotoxic antibodies to cultured melanoma cells in the sera of melanoma patients, J. Natl. Cancer Inst. 58:1201.

Ferrone, S., and Pellegrino, M. A., 1978, Antigens and antibodies in malignant melanoma, in: Handbook of Cancer Immunology, Vol. 3 (H. Waters, ed.), pp. 291–327, Garland, New York.

Ferrone, S., and Pellegrino, M. A., 1979, Serological detection of human melanoma associated antigens, in: Immunodiagnosis of Cancer (R. B. Herberman and K. R. McIntire, eds.), pp. 588–632, Marcel Dekker, New York.

Ferrone, S., Allison, J. P., and Pellegrino, M. A., 1978, Human DR (Ia-like) antigens: Biological and molecular profile, Contemp. Top. Mol. Immunol. 7:239.

Ferrone, S., Imai, K., McCabe, R. P., Molinaro, G. A., Galloway, D. R., and Reisfeld, R. A., 1980, Production, characterization, and use of xenoantisera to human melanoma-associated antigens, in: Serologic Analysis of Human Cancer Antigens (S. Rosenberg, ed.), p. 445, Academic Press, New York.

Fidler, I. J., Gersten, D. M., and Hart, I. R., 1978, The biology of cancer invasion and metasteses, in: Advances in Cancer Research (G. Klein and S. Weinhouse, eds.), pp. 194–250, Academic Press, New York.

Forni, G., Shevach, E. H., and Green, I., 1975, Mutant lines of guinea pig L2C leukemia. I. Deletion of Ia alloantigens is associated with loss in immunogenicity of tumor-associated transplantation antigens, J. Exp. Med. 143:1067.

Fujiwara, H., Aoki, H., Tsuchida, T., and Hamaoka, T., 1978, Immunologic characterization of tumor-associated transplantation antigens on mM102 mammary tumor eliciting preferentially helper T cell activity, J. Immunol. 121:1591.

Galloway, D. R., McCabe, R. P., Pellegrino, M. A., Ferrone, S., and Reisfeld, R. A., 1981, Tumor-associated antigens in spent medium of human melanoma cells: Immunochemical characterization with xenoantisera, J. Immunol. 126:62.

Hakomori, S.-I., 1975, Structures and organization of cell surface glycolipids dependency on cell growth and malignant transformation, Biochim. Biophys. Acta 414:55.

Hellström, K. E., and Hellström, I., 1974, Lymphocyte mediated cytotoxicity and blocking serum activity to tumor antigens, Adv. Immunol. 18:209.

Herlyn, M., Clark, W. H., Mastrangelo, M. J., Guerry, D., Elder, D. E., La Rossa, D., Hamilton, R., Bondi, E., Tuthill, R., Steplewski, Z., and Koprowski, H., 1980, Specific immunoreactivity of hybridoma secreted monoclonal anti-melanoma antibodies to cultured cells and freshly derived human cells, Cancer Res. 40:3602.

Heron, I., Hokland, M., and Berg, K., 1978, Enhanced expression of β_2-microglobulin and HLA antigens on human lymphoid cells by interferon, Proc. Natl. Acad. Sci. U.S.A. 75:6215.

Hersey, R., Murry, E., Werkmeister, J., and McCarthy, W., 1979, Detection of a low molecular weight antigen on melanoma cells by a human antiserum in leukocyte-dependent antibody assays, Br. J. Cancer 40:615.

Howe, A. J., Seeger, R. C., Molinaro, G. A., and Ferrone, S., 1981, Analysis of human tumor cells for HLA-DR antigens with monoclonal antibodies, J. Natl. Cancer Inst. 66:827.

Hunt, L. A., 1979, Biosynthesis and maturation of cellular membrane glycoproteins, J. Supramol. Struct. 12:209.

Hunt, L. A., Etchison, J. R., and Summers, D. F., 1978, Oligosaccharide chains are trimmed during synthesis of the envelope glycoprotein of vesicular stomatitis virus, Proc. Natl. Acad. Sci. U.S.A. 75:754.

Imai, K., and Ferrone, S., 1980, An indirect rosette microassay to characterize human melanoma associated antigens (MAA) recognized by operationally specific xenoantisera, Cancer Res. 40:2252.

Imai, K., Molinaro, G. A., and Ferrone, S., 1980, Monoclonal antibodies to human melanoma associated antigens, Transplant. Proc. 12:380.

Imai, K., Galloway, D. R., and Ferrone, S., 1981a, Serological and immunochemical analysis of the specificity of xenoantiserum 8986 elicited with hybrids between human melanoma cells and murine fibroblasts, Cancer Res. 41:1028.

Imai, K., Ng, A. K., and Ferrone, S., 1981b, Characterization of monoclonal antibodies to human melanoma-associated antigens, J. Natl. Cancer Inst. 66:489.

Imai, K., Ng, A. K., Glassy, M. C., and Ferrone, S., 1981c, Differential effect of interferon on the expression of tumor-associated antigens and histocompatibility antigens on human melanoma cells: Relationship to susceptibility to immune lysis mediated by monoclonal antibodies, J. Immunol. 127:505.

Imai, K., Pellegrino, M. A., Ng, A. K., and Ferrone, S., 1981d, Role of antigen density in immune lysis of inteferon treated human lymphoid cells: Analysis with monoclonal antibodies to the HLA-A, B antigenic molecular complex and to Ia-like antigens *Scand. J. Immunol.* **14**:529.

Imai, K., Ng, A. K., Glassy, M. C., and Ferrone, S., 1981e, ADCC of cultured human melanoma cells: Analysis with monoclonal antibodies to human melanoma associated antigens, *Scand. J. Immunol.* **14**:369.

Imai, K., Wilson, B. S., Kay, N. E., and Ferrone, S., 1981f, Monoclonal antibodies to human melanoma cells: Comparison of serological results of several laboratories and molecular profile of melanoma-associated antigens, in: *Monoclonal Antibodies and T Cell Hybrids* (G. J. Hammerling, ed.), Elsevier, New York (in press).

Indiveri, F., Wilson, B. S., Pellegrino, M. A., and Ferrone, S., 1979, Detection of human histocompatibility antigens with an indirect rosette microassay, *J. Immunol. Methods* **29**:101.

Irie, R. F., Irie, K., and Morton, D. L., 1976, A membrane antigen common to human cancer and fetal brain cells, *Cancer Res.* **36**:3510.

Köhler, G., and Milstein, C., 1975, Continuous cultures of fused cells secreting antibody of predefined specificity, *Nature (London)* **256**:495.

Kurpey, J., Gold, P., and Freedman, S. D., 1978, Physiochemical studies of the carcinoembryonic antigens of the human digestive system, *J. Exp. Med.* **128**:387.

Laemmli, U. K., 1970, Clevage of structural proteins during assembly of the head of bacteriophage T4, *Nature (London)* **222**:680.

Lee, P.-K., Mari, T., Fujimoto, N., Nakamura, T., Maxuzawa, M., and Kosaki, G., 1979, Relationship of AFP-producing cells in gastric cancer, heptocellular cancer and fetal tissues, in: *Carcino-Embryonic Proteins*, Vol. 2 (F. G. Lehmann ed.), pp. 373–381, Elsevier/North-Holland, New York.

Lewis, M. G., and Phillipps, T. M., 1972, Separation of two distinct tumor-associated antibodies in the serum of melanoma patients, *J. Natl. Cancer Inst.* **49**:915.

Martin, W. J., and Imamura, M., 1980, Variable expression of histocompatibility antigens on tumor cells, *Cancer Immunol. Immunother.* **8**:219.

Mastrangelo, M., Bellet, R. E., and Berd, D., 1979, Immunology and immunotherapy of human cutaneous malignant melanoma, in: *Human Malignant Melanoma* (W. H. Clark, Jr., M. Mastrangelo, and L. I. Goldman, eds.), pp. 355–416, Grune and Stratton, New York.

McCabe, R. P., Ferrone, S., Pellegrino, M. A., Kern, D. H., Holmes, E. C., and Reisfeld, R. A., 1978, Purification and immunologic evaluation of human melanoma-associated antigens, *J. Natl. Cancer Inst.* **60**:773.

McCabe, R. P., Galloway, D. R., Ferrone, S., and Reisfeld, R. A., 1979a, Human melanoma-associated antigens (MAA): Serologic and structural characterization, in: *Current Trends in Tumor Immunology* (S. Ferrone, S. Gorini, R. B. Herberman, and R. A. Reisfeld, eds.), pp. 269–286, Garland STPM Press, New York.

McCabe, R. P., Quaranta, V., Frugis, L., Ferrone, S., and Reisfeld, R. A., 1979b, A radioimmunometric antibody binding assay for the evaluation of xenoantisera to melanoma associated antigens, *J. Natl. Cancer Inst.* **62**:455.

Mitchell, K. F., Fuhrer, J. P., Steplewski, Z., and Koprowski, H., 1980, Biochemical characterization of human melanoma cell surfaces: Dissection with monoclonal antibodies, *Proc. Natl. Acad. Sci. U.S.A.* **77**:7287.

Morton, D. L., Malmgren, R. A., Holmes, E. C., and Ketcham, A. S., 1968, Demonstration of antibodies against human malignant melanoma by immunofluoresence, *Surgery* **64**:233.

Natali, P. G., Cordiali-Fei, P., Cavaliere, R., Di Filippo, F., Quaranta, V., Pellegrino, M. A., and Ferrone, S., 1981, Ia-like antigens on freshly explanted human malignant melanoma, *Clin. Immunol. Immunopathol.* **19**:250.

Parmiani, G., Carbone, G., Invernizzi, G., Pierotti, M. A., Sensi, M. L., Rogers, M. J., and Appella, E., 1979, Alien histocompatibility antigens on tumor cells, *Immunogenetics* **9**:1.

Pellegrino, M. A., Ferrone, S., and Pellegrino, A., 1972, A simple microabsorption technique for HLA typing, *Proc. Soc. Exp. Biol. Med.* **139**:484.

Pellegrino, M. A., Ferrone, S., Brautbar, C., and Hayflick, L., 1976, Changes in HLA antigen profiles on SV$_{40}$ transformed human fibroblasts, *Exp. Cell Res.* **97**:340.

Pellegrino, M. A., Ferrone, S., Reisfeld, R. A., Irie, R. F., and Golub, S. H., 1977, Expression of histocompatibility (HLA) antigens on tumor cells and normal cells from patients with melanoma, *Cancer* **40**:36.

Pellegrino, M. A., Weaver, J. F., Nelson-Rees, W. A., and Ferrone, S., 1982, Ia-like and HLA-A B antigens on tumor cells in long term culture, *Transplant. Proc.* **13**:1939.

Pollack, M. S., Heagney, S., and Fogh, J., 1980a, HLA typing of cultured human tumor cell lines: The detection of genetically appropriate HLA-A, B, C and DR alloantigens, *Transplant. Proc.* **12**:134.

Pollack, M. S., Livingston, P. O., Fogh, J., Carey, T. E., Oettgen, H. F., and Dupont, B., 1980b, Genetically appropriate expression of HLA and DR (IA) alloantigens on human melanoma cell lines, *Tissue Antigens* **15**:249.

Quaranta, V., Walker, L. E., Pellegrino, M. A., and Ferrone, S., 1980, Purification of immunologically functional subsets of human Ia-like antigens on a monoclonal antibody (Q5/13) immunoadsorbent, *J. Immunol.* **125**:1421.

Quaranta, V., Pellegrino, M. A., and Ferrone, S., 1981a, Serologic and immunochemical characterization of the specificity of four monoclonal antibodies to distinct antigenic determinants expressed on subpopulations of human Ia-like antigens, *J. Immunol.* **126**:548.

Quaranta, V., Walker, L. E., Ruberto, G., Pellegrino, M. A., and Ferrone, S., 1981b, The free and the β_2-microglobulin-associated heavy chain of HLA-A, B alloantigens share the antigenic determinant recognized by the monoclonal antibody Q1/28, *Immunogenetics* **13**:285.

Robbins, P. W., Hubbard, S. C., Turco, S. J., and Wirth, D. F., 1977, Proposal for a common oligosaccharide intermediate in the synthesis of membrane glycoproteins, *Cell* **12**:895.

Rogers, M. J., Appella, E., Pierotti, M. A., Invernizzi, G., and Parmiani, G., 1979, Biochemical characterization of alien H-2 antigens expressed on a methylcholanthrene-induced tumor, *Proc. Natl. Acad. Sci. U.S.A.* **76**:1415.

Ruoslahti, E., Pihko, H., and Seppala, M., 1974, Alpha-fetoprotein: Immunochemical purification and chemical properties, expression in normal state and in malignant and non-malignant liver disease, *Transplant. Rev.* **20**:38.

Salisbury, J. G., and Graham, J. M., 1981, Cell surface radioiodination with the sparingly soluble catalyst Iodogen: Differences between dividing and non-dividing populations of rodent thymocytes, *Biochem. J.* **194**:351.

Seibert, E., Sorg, C., Happle, R., and Macher, E., 1977, Membrane-associated antigens of human malignant melanoma. III. Specificity of human sera reacting with cultured melanoma cells, *Int. J. Cancer* **19**:172.

Shearman, P. J., Gallatin, W. M., and Longenecker, B. M., 1980, Detection of a cell-surface antigen correlated with organ-specific metastasis, *Nature (London)* **286**:267.

Shiku, H., Takahasi, T., Oettgen, F., and Old, L. J., 1976, Cell surface antigens of human malignant melanoma. II. Serological typing with immune adherence assays and definition of two new surface antigens, *J. Exp. Med.* **144**:873.

Singer, S. J., 1974, The molecular organization of membranes, *Annu. Rev. Biochem.* **43**:805.

Stuhlmiller, G. M., and Seigler, H. F., 1975, Characterization of a chimpanzee anti-human melanoma antiserum, *Cancer Res.* **35**:2132.

Stuhlmiller, G. M., Boylston, J. A., Seigler, H. F., and Fetter, B. F., 1977, Immunodiagnosis of melanoma using chimpanzee anti-human melanoma antiserum, *Am. J. Clin. Pathol.* **67**:573.

Stuhlmiller, G. M., Green, R. W., and Seigler, H. F., 1978, Solubilization and partial isolation of human melanoma tumor-associated antigens, *J. Natl. Cancer Inst.* **61**:61.

Tabas, I., Schlesinger, S., and Kornfeld, S., 1978, Processing of high mannose oligosaccharides to form complex type oligosaccharides on the newly synthesized polypeptides of the vesicular stomatitis virus G protein and the IgG heavy chain, *J. Biol. Chem.* **253**:716.

Takasugi, M., and Terasaki, P. I., 1972, Detection of HL-A and other cell-surface antigens on cultured cells by a cytotoxic plating inhibition test, *J. Natl. Cancer Inst.* **49**:1229.

Thorsby, E., Bergholtz, B., and Nousiainen, H., 1981, Self-HLA-D-region products restrict human T-lymphocyte activation by antigen, in: *Current Trends in Histocompatibility*, Vol. 2 (R. A. Reisfeld and S. Ferrone, eds.), Plenum Press, New York (in press).

Truax, H., Barnett, R. N., Hukill, P. B., Campbell, P. C., and Eisenberg, H., 1966, Effect of inaccurate pathological diagnosis on survival statistics for melanoma, *Cancer* **19**:1543.

Werkmeister, J., Edwards, A., McCarthy, W., and Hersey, P., 1980, Prognostic significance of expression of antigens on melanoma cells, *Cancer Immunol. Immunother.* **9**:233.

Wilson, B. S., Indiveri, F., Pellegrino, M. A., and Ferrone, S., 1979, DR (Ia-like) antigens on human melanoma cells: Serological detection and immunochemical characterization, *J. Exp. Med.* **149**:658.

Wilson, B. S., Indiveri, F., Molinaro, G. A., Quaranta, V., and Ferrone, S., 1980, Characterization of DR antigens on cultured melanoma cells by using monoclonal antibodies, *Transplant. Proc.* **12**:125.

Wilson, B. S., Ng, A. K., Quaranta, V., and Ferrone, S., 1981a, HLA polyclonal and monoclonal xenoantibodies: Production, characterization and application to the study of HLA antigens, in: *Current Trends in Histocompatibility*, Vol. 2 (R. A. Reisfeld and S. Ferrone, eds.), Plenum Press, New York (in press).

Wilson, B. S., Glassy, M. C., Quaranta, V., Ng, A. K., and Ferrone, S., 1981b, Effect of tunicamycin on the assembly and antigenicity of HLA antigens: Analysis with monoclonal antibodies, *Scand. J. Immunol.* **14**:201.

Wilson, B. S., Ruberto, G., and Ferrone, S., 1981c, Sulfation and molecular weight of fibronectin shed by human melanoma cells, *Biochem. Biophys. Res. Commun.* **101**:1047.

Wilson, B. S., Kay, N. E., Imai, K. and Ferrone, S., 1982, Heterogeneity of human melanoma-associated antigens defined by monoclonal antiodies and conventional xenoantigens, *Cancer Immunol. Immunother.* (in press).

Wilson, N. I., Cochran, A. J., Ross, C. E., Mackie, R. M., Ogg, L. J., and Todd, G., 1979, Immunological aspects of benign melanotic tumors and melanoma *in situ, Cancer Immunol. Immunother.* **6**:27.

Winchester, R. J., Wang, C. Y., Gibofsky, A., Kunkel, H. G., Lloyd, K. O., and Old, L. J., 1978, Expression of Ia-like antigens on cultured human malignant melanoma cell lines, *Proc. Natl. Acad. Sci. U.S.A.* **75**:6235.

Woodbury, R. G., Brown, J. P., Yeh, M. Y., Hellström, I., and Hellström, K. E., 1980, Identification of a cell surface protein, p97, in human melanoma and certain other neoplasms, *Proc. Natl. Acad. Sci. U.S.A.* **77**:2813.

Index